Brief Table of Contents

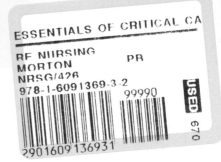

Essentials of Critical Care Nursing

A Holistic Approach

Patricia Gonce Morton, RN, PhD, ACNP-BC, FAAN
Professor and Associate Dean for Academic Affairs
University of Maryland School of Nursing
Acute Care Nurse Practitioner
University of Maryland Medical Center
Baltimore, Maryland

Dorrie K. Fontaine, RN, PhD, FAAN
Dean, School of Nursing, University of Virginia
Sadie Health Cabaniss Professor of Nursing
Charlottesville, Virginia

 Wolters Kluwer | Lippincott Williams & Wilkins
Health

Philadelphia • Baltimore • New York • London
Buenos Aires • Hong Kong • Sydney • Tokyo

Executive Acquisitions Editor: Elizabeth Nieginski
Senior Product Manager: Helen Kogut
Editorial Assistant: Zachary Shapiro
Design Coordinator: Joan Wendt
Illustration Coordinator: Brett MacNaughton
Manufacturing Coordinator: Karin Duffield
Prepress Vendor: SPi Global

9 8 7 6 5 4 3 2 1

Printed in China

Library of Congress Cataloging-in-Publication Data
Morton, Patricia Gonce, 1952-
  Essentials of critical care nursing : a holistic approach / Patricia Gonce Morton, Dorrie K. Fontaine.
    p. ; cm.
  Related work: Critical care nursing / [edited by] Patricia Gonce Morton, Dorrie K. Fontaine. 9th ed. c2009.
  Includes bibliographical references and index.
  ISBN 978-1-60913-693-2
 I. Fontaine, Dorrie K. II. Critical care nursing. III. Title.
  [DNLM: 1. Critical Care. 2. Holistic Nursing—methods.   WY 154]
  616.02'8—dc23
                                                                    2011040475

Care has been taken to confirm the accuracy of the information presented and to describe generally accepted practices. However, the author, editors, and publisher are not responsible for errors or omissions or for any consequences from application of the information in this book and make no warranty, expressed or implied, with respect to the currency, completeness, or accuracy of the contents of the publication. Application of this information in a particular situation remains the professional responsibility of the practitioner; the clinical treatments described and recommended may not be considered absolute and universal recommendations.

The author, editors, and publisher have exerted every effort to ensure that drug selection and dosage set forth in this text are in accordance with the current recommendations and practice at the time of publication. However, in view of ongoing research, changes in government regulations, and the constant flow of information relating to drug therapy and drug reactions, the reader is urged to check the package insert for each drug for any change in indications and dosage and for added warnings and precautions. This is particularly important when the recommended agent is a new or infrequently employed drug.

Some drugs and medical devices presented in this publication have Food and Drug Administration (FDA) clearance for limited use in restricted research settings. It is the responsibility of the health care provider to ascertain the FDA status of each drug or device planned for use in his or her clinical practice.

RRS1202

To the students and the nurses who will learn from this book. May you provide holistic, patient-centered care to all critically ill patients and their families.
Never lose site of the difference you make in their lives.

Trish and Dorrie

Clinical Consultant

Kendra Menzies Kent, RN, MS, CCRN, CNRN
ICU Staff Nurse
St. Mary's Hospital
West Palm Beach, Florida

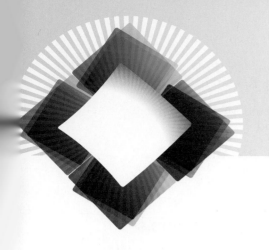

Thank You

The authors and Lippincott Williams & Wilkins extend a special, heartfelt thank you to the contributors of the ninth edition of *Critical Care Nursing: A Holistic Approach* whose work served as the basis for the content in this book.

Contributors

Susan E. Anderson, RN, MSN
Senior Quality Assurance Specialist
United States Army Graduate Program
    in Anesthesia Nursing
Fort Sam Houston, Texas

Sue Apple, RN, PhD
Assistant Professor
Department of Professional Nursing
School of Nursing and Health Studies
Georgetown University
Washington, District of Columbia

Carla A. Aresco, RN, MS, CRNP
Nurse Practitioner, Shock Trauma
R Adams Cowley Shock Trauma Center
University of Maryland Medical Center
Baltimore, Maryland

Mona N. Bahouth, MSN, CRNP, MD
Neurology Resident
Johns Hopkins Hospital
Baltimore, Maryland

Kathryn S. Bizek, MSN, ACNS-BC, CCRN
Nurse Practitioner, Cardiac Electrophysiology
Henry Ford Heart and Vascular Institute
Henry Ford Health System
Detroit, Michigan

Kay Blum, PhD, CRNP
Nurse Practitioner and Assistant Professor
University of Maryland Medical System
University of Maryland School of Nursing
Baltimore, Maryland

Eileen M. Bohan, RN, BSN, CNRN
Senior Program Coordinator
The Johns Hopkins University
Baltimore, Maryland

Garrett K. Chan, PhD, APRN, FAEN, FPCN
Lead Advanced Practice Nurse
Stanford Hospitals and Clinics
Stanford, California

Donna Charlebois, RN, MSN, ACNP-CS
Lung Transplant Coordinator
University of Virginia
Charlottesville, Virginia

JoAnn Coleman, RN, DNP, ACNP, AOCN
Acute Care Nurse Practitioner and Coordinator
Gastrointestinal Surgical Oncology
John Hopkins Hospital
Baltimore, Maryland

Vicki J. Coombs, RN, PhD, FAHA
Senior Vice President
Spectrum Clinical Research, Inc.
Towson, Maryland

Joan M. Davenport, RN, PhD
Assistant Professor and Vice-Chair
Department of Organizational Systems
    and Adult Health
University of Maryland School of Nursing
Baltimore, Maryland

Marla J. De Jong, RN, PhD, CCNS, Colonel
Dean
United States Air Force School of Aerospace
    Medicine
Wright-Patterson Air Force Base, Ohio

Nancy Kern Feeley, RN, MS, CRNP, CNN
Nephrology Adult Nurse Practitioner
The Johns Hopkins University
Baltimore, Maryland

Charles Fisher, RN, MSN, CCRN, ACNP-BC
Acute Care Nurse Practitioner Medical ICU
University of Virginia Health System
Charlottesville, Virginia

Barbara Fitzsimmons, RN, MS, CNRN
Nurse Educator
Department of Neuroscience Nursing
The Johns Hopkins Hospital
Baltimore, Maryland

Conrad Gordon, RN, MS, ACNP
Assistant Professor
Department of Organizational Systems
    and Adult Health
University of Maryland School of Nursing
Baltimore, Maryland

Christine Grady, RN, PhD
Head, Section on Human Subjects Research
Department of Bioethics
Clinical Center
National Institutes of Health
Bethesda, Maryland

Debby Greenlaw, MS, CCRN, ACNP
Acute Care Nurse Practitioner
Hospitalist Group, Providence Hospital
Columbia, South Carolina

Kathy A. Hausman, RN, C, PhD
Chair, Department of Nursing
Baltimore City Community College
Baltimore, Maryland

Jan M. Headley, RN, BS
Director, Clinical Marketing and Professional
    Education
Edwards Lifesciences LLC
Irvine, California

Janie Heath, PhD, APRN-BC, FAAN
Associate Dean Academic Affairs
University of Virginia School of Nursing
Charlottesville, Virginia

Kiersten N. Henry, MS, APRN-BC, CCNS,
CCRN-CMC
Cardiovascular Nurse Practitioner
Montgomery General Hospital
Olney, Maryland

Gennell D. Hilton, PhD, CRNP, CCNS, CCRN
Nurse Practitioner, Trauma Services
San Francisco General Hospital
San Francisco, California
Faculty, Life Sciences Department
Santa Rosa Junior College
Santa Rosa, California

Dorene M. Holcombe, RN, MS, ACNP, CCRN
Nephrology Acute Care Nurse Practitioner
Johns Hopkins University School of Medicine
Baltimore, Maryland

Christina Hurlock-Chorostecki, PhD(c),
NP-Adult
Nurse Practitioner
St. Joseph's Health Care
London, Ontario, Canada

Karen L. Johnson, RN, PhD
Director of Nursing, Research, and Evidence-Based
    Practice
University of Maryland Medical Center
Baltimore, Maryland

Dennis W. Jones, RN, MS, CFRN
Critical Care Flight Nurse
Johns Hopkins Hospital
Baltimore, Maryland

Kimmith M. Jones, RN, DNP, CCNS
Advanced Practice Nurse
Critical Care and Emergency Center
Sinai Hospital of Baltimore
Baltimore, Maryland

Roberta Kaplow, RN, PhD, AOCNS,
CCNS, CCRN
Clinical Nurse Specialist
Emory University Hospital
Atlanta, Georgia

Jane Kapustin, PhD, CRNP
Associate Professor of Nursing
Assistant Dean for Masters and DNP Programs
University of Maryland School of Nursing
Adult Nurse Practitioner, Joslin Diabetes Center
University of Maryland Medical Center
Baltimore, Maryland

Susan N. Luchka, RN, MSN, CCRN, ET
Director of Clinical Education
Memorial Hospital
York, Pennsylvania

Christine N. Lynch, RN, MS, CCRN, CRNP
Acute Care Nurse Practitioner, Surgical
    Critical Care
Union Memorial Hospital
Baltimore, Maryland

Cathleen R. Maiolatesi, RN, MS
Advanced Practice Nurse
The Johns Hopkins Hospital
Baltimore, Maryland

Sandra W. McLeskey, RN, PhD
Professor
University of Maryland School of Nursing
Baltimore, Maryland

Alexander R. McMullen III, RN, JD, MBA, BSN
Attorney/Principal
McMullen and Drury
Towson, Maryland

Patricia C. McMullen, PhD, JD, CRNP
Associate Provost for Academic Administration
The Catholic University of America
Washington, District of Columbia

Paul K. Merrel, RN, MSN, CCNS
Advanced Practice Nurse 2-CNS, Adult
  Critical Care
University of Virginia Health System
Charlottesville, Virginia

Sandra A. Mitchell, PhD, ARNP, AOCN
Senior Research Nurse, Clinical Center
National Institute of Health
Bethesda, Maryland

Nancy Munro, RN, MN, CCRN, ANCP
Acute Care Nurse Practitioner
Critical Care Medicine Department
National Institutes of Health
Bethesda, Maryland
Clinical Instructor
University of Maryland School of Nursing
Baltimore, Maryland

Angela C. Muzzy, RN, MSN, CCRN, CNS
Clinical Nurse Specialist/CVICU
University Medical Center
Tucson, Arizona

Colleen Krebs Norton, RN, PhD, CCRN
Associate Professor and Director of the
  Baccalaureate Nursing Program
Georgetown University School of Nursing and
  Health Studies
Washington, District of Columbia

Dulce Obias-Manno, RN, BSN, MHSA, CCDS,
CEPS, FHRS
Nurse Coordinator, Cardiac Arrhythmia Center/
  Device Clinic
Medstar/Washington Hospital Center
Washington, District of Columbia

Mary O. Palazzo, RN, MS
Director of Cardiothoracic Surgery, Heart Institute
St. Joseph Medical Center
Towson, Maryland

Suzanne Prevost, RN, PhD, COI
Associate Dean for Practice and Community
  Engagement
University of Kentucky College of Nursing
Lexington, Kentucky

Kim Reck, RN, MSN, CRNP
Clinical Program Manager, CRNP
Division of Cardiology
University of Maryland Medical Center
Baltimore, Maryland

Kathryn P. Reese, RN, BSN, Major
Element Chief, Cardiac Intensive Care Unit
Wilford Hall Medical Center
Lackland Air Force Base, Texas

Michael V. Relf, RN, PhD, CNE, ACNS-BC,
AACRN, FAAN
Associate Professor and Assistant Dean for
  Undergraduate Education
Duke University School of Nursing
Durham, North Carolina

Kenneth J. Rempher, RN, PhD, MBA, CCRN
Assistant Vice President Patient Care Services
Sinai Hospital of Baltimore
Baltimore, Maryland

Valerie K. Sabol, PhD, ACNP-BC, GNP-BC,
CCNS
Specialty Director
Acute Care Nurse Practitioner (ACNP)/Critical Care
  Clinical Nurse Specialist (CCNS) Master's Tracks
Duke University School of Nursing
Durham, North Carolina

Brenda K. Shelton, RN, MS, CCRN, AOCN
Critical Care Clinical Nurse Specialist
The Sidney Kimmel Comprehensive Cancer Center
  at Johns Hopkins
Baltimore, Maryland

Jo Ann Hoffman Sikora, RN, MS, CRNP
Nurse Practitioner, Division of Cardiac Surgery
University of Maryland Medical Systems
Baltimore, Maryland

Kara Adams Snyder, RN, MS, CCRN, CCNS
Clinical Nurse Specialist, Surgical Trauma
  Critical Care
University Medical Center
Tucson, Arizona

Debbi S. Spencer, RN, MS
Chief Nurse, Joint Trauma System
United States Army Institute of Surgical Research
Fort Sam Houston, Texas

Allison G. Steele, MSN, BSN, CRNP
Nurse Practitioner
University Physicians Inc.
University of Maryland Department of Medicine
Division of Gastroenterology and Hepatology
Baltimore, Maryland

Louis R. Stout, RN, MS, CEN
Lieutenant Colonel, United States Army
  Nurse Corps
United States Army Medical Department
Fort Lewis, Washington

Sidenia S. Tribble, RN, MSN, APRN-BC, CCRN
Acute Care Nurse Practitioner
Page Memorial Hospital
Luray, Virginia

Terry Tucker, RN, MS, CCRN, CEN
Critical Care Clinical Nurse Specialist
Maryland General Hospital
Baltimore, Maryland

Mary van Soeren, RN, PhD
Director
Canadian Health Care Innovations
Guelph, Ontario, Canada

Kathryn T. VonRueden, RN, MS, FCCM
Associate Professor, Trauma, Critical Care
Department of Organizational Systems
   and Adult Health
University of Maryland School of Nursing
Clinical Nurse Specialist, Trauma Resuscitation Unit
R Adams Cowley Shock Trauma Center
University of Maryland Medical Center
Baltimore, Maryland

Janet Armstead Wulf, RN, MS, CNL, CHPN
Staff Nurse
Union Memorial Hospital
Baltimore, Maryland

Karen L. Yarbrough, MS, CRNP
Acute Care Nurse Practitioner
Director, Stroke Programs
Stroke and Neurocritical Care
University of Maryland Medical Center
Baltimore, Maryland

Elizabeth Zink, RN, MS, CCRN, CNRN
Clinical Nurse Specialist
Neurosciences Critical Care Unit
The Johns Hopkins Hospital
Baltimore, Maryland

Reviewers

Jane Baltimore, MSN
Clinical Nurse Specialist
Harborview Medical Center
Seattle, Washington

Susan Barnason, PhD, MSN, BSN, MA
Associate Professor
University of Nebraska Medical Center College of
    Nursing
Lincoln, Nebraska

Mali M. Bartges, RN, MSN
Associate Professor
Northampton Community College
Bethlehem, Pennsylvania

Deborah Becker, PhD, ACNP, BC, CCNS
Practice Assistant Professor of Nursing
University of Pennsylvania School of Nursing
Philadelphia, Pennsylvania

Cynthia Gurdak Berry, RN, DNP
Assistant Professor
Ida V. Moffett School of Nursing, Samford University
Birmingham, Alabama

Mary Spitak Bilitski, RN, MSN, CVN
Instructor of Nursing
The Washington Hospital School of Nursing
Washington, Pennsylvania

Kathleen Buck, BSN
Faculty
Huntington University
Huntington, Indiana

Sharon Burke, MSN, APRN, CCRN, BCEN
Instructor
Thomas Jefferson University
Philadelphia, Pennsylvania

Doris Cavlovich, RN, MSN, CCRN
Nursing Instructor II
St. Margaret School of Nursing
Pittsburgh, Pennsylvania

Julie C. Chew, RN, PhD
Faculty
Mohave Community College
Colorado City, Arizona

Patricia Connick, RegN, CNCC(c)
Faculty Health Sciences – Nursing Department
Georgian College of Applied Arts & Technology,
    Barrie Campus
Durham College, Oshawa Campus
Bracebridge, Ontario, Canada

L. Angelise Davis, RN, DSN, MN, AHNP
Associate Professor, Baccalaureate Nursing
    Program
Mary Black School of Nursing, University of South
    Carolina Upstate
Spartanburg, South Carolina

Jack E. Dean, MSN, BSN, BS
Instructor
UPMC Shadyside Hospital School of Nursing
Pittsburgh, Pennsylvania

Daniel Defeo, MSN, MA
West Virginia University School of Nursing
South Morgantown, West Virginia

Theresa Delahoyde, RN, EdD
Associate Professor of Nursing
BryanLGH College of Health Sciences
Lincoln, Nebraska

Hazel Downing, RN, EdD, MN
Assistant Professor of Nursing
Hawaii Pacific University
Kanehoe, Hawaii

Kathleen Evanina, RN, PhDc, CRNP-BC
Professor
Marywood University
Scranton, Pennsylvania

Shelley Gerbrandt, RN, BSN, CCN(C)
Facilitator, Basic Critical Care Program – Casual
Sask Institute of Applied Science and Technology
Regina, Saskatchewan

Kelly Goebel, DNP, ACNP-BC, CCRN
Associate Professor
Nova Southeastern University
Fort Myers, Florida

Linda M. Graham, MSN
Assistant Professor
Department of Nursing
Thomas More College
Crestview Hills, Kentucky

Margaret Gramas, RN, MSN
Nursing Instructor
Morton College
Cicero, Illinois

Cam A. Hamilton, RN, MSN
Instructor
Auburn University at Montgomery
Montgomery, Alabama

Trina R. Hill RN, MAEd, BScN
Faculty
Saskatchewan Institute of Applied Science and
    Technology (SIAST)
Regina, Saskatchewan

Glenda Susan Jones, RN, MSN, CNS, CCRN
Assistant Professor of Nursing
Jefferson College of Health Science
Roanoke, Virginia

Catherine B. Kaesberg, MSN, BSN
Instructional Assistant Professor
Faculty
Illinois State University
Normal, Illinois

Heather Kendall, RN, MSN, CCRN-CMC-CSC
Assistant Professor
Missouri Western State University
St. Joseph, Missouri

Tonia Kennedy, RN, MSN, CCRN
Director of Generic Program and Assistant
    Professor of Nursing
Liberty University
Lynchburg, Virginia

Anita J.K. Langston, MSN, ANP-BC, CCRN,
CCNS
Clinical Associate Professor
University of Memphis
Memphis, Tennessee

Janice Garrison Lanham, RN, MS, CCRN,
CNS, FNP
Nursing Faculty/Lecturer
School of Nursing, Clemson University
Clemson, South Carolina

Karen S. March, RN, PhD, MSN, CCRN,
ACNS-BC
Associate Professor of Nursing
York College of Pennsylvania
York, Pennsylvania

Leigh W. Moore, RN, MSN, CNOR, CNE
Associate Professor of Nursing
Southside Virginia Community College
Alberta, Virginia

Teresa Newby, RN, MSN
Nursing Department Chair
Crown College
St. Bonifacius, Minnesota

Crystal O'Connell-Schauerte, MscN, BscB
Nursing Professor
Algonquin College
Ottawa, Ontario, Canada

Jeanne M. Papa, MSN, MBE, CRNP
Full-time Faculty
Neumann University
Aston, Pennsylvania

Patricia Perry, RN, MSN, BSN
Nursing Instructor
Galveston College
Galveston, Texas

Carrie Pucino, RN, MS,CCRN
Nursing Faculty
York College of Pennsylvania
York, Pennsylvania

Carol Anne Purvis, RN, EdD, MSN, MEd, BSN
Associate Professor of Nursing
Gordon College
Barnseville, Georgia

Stephanie A. Reagan, MSN, CNS
Associate Professor of Nursing
Malone University
Canton, Ohio

Mary Runde, RN, MN-APN
Online Teacher, Critical Care
Durham College
Oshawa, Ontario

Nancy Sarpy, RN, MS
Assistant Professor of Nursing
Loma Linda University School of Nursing
Loma Linda, California

Heidi H. Schmoll, MSN-Ed, BSN, ADN, AA, AS
Simulation Nurse Educator
Medical University of South Carolina
Charleston, South Carolina

Susan Schroeder, RN, MSN
Assistant Professor of Nursing
Marian University School of Nursing
Indianapolis, Indiana

Deborah J. Schwytzer, MS, BSN, BS
Associate Professor of Nursing
University of Cincinnati College of Nursing
Cincinnati, Ohio

Joanne Farley Serembus, RN, EdD, CCRN, CNE
Associate Professor
Drexel University
College of Nursing and Health Professions
Philadelphia, Pennsylvania

Eileen Shackell, RN, MSN, CNCC(c)
Faculty
British Columbia Institute of Technology
Burnaby, British Columbia, Canada

Lora R. Shelton, RN, DNP, FNP-BC
Instructor
Ida V. Moffett School of Nursing, Samford University
Birmingham, Alabama

Susan Shirato, RN, DNP, CCRN
Nursing Instructor
Jefferson School of Nursing, Thomas Jefferson University
Philadelphia, Pennsylvania

Lisa B. Soontupe, RN, EdD
Associate Professor
Nova Southeastern University
Fort Lauderdale, Florida

Amy K. Stoker, RN MSN, CCRN
Faculty Coordinator N304 Complex Health Nursing
UPMC Shadyside School of Nursing
Pittsburgh, Pennsylvania

Donna Talty, RN, MSN, FNP-BC, CNE
Professor of Nursing
Oakton Community College
Des Plaines, Illinois

Stephanie B. Turner, RN, EdD, MSN
Nursing Faculty
Wallace State Community College
Hanceville, Alabama

Ronald S. Ulberg, RN, MSN, CCRN
Assistant Teaching Professor
Brigham Young University
Provo, Utah

Judy Voss, RN, MSN
Lecturer
The University of Texas – Pan American
Edinburg, Texas

Sally A. Weiss, RN, EdD, MSN, CNE, ANEF
Associate Chair Nursing Department/Professor
Nova Southeastern University
Miami, Florida

Rachel Wilburn, RN, MSN, BSN
Assistant Professor
McNeese State University College of Nursing
Lake Charles, Louisiana

Phyllis D. Wille, RN, MS, FNP-C
Nursing Faculty
Danville Area Community College
Danville, Illinois

Jacqueline C. Zalumas, RN, PhD, FNP-BC
Professor of Nursing
Georgia Baptist College of Nursing, Mercer University
Atlanta, Georgia

Preface

In the United States, changes in healthcare delivery and the changing healthcare needs of the population are leading to an increased demand for nurses who are educated to provide care for critically ill patients. Today's critically ill patient is liable to be older and more critically ill than ever before, thus increasing the demand for nurses with the skills to handle complex, life-threatening conditions. Nurses who are educated to provide critical care are highly sought after now, and will be for the foreseeable future.

Essentials of Critical Care Nursing: A Holistic Approach, the newest member of the family of books that started in 1973 with the first edition of *Critical Care Nursing: A Holistic Approach*, has been created as an introduction to the specialty of critical care nursing and focuses on entry-level information a novice would need to care for critically ill patients. Like the classic parent text (now in its 10th edition), *Essentials of Critical Care Nursing* remains true to our commitment to excellence by providing students with the most up-to-date information needed to care for critically ill patients and their families, with a strong emphasis on holistic care. The patient is the center of the healthcare team's efforts, and all interventions must be based on an understanding of the patient's psychosocial, as well as physical, needs. For today's critical care nurse, knowledge of disease processes and competence in using high-tech equipment in the care of critically ill patients is not enough. Today's critical care nurse must also include the family in all aspects of care and demonstrate caring behaviors that address the human aspect of suffering.

Essentials of Critical Care Nursing: A Holistic Approach provides a solid, focused introduction to the discipline of critical care nursing. In writing the text, we assumed a basic knowledge of medical–surgical nursing, anatomy and physiology, pathophysiology, and assessment. However, these areas are reviewed as needed within the context of specific discussions, focusing specifically on the needs of the patient in a critical care setting. A strong emphasis on what the novice nurse needs to know and do in caring for critically ill patients and their families is maintained throughout the book.

Organization

Essentials of Critical Care Nursing: A Holistic Approach is organized into 11 parts:

Part 1: The four chapters that make up Part 1 introduce the reader to the concept of holistic care, as it applies in critical care practice. In Chapter 1, the reader is introduced to issues of particular pertinence to critical care nursing practice, including the benefits of certification, the importance of evidence-based practice, and how a healthy work environment contributes to the well-being of the nurse and facilitates the optimal care of patients and families. Chapter 2 reviews the psychosocial effects of critical illness on the patient and the family, and describes the nurse's role in guiding the patient and family through the crisis. Chapter 3 emphasizes the role of the nurse in providing patient and family education in critical care. In Chapter 4, legal and ethical issues in critical care practice are explored.

Part 2: The seven chapters that comprise Part 2 address essential concepts and interventions that pertain to the care of the critically ill patient. Chapter 5 focuses on strategies for relieving pain and promoting comfort, and Chapter 6 concentrates on the topics of end-of-life and palliative care. Chapter 7 addresses the assessment of nutrition and fluid and electrolyte balance and describes associated nursing interventions. Chapter 8 explores dysrhythmia interpretation and the management of patients with dysrhythmias. Chapter 9 reviews hemodynamic monitoring. Chapter 10 concentrates on airway management and ventilatory support. The unit concludes with Chapter 11, which addresses the management of a patient in cardiopulmonary arrest.

Parts 3 through 10: Parts 3 through 10 take a body systems approach to presenting disorders most commonly seen in critical care. Each part is structured so that general assessment techniques and management modalities that pertain to the organ system under discussion are presented first, followed by a discussion of specific disorders of that organ system that often necessitate admission to the critical care unit. By covering assessment and management modalities in some detail initially, we provide the student with foundational knowledge and avoid the repetition of information that can occur when the same assessment technique or management modality is used in the assessment or management of multiple disorders.

Part 11: The final part of the text, Part 11, focuses on multisystemic disorders, including shock, multisystem organ dysfunction syndrome (MODS), and trauma.

Features

The features of *Essentials of Critical Care Nursing: A Holistic Approach* have been designed to assist readers with practice as well as learning. Many of the features support the quality and safety pre-licensure competencies put forth by the Quality and Safety Education for Nurses (QSEN) initiative, which seeks to develop the knowledge, skills, and attitudes (KSAs) necessary to continuously improve the quality and safety of the healthcare system. Key quality and safety competencies that are supported by the features in this text include patient-centered care, teamwork and collaboration, evidence-based practice, quality improvement, and safety.

- **Evidence-Based Practice Highlights.** These boxes present current evidence-based recommendations related to key nursing interventions. (QSEN competencies: evidence-based practice, quality improvement)
- **Collaborative Care Guides.** These boxes describe how the healthcare team works together to manage a patient's illness and minimize complications. The information is presented in a tabular format, with outcomes in the first column and interventions in the second. (QSEN competencies: patient-centered care, teamwork and collaboration)
- **Red Flag Notes.** These notes highlight clinically important information, such as signs and symptoms of developing complications or life-threatening conditions, and actions the nurse should take to ensure safe care. (QSEN competencies: safety)
- **The Older Patient Notes.** These notes, appearing within the flow of the text, highlight information related to assessing and caring for older patients in the critical care setting. (QSEN competencies: patient-centered care)
- **Drug Therapy Tables.** These tables summarize information related to the safe administration and monitoring of drug therapy. (QSEN competencies: safety)
- **Diagnostic Tests Tables.** These tables summarize information about key diagnostic tests, with a focus on the key information the nurse should be aware of with regard to preparing a patient for a diagnostic test and caring for the patient during or after the test. (QSEN competencies: safety)
- **Health History Boxes.** These boxes summarize aspects of the history that are important to explore to gain insight into the patient's current critical health problem. (QSEN competencies: patient-centered care)
- **Case Studies.** Each chapter concludes with a case study followed by a series of critical thinking questions designed to guide the student's knowledge to practical application.

Ancillary Package

To further facilitate teaching and learning, a carefully designed ancillary package is available.

Resources for Instructors

Tools to assist instructors with teaching the course are available upon adoption of this text on **thePoint** as well as on an Instructor's Resource DVD-ROM for instructors who prefer that method of delivery.

- A **Test Generator** includes a bank of over 600 questions to aid in the creation of quizzes and tests for assessing students' mastery of the material.
- An **Image Bank** contains illustrations and photographs from the book in formats suitable for print or digital use.
- **PowerPoint Presentations** for each chapter facilitate the development of slide shows and handouts, providing an easy way to integrate the textbook with the students' classroom experience.
- **Case Study Questions and Discussion Points.** Discussion points for the case studies that appear in the text are provided to facilitate small group discussions about the clinical scenarios presented in the cases.
- **Guided Lecture Notes** guide instructors through the chapters, objective by objective, and provide corresponding PowerPoint slide numbers.
- **Sample Syllabi** provide guidance for structuring the critical care course.
- A **QSEN Pre-Licensure KSA Competencies Map** identifies content in the textbook that supports QSEN's pre-licensure KSA competencies of patient-centered care, teamwork and collaboration, evidence-based practice, quality improvement, safety, and informatics.
- **Strategies for Effective Teaching** provide tips for preparing the course, meeting students' needs, and helping students to succeed.

Instructors are also given access to all of the student resources.

Resources for Students

An exciting set of free resources is available to help students master the material. These materials are accessible on **thePoint** with the access code printed in the front of the textbook.

- An **E-Book** on **thePoint** provides access to the book's full text and images online.
- **Journal Articles** offer access to current research related to chapter content.
- **Internet Resources** provide links to Web sites of interest that support the topics discussed in the text.
- **Learning Objectives** are supplied for each chapter in the book, to guide teaching and learning.
- **Chapter Review Questions** provide an easy way for students to check their understanding of chapter content.
- **Answers to Chapter Review Questions** with rationales are also accessible to students to allow self-assessment of their mastery of the chapter content.
- **Concepts in Action Animations** bring physiologic and pathophysiologic concepts to life.
- **Monographs of 100 Commonly Prescribed Drugs** provide up-to-date, detailed drug information for 100 commonly prescribed drugs in a quick-review format.
- A **Spanish-English Audio Glossary** provides helpful words and phrases for communicating with Spanish-speaking patients.

It is with great pleasure that we introduce these resources—the textbook and the ancillary package—to you. It is our intent that these resources will provide a solid introduction to, and foundation for, the discipline of critical care nursing. We hope that we have succeeded in that goal, and we welcome feedback from our readers.

Patricia Gonce Morton, RN, PhD, ACNP-BC, FAAN
Dorrie K. Fontaine, RN, PhD, FAAN
Kendra Menzies Kent, RN, MS, CCRN, CNRN

Acknowledgments

This book was made possible through the dedication and hard work of many people. First, we would like to thank Kendra Menzies Kent, RN, MS, CCRN, CNRN, who served as a content expert and reviewer for the entire book. Kendra helped us immeasurably with reducing, refocusing, reorganizing, and updating information to create this new textbook. Our publisher, Lippincott Williams & Wilkins, demonstrated the same commitment to producing an excellent essentials text that they have shown through all editions of the parent text. We especially want to thank Melanie Cann, Director, Product Development, for her editorial insight and direction, and Helen Kogut, Senior Product Manager, for the masterful job she did of coordinating the efforts of authors, content experts, editors, and vendors to make this essentials text a reality. We would also like to acknowledge Matt Skalka, Product Manager at Words & Numbers, for his work on behalf of the project. Finally, we must express our appreciation to Elizabeth Nieginski, Executive Editor, for her encouragement and support throughout the development of the textbook.

Contents

The Concept of Holism Applied to Critical Care Nursing Practice

ONE

Critical Care Nursing Practice

OBJECTIVES

Based on the content in this chapter, the reader should be able to:

1 Describe the value of certification in critical care nursing.
2 Describe the value of evidence-based practice (EBP) in caring for critically ill patients.
3 List the six standards for a healthy work environment and describe how the work environment can affect patient outcomes and employee well-being.
4 Describe the critical care nurse's role in promoting a healthy work environment.
5 Explain the underlying premises of the synergy model.

Critical care nurses routinely care for patients with complex, life-threatening conditions. In addition to managing the physiological alterations brought on by critical illness, critical care nurses must also manage the accompanying psychosocial challenges and ethical conflicts that often arise in the critical care setting. While operating within a highly technological environment, critical care nurses are charged with providing compassionate, patient- and family-focused care.

The overreaching professional goal for the critical care nurse is to promote optimal outcomes for the patients and families who are being cared for in the complex setting of the critical care unit. Becoming certified in the discipline of critical care nursing,

seeking to provide interventions that are based on current evidence, working to create and promote a healthy work environment (HWE), and working to cultivate core nursing competencies (eg, clinical judgment, advocacy, collaboration) are strategies the critical care nurse can use to achieve this goal.

Value of Certification

Specialty certification by the American Association of Critical-Care Nurses (AACN) promotes excellence in the critical care nursing profession by helping nurses achieve and maintain an up-to-date knowledge base and allowing nurses to voluntarily demonstrate their breadth and depth of knowledge of the discipline of critical care nursing.[1] Certification has value for patients and families, employers, and nurses themselves:

- **Value to the patient and family.** Certification validates to patients and families that the nurses caring for them have demonstrated experience and knowledge that exceeds that which is assessed in entry-level licensure examinations.[1] Experience and knowledge enable nurses to recognize and respond to clinical situations more quickly, and research has shown that nurses who have had their knowledge validated through a certification examination make decisions with greater confidence, promoting optimal outcomes.[1] In addition, nurses who are certified in a specialty have demonstrated commitment to continual learning, an attribute that is needed to care for patients with complex multisystem problems.
- **Value to employers.** Certification validates to employers that the nurse is committed to the discipline and has the knowledge and experience to work efficiently to promote optimal patient outcomes. It has been suggested that organizations that support and recognize the value of certification may experience decreased turnover and improved retention rates.[1] In addition, employing nurses who have achieved certification demonstrates to the public (ie, healthcare consumers) and to credentialing organizations (eg, the Joint Commission, the American Nurses Credentialing Center) that the facility has recruited and retained knowledge-validated nurses.[1]
- **Value to nurses.** Certification provides nurses with a sense of professional pride and achievement, and the confidence that comes with certification may give the nurse a competitive edge when seeking a promotion or new career opportunities. In addition, certified nurses can anticipate increased recognition from peers and employers. Certification may have monetary benefits as well. For example, some employers recognize certification with a salary differential, and one of the world's largest insurance brokers offers a discount on malpractice premiums to nurses who are certified in critical care.[1]

Evidence-Based Practice in Critical Care Nursing

Evidence-based practice (EBP) is the use of the best available research data from well-designed studies coupled with experiential knowledge and characteristics, values, and patient preferences in clinical practice to support clinical decision making.[2] The use of research findings in clinical practice is essential to promote optimal outcomes and to ensure that nursing practice is effective.[3] Practice based on intuition or information that does not have a scientific basis is not in the best interest of patients and families.

Although knowledge regarding effectual nursing interventions continues to increase, transfer of evidence into practice can be a long process. Common barriers to implementation are summarized in Box 1-1. Strategies for promoting the incorporation of evidence into clinical practice include

- Use of protocols, clinical pathways, and algorithms[4]
- Increasing clinicians' awareness of available resources (eg, databases such as PubMed, CINAHL, and MEDLINE; Web sites such as UpToDate, which offers real-time evidence-based recommendations for patient care, and the Cochrane Library, a source of high-quality, independent evidence to inform healthcare decision making; and professional nursing organizations, such as the AACN, which publishes research-based Practice Alerts)
- Creating an organizational culture that supports EBP (eg, identifying EBP champions, incorporating EBP activities into nurses' roles, allocating time and money to the process, promoting multidisciplinary collaboration among researchers and practitioners)[4]

Healthy Work Environments

A healthy work environment (HWE) optimizes professional collaboration and nursing practice (thus facilitating quality clinical outcomes) and promotes employee satisfaction. In 2001, in light of data indicating that harmful healthcare working environments exist nationwide and that these environments result in medical errors, poor healthcare delivery, and dissatisfaction among healthcare providers, the AACN helped develop the HWE initiative. The HWE initiative focuses on barriers to patient safety and employee satisfaction and identifies six essential standards for promoting a HWE: skilled communication, true collaboration, effective decision making, appropriate staffing, meaningful recognition, and authentic leadership (Box 1-2).

Skilled Communication

Skilled communication is essential to prevent errors as well as to recruit and retain healthcare providers. Almost 70% of sentinel events reported to the Joint Commission in 2005 were related to communication issues.[5] AACN partnered with VitalSmarts (a

---

BOX 1·1 Barriers to Evidence-Based Practice (EBP)

- Lack of knowledge
- Lack of research skills, resources, or both
- Lack of organizational support and management commitment
- Lack of time
- Lack of incentive to change behavior
- Lack of confidence in personal ability to change practice
- Lack of authority to change practice

BOX 1-2   Critical Elements of the Six Essential Standards of a Healthy Work Environment

Standard 1: Skilled Communication

Nurses must be as proficient in communication skills as they are in clinical skills.

- The healthcare organization provides team members with support for and access to education programs that develop critical communication skills including self-awareness, inquiry/dialogue, conflict management, negotiation, advocacy, and listening.
- Skilled communicators focus on finding solutions and achieving desirable outcomes.
- Skilled communicators seek to protect and advance collaborative relationships among colleagues.
- Skilled communicators invite and hear all relevant perspectives.
- Skilled communicators call on goodwill and mutual respect to build consensus and arrive at common understanding.
- Skilled communicators demonstrate congruence between words and actions, holding others accountable for doing the same.
- The healthcare organization establishes zero-tolerance policies and enforces them to address and eliminate abuse and disrespectful behavior in the workplace.
- The healthcare organization establishes formal structures and processes that ensure effective information sharing among patients, families, and the healthcare team.
- Skilled communicators have access to appropriate communication technologies and are proficient in their use.
- The healthcare organization establishes systems that require individuals and teams to formally evaluate the impact of communication on clinical, financial, and work environment outcomes.
- The healthcare organization includes communication as a criterion in its formal performance appraisal system, and team members demonstrate skilled communication to qualify for professional advancement.

Standard 2: True Collaboration

Nurses must be relentless in pursuing and fostering true collaboration.

- The healthcare organization provides team members with support for and access to education programs that develop collaboration skills.
- The healthcare organization creates, uses, and evaluates processes that define each team member's accountability for collaboration and how unwillingness to collaborate will be addressed.
- The healthcare organization creates, uses, and evaluates operational structures that ensure the decision-making authority of nurses is acknowledged and incorporated as the norm.
- The healthcare organization ensures unrestricted access to structured forums, such as ethics committees, and makes available the time needed to resolve disputes among all critical participants, including patients, families, and the healthcare team.
- Every team member embraces true collaboration as an ongoing process and invests in its development to ensure a sustained culture of collaboration.

- Every team member contributes to the achievement of common goals by giving power and respect to each person's voice, integrating individual differences, resolving competing interests, and safeguarding the essential contribution each must make in order to achieve optimal outcomes.
- Every team member acts with a high level of personal integrity.
- Team members master skilled communication, an essential element of true collaboration.
- Each team member demonstrates competence appropriate to his or her role and responsibilities.
- Nurse managers and medical directors are equal partners in modeling and fostering true collaboration.

Standard 3: Effective Decision Making

Nurses must be valued and committed partners in making policy, directing and evaluating clinical care, and leading organizational operations.

- The healthcare organization provides team members with support for and access to ongoing education and development programs focusing on strategies that ensure collaborative decision making. Program content includes mutual goal setting, negotiation, facilitation, conflict management, systems thinking, and performance improvement.
- The healthcare organization clearly articulates organizational values, and team members incorporate these values when making decisions.
- The healthcare organization has operational structures in place that ensure the perspectives of patients and their families are incorporated into every decision affecting patient care.
- Individual team members share accountability for effective decision making by acquiring necessary skills, mastering relevant content, assessing situations accurately, sharing fact-based information, communicating professional opinions clearly, and inquiring actively.
- The healthcare organization establishes systems, such as structured forums involving all departments and healthcare disciplines, to facilitate data-driven decisions.
- The healthcare organization establishes deliberate decision-making processes that ensure respect for the rights of every individual, incorporate all key perspectives, and designate clear accountability.
- The healthcare organization has fair and effective processes in place at all levels to objectively evaluate the results of decisions, including delayed decisions and indecision.

Standard 4: Appropriate Staffing

Staffing must ensure the effective match between patient needs and nurse competencies.

- The healthcare organization has staffing policies in place that are solidly grounded in ethical principles and support the professional obligation of nurses to provide high-quality care.

(continued on page 4)

BOX 1-2 Critical Elements of the Six Essential Standards of a Healthy Work Environment (continued)

- Nurses participate in all organizational phases of the staffing process from education and planning—including matching nurses' competencies with patients' assessed needs—through evaluation.
- The healthcare organization has formal processes in place to evaluate the effect of staffing decisions on patient and system outcomes. This evaluation includes analysis of when patient needs and nurse competencies are mismatched and how often contingency plans are implemented.
- The healthcare organization has a system in place that facilitates team members' use of staffing and outcomes data to develop more effective staffing models.
- The healthcare organization provides support services at every level of activity to ensure nurses can optimally focus on the priorities and requirements of patient and family care.
- The healthcare organization adopts technologies that increase the effectiveness of nursing care delivery. Nurses are engaged in the selection, adaptation, and evaluation of these technologies.

Standard 5: Meaningful Recognition
Nurses must be recognized and must recognize others for the value each brings to the work of the organization.

- The healthcare organization has a comprehensive system in place that includes formal processes and structured forums that ensure a sustainable focus on recognizing all team members for their contributions and the value they bring to the work of the organization.
- The healthcare organization establishes a systematic process for all team members to learn about the facility's recognition system and how to participate by recognizing the contributions of colleagues and the value they bring to the organization.
- The healthcare organization's recognition system reaches from the bedside to the board table, ensuring individuals receive recognition consistent with their personal definition of meaning, fulfillment, development, and advancement at every stage of their professional career.
- The healthcare organization's recognition system includes processes that validate that recognition is meaningful to those being acknowledged.
- Team members understand that everyone is responsible for playing an active role in the organization's recognition program and meaningfully recognizing contributions.

- The healthcare organization regularly and comprehensively evaluates its recognition system, ensuring effective programs that help to move the organization toward a sustainable culture of excellence that values meaningful recognition.

Standard 6: Authentic Leadership
Nurse leaders must fully embrace the imperative of a healthy work environment (HWE), authentically live it, and engage others in its achievement.

- The healthcare organization provides support for and access to educational programs to ensure that nurse leaders develop and enhance knowledge and abilities in skilled communication, effective decision making, true collaboration, meaningful recognition, and ensuring resources to achieve appropriate staffing.
- Nurse leaders demonstrate an understanding of the requirements and dynamics at the point of care and within this context successfully translate the vision of a HWE.
- Nurse leaders excel at generating visible enthusiasm for achieving the standards that create and sustain HWEs.
- Nurse leaders lead the design of systems necessary to effectively implement and sustain standards for HWEs.
- The healthcare organization ensures that nurse leaders are appropriately positioned in their pivotal role in creating and sustaining HWEs. This includes participation in key decision-making forums, access to essential information, and the authority to make necessary decisions.
- The healthcare organization facilitates the efforts of nurse leaders to create and sustain a HWE by providing the necessary time and financial and human resources.
- The healthcare organization provides a formal comentoring program for all nurse leaders. Nurse leaders actively engage in the comentoring program.
- Nurse leaders role-model skilled communication, true collaboration, effective decision making, meaningful recognition, and authentic leadership.
- The healthcare organization includes the leadership contribution to creating and sustaining a HWE as a criterion in each nurse leader's performance appraisal. Nurse leaders must demonstrate sustained leadership in creating and sustaining a HWE to achieve professional advancement.
- Nurse leaders and team members mutually and objectively evaluate the impact of leadership processes and decisions on the organization's progress toward creating and sustaining a HWE.

From http://www.aacn.org/aacn/pubpolcy.nsf/Files/ExecSum/$file/ExecSum.pdf

company that provides corporate training and organizational performance solutions) to conduct a study of conversations that do not occur in hospitals, to the detriment of patient safety and provider well-being. The "Silence Kills" study used focus groups, interviews, workplace observation, and surveys of nurses, physicians, and administrators in urban, rural, and suburban hospitals nationwide.[6] Overwhelming data indicated that poor communication and collaboration were prevalent among healthcare providers. The study concluded that healthcare providers repeatedly observe errors, breaking of rules, and dangerous levels of incompetence, yet rather than speak up, they consider leaving their respective units because of their concerns. The ability to communicate effectively and assertively and manage conflict is essential for advocating for oneself and others, and fosters a positive workplace environment characterized by an atmosphere of respect and collaboration.

True Collaboration

Collaboration is a multifaceted concept, which has been defined as working together to accomplish a common goal. One researcher has identified collaboration as both a process (blending different points of view to better comprehend a difficult issue) and an outcome (the integration of solutions contributed by more than one person).[7] This researcher has identified 10 lessons in collaboration: (1) know thyself; (2) learn to value and manage diversity; (3) develop constructive conflict resolution skills; (4) create win–win situations; (5) master interpersonal and process skills; (6) recognize that collaboration is a journey; (7) leverage all multidisciplinary forums; (8) appreciate that collaboration can occur spontaneously; (9) balance autonomy and unity in collaborative relationships; and (10) remember that collaboration is not required for all decisions.[7] Other investigators have suggested that collaboration is defined through five concepts: sharing, partnership, power, interdependency, and process.[8]

Results of several studies have supported a high correlation between nurse–physician collaboration and positive patient outcomes and a decreased incidence of medication errors.[9] However, a number of barriers exist that preclude true collaboration in healthcare organizations, including variations in how "collaboration" is conceptualized; the lack of time for communication; the complexity of the skills required to facilitate collaboration; and issues related to autonomy, power, and role confusion.[10]

Effective Decision Making

Because the healthcare environment mandates that nurses be accountable for their practice, they must be able to participate in effective decision making. A high degree of responsibility and autonomy is necessary. An environment that consistently and successfully encourages nurses to participate in decision making promotes quality patient outcomes and improved employee satisfaction.

Appropriate Staffing

There is a significant relationship between inadequate nurse staffing and adverse patient events. According to the Joint Commission, based on database records from 1995 to 2004, staffing levels were a root cause of nearly a quarter of the sentinel events that resulted in death, injury, or permanent loss of function.[5] Adequacy of staffing has traditionally been based primarily on the number of staff assigned to a unit on a given shift. However, appropriate staffing must also consider the competencies of the staff assigned in relation to the needs of the patient and family during that shift. When the needs of patients and families are matched with the competencies of the assigned nurse, optimal outcomes may be achieved. The ability to monitor patient health status, perform therapeutic interventions, integrate patient care to avoid healthcare gaps, and promote optimal patient outcomes is compromised when the number of nurses is inadequate, or when nurses lack the required competencies.

Meaningful Recognition

Employee recognition can have a significant effect on job satisfaction, and can help to retain high-performing nurses and ensure an adequate workforce in the future. Effective recognition programs enhance the nurse's sense of accomplishment and validate the nurse's contributions to quality healthcare. The recognition may be modest in scale but must represent genuine caring and appreciation. In addition to monetary rewards when possible, recognition can take the form of verbal or written praise, appreciation, and acknowledgment of excellent performance.[11,12] Researchers have also suggested that to recruit and retain staff, employers need to recognize staff expectations (eg, the desire to lead balanced lives, receive opportunities for personal and professional growth, or make a meaningful contribution to the world through work).

Authentic Leadership

Nursing leaders play an essential role in creating a healthcare environment that is conducive to promoting quality patient outcomes and employee well-being.[13] Attributes of an authentic leader that are essential for establishing and maintaining a HWE include genuineness, trustworthiness, reliability, compassion, and believability.[14] An effective leader seeks to (1) balance the tension between production and efficiency; (2) create and sustain trust throughout the organization; (3) actively manage the process of change; (4) involve workers in decision making pertaining to work design and work flow; and (5) use knowledge management to establish the organization as a learning organization.[14]

The Synergy Model

The synergy model, developed by the AACN, has served as the foundation for certified practice since the late 1990s.[15] It is the conceptual model for undergraduate and graduate curricula and has been used in a variety of clinical settings as the basis for job descriptions, performance appraisals, and career advancement.[16]

The underlying premises of the synergy model are (1) patients' characteristics are of concern to

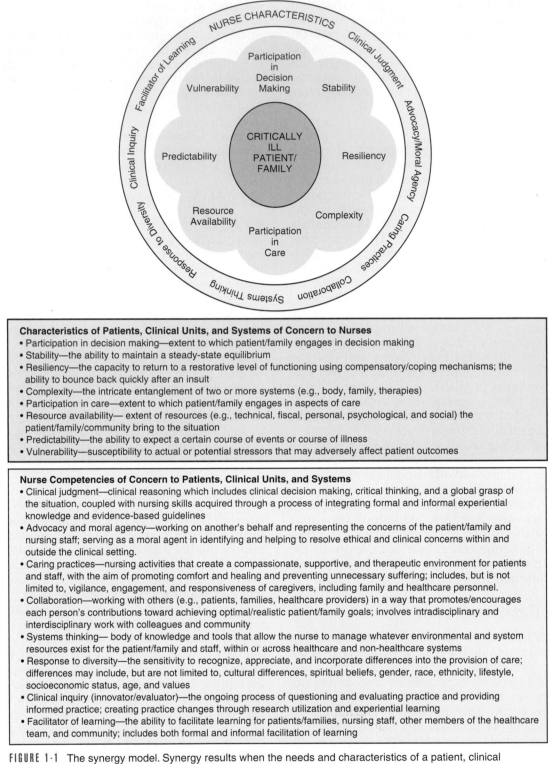

Characteristics of Patients, Clinical Units, and Systems of Concern to Nurses
- Participation in decision making—extent to which patient/family engages in decision making
- Stability—the ability to maintain a steady-state equilibrium
- Resiliency—the capacity to return to a restorative level of functioning using compensatory/coping mechanisms; the ability to bounce back quickly after an insult
- Complexity—the intricate entanglement of two or more systems (e.g., body, family, therapies)
- Participation in care—extent to which patient/family engages in aspects of care
- Resource availability— extent of resources (e.g., technical, fiscal, personal, psychological, and social) the patient/family/community bring to the situation
- Predictability—the ability to expect a certain course of events or course of illness
- Vulnerability—susceptibility to actual or potential stressors that may adversely affect patient outcomes

Nurse Competencies of Concern to Patients, Clinical Units, and Systems
- Clinical judgment—clinical reasoning which includes clinical decision making, critical thinking, and a global grasp of the situation, coupled with nursing skills acquired through a process of integrating formal and informal experiential knowledge and evidence-based guidelines
- Advocacy and moral agency—working on another's behalf and representing the concerns of the patient/family and nursing staff; serving as a moral agent in identifying and helping to resolve ethical and clinical concerns within and outside the clinical setting.
- Caring practices—nursing activities that create a compassionate, supportive, and therapeutic environment for patients and staff, with the aim of promoting comfort and healing and preventing unnecessary suffering; includes, but is not limited to, vigilance, engagement, and responsiveness of caregivers, including family and healthcare personnel.
- Collaboration—working with others (e.g., patients, families, healthcare providers) in a way that promotes/encourages each person's contributions toward achieving optimal/realistic patient/family goals; involves intradisciplinary and interdisciplinary work with colleagues and community
- Systems thinking— body of knowledge and tools that allow the nurse to manage whatever environmental and system resources exist for the patient/family and staff, within or across healthcare and non-healthcare systems
- Response to diversity—the sensitivity to recognize, appreciate, and incorporate differences into the provision of care; differences may include, but are not limited to, cultural differences, spiritual beliefs, gender, race, ethnicity, lifestyle, socioeconomic status, age, and values
- Clinical inquiry (innovator/evaluator)—the ongoing process of questioning and evaluating practice and providing informed practice; creating practice changes through research utilization and experiential learning
- Facilitator of learning—the ability to facilitate learning for patients/families, nursing staff, other members of the healthcare team, and community; includes both formal and informal facilitation of learning

FIGURE 1-1   The synergy model. Synergy results when the needs and characteristics of a patient, clinical unit, or system (*blue*) are matched with a nurse's competencies (*green*)

nurses; (2) nurses' competencies are important to patients; (3) patients' characteristics drive nurses' competencies; and (4) when patients' characteristics and nurses' competencies match and synergize, outcomes for the patient are optimal.[15] Eight characteristics (of patients, units, or systems) and eight nurse competencies that constitute nursing practice form the basis of the model (Fig. 1-1). Patient/unit/system characteristics range depending on the situation and are expressed as level 1, 3, or 5, with 1 being "low" and 5 being "high." Similarly, nurse competencies range depending on the nurse's level of expertise, and are expressed as level 1, 3, or 5, with 1 being "competent" and 5 being "expert."

The synergy model is used to evaluate the relationship between clinical practice and outcomes. Patient-derived outcomes may include functional change, behavioral change, trust, satisfaction, comfort, and quality of life. Nurse-derived outcomes may include physiological changes, absence of complications, and the extent to which care or treatment objectives are attained. Healthcare system–derived outcomes may include reduced recidivism, reduced costs, and enhanced resource utilization.

CASE STUDY

Mrs. C., an 82-year-old woman, is brought by ambulance to the emergency room because she is experiencing left-sided weakness and difficulty with speech. Mrs. C., an insulin-dependent diabetic who had an acute myocardial infarction 2 years ago, lives at home alone but is checked on frequently by family members. Mrs. C. has limited financial support. Today, her granddaughter stopped by to check on her and called 911 when she noticed that Mrs. C. was having trouble speaking.

In the emergency room, the healthcare team assessed Mrs. C.'s neurological status using the National Institutes of Health (NIH) stroke scale. CT studies were negative for hemorrhagic stroke. She was admitted to the critical care unit for ischemic stroke.

The critical care nurse performed a bedside swallow evaluation prior to administering oral medication. Based on this evaluation, the nurse decided to obtain a speech therapy consult to perform a more comprehensive swallow examination. The oral medication was held until the evaluation could be performed. Mrs. C.'s son arrived at the hospital to visit his mother; although he came during non-visiting hours, the nurse allowed him to visit with his mother, and provided him with a pamphlet that provided information regarding the critical care unit environment, what to expect, and visitation hours. Because Mrs. C. is currently unable to make her own healthcare decisions, her son provided the hospital with a copy of his mother's power of attorney for healthcare, which identified him as the primary decision maker.

1. Which patient characteristics are concerns for Mrs. C.?

2. By performing the swallow evaluation and obtaining a speech therapy consult, the critical care nurse demonstrated which nurse competencies?

3. Allowing Mrs. C.'s son to visit even though his visit did not coincide with standard visiting hours demonstrates which nurse competencies?

References

1. Kaplow R: The value of certification. AACN Adv Crit Care 2(1):25–32, 2011
2. Melnyk BM, Fineout-Overholt E: Evidence-Based Practice in Nursing and Healthcare: A Guide to Best Practice. Philadelphia, PA: Lippincott Williams & Wilkins, 2010
3. Staffileno B, McKinney C: Evidence based nursing. Nurs Manag 42(6):10–14, 2011
4. Schulman C: Strategies for starting a successful evidence based nursing program. AACN Adv Crit Care 19(3):301–311, 2008
5. Joint Commission on Accreditation of Healthcare Organizations. Retrieved June 15, 2006, from http://www.jointcommission.org/NR
6. Maxfield D, Grenny J, McMillan R, et al.: Silence kills: The seven crucial conversations for healthcare. Retrieved from http://www.aacn.org/aacn/pubpolcy.nsf
7. Gardner DB: Ten lessons in collaboration. Online J Issues Nurs 10(1):2, 2005
8. D'Amour D, Ferrada-Videla M, San Martin Rodriguez L, et al.: The conceptual basis for interprofessional collaboration: Core concepts and theoretical frameworks. J Interprof Care 19(suppl 1):116–131, 2005
9. LaValley D: Physician-Nurse collaboration and patient safety. Forum 26(2), 2008
10. Schmalenberg C, Kramer M: Clinical units with the healthiest work environments. Crit Care Nurse 28:65–67, 2008
11. Kramer M, Maguire P, Brewer B: Clinical nurses in Magnet hospitals confirm productive healthy unit work environments. J Nurs Management 19(1):5–17, 2011
12. Briggs L, Schriner C: Recognition and support for today's preceptor. J Contin Educ Nurs 41(7):317–322, 2010
13. Mastal M, Joshi M, Schulke K: Nursing leadership: Championing quality and patient safety in boardroom. Nurs Econ 25(6):323–330, 2007
14. Shirey MR: Authentic leaders creating healthy work environments for nursing practice. Am J Crit Care 15(4):256–267, 2006
15. American Association of Critical-Care Nurses Certification Corporation: The AACN Synergy Model for Patient Care. Retrieved June 15, 2006, from http://www.certcorp.org/certcorp/certcorp.nsf/vwdoc/SynModel
16. Reed KD, Cline M, Kerfoot KM: Implementation of the synergy model in critical care. In Kaplow R, Hardin SR (eds): Critical Care Nursing: Synergy for Optimal Outcomes. Sudbury, MA: Jones & Bartlett, 2007

Want to know more? A wide variety of resources to enhance your learning and understanding of this chapter are available on **the Point**. Visit **http://thepoint.lww.com/MortonEss1e** to access chapter review questions and more!

The Patient's and Family's Experience With Critical Illness

OBJECTIVES

Based on the content in this chapter, the reader should be able to:

1 Explain the effects of prolonged stress and anxiety and describe measures the nurse can take to minimize the amount of stress and anxiety patients and family members experience.
2 Describe the critical care nurse's role in assisting the family through the crisis.
3 Describe strategies to promote sleep in critically ill patients.
4 Discuss alternatives to the use of physical restraints in the critical care unit.

The patient's experience in a critical care unit has lasting meaning for the patient and family. Often, it is the caring and emotional support given by the nurse that is remembered and valued. A number of authors have sought to study and describe patients' experiences related to their stay in a critical care unit. Research has found that although many patients recall negative experiences, they also recall neutral and positive experiences. Negative experiences were related to fear, anxiety, sleep disturbance, cognitive impairment, and pain or discomfort. Positive experiences were related to feelings of being safe and secure and were often attributed to the care provided by nurses, specifically nurses' technical competence and effective interpersonal skills.[1] The need to feel safe and the need for information were predominant themes in other research studies as well.[1]

Managing Stress and Anxiety

Patients admitted to the critical care unit are subject to multiple physical, psychological, and environmental stressors, as are their family members. For example, patients and their families frequently perceive admission to critical care as a sign of impending death, based on their own past experiences or the experiences of others. In addition, the near-constant noise (eg, from equipment and alarms), bright lights, and lack of privacy in the critical care unit are intimidating and stress inducing. The body responds to these stressors by activating the hypothalamic–pituitary–adrenal axis. The resultant increase in catecholamine, glucocorticoid, and mineralocorticoid levels leads to a cascade of physiological responses known as the stress response (Fig. 2-1). In critically ill patients, prolonged activation of the stress response can lead to immunosuppression, hypoperfusion, tissue hypoxia, and other physiologic effects that impair healing and jeopardize recovery.

Anxiety, pain, and fear can initiate or perpetuate the stress response. Anxiety is an emotional state of apprehension in response to a real or perceived threat that is associated with motor tension, increased sympathetic activity, and hypervigilance. Feelings of helplessness, loss of control, loss of function or self-esteem, and isolation can produce anxiety, as can a fear of dying. Left untreated or undertreated, anxiety can contribute to the morbidity and mortality of critically ill patients.

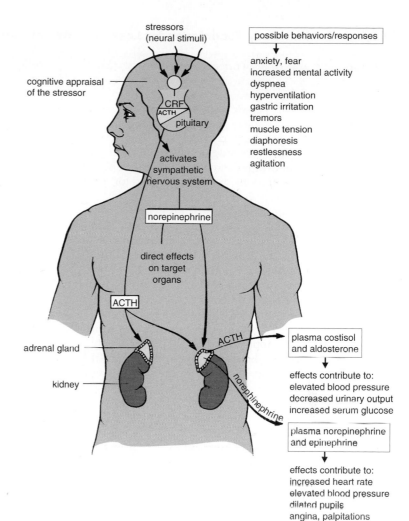

stressors
(neural stimuli)

possible behaviors/responses

anxiety, fear
increased mental activity
dyspnea
hyperventilation
gastric irritation
tremors
muscle tension
diaphoresis
restlessness
agitation

cognitive appraisal
of the stressor

CRF
ACTH
pituitary

activates
sympathetic
nervous system

norepinephrine

direct effects
on target
organs

ACTH

adrenal gland

kidney

ACTH

plasma costisol
and aldosterone

effects contribute to:
elevated blood pressure
decreased urinary output
increased serum glucose

plasma norepinephrine
and epinephrine

effects contribute to:
increased heart rate
elevated blood pressure
dilated pupils
angina, palpitations

norephinephrine

FIGURE 2-1   The stress response. Prolonged stress has far-reaching physiological effects that hinder the body's ability to heal. CRF, corticotropin releasing factor; ACTH, adrenocorticotropic hormone.

RED FLAG! *It is important to assess patients and family members for anxiety. The top five physiological and behavioral indicators of anxiety are agitated behavior, increased blood pressure, increased heart rate, verbalization of anxiety, and restlessness.*[2]

Management of stress and anxiety entails eliminating or minimizing the stressors. For the critically ill patient, providing supportive care (eg, nutrition, oxygenation, pain management, sedatives, and anxiolytics) is indicated.[3] Mind–body strategies that may be employed to lessen stress and anxiety are summarized in Box 2-1. Often, the way the nurse interacts with the patient and family can have a significant impact on the amount of stress and anxiety they experience. Positive actions the nurse can take to minimize stress and anxiety include

- **Fostering trust.** When patients or family members mistrust caregivers, they are more anxious because they are unable to feel safe and secure. A trusting relationship between the nurse and patient can make a difference in the patient's recovery or facilitating a dignified death. Displaying a confident, caring attitude; demonstrating technical competence; and developing effective communication techniques are strategies that help the nurse to foster trusting relationships with both patients and family members.

- **Providing information.** Anxiety can be greatly relieved with simple explanations. Critically ill patients and their family members need to know what is happening at the moment, what will happen to the patient in the near future, how the patient is doing, and what they can expect. Many patients also need frequent explanations of what happened to them. These explanations reorient them, sort out sequences of events, and help them distinguish real events from dreams or hallucinations.

BOX 2-1 Mind–Body Techniques for Lessening Anxiety and Stress

- **Presencing and reassurance.** Presencing, or "just being there," can alleviate distress and anxiety. Nurses practice presencing by adopting a caring attitude, paying attention to the person's needs, and actively listening. Reassurance can be provided verbally or through caring touch. Verbal reassurance is most appropriate for people who are expressing unrealistic or exaggerated fears. It is not valuable when it prevents a person from expressing emotions or stifles the need for further dialogue.
- **Reframing dialogue.** Highly anxious people tend to give themselves messages that perpetuate their anxiety. For example, a patient may be thinking things such as, "I can't stand it in here. I've got to get out." The nurse encourages the person to share his or her internal dialogue, and then helps the person replace the negative thoughts with constructive, reassuring ones (eg, "I've been in tough situations before, and I'm capable of making it through this one!"). A similar method can be applied to external dialogues. By speaking accurately about the situation to others, the person's own misconceptions about the situation will be improved.
- **Cognitive reappraisal.** This technique asks the person to identify a particular stressor and then reframe his or her perception of the stressor in a more positive light so that the stimulus is no longer viewed as threatening.
- **Guided imagery.** Guided imagery is a way of purposefully diverting or focusing a person's thoughts. Guided imagery can be used to promote relaxation through mental escape. The nurse encourages the person to imagine being in a very pleasant place or taking part in a very pleasant experience. The nurse instructs the person to focus and linger on the sensations that are experienced, prompting with questions if necessary (eg, "What colors do you see?" "What do you hear?" "How does the air smell?"). Guided imagery can also be used to mentally prepare to meet a challenge (eg, relearning how to walk) successfully. When applied in this way, the nurse teaches the person to visualize herself moving through the task and successfully completing it.
- **Relaxation training.** In progressive relaxation, the person is directed to find a comfortable position and then to take several deep breaths and let them out slowly. Next, the person is asked to clench a fist or curl the toes as tightly as possible, to hold the position for a few seconds, and then to let go while focusing on the sensations of the releasing muscles. The person progresses in this way, tensing and releasing the muscles in a systematic manner throughout the body.
- **Deep breathing.** People who are acutely anxious tend to hold their breath. Diaphragmatic (abdominal) breathing may be useful as both a distraction and a coping mechanism. To practice diaphragmatic breathing, the person places a hand on the abdomen, inhales deeply through the nose, holds the breath briefly, and exhales through pursed lips.
- **Music therapy.** Music therapy can reduce anxiety, provide distraction, and promote relaxation, rest, and sleep. It has also been shown to be effective for relaxing mechanically ventilated patients. Usually, music sessions are 20 to 90 minutes long, once or twice daily. Most people prefer music that is familiar to them.
- **Humor.** Laughter releases endorphins (the body's natural pain relievers) into the bloodstream, and can relieve tension and anxiety and relax muscles. The use of humor, spontaneous or planned, can help reduce procedural anxiety and provide distraction. The nurse takes cues from the person regarding the appropriate use of humor.
- **Massage.** Nurses have traditionally used effleurage (slow, rhythmic strokes from distal to proximal areas of long muscles such as those of the back or extremities) to promote patient comfort. Massage can be combined with the use of scented oils or lotions (eg, lavender to promote relaxation). Not all patients are good candidates for massage. For example, massage is not appropriate for patients who are hemodynamically unstable.
- **Therapeutic touch.** In therapeutic touch, the practitioner's hands move over a patient in a systematic way to rebalance the patient's energy fields. Therapeutic touch as a complementary therapy has been used successfully in acute care settings to decrease anxiety and promote a sense of well-being.
- **Meridian therapy.** Meridian therapy, which originates from traditional Chinese medicine, refers to therapies that involve an acupoint (eg, acupuncture, acupressure, the activation of specific sites with electrical stimulation and low-intensity laser).
- **Pet (animal-assisted) therapy.** Interacting with animals can provide physical benefits (eg, lowered blood pressure), as well as emotional ones (eg, increased self-esteem). Some facilities allow pets to visits their owners. Other facilities participate in formal programs wherein volunteer owner–dog teams visit patients in the critical care unit.

- **Ensuring privacy.** Ensuring privacy while sensitive or confidential information is being exchanged can markedly reduce the anxiety of a patient or family member. Healthcare providers are not always mindful of their surroundings when discussing confidential details of a patient's case. The nurse can direct healthcare providers and family members to a quiet room away from the general waiting area to afford privacy when discussing specific patient information.
- **Allowing control.** Nursing measures that reinforce a person's sense of control help increase autonomy and reduce the overpowering sense of loss of control that can increase anxiety and stress.

The nurse can help the patient and family exert more control over the environment by providing order and predictability in routines; using anticipatory guidance; allowing the patient and family to make choices whenever possible; involving the patient and family in decision making; and explaining procedures thoroughly, including why the procedure is needed.

Assisting the Family Through the Crisis

A critical illness is a sudden, unexpected, and stressful occurrence for both the patient and the family that threatens the equilibrium of the family unit. During the acute crisis, family members often experience stress, disorganization, and feelings of helplessness that make it difficult for them to mobilize appropriate coping resources.[2] The critical care nurse plays a key role in assisting the family through this stress response and helping them to adapt to the critical care environment. When caring for the family, the nurse seeks to (1) provide a human, caring presence; (2) acknowledge multiple perceptions; (3) respect diversity; and (4) value each person within the context of the family.

The way a family reacts to a crisis is difficult to categorize because reactions depend on the different coping styles, personalities, and stress management techniques of the family. However, the following generalizations usually hold true:

- Whether people emerge stronger or weaker as a result of a crisis is based not so much on their character, as on the quality of help they receive during the crisis.
- People are more open to suggestions and help during an actual crisis.
- With the onset of a crisis, old memories of past crises may be evoked. If maladaptive behavior was used to deal with previous situations, the same type of behavior may be repeated in the face of a new crisis. If adaptive behavior was used, the impact of the crisis may be lessened.
- The primary way to survive a crisis is to be aware of it.

The nurse's initial interaction with family members is extremely important because it helps establish a foundation of trust and respect between the nurse and family. Taking a few minutes to learn the names of family members and their relationship to the patient signifies respect and begins to build a therapeutic and trusting relationship. The primary goal of the nurse is to assist the family as they deal with the crisis phase of this illness by providing consistent and accurate information about the condition of their loved one. Research has demonstrated that up-to-date information is the highest priority for family members who are coping with critical illness.[3]

Frequently, the period of illness extends well beyond the initial crisis phase and creates additional burdens for the patient and the family. The patient may experience a slow and unpredictable course with periods of organ compromise or failure. Recovery is measured in small changes that occur over days and weeks. Over time, it may become increasingly difficult for the family to obtain information and patient status reports from the healthcare team. Often, physician schedules are unpredictable and physician visits may not coincide with family member availability. With protracted critical illness, many families struggle to keep the lines of communication open to the extended family, creating opportunities for conflict and misinformation. Throughout the patient's illness, it is vitally important for the critical care nurse to maintain a link with the family.

 RED FLAG! *The time the critical care nurse can spend with the family is often limited because of the crucial physiological and psychosocial needs of the patient. Therefore, it is important to make every interaction with the family as useful and therapeutic as possible.*

Identifying and Meeting Family Needs

Nursing assessment of the family seeks to identify the family's strengths as well as the problems they are facing. The nursing assessment is comprehensive, exploring family members' physiological, psychological, and spiritual responses to crisis, as well as social, environmental, cultural, and economic factors that influence the family. The family history provides insight into the family's past experience with critical illness, and is helpful for identifying family roles and relationships. Identifying a formal or informal leader of the family facilitates decision making and communication about legal matters (eg, obtaining consent, withdrawing life support).

Numerous assessment tools, such as the Critical Care Family Needs Inventory (CCFNI), are available to aid the nurse in determining the needs and problems the family faces. Nursing research using these tools reveals a great deal of consistency in what needs are important to family members (Box 2-2). Nursing interventions that help to address the needs of a family in crisis are given in Box 2-3. An approach to assisting the family with problem-solving is given in Box 2-4.

Some families will benefit from a referral to another objective professional with experience in critical illness and its impact on the family (eg, a mental health clinical specialist, a social worker, a psychologist, or a chaplain). Many critical care units have such resources available on a 24-hour, on-call basis to ensure prompt interventions. The nurse can best encourage the family to accept help from others by acknowledging the difficulty and complexity of the problem and providing contact information for several professionals who will be able to assist.

BOX 2-2 Commonly Identified Needs of Family Members in Crisis

- The need to feel satisfied with the care given
- The need for courteous caregivers who show an interest in how the family is doing
- The need to receive information about the patient at least once a day, and assurance that someone will call the family with any changes
- The need to see the patient frequently and be in close proximity to the patient
- The need for honest information about the patient's condition, including information about the patient's prognosis
- The need to have understandable explanations of why things are being done
- The need to have physical needs met (eg, a comfortable place to wait with easy access to refreshments and bathroom facilities)
- The need to have emotional needs met (eg, the need to feel that there is hope, the need to share negative feelings)

Facilitating Visitation

Policies regarding visiting hours should be evaluated periodically. Family presence at the bedside has been shown to decrease patient and family anxiety, and can have a positive effect on the patient's physiological parameters (eg, intracranial pressure) as well. Novel approaches to visitation (eg, children accompanied by an adult, animals as part of

BOX 2-3 Nursing Interventions for Care of the Family in Crisis

- Convey feelings of hope and confidence in the family's ability to deal with the situation.
- Try to perceive the feelings that the crisis evokes in the family.
- Demonstrate concern about the patient and family and a willingness to help.
- Speak openly to the patient and the family about the critical illness.
- Discuss all issues as they relate to the patient specifically, avoiding generalizations.
- Be realistic and honest about the situation, taking care not to give false reassurance.
- Ensure that the family receives information about all significant changes in the patient's condition.
- Mitigate feelings of powerlessness and hopelessness by involving families in decision making and patient care.
- Advocate for the adjustment of visiting hours to accommodate the needs of the family.
- Locate space near the unit where the family can be alone and have privacy.
- Recognize the patient's and family's spirituality, and suggest the assistance of a spiritual advisor if there is a need.

BOX 2-4 Assisting the Family in Crisis With Problem-Solving

1. **Identify the problem.** Families in crisis are often overwhelmed and immobilized by acute stress and anxiety. Helping the family to articulate the immediate problem reduces anxiety by giving family members a clearer understanding of what is happening, and facilitates the planning of goal-directed activities.
2. **Identify available support systems.** Asking family members to identify the person to whom they usually turn when they are upset, and encouraging them to seek assistance from that person now, helps direct the family back to the normal mechanisms for handling stressful issues. Few families are truly without resources; rather, they only have failed to recognize and call on them.
3. **Focus on feelings.** During the difficult days of the critical illness, the family may become dependent on the judgment of professionals. It is important that the nurse acknowledges the family's feelings and recognizes the complexity of the problem, while emphasizing the responsibility each member of the family has for his or her feelings, actions, and decisions. The nurse encourages family members to reflect on their feelings and practices by using active listening.
4. **Identify steps.** Once the problem has been defined and the family begins goal-directed activities, the nurse may help further by asking the family members to identify the steps that they must take to achieve those goals. For example, sometimes the nurse must help family members recognize that returning home to rest is an important step for maintaining their own health and ability to help the patient.

an animal-assisted therapy program) have also been shown to have positive effects on patients, including increased feelings of happiness and calmness and reduced feelings of loneliness.[4] These findings support the need for less restrictive and individualized visiting policies for patients and families.

The nurse prepares family members for the initial visit to the unit by providing explanations of the functions of monitors, IV drips, ventilators, and other equipment, as well as the meaning of alarms, before and during the visit. The nurse also introduces the family to the members of the healthcare team involved in the patient's care, providing names, titles, and an explanation of responsibilities. Encouraging family members to provide direct care to the patient (eg, assistance with grooming, eating, or hygiene), if they are interested, can help decrease anxiety and provide the family with some sense of control.

Managing Family Presence During Invasive Procedures and Resuscitation Efforts

Although controversial, family presence during invasive procedures and resuscitation efforts is becoming more common. In light of current research, it has demonstrated positive benefits for family members. When family members were interviewed, 97.5% believed that family presence was a right, 100% said they would repeat family presence in the same situation again, 95% believed that their presence helped the patient, even if the patient was unconscious, and 95% said it helped them realize the seriousness of the patient's condition.[5] In the event of the patient's death, family members have reported that being present during resuscitation efforts was helpful during the bereavement process.[3]

However, many healthcare providers are uncomfortable with family presence during resuscitation efforts, due to concerns about litigation, making a mistake, or that caring for family members may take time and attention away from the patient. The American Association of Critical-Care Nurses (AACN) recommends that each facility establish policies and procedures for handling family presence during resuscitation.[6] Every effort must be made to have a knowledgeable person present to explain to the family what measures are being implemented and the rationale. Protocols must also be in place to escort family members from the room if the healthcare team cannot perform resuscitative measures effectively.

Facilitating Family Conferences

As a patient and family advocate, the nurse provides accurate information and shares the plan of care with the family. The nurse may arrange for a family conference to provide a forum for healthcare providers and family members to share information in an organized way. During the family conference, the healthcare team provides information about the condition of the patient and the patient's prognosis and reviews recommendations for care. Family conferences facilitate open communication and are often useful for dispelling misinformation and misconceptions about the patient's progress. Family conferences also serve as a forum for exploring how family members may wish to participate in determining treatment goals for the patient.[5]

Consensus among providers is an important step before presenting treatment options and recommendations.[3] Providing conflicting information creates confusion for everyone involved and may lead families to request nonbeneficial interventions. Box 2-5 describes the nurse's role before and after the family conference[5] and Box 2-6 describes how to facilitate communication during a family conference. Encouraging the family to be active participants during the family conference increases their level of satisfaction and improves the quality of communication among providers and families.[7]

BOX 2-5 The Nurse's Role Before and After the Family Conference

Before the Conference
- Explain the medical equipment and therapies that are being used in the care of the patient to the family.
- Tell the family what to expect during their conference with the healthcare team members.
- Talk with the family about their spiritual or religious needs and take actions to address unmet spiritual or religious needs.
- Talk with the family about specific cultural needs and take actions to address unmet cultural needs.
- Talk with the family about what the patient values in life.
- Talk with the family about the patient's illness and treatment.
- Talk with the family about their feelings.
- Reminisce with the family about the patient.
- Tell the family it is all right to talk to and touch their loved one.
- Discuss with the family what the patient might have wanted if he or she were able to participate in the treatment decision-making process.
- Locate a private place or room for the family to talk among themselves.

After the Conference
- Talk with the family about how the conference went.
- Talk with any other healthcare team members who were present at the conference about how the conference went.
- Ask the family if they had any questions following the conference.
- Talk with the family about their feelings.
- Talk with the family about any disagreement among the family concerning the plan of care.
- Talk with the family about changes in the patient's plan of care as a result of the conference.
- Support the decisions the family made during the conference.
- Reassure the family that the patient will be kept comfortable.
- Tell the family it is all right to talk to and touch their loved one.
- Locate a private place or room for the family to talk among themselves.

From Curtis JR, Patrick DL, Shannon SE, et al.: The family conference as a focus to improve communication about end-of-life care in the intensive care unit: Opportunities for improvement. Crit Care Med 29(2 suppl):N26–N33, 2001.

RED FLAG! *The nurse should have the patient's permission before giving confidential medical information to family members. If that is not possible because of the patient's condition, the patient's next of kin should be identified as the person who may receive confidential information. The names of those family members approved to receive medical information about the patient should be recorded in the patient's medical record.[8]*

BOX 2·6 Facilitating Communication During a Family Conference

Before the Conference
- Review previous knowledge of the patient and family.
- Review previous knowledge of the family's attitudes and reactions.
- Review your knowledge of the disease—prognosis, treatment options.
- Examine your own personal feelings, attitudes, biases, and grieving.
- Plan the specifics of location and setting: a quiet, private place.
- Discuss with the family in advance about who will be present.

During the Conference
- Introduce everyone present.
- If appropriate, set the tone in a nonthreatening way: "This is a conversation we have with all families…"
- Discuss the goals of the specific conference.
- Find out what the family understands.
- Review what has happened and what is happening to the patient.
- Discuss prognosis frankly in a way that is meaningful to the family.
- Acknowledge uncertainty in the prognosis.
- Review the principle of substituted judgment: "What would the patient want?"

- Support the family's decision.
- Do not discourage all hope; consider redirecting hope toward a comfortable death with dignity if appropriate.
- Avoid the temptation to give too much medical detail.
- Make it clear that withholding life-sustaining treatment is not withholding caring.
- Make explicit what care will be provided including symptom management, where the care will be delivered, and the family's access to the patient.
- If life-sustaining treatments will be withheld or withdrawn, discuss what the patient's death might be like.
- Use repetition to show that you understand what the patient or family is saying.
- Acknowledge strong emotions and use reflection to encourage patients or families to talk about these emotions.
- Tolerate silence.

At the Conclusion of the Conference
- Achieve common understanding of the disease and treatment issues.
- Make a recommendation about treatment.
- Ask if there are any questions.
- Review the follow-up plan and make sure the family knows how to reach you for questions.

From Curtis JR, Patrick DL, Shannon SE, et al.: The family conference as a focus to improve communication about end-of-life care in the intensive care unit: Opportunities for improvement. Crit Care Med 29(2 suppl):N26–N33, 2001.

Practicing Cultural Sensitivity

Culturally competent nursing care is defined as being sensitive to issues related to culture, race, gender, sexual orientation, social class, and economic situation.[3] In addition, culturally competent nursing considers the family structure and gender role as it relates to the patient. Health and illness beliefs are deeply rooted in culture. How a patient or family member responds to the diagnosis or a proposed treatment may be strongly influenced by his or her values and culture. During initial assessment, the critical care nurse obtains several key pieces of information regarding the patient's cultural beliefs (Box 2-7). Astuteness and sensitivity on the part of the critical care nurse are required to ensure that the highly technologic, illness-focused critical care environment does not clash with the patient's and family's cultural beliefs and values. Because individual responses and values may vary within the same culture, the nurse takes care to recognize the patient and family members as individuals within the cultural context.

Supporting Spirituality

Spirituality speaks to the manner by which a person seeks meaning in his or her life, and experiences connectedness with the universe at large. Spirituality is intrinsically related to a person's beliefs and values, and for some people, it has a religious component. The nurse assesses the patient's and family's spiritual belief systems and assists the patient and family in recognizing and drawing on the values and beliefs they already hold. Critical illness may

BOX 2·7 Key Pieces of Information to Obtain as Part of the Cultural Assessment

- Place of birth
- Length of time in this country
  - Does the patient live in an ethnic community?
  - Who are the patient's major support people?
- Primary and secondary languages (speaking and reading ability)
- Religious practices
- Health and illness beliefs and practices
- Communication practices (verbal and nonverbal)
- How decisions are made in the context of the patient and family

Adapted from Lipson JG: Culturally competent nursing care. In Lipson JG, Dibble SL, Mainarik PA (eds): Culture and Nursing Care: A Pocket Guide. San Francisco, UCSF Nursing Press, 2005, pp 1–6.

deepen or challenge existing spirituality. During these times, it may be useful to call on a spiritual or religious leader, hospital chaplain, or pastoral care representative to help the patient and family make meaningful use of the critical illness experience.

Preparing the Patient and Family for Discharge

As the patient's condition improves and plans for transfer to a lower acuity area are discussed with the healthcare team, the critical care nurse must prepare the patient and family for the eventual discharge from the unit. This milestone in recovery is typically viewed by the patient and family in one of two ways. If the patient and family believe that the patient's condition has improved sufficiently and that the intensity of critical care is no longer necessary, then this step is viewed in a positive light. However, if they believe that the depth of nursing support and level of monitoring on a lower acuity unit are inadequate to meet the needs of the patient, there may be resistance to the transfer process. Providing information about the new unit's routine, staffing patterns, and visiting hours before making the transfer can help mitigate some of the negative feelings and anxiety associated with the change.[3]

Once the transfer has been made, it is important that the receiving nurse further assist the patient and family with adjusting to the new routine. The nurse begins by acknowledging the normal anxiety that accompanies the transfer process, and emphasizes that the transition is a positive stage in the recovery process. The nurse also reassures the patient and family that even though the intensity of treatment has changed, staff members are trained to anticipate the patient's needs and will respond appropriately to changes in the patient's status. Once the patient's and family's initial anxiety diminishes, the nurse can begin to set new self-care goals and expectations based on assessment of the patient.

Promoting Rest and Sleep for the Critically Ill Patient

Sleep deprivation is common in critically ill patients, due to environmental factors, anxiety, pain, medication side effects, and therapeutic interventions that disrupt sleep. Secretion of melatonin (a hormone that facilitates sleep) is inhibited by light and stimulated by darkness; the constant, high-intensity lighting typical of the critical care unit disrupts this normal rhythm. Sleep deprivation contributes to stress and, if prolonged, can lead to altered cognition, confusion, and difficulty with ventilator weaning.

BOX 2-8 Nursing Interventions for Promoting Sleep

- Ensure the patient is comfortable (eg, manage pain, use pillows to ensure a comfortable position).
- Schedule care and procedures (eg, labs, x-rays) to disrupt sleep as little as possible.
- Try to orient the patient to normal sleep–wake cycles as much as possible. Provide large clocks and calendars, and dim the lights at bedtime.
- Make an effort to control noise, especially during the evening hours: decrease noise from televisions and talking, post signs to alert others to the need to be quiet (eg, "Patient Sleeping").
- Ensure privacy by closing the door and pulling the curtains (if possible).
- Institute a bedtime routine (eg, brushing teeth, washing face). As part of the bedtime routine, consider providing a 5-minute massage.
- At bedtime, provide information to lower anxiety. Review the day together, remind the patient of progress made toward recovery, and explain what to expect for the next day.
- Employ anxiety-reducing strategies (eg, relaxation techniques, guided imagery, music therapy).

The nurse assesses the amount and quality of the patient's sleep, and intervenes to facilitate rest and sleep (Box 2-8). The patient's own report of sleep quality is the best measure of sleep adequacy. A visual analog scale is recommended to evaluate sleep quality in select patients at high risk for sleep disruption owing to an extended stay on the critical care unit.[9] Some situations (eg, mechanical ventilation) make a self-report of sleep quality difficult to obtain. If a self-report is unobtainable, systematic observation has been shown to be somewhat valid and reliable.[9]

Using Restraints in Critical Care

Physical restraints must occasionally be used for patients in critical care to prevent potentially serious disruptions in therapy resulting from accidental dislodgment of endotracheal tubes, IV lines, and other invasive therapies; to prevent falls; and to manage disruptive behavior. However, the use of restraints can increase agitation and puts the patient at risk for other potentially serious injuries, including falls, fractures, and strangulation. Alternatives to physical restraints must always be sought and tried first (Box 2-9). Standards on physical restraint use are published and monitored by the Joint Commission and the Centers for Medicare and Medicaid Services. These standards are summarized in Box 2-10.

BOX 2-9 Alternatives to Physical Restraints

Environmental Modifications
- Keep the bed in the lowest position.
- Minimize the use of side rails to what is needed for positioning.
- Optimize room lighting.
- Activate bed and chair exit alarms where available.
- Remove unnecessary furniture or equipment.
- Ensure that the bed wheels are locked.
- Position the call light within easy reach.
- Ensure that the patient has needed vision and hearing aids.

Therapeutic Interventions
- Frequently assess the need for treatments and discontinue lines and catheters at the earliest opportunity.
- Orient the patient to invasive medical equipment. Help the patient explore the equipment by guiding the patient's hand over it. Explain the purpose of the equipment, as well as the meaning of any alarms that may sound.
- Disguise treatments, if necessary (eg, keep IV solution bags out of the patient's field of vision, apply a loose stockinette or long-sleeved gown over IV sites).

- Ensure comfort by meeting the patient's physical needs (eg, frequent toileting, skin care, pain management, hypoxemia management, positioning).
- Mobilize the patient as much as possible.
- Allow the patient to make choices and exert some degree of control when possible.

Diversionary Activities
- Enlist family members or volunteers to provide company and diversion.
- Facilitate solitary diversionary activities (eg, music, videos or television, audio books).

Therapeutic Use of Self
- Use calm, reassuring tones.
- Introduce yourself and let the patient know he or she is safe.
- Find an effective method of communicating with intubated or nonverbal patients.
- Reorient patients frequently by explaining treatments, medical devices, care plans, activities, and unfamiliar sounds, noises, or alarms.

BOX 2-10 Summary of Care Standards Regarding Physical Restraints

Initiating Restraints
- Restraints require the order of a licensed independent practitioner who must personally see and evaluate the patient within a specified time period.
- Restraints are used only as an emergency measure or after restraint alternatives have failed. (The restraint alternatives that were tried and the patient's responses to them are documented.)
- Restraints are instituted by staff who are trained and competent to use restraints safely. (A comprehensive training and monitoring program must be in place.)
- Restraint orders must be time limited. (A patient must not be placed in a restraint for longer than 24 hours, with reassessment and documentation of continued need for restraint at more frequent intervals.)
- Patients and families are informed about the rationale for the use of the restraint.

Monitoring Patients in Restraints
- The patient's rights, dignity, and well-being are protected.
- The patient is assessed every 15 minutes by trained and competent staff.
- The assessment and documentation must include evaluation of the patient's nutrition, hydration, hygiene, elimination, vital signs, circulation, range of motion, injury due to the restraint, physical and psychological comfort, and readiness for discontinuance of the restraint.

CASE STUDY

Ms. J. is a 40-year-old pregnant woman who is admitted to the hospital at 34 weeks, 5 days of gestation with complaints of vaginal bleeding, painful contractions, and nausea and vomiting. Until this time, she has received routine prenatal care, and the pregnancy has been uneventful. Before her admission to the hospital, she was eating lunch at work when she felt a "pop" in her abdomen; shortly afterward, her symptoms began. She states that the last time she felt fetal movement was earlier in the morning. At the hospital, an external fetal monitor and portable ultrasound detect no fetal heart tones. There is blood in the vaginal vault and no active bleeding, and the cervix is long and closed.

Ms. J. is admitted to the labor and delivery unit with the diagnosis of a fetal death in utero, probably due to an abruption of the placenta, and the plan is to deliver her by induction of labor. Shortly after admission, she complains of increasing pelvic pressure. Examination reveals that she is fully dilated, and she spontaneously delivers a stillborn male child. Delivery of the placenta, as well as a 250-mL clot, follows, confirming the diagnosis of placental abruption. Despite administration of medications to assist the uterus to contract and control bleeding, Ms. J. begins to bleed steadily. Clinicians decide to perform dilation and curettage (D&C).

Following the D&C, Ms. J.'s uterus becomes well contracted, bleeding decreases, and coagulation parameters begin to improve. Her estimated blood loss is 8000 mL.

Ms. J. begins to bleed again later that evening and is again transferred to the operating room, where a uterine artery embolization is performed. Ventilation becomes difficult, and she is intubated. She is transferred to the critical care unit for closer surveillance, ventilatory support, and fluid resuscitation. Clinicians make an additional diagnosis of disseminated intravascular coagulation (DIC). Ms. J.'s husband stays with Ms. J. throughout the night during her first 2 days the critical care unit. On day 3, Ms. J. is extubated and is hemodynamically stable. She is transferred to the progressive care unit after she is weaned from the ventilator.

1. Mr. J. stayed at his wife's bedside throughout her first 2 days in the critical care unit. How does this demonstrate the critical care staff's commitment to meeting both the patient's and the family's needs?

2. Describe actions the critical care nursing staff can take to ensure that Ms. J. and her husband view this difficult time in their lives in the most positive way possible.

References

1. Curtis R, White D: Practical guidance for evidence based ICU family conference. Chest 134(4):835–843, 2008
2. Borges K, Mello M, David C: Patient families in ICU: Describing their strategies to face the situation. Crit Care 15:P527, 2011
3. Davidson J, et al.: Clinical practice guidelines for support of family in patient centered intensive care unit: An American College of Critical Care Medicine Task Force 2004–2005. Crit Care Med 35(2):605–622, 2007
4. Miracle V: A closing word: Critical care visitation. Dimens Crit Care Nurs 24(1):48–49, 2005
5. Curtis JR, Patrick DL, Shannon SE, et al.: The family conference as a focus to improve communication about end-of-life care in the intensive care unit: Opportunities for improvement. Crit Care Med 29(2 suppl):N26–N33, 2001
6. American Association of Critical-Care Nurses: Family presence during CPR and invasive procedures. Practice alert. Retrieved October 20, 2006, from http://www.aacn.org/AACN/practice Alert.nsf/Files/FP/$file/Family%20 Presence%20During%20CPR%2011–2004.pdf
7. Nelson J: Family meetings made simpler: A toolkit for ICU. J Crit Care 24:626e7–627e14, 2009
8. Jansen MPM, Schmitt NA: Family-focused interventions. Crit Care Nurs Clin N Am 15(3):347–354, 2003
9. Dogan O, Ertekin S, Dogan S: Sleep quality in hospitalized patients. J Clin Nurs 14:107–113, 2005

Want to know more? A wide variety of resources to enhance your learning and understanding of this chapter are available on the**Point**✳. Visit **http://thepoint.lww.com/MortonEss1e** to access chapter review questions and more!

3

Patient and Family Education in Critical Care

Based on the content in this chapter, the reader should be able to:

1 Describe barriers to learning and ways to manage them.
2 Describe the assessment of learning in the critical care environment.
3 Describe how the three domains of learning and the six principles of adult learning can be used when developing a teaching plan.
4 Explain the importance of evaluating the effectiveness of teaching and learning.

In the critical care setting, it is always a challenge to meet the educational needs of patients and families because of the life-threatening nature of critical illness. The nurse must deal with the anxiety and fear that is associated with a diagnosis of critical illness while trying to teach difficult concepts in an environment that is poorly suited to learning. In the current healthcare environment, it is not unusual for a patient to be discharged home directly from the critical care unit, placing even greater responsibility on the patient and family to provide for complex care at home and further increasing the need for adequate patient and family education.

Recognizing and Managing Barriers to Learning

Several factors can present barriers to learning, including the illness itself and interventions to manage it, emotional and environmental distractions, language barriers, and sensory deficits.

Effects of Critical Illness and Therapeutic Interventions

Altered metabolic responses, exposure to general anesthesia, use of cardiopulmonary bypass, episodes of hypoxia, and marked sleep deprivation can compromise mental acuity and decrease a person's learning capacity and recall. In addition, combating a severe illness consumes most of the patient's energy, leaving little energy left to devote to learning.

Emotional and Environmental Distractions

The critical care nurse must be very sensitive to the heightened anxiety that accompanies an admission to the critical care unit. This anxiety can markedly reduce the ability of the patient and family to concentrate and focus attention on learning. Conveying information in a concise, clear manner and avoiding long, tedious explanations can help patients and family members focus on the information they are being given. Even so, intense anxiety may cause patients and families to forget much of this information, so the nurse must be prepared to repeat information and answer identical questions repeatedly.

The environment itself also poses many distractions. Actions such as closing the door to the patient's room, placing a comfortable chair at the bedside, and reducing the alarm volumes on bedside equipment can minimize the number of interruptions and may improve the learner's ability to focus on the topic of a teaching session.

Language Barriers

An inability to speak or read English can pose a major obstacle to patient and family education, especially in the stressful critical care environment. A medical interpreter must be obtained for patients and family members who do not speak English. Asking a friend or family member to translate is inappropriate and can pose many problems:

- Complex medical information and terminology may be unfamiliar to the person translating.
- It may be difficult for a family member or friend to translate without bias.
- In many cultures, decision making is assumed by the eldest member of the family, and asking another family member to interpret medical information may disrupt the social order of the family.[1]
- Having a family member or friend translate personal medical information may be awkward for the patient, the family member or friend, or both. It may also represent a breach of patient confidentiality.

Guidelines for communicating through an interpreter are given in Box 3-1.

Patients and family members who speak English may still struggle with reading the language. The nurse should not assume that a document such as a consent form is clearly understood when it is returned signed and unquestioned; the document may be written beyond the patient's reading and comprehension level. Written educational material should always be in the active voice and targeted for a fifth- to eighth-grade reading level.[2] In addition, the nurse should verbally review any written material with the patient or family in case they are unable to read the document and are too embarrassed to admit it.

Sensory Deficits

Effective education for deaf and hearing-impaired patients and families necessitates planning and additional resources. The nurse asks deaf or hearing-impaired patients or family members about their preferred mode of communication (eg, sign language, written notes, lip reading, oral interpreters, or other assistive devices).[3] To ensure that deaf or hearing-impaired patients or family members can communicate concerns and questions effectively, an oral interpreter should be used for the discussion

---

BOX 3-1 Guidelines for Communication Using an Interpreter

- Before the session, meet with the interpreter to give background information and explain the purpose of the session.
- If possible, have the interpreter meet with the patient or family to determine their educational level, healthcare beliefs, and healthcare attitudes to plan the depth of information needed.
- Speak in short units of speech and avoid long explanations and use of medical jargon, abbreviations, and colloquialisms.
- When speaking, look directly toward the patient and family members, not at the interpreter. Watch the patient's and family members' body language and nonverbal communication response.
- Be aware that interpreted interviews take a long time to complete and may become tiresome for the patient.
- Written instructions should also be translated and reviewed in the presence of an interpreter so that any questions can be addressed immediately.
- Have the patient and family members validate the information given to them through the interpreter, to make sure that they understand the instructions or message that has been given.

---

of treatment options; to provide background information before obtaining informed consent for procedures, blood administration, or surgery; and to explain discharge instructions.

Vision impairment must also be taken into consideration when preparing written resources for the patient and family (Box 3-2).

Providing Patient and Family Education

Patient and family education entails more than just providing an educational brochure or turning on an instructional video; it is an interactive process based

---

BOX 3-2 Guidelines for Preparing Printed Educational Materials

- Use a large font (12 point or greater).
- Use a serif font (eg, M) instead of a sanserif font (eg, M).
- Avoid script or stylized fonts.
- Avoid the use of all uppercase letters, except in headings.
- Keep line lengths short (eg, less than 5 in).
- Use a matte, rather than a glossy, paper to cut down on glare.
- Use black ink on plain white or off-white paper.

BOX 3-3　Content Areas for Patient and Family Education

- The pathophysiology of the patient's illness
- Diagnostic studies (purpose, method of performing, preparation, and follow-up)
- The treatment plan
- Medications (purpose, desired and adverse effects, safe administration)
- Pain management techniques
- Medical equipment (purpose, safe and effective use)
- Rationale for restraint or seclusion
- Future and ongoing care (eg, information about step-down unit, available community resources)

on a therapeutic relationship. Frequently, assessment of learning needs and the provision of information are integrated naturally into the process of providing care. Teachable moments, which often occur during the course of providing routine patient care, are those instances when the nurse and learner together recognize the need for education and the learner is open to hearing information and learning new problem-solving skills.[1] Patient and family teaching encompasses many areas (Box 3-3).

Assessing Learning Needs

Assessment is a dynamic and ongoing process, providing the critical care nurse with many opportunities to meet the learning needs of patients and families. Understanding the learning needs of patients and families does not require a protracted interview or use of formal assessment tools with overly generic questions about health beliefs and learning styles. It is better to use an informal style and open-ended dialogue to establish what the patient and family "need to know." Use of open-ended questions such as "What is your understanding of your mother's condition?" or "What did the physician tell you about the surgery?" gives the nurse a starting point for teaching. It also validates whether the patient or family member clearly understands previous explanations given by other members of the healthcare team. It may be necessary for the nurse to bridge the knowledge gap between the physician's explanation and the patient's or family member's baseline knowledge of medical terminology and concepts. Assessing the person's level of education and degree of "health literacy" can help the nurse tailor information to the patient's or family member's level of understanding. This is particularly important within the critical care setting, where healthcare problems are often complex and patients or family members are often required to make urgent decisions about care.[4]

Developing Effective Teaching Strategies

Successful teaching plans take into account basic principles of adult learning (Table 3-1). Considering the three domains of learning while developing a teaching plan also assists the nurse in selecting suitable teaching methods (Fig. 3-1):

- The **cognitive domain** is concerned with the acquisition and application of knowledge. Teaching methods that are used in the cognitive domain seek to develop the knowledge that

TABLE 3-1　Six Principles of Adult Learning

Principle	Underlying Concept	Teaching Strategy
The need to know	Adults need to understand why they need to learn something before they are willing to commit the energy and time to learn it.	Ensure that the learner understands why the information is important to learn.
The learner's self-concept	Adults are self-directed and responsible for their own decision making. In general, adults resent the feeling that others are making choices for them.	Create learning situations that are more self-directed and independent.
The learner's life experience	Adults have accumulated many experiences over the course of their lives, and these life experiences define and shape adult beliefs, values, and attitudes.	Emphasize experiential techniques (eg, case studies, simulation, problem-solving exercises) and techniques that draw on the experiences of peers (eg, group learning).
Readiness to learn	Adults are ready to learn the things they need to know.	Help the learner see how the information is applicable to real-life situations.
Orientation to learning	Adults are motivated to learn if the information will help them to perform useful tasks or to deal with problems in their life.	Help the learner see how the information is applicable to real-life situations.
Motivation to learn	Adults are more motivated by internal forces such as improved quality of life, increased job satisfaction, and improved self-esteem.	Help the learner see how the information will meet these needs.

Adapted from Meleis A, Isenberg M, Koerner J, et al.: Diversity, Marginalization, and Culturally Competent Health Care: Issues in Knowledge Development. Washington, DC: Academy of Nursing, 2000.

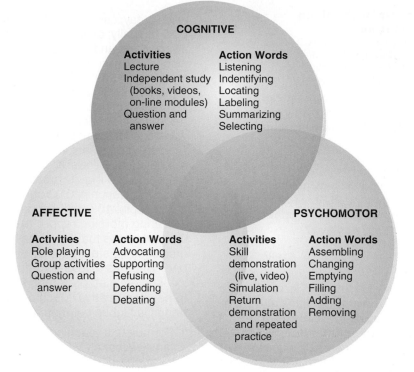

FIGURE 3-1 Teaching methods based on the domains of learning.

provides a basis for understanding the situation or modifying behavior.[5]

- The **affective domain** is concerned with the acquisition or modification of values, attitudes, and behaviors.[5] Values and attitudes influence what the patient considers important enough to learn as well as the patient's willingness to learn. Exercises that allow the learner to consider different points of view or behaviors (eg, role playing, group learning activities) are often used when appealing to the affective domain.

- The **psychomotor domain** is concerned with the development of motor skills (eg, learning how to inject insulin). Step-by-step demonstrations, videos, simulations, and the opportunity to practice and demonstrate the newly acquired skill are teaching methods employed in the psychomotor domain. Learning new skills is intimidating to many adults; therefore, it is important that the nurse provide praise and encouragement with each teaching session.

 RED FLAG! *Learning is best accomplished when the message is consistent and the knowledge progresses from simple to more complex concepts.*

Evaluating Teaching and Learning

Evaluation of teaching and learning is an essential component of the healthcare continuum. Evaluation helps the nurse determine the adequacy of instruction by revealing knowledge gaps and elements of the teaching plan that are not working.[6] Setting

unrealistic educational goals hinders learning and frustrates both the nurse and the learner. A teaching plan that is ineffective, poorly timed, or not meeting the learner's needs must be altered.

Immediate feedback can be gained by asking questions to validate the learner's grasp of the information presented. The nurse avoids using leading questions to achieve a desired answer. Phrasing questions as a request for help (eg, "Can you repeat back to me what I just told you so I can make sure I didn't forget anything?") is often less intimidating than quizzing the learner. Direct observation of newly learned skills is also part of the evaluation. Cultivating a relaxed, positive learning environment and developing a good rapport with the patient or family member can help minimize the self-consciousness many adults feel when asked to perform a newly acquired skill in front of others.

Documenting

The Joint Commission's patient care standards place an emphasis on patient and family education. The goal of these educational standards is to guide hospitals to create an environment in which both the patient and the healthcare team members are responsible for teaching and learning. The medical record should reflect an interdisciplinary approach toward patient education that begins on admission and continues throughout the hospital stay. Components of teaching documentation are given in Box 3-4.

Components of Teaching Documentation

- Participants (Who was taught?)
- Content (What was taught?)
- Date and time (When was it taught?)
- Patient status (What was the patient's condition at the time?)
- Patient's readiness to learn (Was the patient open to receiving the information?)
- Evaluation of learning (How well did the learner appear to understand the information?)
- Teaching methods (How was the patient taught?)
- Follow-up and learning evaluation (If teaching was incomplete, what was the reason? What additional education needs does the patient have?)

Although it may be difficult for critical care nurses to think in terms of teaching plans and interdisciplinary learning because critically ill patients require so much care just to maintain physiological function, it is important to remember that much of the teaching the nurse does is informal. Every time nurses explain what they are doing and why they are doing it, they are providing a form of education! This type of informal instruction meets the Joint Commission standard for patient education, and should be documented.

CASE STUDY

Ms. V. is a 19-year-old Hispanic woman who has been admitted to the critical care unit from the delivery room for an episode of acute pulmonary edema that developed during the birth of her first child. She has recently immigrated to the United States from Central America, and she speaks very little English. Through an interpreter, it is determined that she has received no prenatal care and is taking no medications. She denies any past medical problems, but she has never seen a physician before. She denies using tobacco, alcohol, or drugs.

Physical examination reveals an enlarged heart, presence of an S_3 and S_4, and a murmur of mitral regurgitation. A chest radiograph demonstrates marked cardiac enlargement. A transthoracic echocardiogram reveals severe left ventricular enlargement and dysfunction; ejection fraction is estimated at 35% (normal is 50% to 70%). Based on the results of these tests, Ms. V. is diagnosed with peripartum cardiomyopathy.

Ms. V. is currently on the cardiac step-down unit receiving the following medications: enalapril, 5 mg twice a day; carvedilol, 25 mg twice a day; digoxin, 0.25 mg daily; amlodipine, 5 mg daily; furosemide, 40 mg daily; and milrinone, 0.50 µg/kg/min. She is also on a low-sodium diet and fluid restriction. This morning her vital signs are as follows: temp, 98.2°F (36.8°C); BP, 90/52 mm Hg; HR, 120 beats/min; RR, 28 breaths/min; and pulse oximetry, 92% on 2 L by nasal cannula. Telemetry reveals sinus tachycardia with frequent premature ventricular contractions. Crackles are present in both lung bases. Laboratory results are as follows: K^+, 2.9 mEq/L; BUN, 45 mg/dL; creatinine, 2.0 mg/dL; brain natriuretic peptide, 50 pg/mL; troponin, 0.02 ng/mL; WBCs, 9.0×10^3 mL; hemoglobin, 10.0 g/dL; and hematocrit, 30.3%.

During morning report, the nurse coming onto the unit learns that Ms. V. has been refusing the medications, stating that they are making her "feel bad." She has also been refusing the prescribed low-sodium diet, preferring instead food brought to her by a relative. Much of the food the relative brings is high in calories and sodium.

1. Formulate a teaching plan for Ms. V. and her family. What should the nurse address, and in what order? What measures can the nurse use to evaluate the effectiveness of the teaching plan?

2. What strategies might help the nurse implement the teaching plan effectively?

3. What is the best way for the nurse to communicate through an interpreter?

References

1. Rankin SH, Stallings KD, London F: Patient Education in Health and Illness, 5th ed. Philadelphia, PA: Lippincott Williams & Wilkins, 2005, pp 224–250
2. Irnik M, Jett M: Creating written patient education materials. Chest 133(4):1038–1040, 2008
3. Michigan Association for Deaf, Hearing, and Speech Services: Hospitals' responsibilities to the deaf under the ADA. Retrieved November 1, 2006, from http://www.deaf-talk.com/pdf/ hospitalresponsibilites.pdf
4. Riley JB, Cloonan P, Norton C: Low health literacy: A challenge to critical care. Crit Care Nurs Q 29(2):174–178, 2006
5. Redman BK: The Practice of Patient Education: A Case Study Approach, 10th ed. St. Louis, MO: Mosby Elsevier, 2007, pp 1–26
6. Redman BK: The Practice of Patient Education: A Case Study Approach, 10th ed. St. Louis, MO: Mosby Elsevier, 2007, pp 56–73

Want to know more? A wide variety of resources to enhance your learning and understanding of this chapter are available on thePoint✳. Visit **http://thepoint.lww.com/MortonEss1e** to access chapter review questions and more!

Ethical and Legal Issues in Critical Care Nursing

Based on the content in this chapter, the reader should be able to:

1 Explain the way ethics assists nurses and other clinicians in resolving moral problems.

2 Recognize the applicability of the *Code of Ethics for Nurses* of the American Nurses Association to everyday practice.

3 Identify resources available to nurses to resolve ethical dilemmas.

4 Describe steps in the process of ethical decision making.

5 Discuss examples of ethical issues confronted by critical care nurses in practice.

6 Describe major areas of the law that affect critical care nursing practice.

7 State five legal responsibilities of every registered nurse.

8 Explain the concept of duty and the potential consequences of breach of duty.

9 Explain types of vicarious liability.

10 Discuss laws that are of particular applicability to the critical care nurse.

In the complex arena of critical care, questions regarding the appropriate use of technology and information abound and crucial decisions about life and death are made with striking frequency and urgency. Although advancements in healthcare technology and information provide indisputable benefits, these same advancements also raise profound ethical and legal challenges. The nurse relies on an understanding of ethical principles and legal requirements to make sound decisions.

Ethics in Critical Care

"Ethics" can be defined as a set of principles of right conduct or a system of moral values. Ethics help us to answer questions about what is right or good, or what ought to be done in specific situations. Several general approaches to ethics exist (Box 4-1). Ethical analysis helps the nurse to clarify moral issues and principles involved in a situation, examine his or her responsibilities and obligations, and provide an ethically adequate rationale for any decision made or action taken.

Informed clinicians and clear organizational policies help to prevent and resolve ethical dilemmas in healthcare organizations. The Joint Commission requires policy statements and guidelines addressing issues such as the resolution of ethical dilemmas, informed consent, use of surrogate decision makers, decisions about care and treatment at the end of life, and confidentiality of information.

BOX 4-1 General Approaches to Ethics

Consequentialism: Consequences of actions determine whether an action is right or wrong.
Nonconsequentialism (deontological approach): Conformity to moral rules (not consequences) determines whether an action is right or wrong.
Utilitarianism: The right action is that which offers the greatest benefit with the least amount of burden to all affected.
Paternalism: The right action is that which is believed to bring the best outcome for the person, regardless of the person's autonomous actions or requests.
Ethics of care: The right action is determined based on the characteristics of caring relationships between people.
Principlism: A specific set of principles is used to identify and analyze the ethics of a situation.
Virtue ethics: What matters is not only what a person does but also how the person's actions reflect the person's virtues.

Principles of Bioethics

Bioethics is the study of ethical issues and judgments made within the biomedical sciences, including care of patients, the delivery of healthcare, public health, and biomedical research. Bioethics takes into account the difficult and practical realities that arise in the clinical care of people with illnesses. Six widely accepted bioethical principles, summarized in Box 4-2, are often applied to ethical problems in healthcare and nursing practice.

The Nurse's Ethical Responsibilities

Most professional groups have formal codes of ethics for their members; the nursing profession is guided by the American Nurses Association (ANA)

BOX 4-2 Principles of Bioethics

Nonmaleficence: An obligation to never deliberately harm another
Beneficence: An obligation to promote the welfare of others, to maximize benefits and minimize harms
Respect for autonomy: An obligation to respect, and not to interfere with, the choices and actions of autonomous individuals (ie, those capable of self-determination)
Justice: An obligation to be fair in the distribution of burdens and benefits and in the distribution of social goods, such as healthcare or nursing care
Veracity: An obligation to tell the truth
Fidelity: An obligation to keep promises and fulfill commitments

Code of Ethics for Nurses With Interpretive Statements (Box 4-3).[1] Nursing ethics encompasses the nurse's specific professional roles and responsibilities and the relationships the nurse has with patients, other healthcare providers, the facilities with which he or she is affiliated, and society. A nurse never practices in isolation. Decision making, conflict resolution related to ethical issues, and ethical practice are accomplished through communication and collaboration with patients, peers, and colleagues on the healthcare team.

The code of ethics for nursing is strongly based on the principle of "caring." Caring is considered essential to nursing and has been long valued in the nurse–patient relationship. In caring for patients, nurses are committed to promoting the health and welfare of patients and respecting human dignity. The care ethic is based on the understanding that people are unique, that relationships and their value are crucial in moral deliberations, and that emotions and character traits play a role in moral judgment. Sympathy, compassion, trust, solidarity, fidelity, collaboration, and discernment are emphasized.

Sometimes the desire to "cure" interferes with the ability to "care" and provide relief of suffering. Especially in the critical care setting, aggressive treatments are frequently used in an attempt to stabilize patients and keep them alive. The desire to prevent harm by postponing death is shaped by beneficence. However, physical and psychological suffering caused by aggressive treatment, especially treatment of questionable or slight benefit, sometimes constitutes a greater harm than death, and less aggressive treatment and more comfort may be a more beneficent course. To determine what is best for the patient, the nurse involves the patient or surrogate decision maker in discussions and decisions about treatment goals and the risks and benefits of various treatment options.

Nurses promise to act in their patients' best interests, respect their autonomy, and advocate for them. Communicating honestly with patients and families, discussing and respecting their wishes regarding treatment and care, convening patient care conferences for all involved parties when indicated, and facilitating advance care planning discussions and the use of advance directives are all important methods of fulfilling these obligations.

 RED FLAG! *In the critical care unit, patients frequently are unable to make decisions for themselves due to their clinical status, the effects of treatments they are receiving, or both. The nurse frequently and carefully assesses the patient's ability to understand treatment options and make decisions.*

Ethics Committees and Consultation Services

Many healthcare organizations have an ethics committee or an ethics consultation service. Institutional

BOX 4-3 The American Nurses Association's (ANA) Code of Ethics for Nurses

1. The nurse, in all professional relationships, practices with compassion and respect for the inherent dignity, worth, and uniqueness of every individual, unrestricted by considerations of social or economic status, personal attributes, or the nature of health problems.
2. The nurse's primary commitment is to the patient, whether an individual, family, group, or community.
3. The nurse promotes, advocates for, and strives to protect the health, safety, and rights of the patient.
4. The nurse is responsible and accountable for individual nursing practice and determines the appropriate delegation of tasks consistent with the nurse's obligation to provide optimum patient care.
5. The nurse owes the same duty to self as to others, including the responsibility to preserve integrity and safety, to maintain competence, and to continue personal and professional growth.

6. The nurse participates in establishing, maintaining, and improving healthcare environments and conditions of employment conducive to the provision of quality healthcare and consistent with the values of the profession through individual and collective action.
7. The nurse participates in the advancement of the profession through contributions to practice, education, administration, and knowledge development.
8. The nurse collaborates with other health professionals and the public in promoting community, national, and international efforts to meet health needs.
9. The profession of nursing, as represented by associations and their members, is responsible for articulating nursing values, for maintaining the integrity of the profession and its practice, and for shaping social policy.

Reprinted with permission from American Nurses Association: Code of Ethics for Nurses with Interpretive Statements. Washington, DC: American Nurses Publishing, American Nurses Foundation/American Nurses Association, 2001.

ethics committees are usually multidisciplinary and include representatives from various patient care professions and disciplines (eg, nursing, medicine, social work, spiritual care). They may also include one or more members from the lay community. Ethics committee members may offer education to the professional staff and community on issues related to clinical ethics and serve as a resource for institutional policies concerning ethical matters. Individual committee members may also consult at the bedside, providing education, clarification, or dialogue necessary to assist decision makers in resolving an ethical problem. In more complicated cases or when conflict exists among decision makers, consultation by the entire ethics committee may be appropriate. Some committees aim to make a single recommendation for the resolution of the ethical problem, whereas others attempt to frame the morally acceptable options and assist key decision makers in choosing a course of action.

Ethical Decision Making

Resolving ethical dilemmas can be difficult. Ethical dilemmas are dilemmas precisely because compelling reasons exist for taking each of two or more opposing actions. Systematically applying available codes of ethics and ethical principles can help members of the healthcare team and ethics committee identify ethical obligations and systematically decide which "right" actions can help to meet these obligations. Multidisciplinary collaboration and dialogue are also critical to satisfactorily resolving ethical problems. Ethical decision-making models provide a process for systematically and thoughtfully examining a conflict, ensuring that participants consider all important aspects of a situation before taking action (Box 4-4).

Ethical principles, professional guidelines, personal values, emotions, and judgment help guide the nurse's actions and decisions. How the nurse feels about an issue is a manifestation of his or her moral convictions that should not be ignored. The nurse strives, though, to reach ethical decisions by allowing reason to temper emotions and emotions to tutor reason. Differing personal, professional, and institutional values can compound moral conflict. Awareness of differences in professional and personal values and obligations can provide insight into sources of interprofessional or interpersonal ethical conflict. Ideally, competing values are weighed and assigned priority in light of guiding ethical norms.

Moral distress occurs when nurses cannot turn moral choices into moral action,[2] that is, when the nurse knows the proper course of action to take,

BOX 4-4 Model for Ethical Decision Making

1. Gather the relevant facts and identify the decision maker(s) and the stakeholders.
2. Identify the ethical problem(s). Involve others in the process and use consultation resources as appropriate.
3. Analyze the problem using ethical principles and resources.
4. Identify action alternatives in light of the ethical principles; choose one and justify the choice.
5. Evaluate and reflect.

but institutional or interpersonal constraints make it nearly impossible to pursue it.[2] For example, nurses tend to recognize when therapies are no longer beneficial to a patient sooner than family members, which can be a source of moral distress. *The Four A's to Moral Distress*, a resource developed by the American Association of Critical-Care Nurses (AACN), provides a framework for addressing and resolving moral distress (Fig. 4-1). In addition, hospital ethics committees are available to help staff work through situations in which moral distress is a factor.

Common Ethical Dilemmas in Critical Care

Withholding or Withdrawing Treatment

In some cases, a patient or surrogate decision maker may decide to withhold or withdraw a treatment, especially at the end of life. *Withholding* refers to never initiating a treatment, whereas *withdrawing* refers to stopping a treatment once started. The distinction between not starting a treatment and stopping it is not itself of ethical significance; what matters most is whether the decision is consistent with the patient's interests and preferences. When the patient or surrogate decides in good faith that a proposed treatment will impose undue burdens and refuses such treatment, it is morally correct for the healthcare professional to respect that decision. If the patient or surrogate decides that a treatment in progress and the life it provides have become too burdensome, then the treatment may permissibly be stopped.

To presume to understand the needs of a patient and act against the patient's expressed wishes (or to avoid ascertaining what those wishes might be) can be paternalistic. Discussions about treatment preferences ideally occur when the patient is alert and has a reasonably clear sensorium. The nurse helps to ensure that the patient receives adequate information, has the capacity to understand available options, and can deliberate and make a healthcare decision. If a patient is incapable of making an informed decision, a legally authorized surrogate is asked to consent for the patient. Before making a voluntary and informed decision to accept or to refuse any treatment, the patient or surrogate must understand what the treatment entails and how it will most likely affect the disease process and future quality of life. Healthcare providers are responsible for presenting information in an understandable and sensitive manner and for assessing the level of the patient's or surrogate's understanding.

In some cases, the nurse may have a personal moral conviction contrary to a certain decision or may believe that the particular decision is against the patient's best interests or wishes. The nurse is morally permitted to refuse to participate in withholding or withdrawing treatment from a patient as long as the patient's care is assumed by someone else. The nurse is justified in refusing to participate on moral grounds, but the nurse must communicate the decision in appropriate ways.

Limits to Treatment and "Futility of Care"

In contrast to cases in which healthcare workers want to treat patients against their wishes, sometimes a

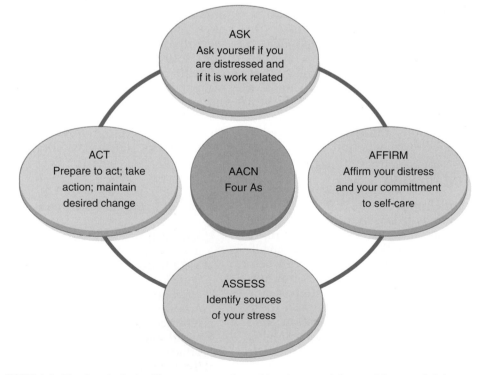

FIGURE 4-1 The four As (ask, affirm, assess, act) provide a framework for resolving moral distress.

patient, family member, or surrogate wants treatment that physicians, nurses, or other members of the healthcare team feel is inappropriate or even futile. Providing care perceived as "excessive," especially for dying patients, is a source of great concern among care providers, especially critical care nurses.[3] There is a great deal of discussion among ethicists, healthcare professionals, and patients' rights groups about when, if ever, a patient's request for treatment can be denied because of futility. Futility is a complex concept that can be understood in at least one of two different ways: (1) when an intervention would be ineffective at producing its intended effect and (2) when an intervention might be physiologically effective but is unlikely to provide meaningful benefit. Lack of consensus on a definition of (and criteria for) futility, coupled with concern about whether healthcare providers can be objective enough to make these determinations, make this a particularly difficult ethical dilemma to resolve.

The Council on Ethical and Judicial Affairs of the American Medical Association recommends that facilities adopt a policy that follows a "fair process approach" to determine futility of interventions.[4] Most such policies require deliberation by multidisciplinary committees, such as ethics committees, rather than unilateral decisions by a physician, and require genuine attempts to transfer the patient's care to another facility if the dilemma cannot be resolved by the facility currently providing care. Some facilities allow a physician, under carefully delineated circumstances and after consultation with others, to write a do-not-resuscitate (DNR) order or withhold certain treatments without the consent of the patient.

Allocation Decisions

The principle of justice comes into play when decisions must be made about the allocation of limited resources, treatments, and even time and attention among patients. Every time a decision is made to transplant a kidney into one person and not another, to respond to one patient's need before another's, or to admit one patient to the critical care unit instead of another, a decision is made about the distribution of resources using justice criteria. Justice requires that decisions about the distribution of healthcare be based on morally significant characteristics, and not on factors such as race, ethnicity, gender, social standing, or religious beliefs. Allocation decisions are ordinarily made independent of the wishes of the patient or family and usually require balancing potential harms and benefits *between* people. Allocation decisions can be very difficult, and not everyone will be happy with the decisions that are made. Two examples of difficult allocation decisions involve the allocation of organs for transplantation and the allocation of beds in the critical care unit.

- **Allocation of organs for transplantation.** The need for organs is greater than the available supply. When a donation occurs, difficult distribution decisions must be made about who receives the organs that are available. In the United States, the Organ Procurement and Transplantation Network maintains a national registry for organ matching[5] and includes all patients on a transplant center's waiting list. When an organ becomes available, information is entered into a computerized organ-matching system that generates a list of potential recipients according to objective criteria. Many factors influence who among those potential recipients actually receives an organ for transplantation.
- **Allocation of beds.** The number of patients that can be cared for on the critical care unit at any given time is limited both by the number of beds and the availability of qualified staff to provide care. Decisions about admitting or discharging patients from critical care often involve some sort of triage to maximize the effective and efficient use of resources. Triage decisions are usually based on considerations of medical utility (ie, a comparative judgment about the probability of success of critical care for the individual patients involved).

Law in Critical Care

Legal issues involving critical care are of increasing concern to the nurse because the number of malpractice suits that name or involve nurses is increasing. There are three areas of the law that affect critical care nursing practice:

- **Administrative law.** Every state legislature has enacted a nurse practice act. Within each of these acts, the practice of nursing is defined, and powers are delegated to a state agency, usually the State Board of Nursing. The state agency develops regulations that dictate how the nurse practice act is to be interpreted and implemented. Practicing nurses are expected to know the provisions of the nurse practice act in their state and any regulations dealing with the practice of nursing. If a citizen feels that he or she has not received reasonable nursing care, the citizen may contact the state agency and file a complaint against the nurse or nurses involved in the care. The state is then responsible for conducting an investigation to determine whether the patient's claim has merit. Due process rights are attached to a nursing license, so certain due process requirements must be met before a state agency can revoke, discipline, or place conditions on a nursing license. Although the nurse's right of due process cannot be abridged, the state agency has the right to temporarily suspend a nurse's license immediately for acts the agency deems dangerous to the welfare of the general public.
- **Civil law.** In civil cases, one private party files a lawsuit against another. One specific area of civil law, tort law, forms the foundation of most civil cases involving nurses. Examples of torts include negligence, malpractice, assault, and battery.

- **Criminal law.** In criminal cases, the local, state, or federal government files a lawsuit against an individual. Criminal offenses, which are extremely rare in nursing situations, include criminal assault and battery, negligent homicide, and murder.

The legal responsibility of the registered nurse in critical care settings does not differ from that of the registered nurse in any work setting. The registered nurse adheres to five principles for the protection of the patient and the practitioner (Box 4-5).

Common Legal Issues in Critical Care

Negligence (Breach of Duty)

The most common lawsuits against nurses and their employers are based on the legal concept of malpractice, known as negligence by a professional. In a malpractice suit, the plaintiff has to show that some type of injury or harm occurred as a result of the nurse's actions or inaction. Malpractice law requires that there be a causal relationship between the conduct of the nurse and the injury to the patient, and that the injury that the patient experienced must be reasonably anticipated.

In a malpractice suit, the first task is establishing duty. A duty is a legal relationship between two or more parties. In most nursing cases, duty arises out of a contractual relationship between the patient and the healthcare facility. A nurse who cares for a patient is legally responsible for providing reasonable care under the circumstances present at the time of the incident. A nurse who fails to provide reasonable care under the circumstances has breached (violated) his or her duty toward the patient. Many different methods are used to determine whether the nurse complied with reasonable standards of care under the circumstances that existed at the time of the incident. The following resources can be used to establish standards of care:

- Testimony from nurse experts in critical care
- The healthcare facility's procedure and protocol manuals
- Nursing job descriptions
- State Board of Nursing standards of care

BOX 4-5   Five Legal Responsibilities of the Registered Nurse

The registered nurse is legally responsible for:

- Performing only those functions for which he or she has been prepared by education and experience
- Performing those functions competently
- Delegating responsibility only to personnel whose competence has been evaluated and found acceptable
- Taking appropriate measures as indicated by observations of the patient
- Being familiar with the employing agency's policies

- Nursing texts, professional journals, and drug reference books
- Standards and guidelines set by professional organizations (eg, AACN, American Heart Association)
- Equipment manufacturers' instructions

Once duty is established, a breach of that duty is required for the nurse to be found negligent. A breach of duty is determined by comparison of the nurse's conduct with the standard of care; that is, the nurse must be found to be negligent. Negligence is found or refuted by a comparison of the nurse's conduct with the standard of care. In general, negligence is either ordinary or gross. Ordinary negligence implies professional carelessness, whereas gross negligence suggests that the nurse willfully and consciously ignored a known risk for harm to the patient. Most cases involve ordinary negligence. Examples of actions that could lead to charges of gross negligence include acting in a way that contradicts sound nursing advice, or providing patient care while under the influence of drugs or alcohol.

The law attempts to return the plaintiff to a position he or she would have been in had an injury not been suffered. Unfortunately, injuries to patients usually cannot be undone. As such, most courts attempt to give monetary awards to compensate for the injuries sustained by the plaintiff. Examples of economic damages (ie, damages that can be calculated within a degree of certainty) include medical costs and lost wages. Noneconomic damages, such as pain and suffering and loss of consortium (services) that occurred as a result of the malpractice, are somewhat more difficult to calculate. Many state and federal governments place monetary limits on the amount a plaintiff can recover for pain and suffering, regardless of the amount that may be awarded by a jury.

Vicarious Liability

In some cases, a person or facility can be held liable for the conduct of another. This is called vicarious liability. There are various types of vicarious liability:

- **Respondeat superior** ("let the master answer for the sins of the servant") is the major legal theory under which hospitals are held liable for the negligence of their employees. In some situations, respondeat superior is not applicable. For instance, hospitals are not usually responsible for temporary agency personnel because they are usually employees of the agency, not the hospital. Similarly, physicians, unless they are employed by the hospital, do not typically come within the sphere of this doctrine.
- **Corporate liability** occurs when a hospital is found liable for its own unreasonable conduct. For example, if it is found that a unit is chronically understaffed and a patient suffers an injury as a result of short staffing, the hospital can be held accountable. Corporate liability may also apply in "floating" situations. A nurse working in a critical care setting must be competent to make

immediate nursing judgments and to act on those decisions. If the nurse does not possess the knowledge and skills required of a critical care nurse, he or she should not be providing critical care. Box 4-6 addresses issues of concern to the floating nurse.

- **Negligent supervision** is claimed when a supervisor fails to reasonably supervise people under his or her direction. For example, if a nurse is rotated to an unfamiliar unit and informs the charge nurse that she has never worked in critical care, it would be unreasonable for the charge nurse to ask her to perform invasive monitoring.

- **Rule of personal liability.** In the past, the nurse was expected to implement the physician's orders without question, and as "the captain of the ship," the physician was legally responsible for these actions. However, the "captain of the ship" doctrine has largely been replaced by the rule of personal liability—that is, nurses are expected to make sound decisions by virtue of their specialized education, training, and experience. If the nurse is unsure about the propriety of a physician's order, the nurse must seek clarification from the physician. When questioning an order, the nurse first shares his or her specific concerns with the physician who wrote the order. This frequently results in an explanation of the order and a medical justification for the order in the patient's medical record. If this approach is unsuccessful, the nurse follows the established chain of command for resolving the issue, per facility policy. Similarly, if a nurse is required to perform medical acts and is not under the direct and immediate supervision of a delegating physician, the activities must be based on established protocols created by the medical and nursing departments and reviewed for compliance with state nurse practice acts. In the event of a malpractice suit, the critical care protocols and procedures can be introduced as evidence to help establish the applicable standard of care.

Laws Affecting Nursing Practice

Laws of particular applicability to the critical care nurse include the following:

- **Informed consent doctrine.** In most instances, the law requires that the patient be given enough information before a treatment to make an informed, intelligent decision. Usually, obtaining informed consent from the patient or the family is the responsibility of the physician, but the nurse is frequently asked to witness signing of the consent form. By witnessing the signing, the nurse is attesting that the signature on the consent form is the patient's or the family member's.

- **Patient Self-Determination Act of 1991.** This federal statute is applicable to facilities that receive Medicare reimbursement for patient care. As a condition of reimbursement, the law requires that

---

BOX 4-6 Commonly Asked Questions When Rotating to an Unfamiliar Unit

1. **If I am asked to go to another unit, must I go?**
   Usually, you will be required to go to the other unit. If you refuse, you can be disciplined under the theory that you are breaching your employment contract or that you are failing to abide by the policies and procedures of the hospital. Some nursing units negotiate with hospitals to ensure that only specially trained nurses rotate to specialty units.

2. **If I rotate to an unfamiliar unit, what types of nursing responsibilities must I assume?**
   You will be expected to carry out only those nursing activities that you are competent to perform. In some instances, this will be the performance of basic nursing care activities (eg, blood pressures) and uncomplicated treatments. If you are unfamiliar with the types of medications used on the unit, you should not be administering them until you are thoroughly familiar with them.

3. **What should I do if I feel unprepared when I get to the unit?**
   Suggest that you assist the unit with basic nursing care requirements and that specialized activities (eg, invasive monitoring, cardiac monitoring, or the administration of unfamiliar drugs) be performed by staff who are adequately prepared.

4. **What if the charge nurse orders me to do something I am not able to do safely?**
   You are obligated to say you are unqualified and request that another nurse carry out the task. The charge nurse can be held liable for negligent supervision if she orders you to do an unsafe activity and a patient injury results.

---

hospitals provide information to adults about their rights concerning decision making in that state. The material distributed must include information about the types of advance directives that are legal in that state. Documentation that the patient has received this information must be placed in the medical record. If the patient is incapacitated on admission, the information must be provided to a family member, if available.

- **Safe Medical Devices Act of 1990.** A medical device, defined as virtually anything used in patient care that is not a drug, includes complex pieces of equipment (eg, intraaortic balloon pumps, pacemakers, defibrillators), along with less complicated ones (eg, endotracheal tubes, suture materials, restraints). Since 1976, medical devices have been regulated by the U.S. Food and Drug Administration (FDA). The Safe Medical Devices Act of 1990 requires user facilities to report to the manufacturer medical device malfunctions that result in serious illness, injury, or death to a patient. Facilities are also required to report to the FDA medical devices that result in a patient's death. Nurses and other staff are required to participate in reporting device malfunctions, including those associated with user error, to a designated hospital department. There is a duty not to use equipment that is patently defective. If the equipment suddenly ceases to do what it was intended to do, makes unusual noises, or has a history of malfunction and has not been repaired, the hospital could be liable for damage caused by it. Likewise, the nurse could be liable if he or she knows or should know of these problems and uses the equipment anyway.

- **Uniform Anatomical Gift Act.** Every state in the United States has a law based on the Uniform Anatomical Gift Act. The laws establish the legality of organ donation by patients and their families and set procedures for making and accepting the gift of an organ. Every state also has some provision to enable people to consent to organ donation using a designated place on a driver's license. Many states have also enacted "required request" laws, which seek to increase the supply of organs for transplantation by requiring hospital personnel to ask patients' families about an organ gift at the time of the patient's death.

References

1. American Nurses Association: Code of Ethics for Nurses With Interpretive Statements. Washington, DC: American Nurses Publishing, 2001. Retrieved July 30, 2006, from http://www.nursingworld.org/ethics/ecode.htm
2. AACN Position statement on Moral Distress. Revised in 2008. American Association of Critical Care Nurses. Retrieved from www.aacn.org.
3. Beckstrand R, Callister L, Kirchhoff K: Providing a "good death": Critical care nurses' suggestions for improving end of life care. Am J Crit Care 15(1):38–45, 2006
4. Council on Ethical and Judicial Affairs, American Medical Association: Medical futility in end-of-life care. JAMA 281:937–941, 1999
5. The Organ Procurement and Transplantation Network: About transplantation. Retrieved July 28, 2006, from http://www.optn.org/about/transplantation

Want to know more? A wide variety of resources to enhance your learning and understanding of this chapter are available on thePoint. Visit **http://thepoint.lww.com/MortonEss1e** to access chapter review questions and more!

CASE STUDY

Mr. R., a 62-year-old triathlete, was riding his bicycle when he lost control and flipped over the front, landing on the pavement headfirst. Mr. R. was wearing a helmet. A bystander called 911. When the paramedics arrived, they intubated Mr. R. and transported him to the hospital, where he was found to have a complete spinal cord injury at the C2 level. Mr. R. was placed on mechanical ventilation and will be ventilator dependent for the rest of his life.

Mr. R. is awake and alert, and it has been determined that he is able to make his own decisions. During the course of Mr. R.'s hospitalization, patient/family conferences are held at regular intervals so that the healthcare team, Mr. R., and Mr. R.'s family can discuss Mr. R.'s status and prognosis. After several weeks pass, Mr. R. states that he wishes to be taken off the ventilator, even though he is aware that this will result in his death. Mr. R.'s family members are supportive of him, and they state that they will agree with any decision Mr. R. makes. The physician is uncomfortable with implementing Mr. R.'s request to be removed from the ventilator and refers Mr. R.'s case to the ethics committee.

1. What ethical dilemma does Mr. R.'s case present?
2. Which of the ethical principles may be used to resolve this dilemma?
3. What role does the nurse have in resolving this ethical dilemma?

Essential Interventions in Critical Care

TWO

Relieving Pain and Providing Comfort

OBJECTIVES

Based on the content in this chapter, the reader should be able to:

1 Differentiate between acute and chronic pain.
2 Identify factors that exacerbate the experience of pain in the critically ill.
3 Prepare patients for the common sources of procedural pain in critical care.
4 Compare and contrast tolerance, physical dependence, and addiction.
5 Discuss national guidelines and standards for pain management.
6 Identify appropriate analgesics for high-risk critically ill patients.
7 Describe nonpharmacological interventions for alleviating pain and anxiety.

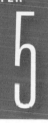

Pain is one of the most common experiences and stressors in critically ill patients. Symptoms of critical illnesses as well as many interventions and procedures in the critical care unit increase pain. Even though pain management has become a national priority in recent years (Table 5-1), pain continues to be misunderstood, poorly assessed, and undertreated in critical care units and many other healthcare settings. Uncontrolled pain triggers physical and emotional stress responses, inhibits healing, increases the risk for other complications, and increases the length of stay in the critical care unit.

Pain Defined

Pain is a complex, subjective phenomenon. The International Association for the Study of Pain defines pain as "an unpleasant sensory and emotional experience associated with actual or potential tissue damage or described in terms of such damage."[1] An operational definition of pain is based on the premise that the individual experiencing the pain is the true authority, pain is subjective and that pain is whatever the experiencing person says it is.

TABLE 5-1   National Standards and Guidelines Related to Pain Management

Agency or Source	Standard or Guideline	Content Highlights
Society of Critical Care Medicine (SCCM) and the American Society of Health-System Pharmacists (ASHP)	Clinical Practice Guidelines for the Sustained Use of Sedatives and Analgesics in the Critically Ill Adult (2002)	The summary contains 28 explicit recommendations related to analgesia and sedation targeted to the critically ill, including the following: • Patient report is the most reliable standard for pain assessment. • Scheduled doses or continuous infusions of opioids are preferred over PRN regimens. • Sedation of agitated patients should be provided only after providing adequate analgesia.
American Geriatric Society	The Management of Persistent Pain in Older Persons	Major recommendations include: • All older persons should be screened for persistent pain on admission to any health care facility. • The verbal 0 to 10 scale is a good first choice for assessment of pain intensity; however, other scales such as word descriptor scales or pain thermometers may be more appropriate for some older patients. • For patients with cognitive impairment, assessment of behaviors and family observations are essential. • Opioid analgesic drugs are effective, with a low potential for addiction, and may have fewer long-term risks than other analgesic drugs.
American College of Cardiology/ American Heart Association Task Force on Practice Guidelines	Guidelines for Cardiovascular Disease Management	Guidelines that are relevant to painful conditions experienced by critically ill patients, including chronic stable angina, unstable angina, peripheral arterial disease, ST-elevation myocardial infarction, and coronary artery bypass graft (CABG) surgery

The pain most critical care unit patients experience is classified as *acute* because it has an identified cause and is expected to resolve within a given time frame. For example, the pain experienced during endotracheal suctioning or a dressing change can be expected to end when the treatment is completed. Similarly, pain at an incision or area of injury is expected to cease once healing has occurred. In contrast, *chronic* pain is caused by physiological mechanisms that are less well understood. Chronic pain differs from acute pain in terms of etiology and expected duration. It may last for an indefinite period and may be difficult or impossible to treat completely. Many critical care unit patients, particularly those who are elderly, experience both acute and chronic pain.

Pain in the Critically Ill

Previously it was thought that critically ill patients were unable to remember their painful experiences because of the acute nature of the illness or injury. Research demonstrates, however, that critical care unit patients do remember painful experiences, and they frequently describe their pain as being moderate to severe in intensity.[2]

Factors Affecting Pain

Multiple factors inherent in the critical care unit environment affect the patient's pain experience (Box 5-1). The effects of each of these factors increase when they are experienced together. For example, pain and anxiety exacerbate each other.

Procedural Pain

Efforts to provide pain relief and comfort measures are complicated by the fact that critical care nurses must continuously perform procedures or treatments that cause pain to the patient, such as chest tube insertion and removal, wound debridement, and even turning a patient in bed. Critical care nurses must be attuned to the pain the patient is experiencing *before* the procedure to provide the best interventions and guidance to help the patient *during* the procedure. Before undergoing procedures known to be associated with pain, patients should be premedicated, and the procedure should be performed only after the medication has taken effect. In addition, the nurse can use interventions such as imagery, distraction, and family support during procedures.

BOX 5-1 Factors Contributing to Pain and Discomfort in the Critically Ill

Physical
- Illnesses and injuries treated in the critical care setting (eg, myocardial infarction, thoracic and neurosurgery, multiple trauma, extensive burns)
- Wounds—post-trauma, postoperative, or postprocedural
- Sleep disturbance and deprivation
- Immobility, inability to move to a comfortable position because of tubes, monitors, or restraints
- Temperature extremes associated with critical illness and the environment—fever or hypothermia

Psychosocial
- Anxiety and depression
- Loss of control
- Impaired communication, inability to report and describe pain
- Fear of pain, disability, or death
- Separation from family
- Unfamiliar and unpleasant surroundings
- Boredom or lack of pleasant distractions

Environment and Routine
- Continuous noise from equipment and staff
- Continuous or unnatural patterns of light
- Awakening and physical manipulation every 1 to 2 hours for vital signs or positioning
- Continuous or frequent invasive, painful procedures
- Competing priorities in care—unstable vital signs, bleeding, dysrhythmias, poor ventilation—may take precedence over pain management

 The Older Patient. *Be aware that arthritis, the most common cause of chronic pain in older patients, can increase the pain of turning in the ICU.*

Consequences of Pain

Patients who have a high level of uncontrolled pain during an acute hospitalization are at risk for delayed recovery and development of chronic pain syndromes after discharge. Pain produces many harmful effects on the body that inhibit healing and recovery from critical illness; these effects are summarized in Table 5-2.

Promoting Effective Pain Control

Barriers to Effective Pain Control

Critical care nurses are often concerned that analgesic administration for pain control may create problems, such as hemodynamic and respiratory compromise, oversedation, or drug addiction. The fear of addiction is one of the greatest concerns and impediments associated with analgesia and pain control. The differences between, and implications of, addiction, tolerance, and dependence are summarized in Table 5-3.

Patient and Family Education

To balance pain control and risks of treatment, communication between nurse, patient, and family is essential. Emphasis is on the prevention of pain because it is easier to prevent pain than to treat it. Patients need to know that most pain can be relieved and that unrelieved pain may have serious consequences for physical and psychological well-being and may interfere with recovery. The nurse helps patients and families understand that pain management is an important part of their care and that the healthcare team will respond quickly to reports of pain.

The nurse discusses plans for pain management with patients when they are best able to understand, such as before surgery rather than during recovery. Also, the patient needs a clear understanding of any specialized pain management technology, such as patient-controlled analgesia (PCA), to alleviate the fear of overdosage. It is necessary to reinforce this information during the course of therapy and encourage patients and family to verbalize questions and concerns. Box 5-2 provides key teaching points for promoting effective pain control.

TABLE 5-2 Effects of Pain

System	Effect	Outcome
Cardiovascular	Increased heart rate, blood pressure, contractility, vasoconstriction	Increases myocardial workload, thereby promoting or exacerbating ischemia
Pulmonary	Splinting; decreased respiration; reduced pulmonary volume and flow	Increased incidence of pulmonary complications (eg, atelectasis, pneumonia)
Neurologic	Increased anxiety and mental confusion; disturbed sleep	Delayed recovery; more pain
Gastrointestinal, nutritional	Decreased gastric emptying and intestinal motility	Impaired function; ileus; inhibits positive nitrogen balance
Musculoskeletal	Muscle contractions, spasms, and rigidity	Inhibits movement and coughing and deep breathing, putting patient at risk for complications of immobility
Immune	Suppressed immune function	Increases risk for pneumonia, wound infections, and sepsis

TABLE 5-3 Tolerance, Physical Dependence, and Addiction

	Definition	Implication
Tolerance	A state of adaptation in which exposure to a drug induces changes that result in a diminution of one or more of the drug's effects over time	Increase dose by 50% and assess effect. Tolerance to side effects, such as respiratory depression, increases as the dose requirement increases.
Physical dependence	A state of adaptation that is manifested by a drug class–specific withdrawal syndrome that can be produced by abrupt cessation, rapid dose reduction, decreasing blood level of the drug, and/or administration of an antagonist	Gradually taper opioid dosage to discontinuation to avoid withdrawal symptoms.
Addiction	A primary, chronic, neurobiological disease, with genetic, psychosocial, and environmental factors influencing its development and manifestations. It is characterized by behaviors that include one or more of the following: impaired control over drug use, compulsive use, continued use despite harm, and craving.	Rarely seen in critical care patients, unless patient is admitted for drug overdose or a history of drug abuse

Definitions from American Pain Society: Definitions related to the use of opioids for the treatment of pain. Retrieved May 12, 2011, from http://www.ampainsoc.org/advocacy/ opioids2.htm

Pain Assessment

The failure of healthcare providers to assess pain and pain relief routinely is one of the most common reasons for unrelieved pain in hospitalized patients.[3] Assessment of pain is as important as any assessment of the other body systems. The patient is assessed at regular intervals to determine the presence of pain or breakthrough pain, the effectiveness of therapy, the presence of side effects, the need for dose adjustment, or the need for supplemental doses to offset procedural pain. In critical care, assessment and treatment of the patient's pain may be hindered by:

- The acuity of the patient's condition
- Altered levels of consciousness
- An inability to communicate pain
- Restricted or limited movement
- Endotracheal intubation

To perform an effective pain assessment, the critical care nurse first attempts to elicit a self-report from the patient. Behavioral observation and changes in physiological parameters are considered along with the patient's self-report.

Patient Self-Report

Because pain is a subjective experience, the patient's self-report is considered the foundation of pain assessment; however, family members and caregivers are often used as proxies for patients unable to self report, which can pose significant communication barriers.[3] A self-report or proxy assessment of pain should be obtained not only at rest, but also during routine activity, such as coughing, deep breathing, and turning. In the conscious and coherent patient, behavioral cues or physiological indicators should never take precedence over the patient's self-report

of pain. If the patient can communicate, the nurse must accept the patient's description of pain as valid. Behavioral and physiological manifestations of pain are extremely individualized and may be minimal or absent, despite the presence of significant pain.

In assessing pain quality, the nurse elicits a specific verbal description of the patient's pain, in their own words, such as "burning," "crushing," "stabbing," "dull," or "sharp," whenever possible. These terms help pinpoint the cause of the pain.

 The Older Patient. *When assessing pain in an older patient, be aware of the following points:*

- *When reporting pain, an older patient may use words such as "aches" or "tenderness," rather than "pain."*
- *Some older patients can experience acutely painful conditions, such as myocardial infarction or appendicitis, without the presence of significant pain.*

BOX 5-2 **Promoting Safe and Effective Pain Control**

- Emphasize the importance of preventing pain before it occurs or becomes severe.
- Help patients and caregivers to understand the difference between tolerance and addiction. This helps to ensure that fears of addiction do not impede necessary analgesic administration.
- Discuss nonpharmacological interventions for minimizing pain (eg, splinting in incision area with a pillow while coughing or ambulating).
- Explain to caregivers the impact of analgesics on pain and respiratory status if they're responsible for administering PCA in the hospital or administering medication after discharge.

Pain scales and rating instruments based on the patient's self-report provide a simple but consistent measure of pain trends over time. Numerical rating scales and visual analog scales are used to measure pain intensity. With these scales, the patient is asked to choose a number, word, or point on a line that best describes the amount of pain he or she is experiencing. The Society of Critical Care Medicine (SCCM) clinical practice guideline suggests that the numerical rating scale is the preferred type of scale for use in critical care units.[4] With this type of scale, the patient is asked to rate the pain, with 0 being no pain and 10 being the worst possible pain imaginable.

Pictures or word boards can also facilitate communication about the patient's pain. The board should include open-ended questions, such as "Do you have pain?", "Where is the pain located?", "How bad is your pain?", and "What helps your pain?"

Observation

Research has demonstrated that nurses can rely on behavioral and physiological indicators of pain in critically ill patients who cannot provide a verbal self-report.[5] Patients who are unable to speak may use eye or facial expressions or movement of hands or legs to communicate their pain. Additionally, protective behaviors (eg, guarding, avoidance of movement, touching or rubbing the area, changing positions, muscular bracing) are suggestive of pain. Other nonverbal behaviors such as frowning, grimacing, clenching the teeth, tightly closing the eyes, and exhibiting restlessness and agitation can indicate pain as well.

Input from family members or other caregivers is helpful in interpreting specific behavioral manifestations of pain based on their knowledge of the patient's behavior before hospitalization.

Physiological Parameters

The observation of the physiological effects of pain assists to some extent in pain assessment; however, much like nonverbal cues, the physiological response to pain is highly individualized. Vital signs, such as heart rate, blood pressure, and respiratory rate, may increase or decrease in the presence of pain. Additionally, it can be difficult to attribute these physiological changes specifically to pain rather than to other causes. For example, an unexpected increase in the severity of the patient's pain may cause hypotension and tachycardia but could also signal the development of life-threatening complications, such as wound dehiscence, infection, or deep venous thrombosis. The absence of physiological or behavioral cues should never be interpreted as absence of pain. If the procedure, surgery, or condition is believed to be associated with pain, the presence of pain should be assumed and treated appropriately.

Contradictions in Pain Assessment

Occasionally, there may be discrepancies between the patient's self-report and behavioral and physiological manifestations. For example, one patient may report pain as 2 out of 10, while being tachycardic, diaphoretic, and splinting with respirations. Another patient may give a self-report of 8 out of 10 while smiling.

These discrepancies can be due to the use of diversionary activities, coping skills, beliefs about pain, cultural background, fears of addiction, or fears of being bothersome to the nursing staff. When these situations occur, they are discussed with the patient, and any misconceptions or knowledge deficits are addressed.

Pain Intervention

Although pharmacological intervention is the most commonly used strategy, nursing management of pain also includes physical, cognitive, and behavioral measures. In addition to administering medications or providing alternative therapies, the nurse's role involves measuring the patient's response to those therapies.

Pharmacological Interventions

Most drug therapy regimens that nurses use in the critical care setting include a combination of nonopioid analgesics, opioids, and sometimes anxiolytics or sedatives. Use of these drugs is explained in the sections that follow; examples, mechanisms of action, and special considerations are outlined in Table 5-4.

Nonopioid Analgesics

Ideally, analgesic regimens should include a nonopioid drug, even if the pain is severe enough to also require an opioid. In many patient populations, nonsteroidal anti-inflammatory drugs (NSAIDs) are the preferred choice for the nonopioid component of analgesic therapy. NSAIDs decrease pain by inhibiting the synthesis of inflammatory mediators (prostaglandin, histamine, and bradykinin) at the site of injury and effectively relieve pain without causing sedation, respiratory depression, or problems with bowel or bladder function. When NSAIDs are used in combination with opioids, the opioid dose can often be reduced and still produce effective analgesia. This decreases the incidence of opioid-related side effects.

Many NSAIDs are supplied only in oral forms but this is not satisfactory in many critically ill patients whose oral intake is restricted. In addition to the concerns about route of administration, a major concern associated with NSAID use is the potential for adverse effects, including gastrointestinal bleeding, platelet inhibition, and renal insufficiency. Second-generation NSAIDs are more selective in their site of action and therefore do not cause these harmful adverse effects, but their slow onset of action may decrease their utility in critically ill patients.

TABLE 5-4 Medications Used in Pain Management

Medication	Mechanism of Action	Nursing Considerations
Acetaminophen	Inhibit prostaglandins	• Lacks anti-inflammatory action • Avoid use in patients with liver or kidney disease • Doses exceeding 4000 mg/d increase risk for hepatic toxicity • Perform routine liver and renal profile testing for patients on a continuous, high-dose regimen
Aspirin	Inhibit prostaglandins and thromboxanes	• Adverse effects include gastrointestinal or postoperative bleeding • Contraindicated in patients with bleeding ulcers, hemorrhagic disorders, asthma, and renal insufficiency

NSAIDs
  Ibuprofen (Motrin)
  Naproxen (Naprosyn)
  Celecoxib (Celebrex)
	Inhibits prostaglandin synthesis by inhibiting the action of the enzyme cyclooxygenase, which is responsible for prostaglandin synthesis	• Adverse effects include gastrointestinal bleeding, platelet inhibition, and renal insufficiency
		• Avoid use in patients with liver or renal disease
		• Perform routine liver and renal profile testing for patients on a continuous, high-dose regimen

Opioid analgesics
  Morphine
  Fentanyl
  Hydromorphone (Dilaudid)
  Codeine
  Methadone (Dolophine)
  Oxycodone
	Bind to receptor sites in the central and peripheral nervous system, changing the perception of pain	• Adverse effects include respiratory depression, oversedation, constipation, urinary retention, and nausea
		• IV administration is usually the preferred route
		• Older patients are often more sensitive to the effects of opioids
		• Patients and families need education about tolerance and the risk of dependence

Local anesthetics
  Bupivacaine
  Chloroprocaine
	Act synergistically with intraspinal opioids and block pain by preventing nerve cell depolarization	• Adverse effects include CNS excitation, drowsiness, respiratory depression, apnea, hypotension, bradycardia, arrhythmias, and/or cardiac arrest
		• Commonly administered by the epidural route in combination with epidural or intrathecal analgesia

Antiemetics
  Promethazine
  Hydroxyzine
	Antagonizes central and peripheral H1 receptors	• Adverse effects include hypotension, restlessness, tremors, and extrapyramidal effects in the older patient
		• In high doses, can create auditory and visual hallucinations causing panic and intense fear
		• During long-term therapy, monitor blood cell counts, liver function studies; perform electrocardiogram and electroencehalogram

Opioid antagonists
  Naloxone
  Naltrexone
	Antagonizes various opioid receptors	• Administering the drug too quickly or giving too much can precipitate severe pain, withdrawal symptoms, tachycardia, dysrhythmias, and cardiac arrest; patients who have been receiving opioids for more than a week are particularly at risk
		• Drug should be diluted and given intravenously, very slowly
		• Monitor for acute withdrawal syndrome patients who are physically dependent on opioids, or who have received large doses of opioids

Benzodiazepines
  Diazepam
  Lorazepam
  Midazolam
	Increase the efficiency of a natural brain chemical, GABA, to decrease the excitability of neurons	• Adverse effects include phlebitis, acidosis, renal failure, prolonged wakening and delayed weaning from ventilator, and pain on injection site
		• Monitor the patient for oversedation and respiratory depression
		• Commonly administered intravenously

Benzodiazepine-specific reversal agent Flumazenil	Antagonizes benzodiazepine receptors	• Adverse effects include CNS manifestations, re-sedation, cardiovascular effects, seizures, and alterations in intracranial pressure and cerebral perfusion pressure • Re-sedation may occur within 1–2 h after administration, so repeated doses or a continuous infusion may be required to maintain therapeutic efficacy
Sedative-hypnotic Propofol		• Adverse effects include low blood pressure, apnea, and pain at the injection site • Monitor the patient's blood pressure • Contraindicated in patients allergic to eggs or soy products

Opioid Analgesics

Opioids are the pharmacological cornerstone of postoperative pain management. They provide pain relief by binding to various receptor sites in the spinal cord, central nervous system (CNS), and peripheral nervous system, thus changing the perception of pain.

Opioids are selected based on individual patient needs and the potential for adverse effects. According to the SCCM, morphine sulfate, fentanyl, and hydromorphone are the preferred agents when IV opioids are needed.[4] Other opioids used in critical care include codeine, oxycodone, and methadone. Even though meperidine continues to be widely used in some settings, national experts and national practice guidelines consider it to be dangerous and do not recommend it for most patients.[4]

The efficacy of analgesia depends on the presence of an adequate and consistent serum drug level. Although opioids may be administered on an "as needed" (PRN) basis, the PRN order poses many barriers to effective pain control. Per the PRN order, the nurse administers a dose of analgesic only when the patient requests it and only after a certain time interval has elapsed since the previous dose. Usually, delays occur between the time of the request and the time the medication is actually administered. PRN orders also pose a problem when the patient is asleep. As serum drug levels decrease, the patient may be suddenly awakened by severe pain, and a greater amount of the drug is needed to achieve adequate serum levels. For these reasons, scheduled opioid doses or continuous infusions are preferred over PRN administration.

Dosing Guidelines

Opioid dosage varies depending on the individual patient, the method of administration, and the pharmacokinetics of the drug. Adequate pain relief occurs once a minimum serum level of the opioid has been achieved. The dosing and titration of opioids must be individualized, and the patient's response and any undesirable effects, such as respiratory depression or oversedation, must be closely assessed. If the patient has previously been taking opioids prior to admission, doses should be adjusted above the previous required dose to achieve an optimal effect. Factors such as age, individual pain tolerance, coexisting diseases, type of surgical procedure, and the concomitant use of sedatives warrant consideration as well. Appropriate dosing and titration can be difficult because many critically ill patients have hepatic or renal dysfunction that result in decreased metabolism of the opioid.

The Older Patient. *Older patients are often more sensitive to the effects of opioids because in older people, opioids achieve higher peak concentrations and have a longer duration of effect. Decreasing the initial opioid dose and slow titration are recommended for older patients.*

Medications should be titrated based on the patient's response, and the drug should be quickly eliminated when analgesia is no longer needed. Most clinicians agree that when using a numerical scale for assessment, pain medications should be titrated according to the following goals:

- The patient's reported pain score is less than his or her own predetermined pain management goal (eg, 3 on a scale of 1 to 10).
- Adequate respiration is maintained.

Because pain may diminish or the pain pattern may change, therapy adjustments may be needed before improvements are seen. Pain reassessment should correspond to the time of onset or peak effect of the drug administered and the time the analgesic effect is expected to dissipate. Response to therapy is best measured as a change from the patient's baseline pain level.

Administration

The two most commonly used routes for opioid administration in the critical care setting are the intravenous route and the spinal route. Other routes that are less commonly used in the critical care setting are reviewed in Box 5-3.

BOX 5·3 Less Commonly Used Methods of Administering Opioids in the Critical Care Setting

Oral route. The oral route is used infrequently in the critical care setting because many patients are unable to take anything by mouth. Serum drug levels obtained after oral administration of opioids are variable and difficult to titrate. In addition, the transformation of oral opioids by the liver causes a significant decrease in serum levels.

Rectal route. The rectal route has many of the same disadvantages as the oral route, including variability in dosing requirements, delays to peak effect, and unstable serum drug levels.

Transdermal route. The transdermal route is used primarily to control chronic cancer pain because it takes 12 to 16 hours to obtain substantial therapeutic effects and up to 48 hours to achieve stable serum concentrations. If used for acute pain, such as postoperative pain, high serum concentrations may remain after the pain has subsided, putting the patient at risk for respiratory depression.[17]

Intramuscular route. The intramuscular route should not be used to provide acute pain relief for the critically ill patient. Intramuscular drug absorption is extremely variable in critically ill patients, due to alterations in cardiac output and tissue perfusion. In addition, intramuscular injections are painful.

Subcutaneous route. In some situations, venous access may be limited or impossible to obtain. When this occurs, continuous subcutaneous infusion and subcutaneous PCA may be used.

IV Administration. IV opioids have the most rapid onset and are easy to administer. Intermittent IV injections may be used when the patient requires short-term acute pain relief—for example, during procedures such as chest tube removal, diagnostic tests, suctioning, or wound care. Continuous IV administration has many benefits for critically ill patients, especially those who have difficulty communicating their pain because of an altered level of consciousness or an endotracheal tube. Continuous IV infusions are easily initiated and maintain consistent serum drug levels compared to intermittent IV injections, which can cause serum levels to fluctuate. When a patient is receiving continuous IV infusions, pain occurring during painful procedures may not be managed unless additional IV bolus injections are given.

PCA is an effective method of pain relief for the critically ill patient who is conscious and able to participate in pain management therapy. With PCA, the patient self-administers small, frequent IV analgesic doses using a programmable infusion device. The PCA device limits the opioid dose within a specific time period, thus preventing oversedation and respiratory depression. PCA produces good-quality analgesia, stable drug concentrations, less sedation, less opioid consumption, and fewer adverse effects.[4] PCA individualizes pain control therapy; and offers the patient greater feelings of control and well-being.

Spinal Administration. Spinal opioids selectively block opioid receptors while leaving sensation, motor, and sympathetic nervous system function intact, resulting in fewer opioid-related side effects. Analgesia from spinal opioids has a longer duration than other routes, and significantly less opioid is needed to achieve effective pain relief. Opioids can be given as a single injection in the epidural or intrathecal space, as intermittent injections, as continuous infusions through an epidural catheter, or through epidural PCA. With epidural or intrathecal analgesia, a local anesthetic can be added to the continuous opioid infusion. Less opioid is needed to provide effective analgesia when used in combination with local anesthetics, and the incidence of opioid-related side effects is decreased.

Epidural Analgesia. Epidural analgesia is noted for providing effective pain relief and improved postoperative pulmonary function. In a classic study, patients whose pain was controlled with epidural anesthesia and epidural analgesia had shorter critical care unit stays, shorter hospital stays, and half as many complications as patients receiving standard anesthesia and analgesia.[5]

This method is especially beneficial for critically ill patients after thoracic, upper abdominal, or peripheral vascular surgery; postoperative patients with a history of obesity or pulmonary disease; and patients with rib fractures or orthopedic trauma. Contraindications to epidural analgesia include systemic infection or sepsis, bleeding disorders, and increased intracranial pressure (ICP).

With epidural analgesia, opioids are administered through a catheter inserted in the spinal canal between the dura mater and vertebral arch. Opioids diffuse across the dura and subarachnoid space and bind with opioid receptor sites. Epidurals may take the form of:

- Intermittent injections given before, during, or after a surgical procedure
- Continuous epidural infusions, which are recommended for more sustained pain relief
- Patient-controlled epidural analgesia (PCEA), which uses the same parameters as IV PCA except in smaller doses

Although the incidence of serious respiratory depression is extremely low with epidural analgesia, respiratory assessments should be performed hourly during the first 24 hours of therapy and every 4 hours thereafter. In addition, because epidural analgesia is invasive, the patient must be closely monitored for signs of local or systemic infections. The insertion site is covered with a sterile dressing, and the catheter is taped securely. To avoid accidental injection of preservative-containing medications (which can be neurotoxic), the epidural catheter, infusion tubing, and pump must be clearly marked.

Intrathecal Analgesia. With intrathecal analgesia, the opioid is injected into the subarachnoid space, located between the arachnoid and pia mater. Intrathecal opioids are significantly more potent than those given epidurally; therefore, less medication is needed to provide effective analgesia. The intrathecal method is usually used to deliver a one-time dose of analgesic, such as before surgery, and is infrequently used as a continuous infusion because of the risk for CNS infection.

Side Effects

Opioids cause undesirable side effects, such as constipation, urinary retention, sedation, respiratory depression, and nausea. These are managed in many ways, including decreasing the opioid dose, avoiding PRN dosing, and adding other medications to supplement opioid doses or to counteract opioid side effects. However, medications commonly prescribed to treat opioid-related adverse effects, such as antiemetics for nausea, can cause other adverse effects, such as hypotension, restlessness, and tremors.

Respiratory depression, a life-threatening complication of opioid administration, is often a concern. However, the incidence of true opioid-induced respiratory depression is low in most patients. In some cases, a respiratory rate as low as 10 breaths/min may not be significant if the patient is still breathing deeply.

RED FLAG! *Patients most at risk for respiratory depression are elderly people who have not recently used opioids and patients with coexisting pulmonary, renal, or hepatic disease.*

If serious respiratory depression does occur, an opioid antagonist can be administered to reverse the adverse effects of the opioid. Antagonists are titrated to effect, which means reversing the oversedation and respiratory depression, not reversing analgesia. This usually occurs within 1 to 2 minutes. After administering an antagonist, the nurse continues to observe the patient closely for oversedation and respiratory depression because the half-life of antagonists is shorter than that of most opioids.

Sedatives and Anxiolytics

Acute pain is frequently accompanied by anxiety, which can increase the patient's perception of pain. When treating acute pain, anxiolytics and hypnotics can be used to complement analgesia and improve the patient's overall comfort.

Anxiolytics

Anxiolytic medications (eg, benzodiazepines) control anxiety and muscle spasms and produce amnesia for uncomfortable procedures. Because these medications have no analgesic effect (except for controlling pain caused by muscle spasm), an analgesic must be administered concomitantly to relieve pain. If an opioid and benzodiazepine are used together, the doses of both medications are usually reduced because of their synergistic effects. The patient must also be closely monitored for oversedation and respiratory depression.

An advantage of benzodiazepines is that they are reversible agents. If respiratory depression occurs because of benzodiazepine administration, benzodiazepine-specific reversal agents can be administered intravenously. These drugs are given reverse the sedative and respiratory depressant effects without reversing opioid analgesics.

Critically ill patients who are receiving repeated doses or continuous infusions of benzodiazepines are given a break from sedation at least once per day. Administration should be interrupted until the patient is fully awake. This helps prevent oversedation, which can inhibit weaning from mechanical ventilation.

Hypnotics

With appropriate airway and ventilatory management, hypnotics can be an ideal agent for patients requiring sedation during painful procedures. Because of their ultrashort half-life, they are reversible simply by discontinuing the infusion, and patients awaken within a few minutes. They also can be used as a continuous infusion for mechanically ventilated patients who require deep, prolonged sedation.

Nonpharmacological Comfort Measures

Research has shown that the combination of nonpharmacological and pharmacological interventions provides better pain control, with less use of opioid analgesics, decreased incidence of anxiety, and increased patient satisfaction.[6,7]

Environmental Modification

Environmental modifications can help to minimize anxiety and agitation. Care should be preplanned to minimize noise and disruptions during normal sleeping hours and to create a pattern of light that mimics normal day–night patterns. Earphones, with music of the patient's choosing, and earplugs have also been recommended for use in the critical care unit.[8]

Distraction

Distraction helps patients direct their attention away from the source of pain or discomfort toward something more pleasant. Initiating a conversation with the patient during an uncomfortable procedure, watching television, and visiting with family are all excellent sources of distraction.

Relaxation Techniques

Relaxation exercises involve repetitive focus on a word, phrase, prayer, or muscular activity, and a conscious effort to reject other intruding thoughts. Most relaxation methods require a quiet environment, a comfortable position, a passive attitude, and concentration.

Breathing exercises have been used with much success in critically ill patients. The quieting reflex is a breathing technique that requires only 6 seconds to complete, calms the sympathetic nervous system, and gives the patient a sense of control over stress and anxiety. The nurse teaches the patient to perform the following steps frequently during the day:

1. Inhale an easy, natural breath.
2. Think "alert mind, calm body."
3. Exhale, allowing the jaw, tongue, and shoulders to go loose.
4. Allow a feeling of warmth and looseness to go down through the body and out through the toes.

Touch

Touch has a positive effect on perceptual and cognitive abilities and can influence physiological parameters, such as respiration and blood flow. Additionally, touch has played a major part in promoting and maintaining reality orientation in patients prone to confusion about time, place, and personal identification. Nursing touch may be most helpful in situations in which people experience fear, anxiety, depression, or isolation.

 The Older Patient. *Older patients often have an increased need for meaningful touch during episodes of crisis.*

Massage

Superficial massage initiates the relaxation response and has been shown to increase the amount of sleep in critical care patients.[9] Hands, feet, and shoulders are good sites for massage in critically ill patients, because the back is less accessible. Family members who wish to provide comfort to a critically ill loved one can be taught the technique of massage.

CASE STUDY

Mr. B., a 28-year-old man, is admitted to the critical care unit. with multiple orthopedic and abdominal injuries sustained in a motorcycle accident. During his third day in the critical care unit., he continues to describe his pain as "intolerable" and says it is not relieved by the combination of oxycodone and acetaminophen that he receives every 4 hours. He is grimacing and continuously asking for more medication before the scheduled dosage interval. The medical resident is frustrated by Mr. B.'s frequent requests and has advised the nurses to be conservative in medicating him because of his history of drug and alcohol abuse.

1. What might be major concerns of the nurse caring for Mr. B.?

2. How could the nurse advocate for Mr. B.?

3. How could the nurse determine whether Mr. B. is seeking drugs for illicit purposes rather than for relief of pain?

4. What approach could the nurse take to convince the medical resident to consider a different analgesic regimen?

References

1. International Association for the Study of Pain: Pain Terminology. Retrieved August 28, 2007, from http://www. iasp-pain.org/AM/Template.cfm?Section=Home&template =/ CM/HTMLDisplay.cfm&ContentID=3088#Pain

2. Puntillo KA, Morris AB, Thompson CL, et al.: Pain behaviors observed during six common procedures: Results from Thunder Project II. Crit Care Med 32(2):421–427, 2004

3. National Cancer Institute: Pain (PDQ). Retrieved September 1, 2007, from http://www.cancer.gov/cancertopics/pdq/supportivecare/pain/HealthProfessional/page1

4. Jacobi J, Fraser G, Coursin D, et al.: Clinical practice guidelines for the sustained use of sedatives and analgesics in the critically ill adult. Crit Care Med 30(1):119–141, 2002

5. Yeager MP, Glass DD, Neff RK, et al.: Epidural anesthesia and analgesia in high-risk surgical patients. Anesthesiology 66(6):729–736, 1987

6. Weintraub M, Mamtani R, Micozzi M: Complimentary and Integrative Medicine in Pain Management. Springer Publishing, 2008

7. Khatta M. A complimentary approach to pain management. Topics Adv Pract Nurs 7(1), 2007

8. Schartz F. Pilot study of patients in postoperative cardiac surgery. Music Med 1(1):70–74, 2009

9. Mitchinson A, et al. Acute postoperative pain management using massage as an adjuvant therapy: a randomized trial. Arch Surg 142(12):1158–1167, 2007

Want to know more? A wide variety of resources to enhance your learning and understanding of this chapter are available on the **Point** ✳. Visit **http://thepoint.lww.com/MortonEss1e** to access chapter review questions and more!

End-of-Life and Palliative Care

OBJECTIVES

Based on the content in this chapter, the reader should be able to:

1 Describe how the integration of palliative care principles into critical care is essential to providing end-of-life care in the critical care setting.
2 Identify common symptoms experienced at the end of life and appropriate measures to address them.
3 Explain the role of advance directives in facilitating end-of-life care.
4 Explain how effective communication among caregivers, patients, and family members can facilitate end-of-life care.
5 Explain aspects of family-centered care that are important during the end-of-life period.
6 Identify strategies caregivers can use for managing their own grief.

Technology, urgency, uncertainty, and conflict are common in critical care practice. These characteristics may inhibit or fragment a coordinated effort that aims to provide good end-of-life care.[1] Critical care nurses play an important role in recognizing opportunities for interventions that support patients, families, and other staff members during the difficult transition period between life and death. "Being with" patients and families in addition to "doing things to" them enables critical care nurses to provide the holistic care that is central to nursing.[1]

The introduction of palliative care principles into critical care practice can provide a framework to address end-of-life issues. Palliative care improves the quality of death and dying for patients and their families by addressing aspects of care that are unrelated to disease-specific treatments, cure, or rehabilitation. According to the World Health Organization,[2] palliative care includes the following interdisciplinary core principles:

- Symptom management
- Advanced care planning
- Family-centered care
- Emotional, psychological, social, and spiritual care
- Facilitating communication
- Awareness of ethical issues
- Caring for the caregiver

In critical care nursing, it is vital to take an interdisciplinary approach to incorporating these core palliative care principles into the patient's daily plan of care. Incorporating palliative care services into critical care leads to improved symptom management, enhanced family support, reduced lengths of hospital stays, increased discharges to home with hospice referrals, and reduced costs.[3] The American Association of Critical-Care Nurses protocols for critical care practice in palliative and end-of-life care provide a good overview of core issues and clinical recommendations for critical care nurses.[4]

Symptom Management

Common symptoms at the end of life include the following.

- **Pain.** The underlying disease pathology, procedures, and interventions are all sources of pain in the dying patient. The assessment and management of pain is discussed in Chapter 5.
- **Dyspnea.** Causes of dyspnea include the underlying disease pathology; anxiety; and environmental issues (eg, feeling crowded). Common interventions used for dyspnea include oxygen, opioids, and anxiolytics. Nonpharmacological interventions such as reducing the room temperature (but not chilling the patient), reducing the number of people in the room at one time, keeping an unobstructed line of sight between the patient and the outside environment, and using a fan to blow air gently across the patient's face have all been found to be effective in decreasing dyspnea.
- **Anxiety and agitation.** Anxiety can be related to any number of physical, emotional, psychological, social, practical, and spiritual issues. Nonpharmacological interventions may include counseling, taking care of practical matters (eg, arranging for the care of a pet), and facilitating resolution of spiritual concerns (eg, arranging for a visit from a clergy member). If medication is needed, short- or long-acting benzodiazepines and antidepressants may be helpful. Additional interventions for anxiety are discussed in Chapter 2, Box 2-1.
- **Depression.** It is a myth that depression is "normal" at the end of life. If feelings of depression persist, appropriate treatment (eg, supportive psychotherapy, cognitive-behavioral therapy, antidepressants) must be initiated.
- **Delirium.** Delirium is an acute change in awareness or cognitive status that may manifest as agitation, withdrawal, confusion, inappropriate behavior, disorientation, or hallucinations. Terminal delirium is common in patients near death and may manifest as day–night reversal. Management of delirium during the end-of-life care is focused more on symptom control and relief of the patient's and family's distress than on diagnosis and treatment of the underlying cause of the delirium. Benzodiazepines or neuroleptics (eg, haloperidol) may be used for symptom control.
- **Nausea and vomiting.** Causes of nausea and vomiting may include physiological factors (eg, intestinal obstruction, constipation, pancreatitis, metabolic disturbances, increased intracranial pressure); emotional factors; treatment-related factors (eg, chemotherapy); and vestibular disturbances. A careful assessment of the source of nausea and vomiting is important in determining the appropriate management. Many classes of drugs are used to provide symptomatic relief. If intestinal obstruction is causing nausea and vomiting, symptomatic relief can also be provided by surgery (to relieve the obstruction) or placement of a nasogastric tube or draining percutaneous endoscopic gastrostomy tube.

Assessing for the presence of symptoms and working collaboratively to intervene and provide relief is crucial in providing good end-of-life care. If symptoms are intractable and cannot be relieved despite appropriate interventions, end-of-life (terminal) sedation may be considered. End-of-life sedation is used when the patient is experiencing unbearable and unmanageable pain or other symptoms and is approaching the last hours or days of life.[5] The goal of end-of-life sedation is to produce a level of obtundation sufficient to relieve suffering without hastening death.[5] Before end-of-life sedation is considered, specialists in other disciplines (eg, pain, palliative care, social services, chaplaincy services, mental health) are consulted to verify that all therapies have been attempted without success.

Advanced Care Planning

Advanced care planning involves making the necessary arrangements so that a person's preferences for end-of-life care are known and can be followed should the person become unable to make decisions or communicate her wishes regarding care at a later time.

Advance Directives

Advance directives are written or oral instructions about future medical care that are to be followed in the event that the person loses the capacity to make decisions. Advance directives can be revised, orally or in writing, at any time. Each state regulates the use of advance directives differently.

Types of advance directives include living wills and durable powers of attorney for healthcare (used to specify a person, called a "healthcare proxy," "surrogate decision maker," or "healthcare agent," who is authorized to make decisions on behalf of the patient in the event that the patient cannot make decisions for himself or herself). The designation of a person as a healthcare proxy must be in written form and should always be up to date. The proxy should know the preferences of the patient and be able to communicate and adhere to those preferences.

When a patient arrives on the unit, the nurse determines if the patient has made an advance directive, and if so, obtains a copy to place in the patient's chart. If the patient does not have an advanced directive but is currently able to make autonomous decisions, the nurse seeks to determine the patient's wishes regarding end-of-life care. If the patient is unable to make decisions or communicate, then the next of kin is used as the proxy for healthcare decisions. The order for determining next of kin is legal guardian, spouse, adult children, parents, adult siblings, other adult relatives, and close friends who are familiar with the patient's activities and beliefs.

Do Not Resuscitate and Do Not Attempt Resuscitation Orders

The standard of care for patients who experience cardiac or respiratory arrest is to initiate cardiopulmonary resuscitation (CPR). The immediate intervention to preserve life without the express consent of the patient is supported by the principle of beneficence. However, patients can request that resuscitation not be attempted, especially when death is imminent and inevitable. Do not resuscitate (DNR) and do not attempt resuscitation (DNAR) orders are orders placed by a physician, most often with the consent of the patient or the healthcare proxy, to alert caregivers that if the patient experiences cardiac or respiratory arrest, no attempts to restore cardiac or pulmonary function should occur. The order is written, signed, and dated by the responsible physician and is reviewed periodically (eg, every 24 to 72 hours) per facility policy.

 RED FLAG! *It is important to recognize that DNR and DNAR orders do not mean "do not give appropriate care." Although resuscitation efforts should not be initiated for a patient with a DNR or DNAR order, the patient should continue to receive appropriate medical and nursing care throughout the duration of the hospitalization.*

 RED FLAG! *If an arrest occurs in a situation in which a formal DNR decision has not been made and written, the presumption of the medical and nursing staffs should be in favor of life, and a code should be called. A "slow code" (one in which the nurse takes excessive time to call the code, or the healthcare team takes an excessive time to respond to it) is never permissible.*

Communication and End-of-Life Care

Communication among the healthcare team, the patient, and family is an important aspect of caregiving in critical care, especially at the end of life. Good communication facilitates a better understanding of how to care for the patient and family and fosters an environment that supports the physical and psychosocial needs of the patient, family, and providers.

Establishing Treatment Goals and Priorities

Establishing treatment goals and priorities is essential to facilitating decision making with regard to care. The way in which options are presented can influence the decisions the patient and family make. For example, if a nurse asks "Do you want the healthcare team to do everything for your loved one?" it sets the family up for a "yes" answer. In the family's mind, the opposite of "everything" is "nothing." It is also important to clearly define terms to ensure understanding and avoid ambiguous language. For example, to the nurse "everything" might include aggressive interventions, whereas to a family member "everything" may include only those interventions that provide comfort and pain relief.

A seven-step approach has been suggested to help negotiate goals in caring for patients[5]:

1. Create the proper setting. Sit down, ensure privacy, and allow adequate time.
2. Determine what the patient and family know. Clarify the current situation and the context in which decisions about goals of care should be made.
3. Explore what the patient and family are expecting or hoping for. Understanding these hopes and expectations will assist the nurse in tailoring communication and reorienting families to what is or might be possible.
4. Suggest realistic goals. To assist with decision making, share your knowledge about the patient's illness, its natural course, the experience of patients in similar circumstances, and the effects that contemporary healthcare may have. Work through unreasonable or unrealistic expectations.
5. Respond empathically to the emotions that may arise.
6. Make a plan and follow through with it.
7. Review and revise the goals and treatments as appropriate.

Delivering Bad News

Critical care nurses must develop effective strategies for delivering bad news. Bad news can range from reporting that a patient is not responding positively to an intervention to telling a family member that a patient has died. Keeping an honest and open line of communication is essential to preserve the trust of the patient and family. Because nurses are at the bedside 24 hours a day, communicating with families early that a patient is not doing well may help avoid a "surprise" announcement of the patient's death. Bad news should be phrased in a way that clearly indicates that the patient is not doing well but the healthcare team is doing its best to help the patient. If discussions regarding withholding or withdrawing life-sustaining measures become necessary, the family may be more receptive because they are more aware of the situation.

Notifying the family members that the patient has died is a special case of delivering bad news. Measures such as being prepared to answer questions about the patient's death, using the person's name (instead of "the patient" or "the deceased"), and being available to provide support can have a positive impact on how the family members remember the last moments of the patient's life. Becoming comfortable with the wording of the message (eg, by practicing phrases before they are needed) allows the nurse to focus on the family and their reaction to the message, instead of the message itself and how that message is delivered.

Family-Centered Care

Serious illness affects not only the patient but also the family.

Visitation

To the greatest extent possible, families should be free to visit a patient who is near death. The ability to see, touch, and communicate with the patient is reassuring for both the patient and family. During this period of closure, cultural or spiritual ceremonies may also take place. The nurse seeks to facilitate visitation while taking into consideration the physical and emotional needs of the patient, as well as the patient's wishes. For example, the nurse must also be alert to signs from the patient (eg, agitation) that a particular family member is unwelcome. If there is tension among certain family members, a visiting schedule may need to be established to allow family members to see the patient without crossing paths.

Bereavement Care

The death of a patient can affect family members in different ways. Previous experiences with death, coping skills, cultural and spiritual beliefs, and the circumstances surrounding the death influence the grief experience. Bereavement support includes providing family members with information about bereavement support services available through the facility, as well as information about how to make arrangements after the death and who can be contacted at the facility if questions arise.

It is important to do everything possible to allow the family sufficient time to go through their leave-taking rituals. Not allowing family members the chance to say goodbye can complicate the grieving process and negatively influence how the family remembers the experience of losing their loved one.

Legal and Ethical Issues in End-of-Life Care

Principle of Double Effect

The principle of double effect involves actions that have two effects, one good and one bad.[6] This principle often applies with the administration of pain medications to patients who are dying. Opioids are used to relieve pain and other symptoms of suffering (ie, the good effect). However, opioids also may cause respiratory and cardiovascular depression that may hasten death (ie, the bad effect). If the primary intention is to relieve pain and suffering with the recognition that it may hasten death, it is morally and legally permissible to administer the opioid.

Withholding or Withdrawing Life-Sustaining Measures

When it becomes clear to the family and healthcare providers that additional treatment will not be beneficial, the decision may be made to withdraw life-support methods (eg, mechanical ventilation, hemodialysis, tube feeding). The healthcare system requires that patients and their proxy decision makers be active in making decisions about healthcare treatment. However, at times, the healthcare team tries to place the responsibility for making a crucial decision, such as withdrawing treatment, on the family. It is important to remember that family members are not healthcare professionals. Even when family members are healthcare professionals, they are family members first and healthcare professionals second, and they may make decisions based more on their relationship with the patient than on sound medical or nursing decisions. The best approach is to help the family understand the benefits and drawbacks of continuing treatment and to make the decision jointly. When the decision is made to withdraw a therapy, measures are taken to reduce the suffering of the patient and to minimize family members' distress. For example opioids or sedatives may be administered to the patient, and the alarms on equipment may be silenced to allow the family to focus on the patient rather than the technology.

Brain Death

All states have laws addressing the definition of death in the state. It is important that the nurse know the legal definition of death in any state where he or she is practicing. A "brain dead" patient (ie, one who has experienced the irreversible loss of all brain function) is legally dead, and there is no legal duty to continue to treat him or her. It is not necessary to obtain court approval to discontinue life support on a patient who is brain-dead. Furthermore, although it can be desirable to obtain family permission to discontinue treatment of a brain-dead patient, there is no legal requirement. However, before terminating life support, physicians and nurses should be sure that organs are not intended for transplantation purposes.

Organ and Tissue Donation

Organs and tissues can be procured after cardiac death or brain death. Both federal law and the Joint Commission require facilities to have written protocols regarding organ and tissue donation, and that family members be given the chance to authorize donation of the patient's tissues and organs.[7] When organ or tissue procurement is a possibility, it is important that all family members are given the information they need to make a decision with which they are comfortable and that their grief is respected.

Caring for the Caregiver

Some deaths affect the nurse more significantly than others. The death of a child, the death of a friend or colleague, mass casualties, or a particularly horrific, traumatic death can have a profound effect on the nurse. Nurses may delay attending to their own grief because the demands of the unit and the needs of the family members may take precedence. It is important for nurses to recognize their grief and take appropriate measures to address it. Self-care strategies include:

- Asking for temporary relief from care responsibilities
- Reflecting on feelings after the event
- Discussing the experience with a colleague, friend, or nurse leader
- Focusing on what was done right
- Maintaining physical health (eg, through regular exercise, proper nutrition, adequate rest, and stress-relieving activities)

References

1. Nelson J, et al.: Integrating palliative care in the ICU. 13(2):89–94, 2011
2. End of Life Care Strategies: Core competencies. Department of Health and NHS End of Life Care Program. July (2008)
3. Campbell ML: Palliative care consultation in the intensive care unit. Crit Care Med 34(11 Suppl):S355–S358, 2006
4. Medina J, Puntillo KA: AACN Protocols for Practice: Palliative Care and End-of-Life Issues in Critical Care. Sudbury, MA: Jones & Bartlett, 2006
5. Emanuel L, von Gunten C, Ferris F, et al. (eds): The Education in Palliative and End-of-Life Care (EPEC) Curriculum: © The EPEC Project. Chicago: Author, 2003.
6. Matzo M, Witt Sherman D: Societal and Professional Issues in Palliative Care. In Palliative Care Nursing: Quality Care to the End of Life. Springer Publishing, 2009
7. Campbell ML, Zalenski R: The emergency department. In Ferrell BR, Coyle N (eds): Textbook of Palliative Care, 2nd ed. New York, NY: Oxford University Press, 2006, pp 861–869

Want to know more? A wide variety of resources to enhance your learning and understanding of this chapter are available on thePoint ✳. Visit **http://thepoint.lww.com/MortonEss1e** to access chapter review questions and more!

CASE STUDY

Mrs. M. is a 35-year-old woman who was in a motor vehicle collision. She sustained a severe brain injury (subdural hematoma and diffuse axonal injury), bilateral pulmonary contusions, and a liver laceration. By hospital day 3, she has received 30 units of packed red blood cells and is beginning to exhibit signs of organ dysfunction (eg, elevated creatinine and blood urea nitrogen levels, coagulopathy). She remains unresponsive. The primary physician is at the bedside and wants to discuss the options for future care with the family. The physician raises the subjects of initiating a do-not-resuscitate (DNR) order and withdrawing life support.

1. What are the nurse's responsibilities toward the family following the conversation with the physician?

2. If the family decides to initiate a do-not-resuscitate (DNR) order, to remove life support, or both, what are the major goals in caring for Mrs. M.?

CHAPTER 7

Providing Nutritional Support, Fluids, and Electrolytes

OBJECTIVES

Based on the content in this chapter, the reader should be able to:

1 Explain how the physiological stressors of illness and injury alter the body's needs for energy.
2 Describe data obtained during assessment of the patient's nutritional status.
3 Describe the nurse's role in providing enteral nutrition.
4 Describe the nurse's role in providing parenteral nutrition.
5 Describe the nurse's role in ensuring fluid balance.
6 Describe the nurse's role in the acute management of electrolyte imbalances.

Physiological stressors, such as illness and injury, alter the body's metabolic and energy demands. Patients can experience considerable weight loss (>10 kg) during and after a stay in the critical care unit. This unintentional weight loss may deplete vital nutrient reserves, which may predispose the patient to malnutrition. Malnutrition from starvation alone can usually be corrected by replacing body stores of essential nutrients. However, malnutrition resulting from critical illness and disease processes that alter metabolism is not as easily rectified and can have serious consequences for the hospitalized patient (Box 7-1). Early identification of nutritional deficiencies and appropriate intervention can lessen morbidity and mortality risks in critically ill patients.

Metabolism has two parts: anabolism and catabolism. Anabolism builds up and repairs the body, which requires energy. Catabolism breaks down food and body tissues to liberate energy. Glucose is the obligatory fuel of the body. The liver, which has the ability to both store and synthesize glucose, regulates glucose entry into the circulatory system. The liver converts and stores excess glucose as either

glycogen or fatty acids (triglycerides). Because there is no pathway for converting fatty acids back to glucose, fatty acids are used directly as a fuel source or are converted to ketones by the liver. After prolonged starvation, the body adapts to preserve vital proteins by using ketones, rather than glucose, as energy. Ketoacidosis occurs when ketone production exceeds utilization.

The pancreatic hormones insulin and glucagon have opposing functions in metabolism. Insulin helps transport glucose for storage into the cells and tissues, prevents fat breakdown, and increases protein synthesis. Glucagon stimulates glycogenolysis (glycogen breakdown) and gluconeogenesis (glucose synthesis from other sources such as proteins), and it increases lipolysis (fat breakdown and mobilization). The catecholamines epinephrine and norepinephrine, which are released from the adrenal medulla in times of stress, also play a role in glycogenolysis. Once glucose and glycogen stores have been exhausted (usually within 8 to 12 hours), hepatic gluconeogenesis increases dramatically to meet metabolic demands in response to glucagon and the glucocorticoid hormone cortisol. If

BOX 7-1 Consequences of Malnutrition for the Hospitalized Patient

- Delayed wound healing
- Increased complications
- Immunosuppression
- Increased length of hospitalization
- Organ impairment
- Increased morbidity and mortality

catabolic processes continue without the support of energy, amino acids, and essential nutrients, existing body stores become depleted and malnutrition may develop.

All tissues require protein to maintain structure and facilitate wound healing. If protein intake is inadequate, the body becomes catabolic, seeking protein from skeletal muscle and vital organs. Protein–calorie malnutrition is typically caused by acute, life-threatening conditions (eg, surgery, trauma, sepsis) and is due to depletion of fat, muscle wasting, and micronutrient deficiencies from acute and chronic illness. Clinical signs of protein-calorie malnutrition include generalized edema (the result of extracellular fluid shifts caused by low-protein oncotic pressures in the intravascular space), hair loss, skin breakdown, poor wound healing and surgical wound dehiscence. Laboratory data reveal low serum albumin levels, and treatment requires aggressive repletion of protein stores.

 RED FLAG! Protein-calorie malnutrition is much easier to prevent than to treat.

Nutritional Assessment

A critically ill patient's nutritional status may fall anywhere on a continuum ranging from optimal nutrition to malnutrition. Nutritional disturbances can be subtle and are frequently nonspecific. The nurse, registered dietician or nutritionist, and other members of the nutritional support team work collaboratively to assess and manage the patient's nutritional status. The nutritional assessment includes:

- A history, including questions aimed at understanding factors that can affect the patient's food intake and the patient's usual eating habits and preferences
- Physical examination (Table 7-1)
- Anthropometric measurements (ie, height, weight, body mass index [BMI], triceps skinfold thickness, and midarm and arm muscle circumference)
- Laboratory studies (Table 7-2)

Serial weight measurement is perhaps the single most important indicator of nutritional status and is the evaluation that the nurse performs most often.

ICU nurses are responsible for obtaining an initial "dry weight" (ie, the patient's weight before fluids are administered), as well as daily weight measurements, vital signs, intake and output measurements, and laboratory data. In addition, the nurse must monitor for clinical signs of dehydration (ie, thirst, dry mucous membranes, tachycardia, poor skin turgor), and fluid excess (ie, peripheral edema, adventitious lung sounds). Early detection and subsequent interventions may prevent the occurrence of excessive fluid shifts and cardiac compromise.

An important factor that influences nutritional status is nitrogen balance, a sensitive indicator of the body's gain or loss of protein. An adult is in nitrogen balance when the nitrogen intake equals the nitrogen output (in urine, feces, and perspiration). A positive nitrogen balance exists when nitrogen intake exceeds nitrogen output and indicates tissue growth (such as occurs during recovery from surgery) and rebuilding of wasted tissue. A negative nitrogen balance indicates that the tissue is breaking down faster than it is being replaced.

Nutritional Support

Goals for nutritional support may include:

- Prevention and treatment of macronutrient and micronutrient deficiencies
- Maintenance of fluid and electrolyte balance
- Reduction in patient morbidity and mortality

In patients unable to meet their nutritional needs with oral intake, nutritional supplementation may be delivered by either enteral or parenteral routes.

Enteral Nutrition

Enteral nutrition refers to any form of nutrition delivered to the gastrointestinal tract through a feeding tube placed into the stomach or the small intestine. Enteral nutrition is considered when the patient cannot or should not eat or intake is insufficient or unreliable.

For patients with an intact gastrointestinal tract, the enteral route is the preferred method of nutritional support ("If the gut works, use it."). The gastrointestinal mucosa depends on nutrient delivery and adequate blood flow to prevent atrophy, thereby maintaining the absorptive, barrier, and immunological functions of the intestine. Gut-associated lymphoid tissue (GALT) lines the gastrointestinal tract and is associated with maintenance of the immunological function of the mucosa. Without food, the gastrointestinal mucosa atrophies, the tissue available to absorb nutrients decreases, and GALT is impaired. Bacterial translocation (ie, the entry of resident gastrointestinal bacteria and endotoxins into the systemic circulation) can trigger immune and inflammatory responses, leading to infection, sepsis, and multisystem organ failure.[1] In addition to helping to preserve gastrointestinal

TABLE 7-1 **Physical Assessment Interpretation in Nutritional Disorders**

Body System or Region	Sign or Symptom	Implications
General	Weakness and fatigue Weight loss	Anemia or electrolyte imbalance, decreased calorie intake, increased calorie use, or inadequate nutrient intake or absorption
Skin, hair, and nails	Dry, flaky skin	Vitamin A, vitamin B complex, or linoleic acid deficiency
	Dry skin with poor turgor	Dehydration
	Rough, scaly skin with bumps	Vitamin A deficiency
	Petechiae or ecchymoses	Vitamin C or K deficiency
	Sore that will not heal	Protein, vitamin C, or zinc deficiency
	Thinning, dry hair	Protein deficiency
	Spoon-shaped, brittle, or rigid nails	Iron deficiency
Eyes	Night blindness; corneal swelling, softening, or dryness; Bitot's spots (gray triangular patches on the conjunctiva)	Vitamin A deficiency
	Red conjunctiva	Riboflavin deficiency
Throat and mouth	Cracks at the corner of mouth	Riboflavin or niacin deficiency
	Magenta tongue	Riboflavin deficiency
	Beefy, red tongue	Vitamin B_{12} deficiency
	Soft, spongy, bleeding gums	Vitamin C deficiency
	Swollen neck (goiter)	Iodine deficiency
Cardiovascular	Edema	Protein deficiency
	Tachycardia, hypotension	Fluid volume deficit
Gastrointestinal	Ascites	Protein deficiency
Musculoskeletal	Bone pain and bow leg	Vitamin D or calcium deficiency
	Muscle wasting	Protein, carbohydrate, and fat deficiency
Neurological	Altered mental status	Dehydration and thiamine or vitamin B_{12} deficiency
	Paresthesia	Vitamin B_{12}, pyridoxine, or thiamine deficiency

From Nutrition Made Incredibly Easy. Philadelphia, PA: Lippincott Williams & Wilkins, Springhouse, 2006.

tract function, enteral feeding is easier, safer, and less costly to administer than parenteral nutrition. Contraindications to enteral nutrition are given in Box 7-2.

A common misconception is that enteral feedings should not be started if bowel sounds are absent. Bowel sounds are an indication of large intestinal motility, not of absorption. After injury and postoperatively, bowel sounds may not be detected for 3 to 5 days owing to gastric atony. The small intestine is less prone to ileus than the stomach or the colon and retains its absorptive and digestive capabilities, making it possible to accept enteral feedings immediately after surgery or trauma.[2]

The ultimate goal is for the patient to resume adequate oral intake. Enteral feeding may be

TABLE 7-2 **Laboratory Studies to Evaluate Nutritional Status**

Study	Clinical Significance
Hemoglobin	Helps identify anemia, protein deficiency, excessive blood loss, hydration status (elevated with dehydration; decreased with overhydration)
Hematocrit	Decreased value with overhydration and increased with dehydration; blood loss; poor dietary intake of iron, protein, certain vitamins
Albumin	Decreased with protein deficiency; blood loss secondary to burns; malnutrition; liver/renal disease; heart failure; major surgery; infections; cancer Elevated with dehydration
Total protein	Decreased with overhydration, malnutrition, liver disease
Prealbumin	Decreased in malnutrition in critically ill patients and those with chronic disease
Transferrin	Reflects current protein status; a more sensitive indicator of visceral protein stores Elevated in pregnancy or iron deficiency Decreased in acute or chronic infection, cirrhosis, renal disease, cancer
Retinol-binding protein	Decreased in overhydration and liver disease
Total lymphocyte count	May indicate malnutrition when no other cause of elevated lymphocyte count apparent; may point to infection, leukemia, or tissue necrosis

BOX 7-2 Contraindications to Enteral Nutrition

Absolute Contraindications
- Mechanical obstruction

Relative Contraindications
- Severe hemorrhagic pancreatitis
- Necrotizing enterocolitis
- Prolonged ileus
- Severe diarrhea
- Protracted vomiting
- Enteric fistulas
- Intestinal dysmotility
- Intestinal ischemia

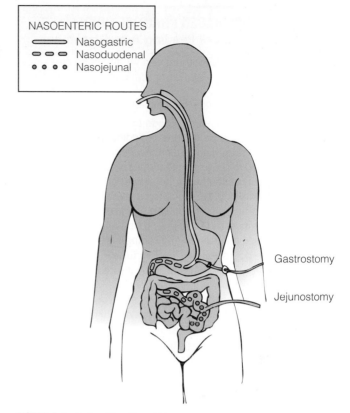

FIGURE 7-1 Enteral feeding routes.

NASOENTERIC ROUTES
Nasogastric
Nasoduodenal
Nasojejunal

Gastrostomy

Jejunostomy

discontinued when the patient can drink enough to maintain hydration and eat enough to meet at least two thirds of her nutritional requirements.

Enteral Feeding Tubes

The expected duration of nutritional support, the placement technique, and the patient's overall condition, aspiration risk, and gastrointestinal tract function are considered when deciding on which type of feeding tube to place.

Nasoenteral Feeding Tubes

Nasoenteral tubes are inserted through the nose or mouth and advanced through the esophagus into the stomach (nasogastric tube), duodenum (nasoduodenal tube), or jejunum (nasojejunal tube) (Fig. 7-1). A nasoenteric tube is indicated for short-term use (ie, less than 4 to 6 weeks). The small diameter of the nasoenteral tube may help prevent reflux and lessen the risk for aspiration because there is less compromise of the lower esophageal sphincter. When placed past the pylorus, nasoduodenal and nasojejunal tubes also carry a reduced risk for aspiration and regurgitation because of the barrier provided by the pyloric sphincter. Potential complications associated with nasoenteral tubes include sinusitis, epistaxis, erosion of the nasal septum or esophagus, otitis, vocal cord paralysis, and distal esophageal strictures.

Nasoenteral tubes can be accidentally placed in the trachea or bronchial tree. Patients with a decreased level of consciousness, poor cough or gag reflex, or an inability to cooperate are at increased risk for pulmonary intubation. Before initiating tube feeding with a nasoenteral tube, proper tube placement must be confirmed by an abdominal radiograph.

 RED FLAG! *Nasoenteral feeding tubes are contraindicated in patients with basilar skull fractures because of the risk for passing the tube through the cribiform fracture and into the brain. For these patients, enteral feeding tubes must be placed orally.*

Because a nasoenteral tube may shift position, ongoing assessment of tube placement is required. After confirming proper positioning radiographically, the tube's exit site from the nose or mouth is marked and documented to facilitate ongoing assessment. An increase in the external length of the tubing can signal that the tube's distal tip has dislocated upward in the gastrointestinal tract (eg, from the intestine into the stomach or esophagus, or from the stomach into the esophagus). Measuring the pH and observing the appearance of fluid withdrawn from the tube may also be used to evaluate tube placement, although this method is not 100% reliable (Table 7-3, p. 51). Injecting air into the tube and auscultating the gastric bubble, although commonly used, is also not 100% accurate and should not be relied on alone to determine tube location.

 RED FLAG! *If at any time tube location is in question, the nurse holds the tube feeding and requests an order for an abdominal radiograph to confirm placement.*

Enterostomal Feeding Tubes

If therapy is expected to last a month or more, a more permanent enterostomal device can be inserted through the abdomen into the stomach (gastrostomy) or jejunum (jejunostomy) (see Fig. 7-1). Various techniques may be used to place enterostomal feeding tubes:

EVIDENCE-BASED PRACTICE GUIDELINES
Verification of Feeding Tube Placement

PROBLEM: Erroneous placement of a feeding tube can cause serious and even fatal complications.

EVIDENCE-BASED PRACTICE GUIDELINES

1. Use a variety of bedside methods to predict tube location during the insertion procedure, including observation for signs of respiratory distress, capnography, measurement of aspirate pH, and observation of aspirate. (level B)
2. Recognize that auscultatory (air bolus) and water bubbling methods of verifying tube location are unreliable. (level B)
3. Obtain radiographic confirmation of correct placement of any blindly inserted tube prior to initiating feedings or medication administration. The radiograph should visualize the entire course of the feeding tube in the gastrointestinal tract and should be read by a radiologist to avoid errors in interpretation. (level A)
4. Mark and document the tube's exit site from the nose or mouth immediately after radiographic confirmation of correct tube placement. (level A)
5. Check tube location at 4-hour intervals after feedings are initiated. (level B)
   Observe for a change in length of the external portion of the feeding tube.
   Review routine chest and abdominal x-ray reports to look for notations about tube location.
   Observe changes in volume of aspirate from the feeding tube.
   Measure pH of feeding tube aspirates if feedings are interrupted for more than a few hours.
   Obtain an x-ray to confirm tube position if there is doubt about the tube's location.

KEY

Level A: Meta-analysis of quantitative studies or metasynthesis of qualitative studies with results that consistently support a specific action, intervention, or treatment

Level B: Well-designed, controlled studies with results that consistently support a specific action, intervention, or treatment

Level C: Qualitative studies, descriptive or correlational studies, integrative review, systematic reviews, or randomized controlled trials with inconsistent results

Level D: Peer-reviewed professional organizational standards with clinical studies to support recommendations

Level E: Multiple case reports, theory-based evidence from expert opinions, or peer-reviewed professional organizational standards without clinical studies to support recommendations

Level M: Manufacturer's recommendations only

■ Adapted from American Association of Critical-Care Nurses (AACN) Practice Alert, revised 12/2009.

• **Percutaneous endoscopy** may be used to place gastrostomy or jejunostomy tubes. Placement is through an abdominal incision using direct endoscopic visualization. Percutaneous endoscopic tube placement may be performed at the bedside or in the endoscopy suite using minimal sedation. Because the endoscope is passed through the mouth and upper gastrointestinal tract, the patient must have an intact oropharynx and an unobstructed esophagus. In addition, the patient must not have any conditions that would result in an inability to bring the gastric wall into apposition with the abdomen. Prior abdominal surgeries, ascites, hepatomegaly, and obesity may impede gastric transillumination and preclude percutaneous endoscopic tube placement. Advantages of percutaneous endoscopy include earlier feeding after tube placement, increased comfort, decreased cost, and decreased recovery time. Complications are infrequent but include wound infection related to bacterial contamination by oral flora during insertion, necrotizing fasciitis, peritonitis, and aspiration. Pneumoperitoneum is common following tube placement by percutaneous endoscopy but is not clinically significant unless accompanied by signs and symptoms of peritonitis.

• **Surgery.** The gastrostomy or jejunostomy tube is inserted through an incision in the abdominal wall under general anesthesia. Disadvantages of surgical placement include the need for general anesthesia, increased recovery time, decreased comfort, and increased cost.

• **Laparoscopy.** A laparoscopically placed gastrostomy tube also requires general anesthesia or IV conscious sedation. Laparoscopic placement is usually used for patients with head, neck, or esophageal cancer. It is less invasive, less painful, and usually involves fewer complications than a surgical gastrostomy.

• **Fluoroscopy.** Direct percutaneous catheter insertion of a gastrostomy tube under fluoroscopy is indicated for patients with high-grade pharyngeal or esophageal obstruction. Disadvantages of fluoroscopic placement include the inability to detect mucosal disease, the potential for prolonged exposure to radiation, the need to transport the patient to a fluoroscopy suite, and increased cost.

Enterostomal tubes are secured to the abdominal wall to prevent dislodgment or migration of the tube and to prevent tension on the tubing (Fig. 7-2). "Buried bumper syndrome" can occur if the retention device is too tight and becomes imbedded in the tissue, leading to mucosal or skin erosion. In-and-out play on the tubing is checked; it should be able to move 1/4 inch to prevent erosion of gastric or abdominal tissue. The length of the external tubing is documented to monitor for migration of the tubing.

Serosanguineous drainage may be expected for 7 to 10 days after insertion. The skin around the insertion site and the retention device is assessed at least daily for skin breakdown, erythema, or drainage. To avoid maceration, the site is kept clean and dry and lifting or adjusting the tube is avoided for several days after the initial insertion. When drainage is present, the amount of dressing

TABLE 7-3 **Characteristics of Aspirate From Enteral Feeding Tubes**

Source of Aspirate	Aspirate pH	Aspirate Appearance	Clinical Significance
Stomach	5 or less	Grassy green or clear and colorless with off-white to tan mucus shreds	Normal if tube is supposed to terminate in stomach
			Abnormal if tube is supposed to terminate in the intestine
Small bowel	6 or greater	Bile-stained (ranging in color from light to golden yellow or brownish-green); thicker and more translucent than fluid withdrawn from a gastric tube	Normal if tube is supposed to terminate in the intestine
			Abnormal if tube is supposed to terminate in stomach
Tracheobronchial tree	6 or greater	Similar to fluid obtained during tracheal suctioning	Abnormal
Pleural space	6 or greater	Straw-colored and watery, possibly blood-tinged	Abnormal

between the external retention device and the skin is limited to avoid pulling the internal retention device taut against the gastric or intestinal mucosa. Cleansing the site with soap and water is adequate. The tissue usually heals within a month. If an enterostomal tube becomes accidentally dislodged, the physician must be notified immediately so that the tube can be reinserted quickly before the tract closes.

Providing Enteral Nutrition

Numerous formulas are available for enteral nutrition, with many designed to assist in the management of specific disease processes (Table 7-4). Enteral formula selection is based on the patient's clinical status, nutrient requirements, fluid and electrolyte restrictions, and gastrointestinal function; the location of enteral access; the expected duration of enteral feeding; and cost. All enteral formulas contain proteins, carbohydrates, fats, vitamins, minerals, trace elements, and water.

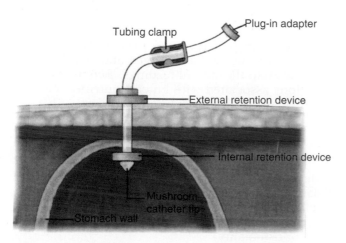

FIGURE 7-2 Percutaneous endoscopic gastrostomy (PEG) tube.

When initiating enteral tube feedings, most clinicians recommend beginning with an isotonic formula at a slow rate (eg, 20 to 30 mL/h), and increasing the rate incrementally until the goal rate is achieved.[1] Dilution of formula may help in tolerance but is not recommended because this may increase the time needed to meet the nutritional requirements.[1]

Methods of administering enteral feedings include the following.

- **Bolus feedings,** considered the most natural physiologically, entail using a syringe to administer a large volume of formula (eg, up to 400 mL) over 5 to 10 minutes, five to six times a day. Alternatively, 300 to 400 mL of formula may be administered by slow gravity drip over a period of 30 to 60 minutes, four to six times a day (this is termed bolus intermittent feeding). Bolus feedings allow for increased patient mobility because the patient is free from a mechanical device between feedings. The stomach is the preferred site for bolus feedings because the stomach and pyloric sphincter regulate the outflow of formula from the stomach. However, because of high residuals, bolus feedings are usually not well tolerated and are often accompanied by nausea, bloating, cramping, diarrhea, or aspiration. The risk for osmotic diarrhea is decreased with bolus intermittent feeding.

- **Continuous feedings** are administered over 24 hours using a feeding pump to ensure a constant flow rate. Continuous feeding is the preferred method when the feeding tube is placed in the intestines because delivery to the intestines that is too rapid may lead to "dumping syndrome" (osmotic diarrhea, abdominal distention, cramps, hyperperistalsis, lightheadedness, diaphoresis, and palpitations). The small intestine can usually tolerate feedings at a rate of 150 mL/h. Continuous feedings are best suited for critically ill patients because they allow more time for nutrients to be absorbed in the intestine and may act prophylactically to prevent stress ulcers and metabolic complications.

TABLE 7-4   Types of Enteral Formulas

Formula	Description	Comments
Polymeric	• Isotonic formulas that can provide enough protein, carbohydrate, fat, vitamins, trace elements, and minerals to prevent nutritional deficiencies • Carbohydrates supplied as oligosaccharides and polysaccharides • Proteins supplied as intact proteins (eg, meat, whey, milk, or soy proteins) • Supply 1–2 kcal/mL	Pancreatic enzymes required for digestion of carbohydrates and proteins
Peptide (elemental)	• Proteins supplied as dipeptides, tripeptides, or oligopeptides and free amino acids (from hydrolysis of whey, milk, or soy protein)	Used when digestion is impaired (eg, pancreatic insufficiency, radiation enteritis, Crohn's disease, short bowel syndrome secondary to surgical resection)
Modular	• Contain individual nutrient components (eg, protein, carbohydrate, fat)	Added to other formulas to meet the patient's individualized needs
Immunonutrition (immune-enhancing)	• Contain addition nutrients purported to enhance immune function (eg, glutamine, arginine, omega-3-polyunsaturated fatty acids)	Immune-enhancing benefits have not been proven

 RED FLAG! *Tube feeding should be held if the patient demonstrates overt signs of regurgitation, vomiting, or aspiration.*

The nurse checks gastric residual volumes every 4 to 6 hours during continuous feedings and before initiating intermittent feedings. Food normally passes through the stomach at a rate of 2 to 10 mL/min; however, gastric emptying is delayed or absent in many critically ill patients. To allow time for normal gastric emptying and reduce the risk for aspiration, it is common to hold the feeding for 1 to 2 hours if the residual volume is greater than 250 mL. The residual volume should be rechecked every 1 to 2 hours until it is less than 200 to 250 mL from a nasogastric tube or less than 100 mL from a gastrostomy tube. The residuals should be replaced and not discarded.

Withholding feedings based on a single high residual volume measurement can be problematic.[3] A high residual volume should raise suspicion of intolerance, but one high value does not mean feeding failure, and automatic cessation of feeding can delay the patient's ability to meet his nutritional goals. When evaluating residual volumes, the following points should be kept in mind:

• There is no concensus about what constitutes a "high" residual volume. Amounts ranging from 100 to 400 mL may be considered "high."
• High infusion rates result in higher residual volumes.
• It is difficult to determine whether gastric contents have been completely removed, so the measured residual volume may be less than the actual residual volume.
• High residual volumes do not always correlate with an increased risk for aspiration, and low residual volumes do not preclude aspiration.[2]

Precipitation of medications, pill fragments, or coagulation of formula may cause obstruction of the feeding tube. To avoid clogging, the feeding tube is flushed with tepid water every 4 to 6 hours during continuous feeds, before and after medication administration, after checking residuals, and when turning off feedings. Obstructions are cleared by flushing the tube with warm water using a large piston syringe and a gentle push–pull motion. Pancreatic enzymes have been effective in unclogging a tube when water is unsuccessful, as long as the enzymes are activated before instillation.[4]

 RED FLAG! *A stylet should never be used to unclog a tube because of the risk for rupturing the tube and perforating the esophagus, stomach, or small intestine.*

Complications of Enteral Nutrition

Although enteral nutrition is associated with fewer complications than parenteral nutrition, complications may still occur (Box 7-3). Many of these complications can be prevented by closely observing residuals and watching for signs and symptoms of intolerance to the enteral feedings. Two major complications associated with enteral nutrition include diarrhea and aspiration.

Diarrhea
Diarrhea in a patient receiving enteral feeding has a myriad of causes:

• Medications (eg, antibiotics)
• Bacterial overgrowth (eg, due to reduced motility, acid suppression)
• Formula composition (eg, intolerance to lactose, fat, or osmolality)
• High infusion rates

BOX 7-3 Complications of Enteral Nutrition

- Diarrhea
- Nausea
- Vomiting
- Bloating
- Abdominal discomfort
- Constipation
- Fluid and electrolyte imbalance
- Hyperglycemia
- Hypoglycemia (if feedings are abruptly terminated)
- Aspiration

- Hypoalbuminemia
- Contamination of the formula or administration set

Measures such as reducing the infusion rate, using a peptide-based formula that is easier to digest or a fiber-containing formula to bulk stools, and giving an absorbing product (eg, Metamucil), may resolve the diarrhea. The risk for diarrhea caused by contamination of the formula or administration set can be reduced by:

- Minimizing breaks in the system
- Using formula in closed, prefilled, ready-to-hang containers
- Hanging no more than 4 hours of formula at one time and using any open formula within 24 hours
- Discarding expired formula
- Changing the administration set daily, and rinsing between bolus feedings
- Using good handwashing technique and wearing gloves when administering feedings or handling the equipment

Aspiration

Aspiration of formula can result in hypoxia or pneumonia. Many critically ill patients have multiple risk factors for aspiration, in addition to enteral feeding (eg, endotracheal intubation, mechanical ventilation, altered level of consciousness). In patients with endotracheal tubes who are receiving enteral nutrition, the incidence of aspiration is as high as 50% to 75%.[2] Intermittent feedings allow the restoration of gastric pH, which can minimize gastric bacterial colonization and the risk for aspiration pneumonia. Other measures to reduce the risk for aspiration in patients who are receiving enteral nutrition include:

- Maintaining the head of the bed at a 30- to 45-degree angle, unless medically contraindicated (if elevating the head of the bed is contraindicated, a reverse Trendelenburg position may be used unless medically contraindicated)
- Discontinuing feedings at least 30 minutes before any procedure for which the patient must lay flat
- Checking residuals frequently, and assessing for signs of feeding intolerance (through subjective reports, if the patient is awake and alert, and abdominal examination to assess bowel sounds and changes in abdominal girth)

- Maintaining endotracheal cuff pressures at 20 to 30 cm H_2O and performing subglottic suctioning prior to deflating the cuff

 RED FLAG! *Signs of pulmonary aspiration include a low-grade fever, coughing, shortness of breath, rhonchi during or after enteral feeding infusions, and tracheal or oral secretions with a sweet formula odor.*

Parenteral Nutrition

Parenteral nutrition is indicated when oral or enteral nutrition is not possible or when absorption or function of the gastrointestinal tract is not sufficient to meet the nutritional needs of the patient. There are two types of parenteral nutrition:

- **Peripheral parenteral nutrition (PPN)** is infused into a small peripheral vein and is often used for short-term nutrition support or as a supplement during transitional phases to enteral or oral nutrition. Because of the risk for phlebitis, concentrations of PPN formulas must not exceed 900 mOsm/L.
- **Total parenteral nutrition (TPN),** also known as central parenteral nutrition, is infused through a large central vein. The TPN formula is highly concentrated. The greater blood volumes in large central veins facilitate dilution and dispersion of the highly osmotic formula.

Formula Composition

TPN delivers all daily required nutrients to the patient in the form of macronutrients (carbohydrates, lipids, and amino acids) and micronutrients (electrolytes, vitamins, and trace minerals). When all three macronutrients are combined together in one TPN bag, the admixture is referred to as a "3 in 1." Sometimes lipids are infused separately. TPN formulation is based on the specific needs of each patient; standard formulas are no longer widely prescribed. While preparing the TPN formula, the pharmacist can also add medications.

Carbohydrates

The primary energy source is carbohydrates. The most common and preferred source of carbohydrates is dextrose (D-glucose) because it is readily metabolized, stimulates the secretion of insulin, and is usually well tolerated in large quantities. The amount of dextrose prescribed in TPN is based on metabolic needs and contributes the most to the osmolality (concentration) of the TPN solution. Once the patient's metabolic needs are met, amino acids can be used for protein synthesis rather than solely as an energy source.

Excessive dextrose concentrations can lead to hyperglycemia, requiring the use of insulin. In addition, because carbon dioxide is an end product of carbohydrate metabolism, excessive dextrose concentrations can lead to carbon dioxide retention and respiratory acidosis, which in turn lead to an increased minute ventilation and work of breathing, making weaning from mechanical ventilation difficult.

Lipids

Lipid emulsions contain essential fatty acids from safflower and soybean vegetable oils. Egg yolk phospholipids are used as emulsifiers, so it is important to check the patient's food allergy history before administration. Before infusion, lipid-containing TPN solutions must be inspected for separation. Loss of emulsion can be identified by yellow-brown marbling of the entire solution or as layering of oil at the surface of the TPN bag. Emulsions that have separated are not safe for infusion and must be returned to the pharmacy for replacement. Lipid emulsions provide an excellent medium for bacterial growth, so excessive manipulation and prolonged hang times are avoided.

Lipid emulsions are isotonic and available in 10%, 20%, and 30% concentrations, providing 1.1, 2.0, and 2.9 kcal/mL, respectively. Higher concentrations provide a greater concentration of calories in less total fluid volume, an important consideration for many patients. In situations in which hyperglycemia has become problematic, dextrose concentrations and volumes may be reduced, and unless contraindicated, lipid concentrations and volumes can be increased.

Baseline and weekly triglyceride trends are used to monitor lipid tolerance. Triglyceride levels exceeding 400 mg/dL suggest impaired lipid clearance and an increased risk for pancreatitis; in this situation, lipid emulsions should be held until levels return to normal. Lipid concentrations may need to be adjusted for patients who are receiving lipids from sources other than TPN (eg, continuous infusion of propofol, a sedative delivered as a lipid emulsion).

 RED FLAG! *Adverse reactions to lipids include fever, chills, chest or back tightness, dyspnea, tachycardia, headache, nausea, and vomiting. If such reactions occur, the infusion should be stopped immediately and the reaction reported to the physician and pharmacist.*

Amino Acids

In TPN, protein is provided as a mixture of essential and nonessential crystalline amino acids in concentrations that supply approximately 15% to 20% of daily caloric needs. Patients with burns, wounds, draining fistulas, renal failure, or hepatic failure may need frequent adjustments in the amount of amino acids they receive. For patients with renal disease, solutions with a higher concentration of essential amino acids are available. For patients with hepatic failure or hypercatabolic conditions, formulas with branched-chain amino acids may be used. Branched-chain amino acids spare the breakdown of other muscle proteins to use as energy, possibly reducing the incidence of hepatic encephalopathy.

Micronutrients

- **Vitamins.** Standard aqueous multivitamin preparations created for TPN provide high levels of thiamine, pyridoxine, ascorbic acid, and folic acid. Concentrations of vitamins in TPN formulas are usually increased over standard U.S. Recommended Dietary Allowance requirements because in TPN, many vitamins are destroyed (by exposure to light and oxygen), lost (due to adherence to plastic tubing and bags), or excreted in the urine before the body can use them. Hypermetabolic conditions of critical illness can exacerbate deficiencies (eg, of vitamin K), necessitating additional monitoring and potentially supplementation. Patients with liver or kidney disease may require lower doses of certain vitamins.
- **Minerals.** Trace minerals are required to maintain biochemical homeostasis. Most commercial mixtures contain chromium, copper, manganese, selenium, and zinc.
- **Electrolytes.** Most electrolyte standard mixtures contain sodium, potassium, calcium, magnesium, phosphorus, chloride, and acetate. Depending on the patient's underlying disease process and physical assessment findings, specific electrolyte concentrations can be adjusted daily in the TPN solution.

 RED FLAG! *Electrolyte supplements or medications should never be added to the TPN bag after the pharmacist has formulated it. Doing so compromises the sterility of the solution and may cause the solution to precipitate.*

Providing Parenteral Nutrition

TPN is usually administered into a central venous catheter. If TPN is expected to be needed for more than a few weeks, a more permanent device (eg, a subcutaneously tunneled Hickman catheter, Port-a-Cath, or peripherally inserted central catheter [PICC]) can be placed. Radiologic confirmation of catheter tip placement is required before the initial infusion. Per facility protocol, the nurse changes the TPN solution bag and tubing (usually every 24 hours) and redresses the catheter insertion site using either a sterile transparent or gauze dressing (usually every 24 to 72 hours).

When administering, use a lumen devoted to the TPN only. Infusing TPN along with other IV therapies (eg, fluids, medications, blood products) into the same lumen carries a high risk for formula contamination and precipitation, and should be avoided. Typically, the solution is infused at a constant rate over a 24-hour period to achieve maximal assimilation of the nutrients and to prevent hyperglycemia or hypoglycemia. During TPN administration, the patient is at risk for hyperglycemia and insulin is often administered to maintain glucose control. Once the TPN infusion is discontinued, insulin requirements become notably less or nonexistent. If new TPN solution is temporarily unavailable, administration of 10% dextrose in water ($D_{10}W$) is recommended to prevent rebound hypoglycemia.

RED FLAG! *If a solution is "behind schedule," the infusion rate should not be increased to make up time because this may cause sudden metabolic fluctuations and fluid overload.*

Tapering TPN is often initiated once the patient is able to safely resume (and tolerate) enteral or oral nutrition sufficient to meet approximately 50% to 75% of his nutritional needs. A calorie count is essential to ensure that the patient's nutritional needs are being met. Before TPN is discontinued, the infusion rate is decreased by half for 30 to 60 minutes to allow a plasma glucose response and prevent rebound hypoglycemia. Checking blood glucose for 30 to 60 minutes after discontinuation facilitates identification and management of immediate glucose abnormalities.

Complications of Parenteral Nutrition

Complications of parenteral nutrition are summarized in Box 7-4. Two major complications include hyperglycemia and refeeding syndrome.

Hyperglycemia
Although hyperglycemia can be caused by either enteral or parenteral feedings, it is more common in patients receiving parenteral nutrition. Even slightly elevated blood glucose levels can impair lymphocyte function, leading to immunosuppression and increased risk for infection. If the renal threshold for glucose reabsorption is exceeded, osmotic diuresis can occur, resulting in dehydration and electrolyte imbalances. To manage hyperglycemia, the pharmacist may add insulin to the TPN solution. Alternatively, insulin may be administered by continuous infusion during TPN administration, or subcutaneously at regular intervals or according to sliding scales.

 RED FLAG! *Many patients receiving parenteral or enteral nutrition are also on insulin drips. To prevent a dangerous hypoglycemic episode from occurring, the nurse must stop the insulin drip any time the nutrition is interrupted.*

BOX 7-4 Complications of Parenteral Nutrition

- Hepatic dysfunction (eg, hepatic steatosis, extrahepatic cholestasis, cholelithiasis)
- Gastrointestinal atrophy
- Metabolic complications (eg, hyperglycemia, hypoglycemia, hypophosphatemia, hypokalemia, hypomagnesemia, hypocalcemia)
- Refeeding syndrome
- Local infection at the catheter insertion site
- Systemic bloodstream infection and sepsis
- Mechanical complications related to catheter insertion (eg, vascular trauma, pneumothorax, thrombosis, venous air embolism)

Refeeding Syndrome
Refeeding syndrome, characterized by rapid shifts in electrolytes, glucose, and volume status within hours to days of nutrition implementation, is one of the most critical complications that occurs with the initiation of TPN. Rapid refeeding, excessive dextrose infusion, severe protein–calorie malnutrition, and conditions such as chronic alcoholism and anorexia nervosa increase the patient's risk for developing refeeding syndrome.

In refeeding syndrome, parenterally delivered glucose loads stimulate insulin release, which in turn stimulates intracellular uptake of phosphorus, glucose, and other electrolytes for anabolic processes. Despite relatively normal serum phosphorus levels on standard laboratory reports, intracellular stores are markedly depleted in malnourished catabolic patients. Severe hypophosphatemia (<1 mg/dL) can lead to neuromuscular, respiratory, and cardiac dysfunction. Low serum levels of potassium, magnesium, and calcium can precipitate cardiac dysrhythmias. The increased intravascular fluid volumes associated with parenteral nutrition can strain the heart, possibly inducing heart failure and myocardial damage.

Prevention of refeeding syndrome includes repletion of phosphorus, potassium, magnesium, and calcium before TPN initiation, limiting the initial concentration of dextrose in the TPN solution, and titrating total volume and rate to evaluate for fluid overload and potential cardiac decompensation. Daily monitoring of phosphorous, potassium, and magnesium is recommended. Weight-based phosphorus repletion algorithms have been shown to be highly efficacious in correcting hypophosphatemia during nutrition support therapy.[5]

Fluids

Critically ill patients often have fluid imbalances related to their primary underlying disease. Assessment of fluid balance and careful management are mainstays of patient care in the critical care setting. The most sensitive indices of changes in body water content are serial weights and intake and output patterns.

- **Weight.** Admission weight is compared with that obtained in the history. Of note is whether the weight has changed significantly over the past 1 to 2 weeks. One liter of fluid equals 1 kg of body weight, equivalent to 2.2 lb. An increase in weight does not specify where the weight is gained. For example, a patient may have depleted intravascular volume yet show an increase in weight because of third-spacing of fluid (ie, movement of fluid to the interstitial space). Rapid daily gains and losses of weight usually are associated with changes in fluid volume and not nutritional factors. Critically ill patients often experience unmeasured insensible losses (eg, through ventilation, fever, and wounds).

- **Intake and output.** The nurse monitors the critically ill patient's intake and output every 1 to 2 hours. The intake and output values are summed to provide an overall balance at the end of a 24-hour period. Accurate intake and output is important in care of a critically ill patient. In the event that renal function decreases, this information may aid in the diagnosis and possible prevention of prerenal azotemia or acute renal failure.

Fluid Volume Deficit

When fluid loss exceeds intake, a fluid volume deficit exists. A fluid volume deficit is a physiological situation in which fluids are lost in an isotonic fashion (both fluid and electrolytes are lost together). Dehydration is the loss of water alone, resulting in a hyperosmolar state. Although a fluid volume deficit and dehydration can coexist, this discussion is limited strictly to disorders of fluid volume deficit.

Fluid volume deficits can occur from:

- **Fever.** As much as 2,500 mL of fluid can be lost in a 24-hour period from a patient with a body temperature of 40°C (104°F) and a respiratory rate of 40 breaths/min.
- **Hyperventilation** Either from disease or use of nonhumidified oxygen delivery systems, can result in substantial fluid loss.
- **Gastrointestinal tract.** Losses can occur as a result of vomiting, nasogastric suction, diarrhea, or enterocutaneous drainage or fistulas.
- **Third-spacing** can result from pleural or peritoneal effusions; edema from liver, renal, or hepatic disease; or diffuse capillary leak.
- **Burns.** Both evaporative and transudative losses through burned skin can result in very large losses of fluid daily.
- **Renal losses.** Renal losses are seen in the diuretic phase of acute tubular necrosis, as a result of excessive diuretic administration, and in patients with cerebral salt wasting syndrome. Renal losses also may occur as a result of solute diuresis from high-protein or high-saline enteral and parenteral nutrition and from administration of osmotic agents (eg, mannitol, radiocontrast). Fluid can also be lost during metabolic alkalosis, in which compensatory urinary bicarbonate excretion obligates renal sodium excretion, frequently resulting in volume depletion.

 RED FLAG! *Elderly patients are at particular risk for a fluid volume deficit because of the multisystem changes associated with aging.*

To correct a fluid volume deficit, it is necessary to treat the underlying cause and replace the lost fluid. Several types of fluids, which have different physiological effects, are available.

Maintenance Fluids

Under normal conditions, the average healthy adult requires about 2.5 L/d. This volume replaces fluids lost through the feces, the respiratory tract, sweating, and urine. When determining the rate of administration of maintenance fluid, factors such as the patient's medical history and age must be considered.

Replacement Fluids

The type of fluid given to a critically ill patient depends on the type of fluid lost. When blood is lost, as in trauma or surgery, blood products may be administered. When intravascular volume is depleted, as in diarrhea, isotonic solutions may be administered. The depletion of extravascular fluids (dehydration) may require replacement with hypotonic solutions. The rate of administration depends on the patient's medical history and amount of volume lost.

Crystalloids

Crystalloid solutions (Box 7-5) are prepared with a specified balance of water and electrolytes. Crystalloids are classified as hypotonic (osmolarity < 250 mEq/L), isotonic (osmolarity approximately 310 mEq/L), or hypertonic (osmolarity > 376 mEq/L). When pure dextrose solutions such as 5% dextrose in water (D_5W) are administered, the dextrose is metabolized, resulting in the administration of free water. When given intravenously, free water decreases the plasma osmolarity, thereby promoting the movement of water evenly into all body compartments. Free water, which is hypotonic, does not stay in the vascular space.

Normal (0.9%) saline is an isotonic solution. Approximately one third of the fluid administered remains in the vascular space, and the remaining fluid moves into the extracellular space or is lost through the renal system. When hypertonic solutions are administered (such as 3% or 7.5% saline), the hypertonicity pulls fluid from the extravascular space to the vascular space, increasing the intravascular volume.

Colloids

Colloids are high-molecular-weight substances that do not cross the capillary membrane under normal conditions (Table 7-5). The starches dextran and hetastarch and the protein albumin differ from each other only slightly but exert similar oncotic pressure.

Fluid Volume Excess

Fluid volume excess occurs when there is retention of sodium, resulting in the reabsorption of water. Electrolytes typically remain unchanged when there is an increase in total body water and electrolytes increase in parallel. Many critically ill patients may have mixed disturbances with manifestations of the confounding compensatory mechanisms. Causes

BOX 7-5 Common Crystalloid Solutions

5% Dextrose in water (D₅W): no electrolytes, 50 g dextrose

- Supplies about 170 cal/L and free water to aid in renal excretion of solutes
- Should not be used in excessive volumes in patients with increased antidiuretic hormone (ADH) activity or to replace fluids in hypovolemic patients

0.9% NaCl (isotonic saline): Na⁺ 154 mEq/L, Cl⁻ 154 mEq/L

- Isotonic fluid commonly used to expand the extracellular fluid in presence of hypovolemia
- Because of relatively high chloride content, it can be used to treat mild metabolic alkalosis

0.45% NaCl (½ strength saline): Na⁺ 77 mEq/L, Cl⁻ 77 mEq/L

- A hypotonic solution that provides sodium, chloride, and free water (sodium and chloride provided in fluid allow kidneys to select and retain needed amounts)
- Free water desirable as aid to kidneys in elimination of solutes

0.33% NaCl (⅓ strength saline): Na⁺ 56 mEq/L, Cl⁻ 56 mEq/L

- A hypotonic solution that provides sodium, chloride, and free water

- Often used to treat hypernatremia (because this solution contains a small amount of sodium, it dilutes the plasma sodium while not allowing the level to drop too rapidly)

3% or 7.5% Saline

- Grossly hypertonic solution used to treat severe hyponatremia or to decrease intracranial pressure (ICP); may also be used to resuscitate trauma patients
- Used only in settings where the patient can be closely monitored

Lactated Ringer's solution: Na⁺ 130 mEq/L, K⁺ 4 mEq/L, Ca²⁺ 3 mEq/L, Cl⁻ 109 mEq/L, lactate (metabolized to bicarbonate) 28 mEq/L

- Approximately isotonic solution that contains multiple electrolytes in about same concentrations as found in plasma (note that this solution is lacking magnesium and phosphate)
- Used in the treatment of hypovolemia, burns, and fluid lost as bile or diarrhea
- Useful in treating mild metabolic acidosis

Adapted from Metheny NM: Fluid and Electrolyte Balance: Nursing Considerations. Philadelphia, PA: Lippincott Williams & Wilkins, 2000, p 181, with permission.

TABLE 7-5 Common Colloid Solutions

Solution	Contents	Indications	Comments
Albumin	Available in two concentrations: 5%: oncotically similar to plasma 25%: hypertonic Both 5% and 25% solutions contain about 130–160 mEq/L of sodium	Used as volume expander in treatment of shock May be useful in treating burns and third-spacing shifts	Cost is approximately 25–30 times more than for crystalloid solutions. Increased interstitial oncotic pressure in disease states in which there is increased capillary leaking (eg, burns, sepsis) may occur; this may result in increased vascular loss of fluid. Use caution with rapid administration; watch for volume overload.
Hetastarch	Synthetic colloid made from starch (6%) and added to sodium chloride solution	May be used to expand plasma volume when volume is lost from hemorrhage, trauma, burns, and sepsis	Plasma volume expansion effects decrease over 24–36 h. Starch is eliminated by kidneys and liver; therefore, use with caution in patients with liver and kidney impairment. Mild, transient coagulopathies may occur. Transient rise in serum amylase may occur.
Dextran	Glucose polysaccharide substance, available as low-molecular-weight dextran (dextran 40) or high-molecular-weight dextran (dextran 70) No electrolyte content	May be used to expand plasma volume when volume is lost from hemorrhage, trauma, burns, and sepsis	Has been associated with greater risk for allergic reaction than albumin or hetastarch. Interference with blood cross-matching may occur. May cause coagulopathy; has more profound effect on coagulation than hetastarch.

of fluid volume excess include overadministration of fluids; heart, kidney, or liver failure; excessive sodium intake; and medications (eg, steroids, desmopressin acetate [DDAVP]).

Management of fluid volume excess is directed toward correction of the underlying disorder. Diuretics are the mainstay of treatment for acute resolution of fluid volume excess. Sodium restriction reduces the amount of water reabsorption and can contribute to acute correction of volume overload.

Electrolytes

Electrolyte disorders commonly occur in critically ill patients, typically in combination with other conditions. Management of the underlying problem ensures long-term restoration of balance. However, acute management of electrolyte disorders is often required to maintain cellular integrity. Common causes and interventions for electrolyte imbalances are summarized in Table 7-6.

TABLE 7-6　Electrolyte Imbalances: Common Causes and Interventions

Selected Medical Conditions		
Electrolyte	Associated With Disturbance	Collaborative Interventions
Sodium		
Hyponatremia	Heart failure Liver failure Kidney failure Hyperlipidemia Hypoproteinemia Syndrome of inappropriate antidiuretic hormone (SIADH) Gastrointestinal loss Adrenal insufficiency Thiazide diuretics Drugs: nonsteroidal anti-inflammatory drugs (NSAIDs), tricyclic antidepressants, selective serotonin reuptake inhibitor (SSRIs), chlorpropamide, omeprazole Tumors associated with ectopic excessive antidiuretic hormone (ADH) production: oat cell carcinoma, leukemia, lymphoma Pulmonary disorders: pneumonia, acute asthma AIDS	Review medication profile and patient history. Monitor for sites of fluid losses or gains. Monitor fluid balance and for signs and symptoms of electrolyte disturbance. Attempt to manage underlying cause. Correction of imbalance may require sodium replacement (3% saline) or water restriction, depending on underlying cause.
Hypernatremia	Profound dehydration usually in patients not able to ask for water (eg, debilitated elderly or children), in those with impaired thirst regulation (eg, elderly), or in those with heatstroke Hypertonic tube feedings without water supplementation Increased insensible water loss (eg, excessive sweating, second- and third-degree burns, hyperventilation) Excessive administration of sodium-containing fluids (3% saline, sodium bicarbonate) Diabetes insipidus Hyperaldosteronism, Cushing's syndrome	Monitor patients at particular risk for hypernatremia, including debilitated or elderly patients, acutely or critically ill children, and patients receiving tube feedings. Monitor laboratory values closely in patients with insensible fluid losses and in those receiving parenteral administration of sodium-containing fluids. Administer therapeutic medications, including vasopressin, desmopressin acetate (DDAVP). Administer hypotonic fluids (1/2 saline to free water, D_5W).
Potassium		
Hypokalemia	Gastrointestinal loss: diarrhea, laxatives, gastric suction Renal loss: potassium-losing diuretics, hyperaldosteronism, osmotic diuresis, steroids, some antibiotics Intracellular shifts: alkalosis, excessive secretion or administration of insulin, hyperalimentation Poor intake: anorexia nervosa, alcoholism, debilitation	Monitor laboratory values closely in patients at particular risk for hypokalemia. Pay particular attention to potassium level in patients receiving digoxin. Administer potassium either PO or IV. Monitor magnesium levels in patients who are refractory to potassium replacement.
Hyperkalemia	Pseudohyperkalemia: prolonged tight application of tourniquet; fist clenching and unclenching immediately before or during blood draws; hemolysis of blood sample	Ensure that minimal negative pressure is used to obtain all laboratory samples, particularly when drawn through small-gauge needles. Restrict potassium-sparing diuretics.

TABLE 7-6 Electrolyte Imbalances: Common Causes and Interventions (continued)

Selected Medical Conditions		
Electrolyte	Associated With Disturbance	Collaborative Interventions
	Decreased potassium excretion: oliguric renal failure, potassium-sparing diuretics, hypoaldosteronism High potassium intake: improper use of oral potassium supplements; rapid IV potassium administration Extracellular shifts: acidosis, crush injuries, tumor cell lysis after chemotherapy	Promote excretion: sodium polystyrene sulfonate PO or per rectum, dialysis, potassium-losing diuretics (eg, furosemide) Emergency management measures: calcium IV, sodium bicarbonate, IV insulin with glucose, β_2-adrenergic agonists
Calcium		
Hypocalcemia	Surgical hypoparathyroidism Primary hypoparathyroidism Malabsorption (alcoholism) Acute pancreatitis Excessive administration of citrated blood Alkalotic states Drugs (loop diuretics, mithramycin, calcitonin) Hyperphosphatemia Sepsis Hypomagnesemia Medullary carcinoma of thyroid Hypoalbuminemia	Monitor for signs and symptoms associated with low calcium, especially for seizures, and stridor. Administer calcium IV for acute replacement. Ensure adequate dietary intake for patients at particular risk.
Hypercalcemia	Hyperparathyroidism Malignant neoplastic disease Drugs (thiazide diuretics, lithium, theophylline) Prolonged immobilization Dehydration	Administer bisphosphonates, such as etidronate or mithramycin, especially when disorder is related to malignancy. Administer diuretics, such as loop diuretics, to promote renal excretion. Provide fluid replacement with 0.9% saline.
Magnesium		
Hypomagnesemia	Inadequate intake: starvation, TPN without adequate Mg^{2+} supplementation, chronic alcoholism Increased GI loss: diarrhea, laxatives, fistulas, nasogastric tube suction, vomiting Increased renal loss: drugs (loop and thiazide diuretics, mannitol, amphotericin B), diuresis (uncontrolled diabetes mellitus, hypoaldosteronism) Changes in magnesium distribution: pancreatitis, burns, insulin, blood products	Monitor for hypokalemia in patients with low magnesium because kidneys are not able to conserve potassium when magnesium level is low. Administer magnesium IV for acute replacement. Administer PO preparations for long-term replacement.
Hypermagnesemia	Renal failure Excessive intake of magnesium-containing compounds (eg, antacids, mineral supplements, laxatives)	Avoid administration of magnesium-containing compounds to patients in renal failure. In extreme cases, dialysis may be indicated.
Phosphorus		
Hypophosphatemia	Refeeding syndrome Alcoholism Phosphate-binding antacids Respiratory alkalosis Administration of exogenous insulin IV Burns	Ensure nutritional intake. Monitor phosphorus for the first few days after initiation of enteral or parenteral nutrition. Administer by oral supplementation (Neutra-Phos capsules) or IV.
Hyperphosphatemia	Renal failure Chemotherapy Excessive administration of phosphate compounds	Avoid administration of phosphorus to patients in renal failure. Administer calcium acetate. Administer IV fluids to promote renal excretion. In severe cases, administration of high levels of glucose with insulin may help shift phosphorus intracellularly.

ADH, antidiuretic hormone; AIDS, acquired immunodeficiency syndrome; DDAVP, desmopressin acetate; NSAID, nonsteroidal anti-inflammatory drug; SIADH, syndrome of inappropriate antidiuretic hormone; SSRI, selective serotonin reuptake inhibitor.

Sodium

Sodium is the major extracellular cation. It is a major contributor of serum osmolarity and controls movement of water. Low serum sodium usually indicates water intake in excess of sodium and is characterized by an increase in body weight. It may also be due to a renal loss of sodium with a normal intravascular volume. High serum sodium usually indicates water loss in excess of sodium and is reflected in weight loss.

Potassium

Potassium is the major intracellular cation. Potassium plays a key role in neuromuscular functioning and maintaining the myocardial resting potential. Both high and low levels may result in alterations in the cardiac rhythm. Because of the narrow range of extracellular potassium balance, renal function is essential to regulation of potassium. In critically ill patients, disorders of potassium are common and have numerous causes. Box 7-6 presents nursing considerations in potassium replacement.

BOX 7-6 Nursing Considerations for Intravenous Potassium Replacement

Dilution
- Do not administer undiluted potassium directly IV.
- Keep all vials of undiluted potassium away from patient care area.
- Dilution of potassium depends on the amount of fluid the patient can tolerate. Highly concentrated potassium solutions can cause irritation, pain, and sclerosing of vein.
- Typical concentrations of potassium are 10 to 40 mEq/100 mL. Premixed bags are available.

Peripheral IV Administration
- In collaboration with prescribing provider, consider the addition of a small volume of lidocaine to minimize pain.
- Administer in central vein if available.
- For mild to moderate hypokalemia, rates of 10 to 20 mEq/h are recommended.
- Rates >40 mEq/h are not recommended.
- Use infusion pump to administer replacement.

Monitoring
- Monitor urinary output, blood urea nitrogen, and creatinine in patients receiving potassium replacement. Patients with impaired renal function or oliguric renal failure may experience transient hyperkalemia. Consider smaller replacement dosages and periodic reevaluation.
- When rate of administration exceeds 10 mEq/h, monitoring of cardiac rhythm is recommended.
- Assess magnesium level because correction of potassium may be refractory to potassium replacement with concurrent hypomagnesemia.

BOX 7-7 Nursing Considerations for Intravenous Calcium Replacement

Dilution
- Calcium can be delivered as calcium gluconate (4.5 mEq of elemental Ca^{2+}) or calcium chloride (13.5 mEq of elemental Ca^{2+}).
- Calcium can be irritating to veins. If peripheral administration is required, calcium gluconate is recommended because damage can occur to surrounding soft tissues.

Administration
- Administer by slow IV push through central vein or administer by mixing with compatible IV fluids.
- Administer slowly (over 1 to 2 hours) for patients receiving digoxin.

Calcium

Almost all (99%) of the calcium in the body is contained in the bone. The remaining 1% is intravascular, either bound to albumin or in an ionized (free) form. The primary function of calcium is promotion of the neuromuscular impulse. Several clotting factors also depend on calcium. Hypocalcemia in the critically ill has numerous causes. Nursing considerations for calcium replacement are given in Box 7-7.

Many critically ill patients have low albumin, which will result in a low serum calcium level. This laboratory finding does not necessarily mean that the patient's ionized calcium (ie, readily available calcium) is low. It is necessary to either assess ionized calcium (if available) or to correct the serum calcium for the albumin level, using the following formula:

$$\text{Corrected calcium} = [0.8 \times (\text{normal albumin} - \text{patient's albumin})] + \text{serum}$$

Magnesium

Most of the magnesium in the body is in the skeletal system and in the intracellular space. About 1% circulates in the intravascular space. Magnesium is a catalyst for hundreds of enzymatic reactions and plays a role in neurotransmission and cardiac contraction. Magnesium is primarily excreted by the kidneys. Nursing considerations for magnesium replacement are summarized in Box 7-8.

Phosphorus

Phosphorus is the major intracellular anion. The source of adenosine triphosphate (ATP), phosphorus is critical to many life-sustaining processes, such as muscle contraction, neuromuscular impulse conduction, and the regulation of several intracellular and extracellular electrolyte balances. Nursing considerations for phosphorus replacement are summarized in Box 7-9.

BOX 7-8 Nursing Considerations for Intravenous Magnesium Replacement

Administration
- Administer with caution to patients with renal failure because magnesium is primarily excreted by the kidneys.
- During emergencies, such as torsades de pointes, magnesium may be injected directly.
- In mild to moderate hypomagnesemia, a rate of infusion of 1 to 2 g over 1 hour is advisable.

Monitoring
- Monitor for hypotension or flushing during administration.
- Monitor deep tendon reflexes periodically during administration.

BOX 7-9 Nursing Considerations for Intravenous Phosphorus Replacement

Phosphorus IV replacement is available as sodium or potassium phosphate. Phosphorus is dosed in millimoles, whereas sodium and potassium are dosed in milliequivalents.

- Administer sodium phosphate for patients with renal failure.
- Do not administer with calcium.
- Administer over several hours, typically 15 to 30 mmol phosphorus over 4 to 6 hours.

CASE STUDY

Mr. P. is a 62-year-old executive who is status post cerebrovascular accident with severe dysphagia. He has a medical history of gastroesophageal reflux disease, coronary artery disease, hypertension, hypercholesterolemia, and type 2 diabetes mellitus. He is currently prescribed pantoprazole, 40 mg daily; aspirin, 81 mg daily; clopidogrel, 75 mg daily; metoprolol, 50 mg twice daily; simvastatin, 20 mg daily; and 15 units Lantus insulin subcutaneously at bedtime. Because of Mr. P.'s severe dysphagia, swallowing studies and calorie counts are ordered to determine whether he will be able to resume safe and adequate oral nutrition. In the meantime, to ensure that Mr. P.'s nutritional needs are met, he is receiving enteral nutrition 400 mL every 4 hours through a small-bore nasogastric tube.

Physical examination reveals a nontender, nondistended, obese abdomen with positive bowel sounds. However, before the instillation of a scheduled feeding, the gastric residual volume is found to be 300 mL. Subsequently, the nurse decides to hold the enteral feedings for the remainder of the day. The following morning, Mr. P. resumes his scheduled enteral bolus feeds of 400 mL every 4 hours, and he is found to have minimal gastric residuals. However, Mr. P. now reports abdominal cramps, bloating, and diarrhea after each bolus feeding; abdominal examination reveals positive bowel sounds with mild abdominal distention.

Because of these multiple issues, the nurse recommends to the physician that a central line be placed and that Mr. P. be started on total parenteral nutrition (TPN) to meet his long-term nutritional requirements.

1. Initially the nurse held the enteral tube feedings based on the residual volume measurement. Was this an appropriate action to take? Why or why not?

2. What was the most likely etiology of the patient's diarrhea? What interventions are needed, if any?

3. Is total parenteral nutrition (TPN) appropriate for this patient? Why or why not?

References

1. McClave S, Martindale R, Varek V, et al.: Guidelines of parenteral and enteral nutrition. American Society for Parenteral and Enteral Nutrition and Society of Critical Care Medicine. J Parenter Enteral Nutr 33(3):277–316, 2009.
2. A guide to enteral access procedures and enteral nutrition. Nat Rev Gastroenterol Hepatol Medscape Nurses, 2009.
3. Montejo J, Minambres E, Bordeje L: Residual volume during enteral nutrition in ICU patients: The REGANE study. Intensive Care Med 36:1386–1393, 2010.
4. Williams N: Medication administration through enteral feeding tubes. Am J Health-Syst Pharm 65(24):2347–2357, 2008.
5. Marino P, Sutin K. The ICU Book. Lippincott Williams & Wilkins, 2008.

Want to know more? A wide variety of resources to enhance your learning and understanding of this chapter are available on **thePoint**. Visit **http://thepoint.lww.com/MortonEss1e** to access chapter review questions and more!

Dysrhythmia Interpretation and Management

Standard 12-Lead Electrocardiogram

An electrocardiogram (ECG) is a graphic recording of the heart's electrical activity. The paper consists of horizontal and vertical lines, each 1 mm apart. The horizontal lines denote time measurements. When the paper is run at a sweep speed of 25 mm/s, each small square measured horizontally is equal to 0.04 second, and each large square (five small squares) equals 0.2 second. Height (voltage) is measured by counting the lines vertically. Each small square measured vertically is 1 mm, and each large square is 5 mm (Fig. 8-1).

Waveforms and Intervals

The heart's normal route of depolarization moves from the sinoatrial (SA) node and atria, downward through the atrioventricular (AV) node, His–Purkinje

system, and ventricles. During the cardiac cycle, the following waveforms and intervals are produced on the ECG surface tracing (see Fig. 8-1):

- *P wave:* The P wave is a small, usually upright and rounded deflection representing depolarization of the atria. It normally is seen before the QRS complex at a consistent interval.
- *PR interval:* The PR interval represents the time from the onset of atrial depolarization until the onset of ventricular depolarization. Included in the interval is the brief delay at the AV node that allows time for atrial contraction before the ventricles are depolarized. The interval is measured from the beginning of the P wave to the beginning of the QRS complex. A normal PR interval is 0.12 to 0.2 second.
- *QRS complex:* The QRS complex represents ventricular depolarization. A normal QRS complex is

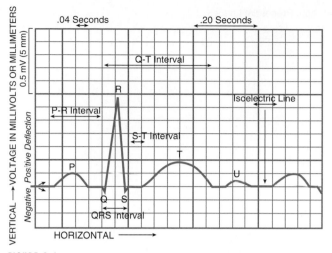

FIGURE 8-1 The waveforms and intervals of the electrocardiogram (ECG) represent the electrical impulse as it traverses the conduction system, resulting in depolarization and repolarization of the myocardium.

0.06 to 0.11 second in width (Fig. 8-2). Atrial repolarization, which occurs during the QRS complex, is not represented by a wave on the ECG.

- *ST segment:* The ST segment is the portion of the tracing from the end of the QRS complex to the beginning of the T wave. It represents the time from the end of ventricular depolarization to the beginning of ventricular repolarization. Normally, it is isoelectric (ie, the ST segment joins the QRS complex at the baseline). ST segments may be elevated or depressed in acute myocardial injury or ischemia (see Chapter 14).
- *T wave:* The T wave is the deflection representing ventricular repolarization and appears after the QRS complex.
- *U wave:* A U wave is a small, usually positive deflection after the T wave that is typically seen only in hypokalemia.

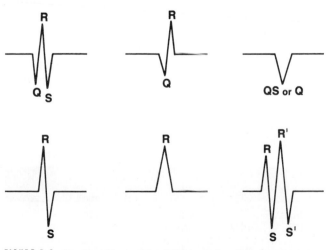

FIGURE 8-2 Configurations of the QRS complex. A Q wave is a negative deflection before an R wave, an R wave is a positive deflection, and an S wave is a negative deflection after an R wave.

- *QT interval:* The QT interval is the period from the beginning of ventricular depolarization to the end of ventricular repolarization. The QT interval is measured from the beginning of the QRS complex to the end of the T wave.

Views (Leads)

A standard 12-lead ECG produces 12 electrical views of the heart using 10 electrodes (Fig. 8-3). For the limb leads, the recording device alternates the combination of electrodes that are active during recording of electrical signals from the heart (Fig. 8-4). This produces six standard views (leads) that are recorded in the heart's frontal plane: I, II, III, augmented voltage of the right arm (aVR), augmented voltage of the left arm (aVL), and augmented voltage of the left foot (aVF). The six precordial leads (V_1, V_2, V_3, V_4, V_5, and V_6) are arranged across the left side of the anterior chest to record electrical activity in the heart's horizontal plane (see Fig. 8-3). Additional horizontal plane leads may be recorded by placing precordial electrodes on the right side of the chest to view right ventricular activity or the back of the chest to view left ventricular posterior wall activity (see Fig. 8-3). The positive electrode acts as a camera, providing a view of the heart from that perspective (Table 8-1). The appearance of the intervals and waveforms on the ECG varies slightly according to which lead is being viewed (Table 8-2).

 RED FLAG! *Proper placement of the electrodes is very important. Misplacement of an electrode by as little as one intercostal space can cause QRS morphology to change, leading to misdiagnoses.*

Uses of the 12-Lead Electrocardiogram

In addition to being used to detect dysrhythmias, the 12-lead ECG is used to determine the electrical axis of the heart; detect atrial or ventricular enlargement; and detect patterns of ischemia, injury, or infarction.

Detection of Dysrhythmias

The 12-lead ECG provides a visual representation of the major events of the cardiac cycle, and therefore is useful for detecting dysrhythmias and estimating atrial and ventricular rates (Box 8-1). A systematic approach to assessing a rhythm strip is given in Box 8-2 on page 66. It is important to take the time to complete each step because many dysrhythmias are not as they first appear. Specific dysrhythmias are discussed in more detail later in this chapter. Because of the effects of electrolytes on the electrical impulse of the heart, ECG changes may also raise suspicion for serum electrolyte imbalances (Table 8-3, p. 66).

Determination of Electrical Axis

Electrical axis refers to the general direction of the wave of excitation as it moves through the heart.

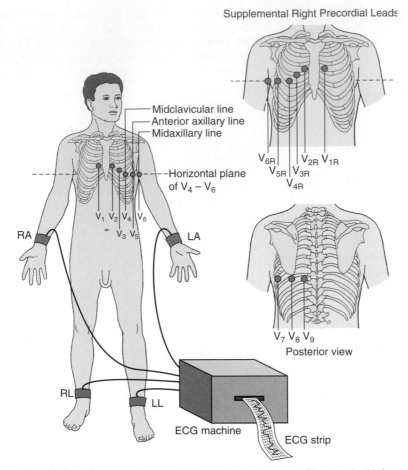

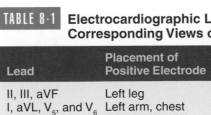

FIGURE 8-3 • Electrocardiogram (ECG) electrode placement. The standard left precordial leads are V₁ through V₆. The right precordial leads, placed across the right side of the chest, are the mirror opposite of the left leads. The posterior leads (V₇ through V₉) are placed on the back to the left of the spine on the same horizontal line as V₆.

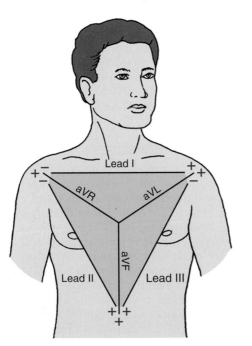

FIGURE 8-4 Frontal plane leads: standard limb leads, I, II, III, plus augmented leads aVR, aVL, and aVF. This allows an examination of electrical conduction across a variety of planes (eg, left arm to leg, right arm to left arm).

In the normal heart, the flow of electrical forces is downward and to the left, a pattern known as normal axis. Because the ventricles make up the largest muscle mass of the heart and therefore make the most significant contribution to the determination of the direction of the flow of forces, the QRS complex is examined in leads I and aVF to determine the electrical axis (Fig. 8-5, p. 67). The direction of the flow of forces in the heart can shift to the left or to the right as a result of an anatomical shift of the heart (eg, in very obese patients and in patients with large abdominal tumors or abdominal ascites),

TABLE 8-1 Electrocardiographic Leads and Corresponding Views of the Heart

Lead	Placement of Positive Electrode	View of the Heart
II, III, aVF	Left leg	Inferior
I, aVL, V₅, and V₆	Left arm, chest	Left lateral
V₁ through V₄	Chest (left side)	Anteroseptal
V₄R through V₆R	Chest (right side)	Right ventricle
V₇ through V₉	Chest	Posterior

TABLE 8-2 **The Normal 12-Lead Electrocardiogram (ECG)**

Lead	Waveform or Interval					
	P	Q	R	S	ST	T
I	Upright	Small, 0.04 s, or none	Dominant	Less than R or none	Isoelectric +1 to −0.5 mm	Upright
II	Upright	Small or none	Dominant	Less than R or none	+1 to −0.5 mm	Upright
III	Upright Flat Diphasic Inverted	Small or none	None to dominant	None to dominant	+1 to −0.5 mm	Upright Flat Diphasic Inverted
aVR	Inverted	Small, none, or large	Small or none	Dominant	+1 to −0.5 mm	Inverted
aVL	Upright	Small, none, or large	Small, none, or dominant	Small, none, or dominant	+1 to −0.5 mm	Upright
	Flat Diphasic Inverted					Flat Diphasic Inverted
aVF	Upright Flat Diphasic Inverted	Small or none	Small, none, or dominant Dominant	None to dominant	+1 to −0.5 mm	Upright
V₁	Upright Flat Diphasic	None May be QS	Small	Deep	0 to +3 mm	Inverted Flat Upright Diphasic
V₂	Upright	None			0 to +3 mm	Upright Diphasic Inverted
V₃	Upright	Small or none			0 to +3 mm	Upright
V₄	Upright	Small or none			+1 to −0.5 mm	Upright
V₅	Upright	Small			+1 to −0.5 mm	Upright
V₆	Upright	Small	Tall	Small or none	+1 to −0.5 mm	Upright

BOX 8-1 **Estimating Heart Rate Using the Electrocardiogram (ECG)**

- Method 1. This method works for regular or irregular rhythms. Count the number of QRS complexes in a 6-second strip and multiply by 10 (to estimate the ventricular rate). Count the number of P waves in a 6-second strip and multiply by 10 (to estimate the atrial rate).
- Method 2. If the rhythm is regular, divide 300 by the number of large boxes on the ECG paper between two R waves (ventricular rate) and between two P waves (atrial rate).
- Method 3. Find a QRS complex that falls directly on a dark line of the ECG paper. This dark line becomes the reference point, and the next six dark lines of the paper are labeled 300, 150, 100, 75, 60, and 50.

  The QRS complex immediately after the reference point is used to estimate ventricular rate (eg, in the figure above, the ventricular rate is approximately 85 beats/min). The same method can be used for estimating atrial rate by using the P waves.

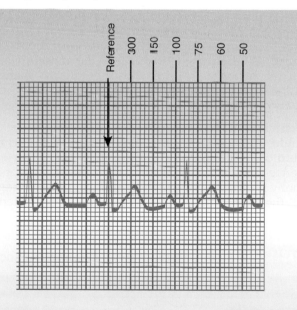

RED FLAG! Estimating the heart rate using the ECG strip or cardiac monitor should never be substituted for determining the heart rate by palpating the pulse. In some situations, electrical activity can occur without contraction. Therefore, palpation of the pulse is a more accurate method of determining heart rate.

BOX 8-2   Assessing a Rhythm Strip

1. Determine the atrial and ventricular heart rates.
   • Are they within normal limits?
   • If not, is there a relationship between the two (ie, one a multiple of the other)?
2. Examine the rhythm to see if it is regular.
   • Is there an equal amount of time between each QRS complex (RR interval)?
   • Is there an equal amount of time between each P wave (PP interval)?
   • Are the PP and RR intervals the same?
3. Look for the P waves.
   • Are they present?
   • Are they upright?
   • Is there one or more P waves for each QRS complex?
   • Do all P waves have the same configuration?
4. Measure the PR interval.
   • Is it normal?
   • Is it the same throughout the strip, or does it vary?
   • If it varies, is there a pattern to the variation?
5. Evaluate the QRS complex.
   • Is it normal in width, or is it wide?
   • Are all complexes of the same configuration?
6. Examine the ST segment.
   • Is it isoelectric, elevated, or depressed?
7. Identify the rhythm and determine its clinical significance.
   • Is the patient symptomatic? (Check skin, neurological status, renal function, coronary circulation, and hemodynamic status or blood pressure.)
   • Is the dysrhythmia life threatening?
   • What is the clinical context?
   • Is the dysrhythmia new or chronic?

conduction defects (eg, left or right bundle branch block), ventricular enlargement (left or right), or myocardial infarction (eg, inferior wall or anterior wall).

Enlargement Patterns

Enlargement of a cardiac chamber may involve hypertrophy of the muscle or dilation of the chamber. The term "ventricular hypertrophy" is commonly used to describe ventricular changes because hypertrophy is the most frequent cause of ventricular enlargement. However, the term "atrial enlargement" is often used (instead of the more specific "atrial hypertrophy") to describe atrial changes because atrial changes on the ECG may result from a variety of causes.

Ventricular Hypertrophy

Right ventricular hypertrophy, often seen in chronic pulmonary conditions, may exist without clear evidence on the ECG because the left ventricle normally is larger than the right and can mask changes in the size of the right ventricle. ECG evidence suggestive of right ventricular hypertrophy includes right atrial enlargement and right axis deviation. In addition, the normal QRS complex pattern across the precordial leads is reversed. Normally, R waves are small in V_1 and gradually grow tall by V_6. With right ventricular hypertrophy, the R wave is tall in V_1 and progresses to small by V_6. Precordial S waves persist rather than gradually disappear.

Left ventricular hypertrophy, often seen in chronic systemic hypertension or aortic stenosis, can be detected on the ECG by adding the deepest S wave in either lead V_1 or V_2 to the tallest R wave in either lead V_5 or V_6. If the sum is 35 mm or more and the patient is older than 35 years of age, left ventricular hypertrophy is suspected. In addition, the T waves in leads V_5 and V_6 may be asymmetrically inverted, and a left axis shift is likely.

Atrial Enlargement

When the atria enlarge, changes are seen in the P wave because the P wave represents atrial depolarization (Fig. 8-6). Right atrial enlargement (P pulmonale) often has an underlying pulmonary cause

TABLE 8-3   Electrocardiographic Changes Associated With Electrolyte Imbalances

Electrolyte Imbalance	Possible Electrocardiographic Findings	Possible Resultant Dysrhythmias
Hyperkalemia	Tall, narrow, peaked T waves; flat, wide P waves; widening of the QRS complex	Sinus bradycardia; sinoatrial block; junctional rhythm; idioventricular rhythm; ventricular tachycardia; ventricular fibrillation
Hypokalemia	Prominent U waves; ST-segment depression; T-wave flattening or inversion	Premature ventricular beats; supraventricular tachycardia; ventricular tachycardia; ventricular fibrillation
Hypercalcemia	Shortened QT interval	Premature ventricular contractions (PVCs)
Hypocalcemia	Lengthened QT interval; T-wave flattening or inversion	Ventricular tachycardia

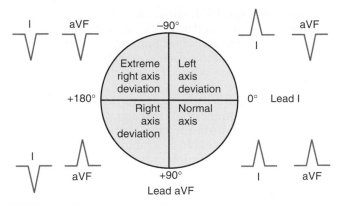

FIGURE 8-5 The electrical axis of the heart is determined by examining the direction of the QRS complex (negative or positive) in leads I and aVF.

and is often seen in association with right ventricular hypertrophy. It is noted on the ECG by the presence of tall, pointed P waves in leads II, III, and aVF. The P wave in lead V_1 may show a diphasic wave with an initial upstroke that is larger than the downstroke (see Fig. 8-6B). Left atrial enlargement (P mitrale) is often associated with mitral valve stenosis. It is noted on the ECG by the presence of broad, notched P waves in leads I, II, and aVL. The P wave in lead V_1 may show a diphasic wave with a terminal downstroke that is larger than the initial upstroke (see Fig. 8-6C).

Ischemia, Injury, and Infarction Patterns

The 12-lead ECG can be useful in detecting myocardial ischemia, injury, or infarction. Ischemia is seen on the ECG as ST-segment depressions and T-wave inversions. Acute patterns of injury are noted by ST-segment elevations. The presence of significant Q waves indicates a myocardial infarction. A more detailed discussion of patterns of ischemia, injury, and infarction is provided in Chapter 14.

Cardiac Monitoring

Cardiac monitoring is used when it is necessary to monitor continuously a patient's heart rate and rhythm. All monitoring systems have three basic components: electrodes, a monitoring cable, and a display screen (cardiac monitor). Electrodes are placed on the patient's chest to receive the electrical current from the cardiac muscle tissue. The electrical signal is then carried by the monitoring cable to the cardiac monitor.

Cardiac monitoring systems may incorporate several advanced features, such as

• Computer systems that store, analyze, and trend monitored data, facilitating retrieval of information to aid in diagnosis and to track trends in the patient's status
• Automatic chart documentation (the ECG recorder is activated by alarms or at preset intervals)
• Expanded alarm systems
• Multilead or 12-lead ECG displays to facilitate complex dysrhythmia interpretation
• ST-segment analysis for monitoring ischemic events[1]
• QT-interval monitoring[2]
• Wireless communication devices that provide data and alarms and can be carried by the nurse

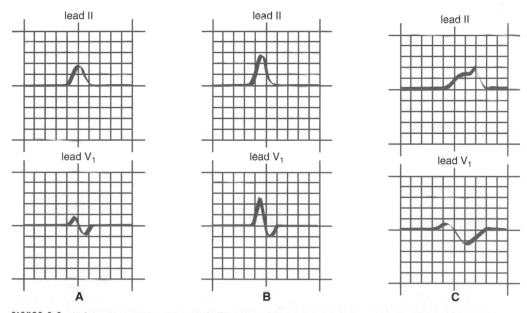

FIGURE 8-6 Atrial enlargement patterns. **A:** The normal P wave in leads II and V_1. **B:** Right atrial enlargement. Note the tall, pointed P wave in lead II and the increased amplitude of the early, right atrial component of the P wave in V_1. **C:** Left atrial enlargement. Note the broad, notched P wave in lead II and the increased amplitude and duration of the P wave in V_1.

EVIDENCE-BASED PRACTICE GUIDELINES
ST-Segment Monitoring

PROBLEM: Research demonstrates that monitoring for ST-segment changes in multiple leads, preferably 12 leads, substantially improves the chance of identifying ischemic events, including silent (asymptomatic) ischemia.

EVIDENCE-BASED PRACTICE GUIDELINES

1. If 12-lead electrocardiography is available, ST-segment monitoring should be performed using all 12 leads. (level V)

2. If 12-lead electrocardiography is not available, leads for ST-segment monitoring are selected based on the patient's needs and risk for ischemia.

   Patients with acute coronary syndrome (ACS) and a known "ST fingerprint" (ie, a pattern of ST-segment elevation, depression, or both that is unique to the patient based on the site of coronary occlusion, obtained during a known ischemic event): Use the lead that best displays the patient's ST finger-print when monitoring. (level V)

   Patients with ACS but no known ST fingerprint: Use leads III and V_3. (level IV)

   Patients without definitive ACS, but in whom ACS is suspected or being ruled out: Use leads III and V_5.

   Noncardiac patients undergoing surgical procedures: Use lead V_5 (useful for identifying demand-related ischemia). (level IV)

3. Once proper lead placement has been determined, mark the skin electrode placement with indelible ink. Do not alter the location of the skin electrodes during monitoring because this can cause false-positive ST-segment changes. (level II)

4. Set the ST alarm parameter 1 to 2 mm above and below the patient's baseline ST segment. (level II)

5. Evaluate the ST segment with the patient in the supine position. (level IV)

6. Recognize that ST depression or elevation of 1 to 2 mm that lasts for 1 minute or more can be clinically significant and requires further assessment. (level II)

KEY

Level I: Manufacturer's recommendations only

Level II: Theory based, no research data to support recommendations, but recommendations from expert consensus group may exist

Level III: Laboratory data, no clinical data to support recommendations

Level IV: Limited clinical studies to support recommendations

Level V: Clinical studies in more than one or two patient populations and situations to support recommendations

Level VI: Clinical studies in a variety of patient populations and situations to support recommendations

■ Adapted from American Association of Critical-Care Nurses (AACN) Practice Alert, revised 5/2009.

There are two types of cardiac monitoring systems:

- Hard-wire monitoring systems, commonly used in critical care units, require the patient to be linked directly to the cardiac monitor via the monitoring cable. Information is displayed and recorded at the bedside and at a central station simultaneously. Because patient mobility is limited, hard-wire monitoring systems can only be used for patients who are on bedrest or confined to the bedside.

- Telemetry monitoring systems do not require a direct wire connection between the patient and the cardiac monitor. Electrodes are connected by a short monitoring cable to a small battery-operated transmitter, which sends radiofrequency signals to a receiver that picks up and displays the signal on a monitor either at the bedside or at a central station. Although telemetry monitoring systems allow for more patient mobility, because the patient is mobile, stable ECG tracings often are more difficult to obtain.

Some hard-wire systems have built-in telemetry capability so that patients may be switched easily from one system to another as monitoring needs change.

Commonly used cardiac monitoring systems include a three-electrode system and a five-electrode system (Fig. 8-7). The three-electrode system allows monitoring of leads I, II, or III with only a single lead viewed on the monitor at one time (single-channel recording) (Fig. 8-8). The three-electrode system can also be used to obtain a modified version of any of the six chest leads, referred to as MCL_1 through MCL_6. Five-electrode systems allow monitoring of any of the 12 leads, with two or more leads viewed on the monitor simultaneously (multichannel recording). Lead selection depends on the clinical situation (Table 8-4, p. 70). Often, multichannel recording is desirable.

Troubleshooting cardiac monitoring problems is summarized in Box 8-3 on page 70.

Common Dysrhythmias

Dysrhythmias Originating at the Sinus Node

Box 8-4 on page 71 summarizes and compares ECG characteristics of sinus rhythms.

Sinus Tachycardia

In sinus tachycardia, the sinus node initiates an impulse at a rate of 100 beats/min (up to 160 to 180 beats/min). Stress, exercise, stimulants (eg, caffeine, nicotine), clinical conditions (eg, fever, anemia, hyperthyroidism, hypoxemia, heart failure, shock), and medications (eg, atropine, epinephrine, dopamine) can cause sinus tachycardia. The rapid rate of sinus tachycardia increases oxygen demands on the myocardium and decreases the filling time of the ventricles, and if allowed to persist, may worsen underlying conditions such as heart failure or ischemia. Treatment is directed at eliminating the underlying cause.

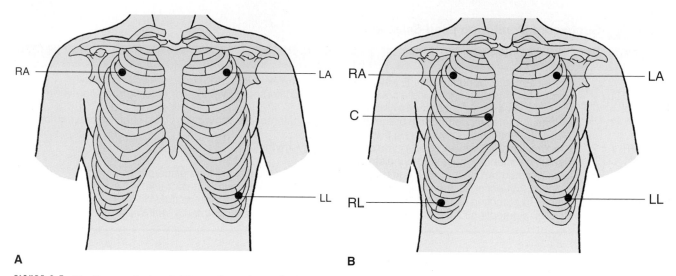

FIGURE 8-7 Cardiac monitoring. **A:** Three-electrode monitoring system. Leads placed in this position allow the nurse to monitor leads I, II, and III. The left leg electrode must be placed below the level of the heart. **B:** Five-electrode monitoring system. Using a five-electrode system allows the nurse to monitor any of the 12 leads of the electrocardiogram (ECG). The chest electrode must be moved to the appropriate chest location when monitoring the precordial leads. C, chest; LA, left arm; LL, left leg; RA, right arm, RL, right leg.

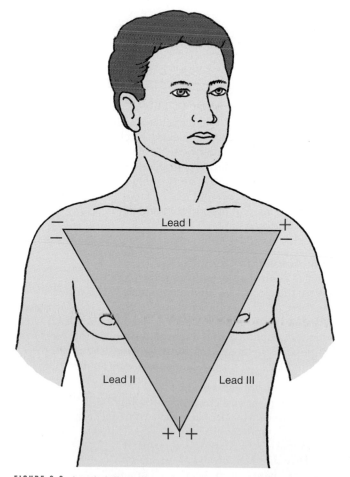

FIGURE 8-8 Leads I, II, or III may be viewed with a three-electrode system.

Sinus Bradycardia

In sinus bradycardia, the sinus node initiates impulses at a rate of less than 60 beats/min. Sinus bradycardia is present in both healthy and diseased hearts. It may be associated with sleep, severe pain, inferior wall myocardial infarction, acute spinal cord injury, and certain drugs (eg, digoxin, β-adrenergic blockers, verapamil, diltiazem). In people with healthy hearts, slow heart rates are tolerated well. However, in those with severe heart disease, the heart may not be able to compensate for a slow rate by increasing the stroke volume. In this situation, sinus bradycardia leads to a low cardiac output. No treatment is indicated unless symptoms are present. If the pulse is very slow and the patient is symptomatic, appropriate measures include atropine or cardiac pacing.

Sinus Dysrhythmia

Sinus dysrhythmia is caused by an irregularity in sinus node discharge, often in association with phases of the respiratory cycle (ie, the sinus node rate gradually increases with inspiration and gradually decreases with expiration). On the ECG, the RR intervals (from the shortest to the longest) vary by more than 0.12 second. Sinus dysrhythmia is often normal, especially in young people with lower heart rates. It also occurs after enhancement of vagal tone (eg, with digoxin or morphine). Symptoms are uncommon unless there are excessively long pauses between heartbeats; usually no treatment is required.

TABLE 8-4 Suggested Monitoring Lead Selection

Lead	Rationale for Use
II	Produces large, upright visible P waves and QRS complexes for determining underlying rhythm
V_1 or MCL_1	Helpful for detecting right bundle branch block and to differentiate ventricular ectopy from supraventricular rhythm aberrantly conducted in the ventricles
V_6 or MCL_6	Helpful for detecting left bundle branch block and to differentiate ventricular ectopy from supraventricular rhythm aberrantly conducted in the ventricles
III, aVF, V_1	Produce visible P waves; useful in detecting atrial dysrhythmias
I	Useful in patients with respiratory distress Less affected by chest motion compared with other leads due to the lead placement
II, III, aVF	Helpful in detecting ischemia, injury, and infarction in the inferior wall left ventricle
I, aVL, V_5, V_6	Helpful in detecting ischemia, injury, and infarction in the lateral wall left ventricle
V_1 through V_4	Helpful in detecting ischemia, injury, and infarction in the septal and anterior wall left ventricle

Sinus Arrest and Sinoatrial Block

In sinus arrest, the sinus node fails to form a discharge, producing pauses of varying lengths because of the absence of atrial depolarization (P wave). The pause ends either when another pacemaker (eg, the AV node or the ventricles) takes over or when sinus node function returns. In SA block, the sinus node fires, but the impulse is delayed or blocked from exiting the sinus node. SA block often is difficult to differentiate from sinus arrest on the ECG.

BOX 8-3 Troubleshooting Cardiac Monitoring Problems

Excessive Triggering of Heart Rate Alarms
- Is the high–low alarm set too close to the patient's heart rate?
- Is the monitor sensitivity level set too high or too low?
- Is the patient cable securely inserted into the monitor receptacle?
- Are the lead wires or connections damaged?
- Has the monitoring lead been properly selected?
- Were the electrodes applied properly?
- Are the R and T waves the same height, causing both waveforms to be sensed?
- Is the baseline unstable, or is there excessive cable or lead wire movement?

Baseline but No Electrocardiogram (ECG) Trace
- Is the size (gain or sensitivity) control properly adjusted?
- Is an appropriate lead selector being used on the monitor?
- Is the patient cable fully inserted into the ECG receptacle?
- Are the electrode wires fully inserted into the patient cable?
- Are the electrode wires firmly attached to the electrodes?
- Are the electrode wires damaged?
- Is the patient cable damaged?
- Call for service if the trace is still absent.
- Is the battery dead (for telemetry system)?

Intermittent Trace
- Is the patient cable fully inserted into the monitor receptacle?
- Are the electrode wires fully inserted into the patient cable?

- Are the electrode wires firmly attached to the electrodes?
- Are the electrode wire connectors loose or worn?
- Have the electrodes been applied properly?
- Are the electrodes properly located and in firm skin contact?
- Is the patient cable damaged?

Wandering or Irregular Baseline
- Is there excessive cable movement? This can be reduced by clipping to the patient's clothing.
- Is the power cord on or near the monitor cable?
- Is there excessive movement by the patient? Are there muscle tremors from anxiety or shivering?
- Is site selection correct?
- Were proper skin preparation and application procedures followed?
- Are the electrodes still moist?

Low-Amplitude Complexes
- Is size control adjusted properly?
- Were the electrodes applied properly?
- Is there dried gel on the electrodes?
- Change electrode sites. Check 12-lead ECG for lead with highest amplitude, and attempt to simulate that lead.
- If none of the preceding steps remedies the problem, the weak signal may be the patient's normal complex.

Sixty-Cycle Interference
- Is the monitor size control set too high?
- Are there nearby electrical devices in use, especially poorly grounded ones?
- Were the electrodes applied properly?
- Is there dried gel on the electrodes?
- Are lead wires or connections damaged?

BOX 8-4 Dysrhythmias Originating at the Sinus Node

	Normal Sinus Rhythm	Sinus Tachycardia	Sinus Bradycardia	Sinus Dysrhythmia
Rate	60 to 100 beats/min	Greater than 100 beats/min	Less than 60 beats/min	60 to 100 beats/min
Rhythm	Regular	Regular	Regular	Irregular
P waves	Present, one per QRS	Present, one per QRS	Present, one per QRS	Present, one per QRS
PR interval	Less than 0.20 s, equal	Less than 0.20 s, equal	Less than 0.20 s, equal	Less than 0.20 s, equal
QRS complex	Less than 0.12 s	Less than 0.12 s	Less than 0.12 s	Less than 0.12 s

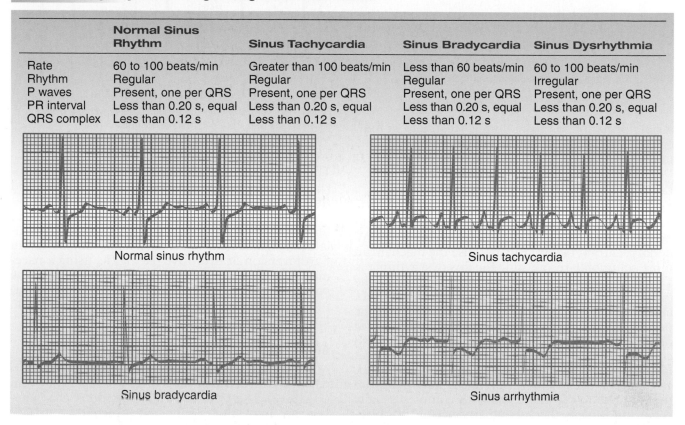

Normal sinus rhythm

Sinus tachycardia

Sinus bradycardia

Sinus arrhythmia

Both dysrhythmias may result from disruption of the sinus node by infarction, degenerative fibrotic changes, drugs (eg, digoxin, β-adrenergic blockers, calcium channel blockers), or excessive vagal stimulation. These rhythms usually are transient and insignificant unless a lower pacemaker fails to take over to pace the ventricles. Treatment to increase the ventricular rate is indicated if the patient is symptomatic. In the presence of serious hemodynamic compromise, a pacemaker may be required.

Sick Sinus Syndrome

Sick sinus syndrome is a chronic form of sinus node disease. Patients exhibit severe degrees of sinus node depression, including marked sinus bradycardia, SA block, or sinus arrest. Often, rapid atrial dysrhythmias, such as atrial flutter or fibrillation ("tachycardia–bradycardia syndrome"), coexist and alternate with periods of sinus node depression (Fig. 8-9).

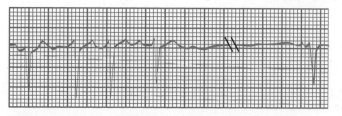

FIGURE 8-9 Sick sinus syndrome. Atrial fibrillation is followed by atrial standstill. A sinus escape beat is seen at the end of the strip.

Management entails control of the rapid atrial dysrhythmias with drug therapy and, in some cases, control of very slow heart rates with implantation of a permanent pacemaker.

Atrial Dysrhythmias

Premature Atrial Contraction

A premature atrial contraction (PAC) occurs when an ectopic atrial impulse discharges prematurely and, in most cases, is conducted in a normal fashion to the ventricles. On the ECG tracing, the P wave is premature and may even be buried in the preceding T wave; it often differs in configuration from the sinus P wave (Fig. 8-10). The QRS complex usually is of normal configuration. A short pause, usually less than "compensatory," is present. (A pause is considered fully "compensatory" if the cycles of the normal and premature beats equal the time of two normal heart cycles.) Patients may have the sensation of a "pause" or "skip" in a heartbeat when PACs are present.

PACs may occur in healthy people as a result of emotions or stimulants (eg, tobacco, alcohol, caffeine). PACs also may be associated with rheumatic heart disease, ischemic heart disease, mitral stenosis, heart failure, hypokalemia, hypomagnesemia, medications, and hyperthyroidism. In some patients, PACs are indicative of increasing atrial irritability and are a precursor to atrial tachycardia,

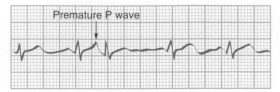

FIGURE 8-10   Premature atrial contraction (PAC).

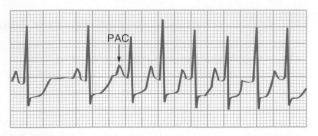

FIGURE 8-11 • Paroxysmal supraventricular tachycardia (PSVT), which begins with a premature atrial contraction (PAC).

atrial fibrillation, or atrial flutter. Treatment, if indicated, is aimed at identifying and addressing the underlying cause.

Paroxysmal Supraventricular Tachycardia

Paroxysmal supraventricular tachycardia (PSVT) is a rapid atrial rhythm occurring at a rate of 150 to 250 beats/min (Fig. 8-11). PSVT is also known as AV nodal reentrant tachycardia because the mechanism most commonly responsible for this dysrhythmia is a reentrant circuit at the level of the AV node. The tachycardia begins abruptly, usually with a PAC, and it ends abruptly. The rhythm is regular, and the paroxysms may last from a few seconds to several hours or even days. P waves may precede the QRS complex but also may be hidden in the T waves at faster rates. The P waves may be negative in leads II, III, and aVF because of retrograde conduction from the AV node to the atria. The QRS complex usually is normal unless there is an underlying intraventricular conduction problem. PSVT must be differentiated from other supraventricular narrow QRS complex tachycardias (Table 8-5).

Like PACs, PSVT often occurs in adults with healthy hearts in response to emotions or stimulants. Patients without underlying heart disease may experience palpitations and some light-headedness, depending on the rate and duration of the PSVT. Rheumatic heart disease, acute myocardial infarction, and digoxin toxicity may also produce PSVT.

These patients may develop dyspnea, angina pectoris, and heart failure as ventricular filling time, and thus cardiac output, is decreased.

A vagal maneuver (eg, carotid sinus massage) may be used to terminate the PSVT. If vagal stimulation is unsuccessful, IV adenosine may be given. Cardioversion or overdrive pacing (ie, using a pacemaker to pace the heart at a rate faster than the patient's intrinsic rate to suppress the tachycardia) may be required if drug therapy is unsuccessful. Long-term prophylactic therapy may be indicated.

Atrial Flutter

Atrial flutter is a rapid atrial ectopic rhythm in which the atria fire at rates of 250 to 350 beats/min (Fig. 8-12). The AV node, which functions as a "gatekeeper," may allow only every second, third, or fourth atrial stimulus to proceed to the ventricles, resulting in what is known as a 2:1, 3:1, or 4:1 flutter block. The rapid and regular atrial rate produces "sawtooth" or "picket-fence" P waves on the ECG. It is usual for a flutter wave to be partially concealed in the QRS complex or T wave. The QRS complex exhibits a normal configuration except when aberrant conduction is present. When the ventricular rate is rapid, the diagnosis of atrial flutter may be difficult. Vagal maneuvers or administration of

TABLE 8-5   Differential Diagnosis of Narrow QRS Tachycardia

Type of Supraventricular Tachycardia	Onset	Atrial Rate	Ventricular Rate	RR Interval	Response to Carotid Massage
Sinus tachycardia	Gradual	100–180 beats/min	Same as sinus rate	Regular	Gradual slowing
Paroxysmal supraventricular tachycardia (PSVT)	Abrupt	150–250 beats/min	Usually same as atrial rate; block seen with digoxin toxicity and AV node disease	Regular, except at onset and termination	May convert to normal sinus rhythm
Atrial flutter	Abrupt	250–350 beats/min	Occurs with 2:1, 3:1, 4:1, or varied ventricular response	Regular or regularly irregular	Abrupt slowing of ventricular response; flutter waves remain
Atrial fibrillation	Abrupt	400–650 beats/min	Depends on ability of AV node to conduct atrial impulse; decreased with drug therapy	Irregularly irregular	Abrupt slowing of ventricular response; fibrillation waves remain

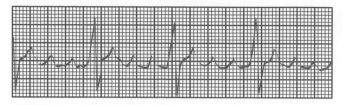

FIGURE 8-12 Atrial flutter. P waves show a characteristic "saw-toothed" pattern.

adenosine increase the degree of AV block and allow recognition of flutter waves.

Atrial flutter often is seen in the presence of underlying cardiac disease, including coronary artery disease (CAD), right-sided heart failure, and rheumatic heart disease. Treatment goals are to reestablish sinus rhythm or, when the ventricular rate is rapid, to achieve ventricular rate control. Drugs may be selected to slow the conduction of the impulses through the AV node or to achieve pharmacological conversion of the rhythm. If pharmacological conversion is not successful, electrical cardioversion can be used. If the patient has been experiencing atrial flutter for more than 72 hours, anticoagulation may be needed before pharmacological or electrical conversion of the rhythm is attempted. Other therapies that may be indicated for the long-term management of atrial flutter include ablation, pacing, and use of an implantable cardioverter–defibrillator (ICD).

Atrial Fibrillation

Atrial fibrillation is a rapid atrial ectopic rhythm, occurring with atrial rates of 350 to 500 beats/min (Fig. 8-13). It is characterized by chaotic atrial activity with small, quivering fibrillatory waves. As in atrial flutter, the ventricular rate and rhythm depend on the ability of the AV junction to function as a gatekeeper. The ventricular rhythm is characteristically irregular.

Although atrial fibrillation may occur as a transient dysrhythmia in healthy young people, the presence of chronic atrial fibrillation is usually associated with atrial muscle disease or atrial distention together with disease of the sinus node. This rhythm commonly occurs in heart failure, ischemic or rheumatic heart disease, congenital heart disease, pulmonary disease, and after open heart surgery.

The immediate clinical concern in patients with atrial fibrillation is the rate of the ventricular

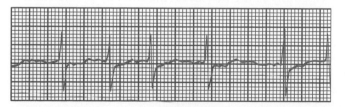

FIGURE 8-13 Atrial fibrillation. Characteristic atrial fibrillatory waves seen with a variable ventricular response.

response and the formation of emboli. If the ventricular rate is too fast, end-diastolic filling time is decreased, and cardiac output is compromised. A ventricular rate that is too slow can also decrease cardiac output. Patients are at risk for the formation of mural thrombi in the fibrillating atrium and embolic events (eg, stroke, myocardial infarction, pulmonary embolus). The treatment principles for atrial fibrillation are the same as those for atrial flutter.

Junctional Dysrhythmias

Junctional (Nodal) Rhythm

A junctional (nodal) rhythm originates in the AV node. When the SA node fails to fire, the AV node usually takes control, but the rate is slower. The rate of a junctional rhythm ranges between 40 and 60 beats/min. The P wave in the dysrhythmia can have one of three possible configurations:

1. The AV node fires, and the wave of depolarization travels backward (retrograde conduction) into the atria. The impulse from the AV node then moves forward into the ventricle. On the ECG, the P wave appears as an inverted wave before a normal QRS complex (Fig. 8-14A).
2. The retrograde conduction into the atria occurs at the same time as the forward conduction into the ventricles. The resulting rhythm strip shows an absent P wave with a normal QRS complex (see Fig. 8-14B). In reality, the P wave is not absent; it is buried inside the QRS complex.
3. Forward conduction into the ventricles precedes retrograde conduction into the atria. On the ECG, a normal QRS complex is followed by an inverted P wave (see Fig. 8-14C).

A junctional rhythm may be the result of hypoxia, hyperkalemia, myocardial infarction, heart failure, valvular disease, drugs (digoxin, β-adrenergic blockers, calcium channel blockers), or any cause of SA node dysfunction. Patients with a junctional rhythm may develop hypotension, decreased cardiac output, and decreased perfusion as a result of the slower rate. The benefit of AV synchrony and the atrial kick (which provides 20% of the cardiac output) is lost when the atria are stimulated with or after ventricular depolarization.

Symptomatic patients may require immediate treatment, which is directed at the underlying cause. Interventions are also directed toward improving the heart rate (eg, through the use of atropine or cardiac pacing) and improving cardiac output.

Premature Junctional Contractions

A premature junctional contraction (PJC) is an ectopic impulse initiated at the AV junction that occurs prematurely, before the next sinus impulse (Fig. 8-15). As in all rhythms originating in the AV

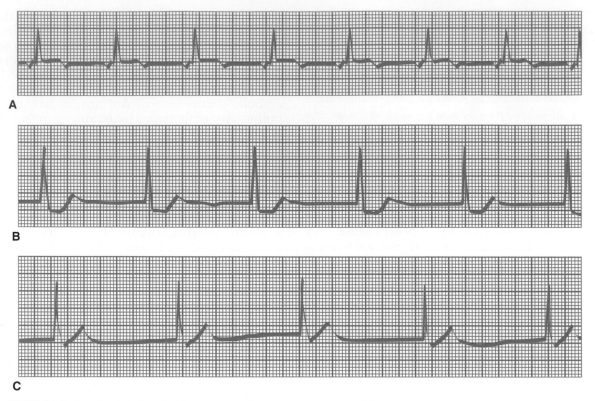

A

B

C

FIGURE 8-14   Junctional rhythm. **A:** A junctional rhythm in which the inverted P wave appears before a normal QRS complex. **B:** A junctional rhythm in which the inverted P wave is buried inside the QRS complex. **C:** A junctional rhythm in which the inverted P wave follows the QRS complex.

junction, the QRS complex is narrow (less than 0.12 second), reflecting normal AV conduction. Rarely, the QRS complex may be wide if the impulse is conducted aberrantly. The atria are depolarized in a retrograde fashion before, during, or after ventricular excitation, producing inverted P waves that may occur before, during, or after the QRS complex. As with PACs, PJCs may occur in healthy people or in those with underlying heart disease. Ischemia or infarction may activate an ectopic focus in the AV junction, as may stimulants or pharmacological agents (eg, digoxin). Although usually asymptomatic, patients may experience a feeling of a "skipped beat." Treatment for PJCs is not necessary.

 RED FLAG! Frequent PJCs may indicate increasing irritability and may be a precursor to a junctional rhythm.

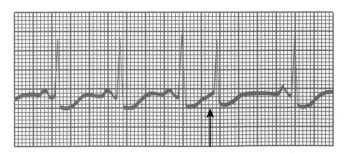

FIGURE 8-15   Premature junctional contraction.

Ventricular Dysrhythmias

Premature Ventricular Contractions

A premature ventricular contraction (PVC) is an ectopic beat originating prematurely at the level of the ventricles. Because the beat originates in the ventricles, there is no atrial electrical activity, and thus no P waves on the ECG (Fig. 8-16A). Rather than traveling through the normal ventricular conduction system, the ventricular depolarization spreads more slowly through the Purkinje system, producing a wide QRS complex with a T wave that is opposite in direction to the QRS complex. A compensatory pause often follows the premature beat as the heart awaits the next stimulus from the sinus node.

Premature ventricular beats can be described by their frequency (number of PVCs per minute) and pattern. Ventricular bigeminy is a PVC that occurs after each sinus beat (see Fig. 8-16A). Ventricular trigeminy is a PVC occurring after two consecutive sinus beats. When PVCs originate from one ventricular site, each of the PVCs has the same configuration and is referred to as "uniform." When PVCs originate from more than one ventricular site, two or more shapes of the QRS complex appear and the PVC is said to be "multiform" (see Fig. 8-16B). Two PVCs in a row are a couplet (see Fig. 8-16C). Three in a row are a triplet, and constitute a short run of ventricular tachycardia (see Fig. 8-16D).

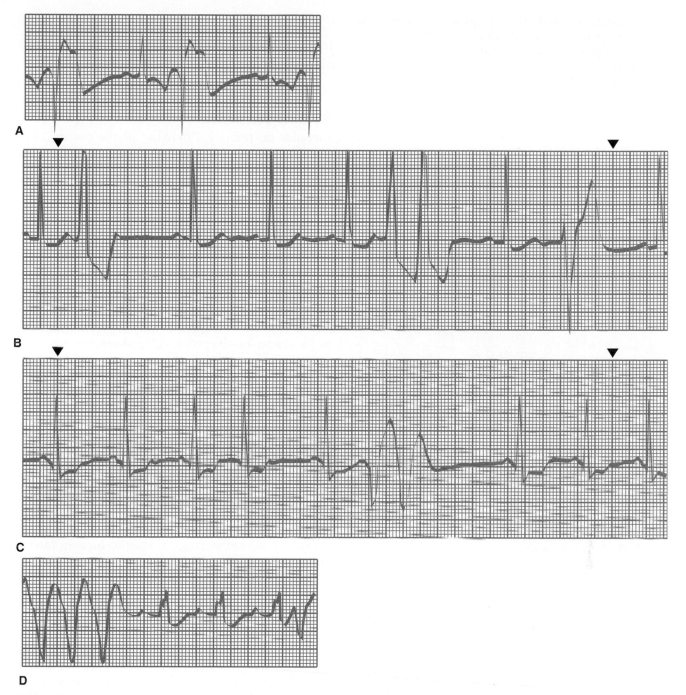

FIGURE 8-16 Various forms and patterns of premature ventricular contractions (PVCs). **A:** Ventricular bigeminy. (Every other beat is a PVC.) **B:** Multiformed PVCs. **C:** Couplet (two PVCs in a row). **D:** Triplet, constituting a run of ventricular tachycardia. The rhythm then converts to sinus rhythm with first-degree heart block.

The most common of all ectopic beats, PVCs can occur with or without heart disease in any age group. They are especially common in people with myocardial disease (ischemia or infarction) or with myocardial irritability (eg, as a result of hypokalemia, increased levels of catecholamines, or mechanical irritation by a wire or catheter). Because of their association with ventricular myocardial irritability, PVCs may lead to ventricular tachycardia or ventricular fibrillation in some patients. In patients with serious heart disease, numerous and multiformed PVCs worsen the prognosis.

Infrequent, isolated PVCs require no treatment. Multiple or consecutive PVCs may be managed with antidysrhythmic agents. In the emergency setting, amiodarone and lidocaine are the drugs of choice. Other antidysrhythmic agents are available for chronic therapy. Treatment of the underlying cause (eg, hypokalemia, digoxin toxicity) may also correct the dysrhythmia.

 RED FLAG! *PVCs approaching the preceding T wave (R-on-T phenomenon) are of clinical concern. The T wave represents ventricular repolarization. If stimulation occurs during this vulnerable period, ventricular fibrillation and sudden death may result (see figure below).*

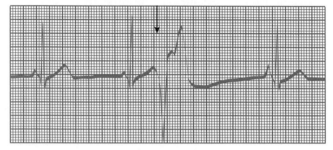

Ventricular Tachycardia

Ventricular tachycardia is defined as three or more PVCs in a row. Ventricular tachycardia is recognized by wide, bizarre QRS complexes occurring in a fairly regular rhythm at a rate greater than 100 beats/min (Fig. 8-17). P waves, if seen, are not related to the QRS complex. Ventricular tachycardia may be a short, nonsustained rhythm or longer and sustained. Dysrhythmia progression depends on the underlying heart disease.

Ventricular tachycardia is a common complication of myocardial infarction. Other causes are the same as those described for PVCs. Signs and symptoms of hemodynamic compromise (eg, ischemic chest pain, hypotension, pulmonary edema, loss of consciousness) may be seen if the tachycardia is sustained. The patient may or may not have a pulse and cardiac output.

If the patient is hemodynamically stable, amiodarone may be administered intravenously. If the patient becomes unstable, synchronized cardioversion (or in emergency situations, unsynchronized defibrillation) is indicated. Long-term treatment for this dysrhythmia may involve the use of an ICD.

 RED FLAG! *Ventricular tachycardia is often a precursor to ventricular fibrillation.*

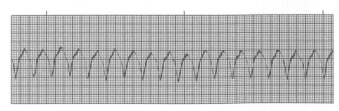

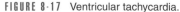
FIGURE 8-17 Ventricular tachycardia.

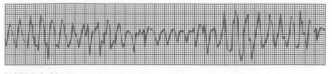

FIGURE 8-18 Torsades de pointes.

Torsades de Pointes

Torsades de pointes ("twisting of the points") is a specific type of ventricular tachycardia (Fig. 8-18). The dysrhythmia is characterized by large, bizarre, polymorphous, or multiformed QRS complexes of varying amplitude and direction, frequently varying from beat to beat and resembling torsion around an isoelectric line (hence the name, "twisting of the points"). The rate of the tachycardia is 100 to 180 beats/min but can be as fast as 200 to 300 beats/min. The rhythm is highly unstable; it may terminate in ventricular fibrillation or revert to sinus rhythm.

Torsades de pointes is most likely to develop in patients with myocardial disease when the refractory period (ie, the QT interval) is prolonged, such as in severe bradycardia, drug therapy (especially with type IA antidysrhythmic agents), and electrolyte disturbances (eg, hypokalemia, hypocalcemia). Other factors that can precipitate this dysrhythmia include familial QT-interval prolongation, central nervous system disorders, and hypothermia.

 RED FLAG! *In patients who are at high risk for torsades de pointes, dysrhythmia monitoring should include measurement of the QT interval and calculation of the QTc (ie, the QT interval corrected for heart rate) using a consistent lead.[2]*

Treatment focuses on shortening the refractory period by administering IV magnesium sulfate or initiating overdrive pacing. Emergency cardioversion or defibrillation is indicated if the dysrhythmia does not revert spontaneously to sinus rhythm.

Ventricular Fibrillation

Ventricular fibrillation is rapid, irregular, and ineffectual depolarizations of the ventricle. On ECG, only irregular oscillations of the baseline are apparent; these may be either coarse or fine in appearance (Fig. 8-19). Loss of consciousness occurs within seconds. There is no pulse and no cardiac output. Causes of ventricular fibrillation include myocardial ischemia and infarction, catheter manipulation in the ventricles, electrocution, terminal rhythms in circulatory failure, and conditions that prolong the refractory period (QT interval).

RED FLAG! *Ventricular fibrillation is fatal if rapid defibrillation is not instituted immediately. If there is no response to defibrillation, support with cardiopulmonary resuscitation (CPR) and drugs is required.*

Accelerated Idioventricular Rhythm

Accelerated idioventricular rhythm (AIVR) occurs when the ventricular pacemaker cells increase their

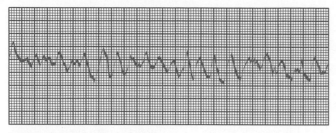

FIGURE 8-19 Ventricular fibrillation.

rate beyond their normal rate of 20 to 40 beats/min. AIVR is characterized by wide QRS complexes occurring regularly at a rate of 50 to 100 beats/min (Fig. 8-20). When the idioventricular rate exceeds the sinus rate, the ventricular pacemaker becomes the primary pacemaker. AIVR may last for a few beats or may be sustained. Typically, AIVR is seen with acute myocardial infarction, often in the setting of coronary artery reperfusion after thrombolytic therapy. It may occur less commonly as a result of ischemia or digoxin toxicity. Patients usually are asymptomatic. Adequate cardiac output can be maintained, and degeneration into ventricular tachycardia is rare. If a patient is hemodynamically compromised, the sinus rate is increased with atropine or atrial pacing to suppress the AIVR.

Atrioventricular Blocks

Atrioventricular (AV) blocks occur when the sinus-initiated beat is delayed or completely blocked from activating the ventricles. The block may occur at the AV node, the bundle of His, or the bundle branches. In first- and second-degree AV block, the block is incomplete; some or all of the impulses eventually are conducted to the ventricles. In third-degree (complete) heart block, none of the sinus-initiated impulses are conducted. Box 8-5 summarizes the ECG characteristics of heart blocks.

First-Degree Atrioventricular Block

In first-degree block, AV conduction (represented by the PR interval) is prolonged and equal in length per beat. All impulses eventually are conducted to the ventricles. First-degree block occurs in people of all ages and in healthy and diseased hearts. Causes may include medications

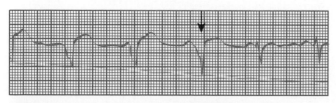

FIGURE 8-20 Accelerated idioventricular rhythm (AIVR). The first three beats are of ventricular origin. The fourth beat (*arrow*) represents a fusion beat. The subsequent two beats are of sinus origin.

(eg, digoxin, β-adrenergic blockers, calcium channel blockers); CAD; infectious disease; and congenital lesions. First-degree block is of no hemodynamic consequence but is an indicator of a potential AV conduction system disturbance and may progress to second- or third-degree AV block. Management entails monitoring the PR interval closely for further block, and exploring underlying causes (eg, drug effect).

Second-Degree Atrioventricular Block—Mobitz I (Wenckebach)

Mobitz type I (Wenckebach) block occurs when AV conduction is delayed progressively with each sinus impulse until eventually the impulse is completely blocked from reaching the ventricles. The cycle then repeats itself. Of the two types of second-degree block, Mobitz type I is the more common. A Mobitz type I block usually is associated with block above the bundle of His; therefore, any medication or disease process that affects the AV node (eg, digoxin, myocarditis, inferior wall myocardial infarction) may produce this type of second-degree block. Patients with a Mobitz type I block rarely are symptomatic because the ventricular rate usually is adequate. The block often is temporary, and if it progresses to third-degree block, a junctional pacemaker at a rate of 40 to 60 beats/min usually takes over to pace the ventricles. No treatment is required except patient monitoring and discontinuation of pharmacotherapy, if a drug is the offending agent.

Second-Degree Atrioventricular Block—Mobitz II

Mobitz type II block is an intermittent block in AV conduction, usually in or below the bundle of His. This type of block is seen in the setting of an anterior wall myocardial infarction and various diseases of the conducting tissue, such as fibrotic disease. A Mobitz type II block is potentially more dangerous than a Mobitz type I block. Mobitz type II block often is permanent, and it may deteriorate rapidly to third-degree heart block with a slow ventricular response of 20 to 40 beats/min. Constant monitoring and observation for progression to third-degree heart block are required. Medications (eg, atropine) or cardiac pacing may be required if the patient becomes symptomatic or if the block occurs in the setting of an acute anterior wall myocardial infarction. Permanent pacing often is indicated for long-term management.

Third-Degree (Complete) Atrioventricular Block

In third-degree (complete) heart block, the sinus node continues to fire normally, but the impulses do not reach the ventricles. The ventricles are stimulated by pacemaker cells either in the junction (at a rate of 40 to 60 beats/min) or in the ventricles (at a rate of 20 to 40 beats/min), depending on the level of the AV block. The causes of complete heart block are the same as for lesser degrees of AV block.

BOX 8-5   Heart Block Rhythms

	First-Degree Heart Block	Second-Degree Heart Block—Mobitz Type I (Wenckebach)	Second-Degree Heart Block—Mobitz Type II	Third-Degree Heart Block
Rate	Usually 60 to 100 beats/min	Usually 60 to 100 beats/min	May be slow depending on number of blocked P waves	Rate determined by ventricular focus, usually very slow
Rhythm	Regular	Irregular due to dropped QRS	Often regular but depends on pattern of block; PP interval regular	May be regular or irregular ventricular focus; PP and RR intervals regular
P waves	Present, one per QRS (1:1)	Present, one per QRS until QRS is missed	Present, more than one P wave per QRS (2:1, 3:1, or 4:1 block)	Present, more than one P wave per QRS; P waves no relationship to QRS complexes
PR interval	Greater than 0.20 s, equal throughout; constant	Progressively gets longer until QRS is missed; pattern repeats	May be normal or prolonged, equal throughout (fixed)	May be normal or prolonged, unequal throughout (variable)
QRS complex	Less than 0.12 s	Less than 0.12 s	Usually greater than 0.12 s (due to BBB)	Greater than 0.12 s

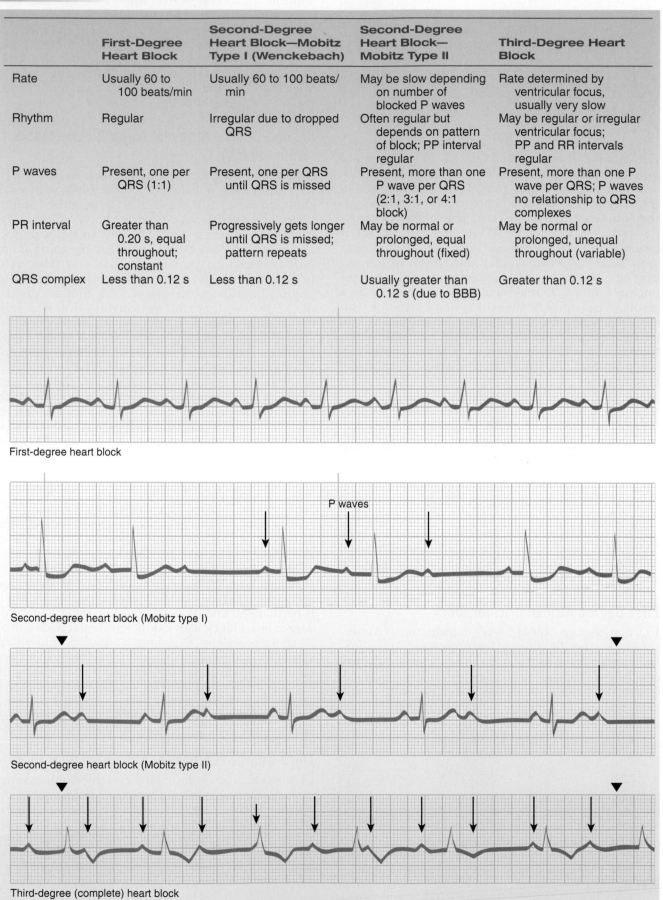

First-degree heart block

P waves

Second-degree heart block (Mobitz type I)

Second-degree heart block (Mobitz type II)

Third-degree (complete) heart block

Complete heart block is often poorly tolerated. If the rhythm is ventricular in origin, the rate is slow, and the pacemaker site is unreliable. The patient may be symptomatic because of a low cardiac output. A pacemaker site high in the bundle of His may provide an adequate rate to sustain cardiac output and is more dependable. A temporary pacing wire is usually inserted immediately, and when the patient is stabilized, a permanent pacemaker is implanted.

Bundle Branch Block

A bundle branch block develops when there is a block in one of the major branches of the intraventricular conduction system. The right ventricle has a single bundle branch and the left ventricle has two bundle branches. The impulse travels along the unaffected bundle and activates one ventricle normally. However, because the impulse must then travel outside the normal conduction system to reach the other ventricle, depolarization of the other ventricle is delayed. The right and left ventricles are thus depolarized sequentially instead of simultaneously. The abnormal activation produces a wide QRS complex (representing the increased time it takes for ventricular depolarization) with two peaks (indicating that depolarization of the two ventricles was not simultaneous).

A bundle branch block is determined by viewing the 12-lead ECG. In right bundle branch block, depolarization of the right ventricle is delayed, which alters the configuration of the QRS complex in the right-sided chest leads, V_1 and V_2. Normally, these leads have a small, single-peaked R-wave and deep S-wave configuration. A right bundle branch block is evidenced by an RSR' configuration in V_1 (Fig. 8-21A) If the initial peak of the QRS complex is smaller than the second peak, the pattern would be described as rSR'. Likewise, if the initial peak of the QRS complex is taller than the second peak, the pattern is described as an RSR'. Whenever ventricular depolarization is abnormal, so is ventricular repolarization. As a result, ST-segment and T-wave abnormalities may be seen in leads V_1 and V_2 for patients with a right bundle branch block.

A left bundle branch block changes the QRS complex pattern in the left-sided chest leads, V_5 and V_6. Normally, these leads have a tall, single-peaked R wave and a small or absent S wave. Instead, the double-peaked RSR' pattern is noted (see Fig. 8-21B). In addition, V_1 shows a small R wave with a widened S wave, indicating delayed conduction through the ventricles. As in right bundle branch block, the ST segments and T waves may be abnormal in leads V_5 and V_6.

The most common causes of bundle branch block are myocardial infarction, hypertension, heart failure, and cardiomyopathy. Right bundle branch block may be found in healthy people with no clinical evidence of heart disease, in patients with congenital lesions involving the septum, and in patients with right ventricular hypertrophy. Left bundle branch block is usually associated with some type of underlying heart disease. Long-term cardiovascular

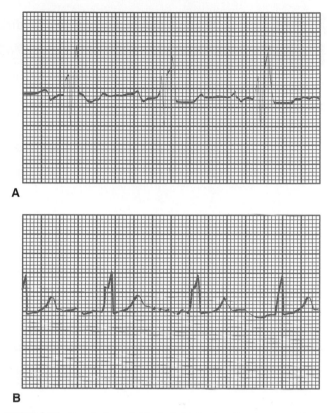

A

B

FIGURE 8-21 Bundle branch block. **A:** V_1 tracing showing the wide QRS complex and double-peaked R wave characteristic of right bundle branch block. **B:** A V_6 tracing showing the wide QRS complex and double-peaked R wave characteristic of left bundle branch block.

disease in the older patient is a common cause of left bundle branch block.

The patient is monitored for involvement of the other bundles or for progression to complete heart block. Progression of block may be very slow or rapid, depending on the clinical setting. A temporary pacemaker may be inserted until a permanent pacemaker can be placed, if indicated.

Management of Dysrhythmias

Pharmacotherapy

Antidysrhythmic drugs are used to restore the heart to a regular rhythm. The therapeutic window is small, and these drugs may have a toxic effect, especially when used in combination with other antidysrhythmic agents. Many antidysrhythmics are classified by their effect on the cardiac action potential—whether they block β-adrenoreceptors or sodium, potassium, or calcium channels (Table 8-6). Table 8-7 summarizes antidysrhythmic drugs that are commonly used in critical care settings.

Class I Antidysrhythmics (Sodium Channel Blockers)

Because many class I antidysrhythmics may cause life-threatening dysrhythmias and often interact

TABLE 8-6 Classification of Antidysrhythmic Medications

Class	Action	Examples
IA	Inhibits fast sodium channel, decreases automaticity, depresses phase 0, and prolongs the action potential duration	Quinidine Procainamide Disopyramide
IB	Inhibits fast sodium channel, depresses phase 0 slightly, and shortens action potential duration	Lidocaine Mexiletine
IC	Inhibits fast sodium channel, depresses phase 0 markedly, slows His–Purkinje conduction profoundly leading to a prolonged QRS duration	Flecainide Moricizine Propafenone
II	Depresses phase 4 depolarization, blocks sympathetic stimulation of the conduction system	Esmolol Propranolol Sotalol (plus class III effects) Acebutolol
III	Blocks potassium channel, prolongs phase 3 repolarization, prolongs action potential duration	Amiodarone Sotalol Ibutilide Dofetilide
IV	Inhibits inward calcium channel, depresses phase 4 depolarization, lengthens repolarization in phases 1 and 2	Verapamil Diltiazem

TABLE 8-7 Selected Antidysrhythmic Medications

Drug	Antidysrhythmic Indications	Major Adverse Effects
Class I		
Procainamide	Ventricular tachycardia, ventricular fibrillation, supraventricular tachycardias, atrial fibrillation, atrial flutter	Hypotension with IV use, asystole, ventricular fibrillation, heart block, torsades de pointes
Lidocaine	Ventricular tachycardia, ventricular fibrillation	Bradycardia, hypotension, tremors, dizziness, tinnitus, convulsions, mental status changes
Flecainide	Atrial fibrillation and paroxysmal supraventricular tachycardia (PSVT) in patients without structural heart disease; ventricular tachycardia	Ventricular dysrhythmias, palpitations, dizziness, dyspnea, headache, fatigue, nausea
Class II		
Esmolol	Supraventricular tachycardias including atrial fibrillation and atrial flutter; noncompensatory sinus tachycardia	Hypotension, heart block, bronchospasm
Propranolol	Supraventricular tachycardias; ventricular dysrhythmias; digoxin-induced tachydysrhythmias; premature ventricular contractions (PVCs)	Hypotension, heart block, bradycardia, heart failure, bronchospasm, gastrointestinal upset
Sotalol	Ventricular tachycardia, ventricular fibrillation, maintenance of normal sinus rhythm in patients with symptomatic atrial fibrillation or atrial flutter	Bradycardia, AV block, heart failure, bronchospasm, gastric pain
Class III		
Ibutilide	Atrial fibrillation, atrial flutter	Hypotension, torsades de pointes, ventricular tachycardia, bundle branch block, bradycardia
Dofetilide	Atrial fibrillation, atrial flutter; maintenance of normal sinus rhythm after conversion	Torsades de pointes, bradycardia
Amiodarone	Ventricular fibrillation, ventricular tachycardia, pulseless ventricular tachycardia, atrial fibrillation, atrial flutter; wide-complex tachycardia, and preexcited atrial fibrillation	Heart block, cardiac arrest, bradycardia, hypotension, ventricular tachycardia
Class IV		
Verapamil	PSVT, ventricular rate control in atrial fibrillation, atrial flutter	Hypotension, heart block, heart failure, bradycardia
Diltiazem	Ventricular rate control in atrial fibrillation, atrial flutter; PVST	Bradycardia, heart block, hypotension
Unclassified		
Adenosine	PSVT; idiopathic ventricular tachycardia; evaluation of ventricular tachycardia, supraventricular tachycardia, latent preexcitation	Bradycardia, heart block, asystole, chest pain
Atropine	Symptomatic sinus bradycardia, AV block, asystole, bradycardic pulseless electrical activity	Palpitations, tachycardia
Digoxin	Ventricular rate control in atrial fibrillation	Heart block, bradycardia, digoxin toxicity
Magnesium sulfate	Torsades de pointes; refractory ventricular tachycardia and ventricular fibrillation; life-threatening dysrhythmias caused by digoxin toxicity	Hypotension, nausea, depressed reflexes, and flushing

with other drugs commonly used for cardiovascular disease, these agents are used only in select cases. In general, research data do not support the effectiveness of class I antidysrhythmics.

Class II Antidysrhythmics (β-Adrenergic Blockers)

This class of drugs has a broad spectrum of activity and an established safety record and is currently the best class of antidysrhythmics for *general* use. Acebutolol, esmolol, propranolol, and sotalol are approved to treat dysrhythmias.

Class III Antidysrhythmic Drugs (Potassium Channel Blockers)

Amiodarone is indicated for the treatment of ventricular tachycardia, atrial fibrillation, and atrial flutter. The advanced cardiac life support (ACLS) algorithms include amiodarone as a first-line option for treating ventricular fibrillation, pulseless ventricular tachycardia, wide-complex tachycardia (either supraventricular or ventricular), and atrial fibrillation.[3] Limitations of amiodarone include its variable onset of action, intolerable adverse effects, dangerous drug interactions, and life-threatening complications associated with chronic therapy.

Ibutilide and dofetilide are indicated for atrial fibrillation and atrial flutter. Ibutilide inhibits potassium current and enhances sodium current, prolonging repolarization. Dofetilide blocks the rapid potassium current channel, prolonging the action potential duration and refractory period. Although these agents may cause a prolonged QT interval and torsades de pointes, they have fewer systemic adverse effects than other class III agents.

Class IV Antidysrhythmics (Calcium Channel Blockers)

Class IV agents are primarily indicated for the treatment of supraventricular tachycardia. In general, calcium channel blockers are only used when β-adrenergic blockers are contraindicated or maximal dosage has been reached without effect. Adverse effects include hypotension, decreased myocardial contractility (except with diltiazem), and bradycardia.

Adenosine

Adenosine is a first-line antidysrhythmic that effectively converts narrow-complex PSVT to normal sinus rhythm by slowing conduction through the AV node. This agent is effective in terminating dysrhythmias caused by reentry involving the SA and AV nodes; however, it does not convert atrial fibrillation, atrial flutter, or ventricular tachycardia to sinus rhythm. Adenosine is also used to differentiate between ventricular tachycardia and supraventricular tachycardia, and treat rare forms of idiopathic ventricular tachycardia. The half-life of adenosine is less than 10 seconds; therefore, adverse effects (which include a brief period of asystole) are short-lived.

Magnesium Sulfate

Magnesium sulfate is the drug of choice for treating torsades de pointes. Magnesium is also used for refractory ventricular tachycardia and ventricular fibrillation, as well as for life-threatening dysrhythmias caused by digoxin toxicity. Its mechanism of action is unclear; however, it has calcium channel blocking properties and inhibits sodium and potassium channels.

Atropine

Atropine reduces the effects of vagal stimulation, thus increasing heart rate and improving cardiac function. It is a first-line drug used to treat symptomatic bradycardia and slowed conduction at the AV node.

 RED FLAG! *It is important not to increase the heart rate excessively in patients with ischemic heart disease because doing so may increase myocardial oxygen consumption and worsen ischemia.*

Digoxin

Digoxin is a mild positive inotrope with antidysrhythmic and bradycardic actions. It is primarily indicated for patients with both heart failure and chronic atrial fibrillation. It may also be used to control a rapid ventricular rate associated with atrial fibrillation or atrial flutter and in combination with calcium channel blockers or β-adrenergic blockers for patients without heart failure. Because of its narrow therapeutic window, toxicity is common and is frequently associated with serious dysrhythmias. Other signs and symptoms of toxicity include palpitations, syncope, gastrointestinal upset, and neurologic changes.

Electrical Cardioversion

In electrical cardioversion, a defibrillator is used to deliver a shock that is synchronized with ventricular depolarization by detecting the patient's R wave; this minimizes the risk for causing ventricular fibrillation, which can occur if a shock is delivered during ventricular repolarization (on the T wave). Cardioversion is indicated to convert sustained supraventricular or ventricular tachydysrhythmias to sinus rhythm, especially when the patient is hemodynamically unstable. It may be used electively for recent-onset dysrhythmias that do not respond to antidysrhythmic agents.

Although recommendations are made for the amount of joules needed to convert various rhythms (Table 8-8), the actual energy needed may vary

TABLE 8-8   Energy Requirements for Cardioversion

Dysrhythmia	Energy Requirements in Joules (J)[a]
Monomorphic ventricular tachycardia with a pulse	100–360
Atrial flutter	50
Atrial fibrillation	200 initially

[a]Energy requirements given are for a monophasic defibrillator. Energy requirements for a biphasic defibrillator vary but are usually less.

depending on the duration of the dysrhythmia, transthoracic impedance, and the type of defibrillator (ie, monophasic or biphasic). Monophasic defibrillators deliver a current of electricity that travels in a single direction between the two paddles that are placed on the patient's chest, whereas biphasic defibrillators deliver a current of electricity that travels back and forth between the two paddles, thus requiring fewer joules.

Precautions and relative contraindications for cardioversion are listed in Table 8-9. The patient should have nothing by mouth before the procedure and receive sedation. After conversion to sinus rhythm, antidysrhythmic therapy may be initiated for rhythm maintenance.

Radiofrequency Ablation

In radiofrequency ablation, a percutaneous catheter is inserted through a vein or artery and positioned in the heart to deliver radiofrequency energy to a localized area of the myocardium, creating a small area of irreversible tissue injury. The localized area of damage prevents the dysrhythmia by eliminating its point of origination (ie, its focus) or by interrupting its conduction (accessory pathway). Radiofrequency ablation is used to treat tachydysrhythmias (eg, PSVT, AV nodal reentrant tachycardia, atrial fibrillation, or flutter).[4]

Before ablation, the patient undergoes an electrophysiological study (EPS). During the EPS, catheters are placed in the heart to record intracardiac electrograms (IC-EGMs). The test provides information about the sequence of electrical activation of the heart in sinus rhythm and any abnormal sequence of activation during an induced dysrhythmia. The recordings are used to create a map that is used to guide the placement of the ablating catheter by identifying the focus of the dysrhythmia or the location of an accessory pathway. When the appropriate site is identified, an ablating catheter is positioned in the targeted area of the heart and the radiofrequency current is applied. Elimination of the target site is evaluated by examining the ECG and IC-EGM tracings and confirmed when the dysrhythmia is no longer inducible on a postprocedure EPS.

Cardiac Pacing

Cardiac pacing is most commonly indicated for conditions that result in failure of the heart to initiate or conduct an intrinsic electrical impulse at a rate adequate to maintain perfusion (eg, dysrhythmias, atherosclerotic heart disease, acute myocardial infarction). Cardiac pacing can be used to treat bradydysrhythmias and tachydysrhythmias. Common terms associated with cardiac pacing are defined in Box 8-6.

Types of Pacing Systems

Pacing systems consist of a pulse generator and one to three leads with electrodes. The electrodes at the distal end of the lead provide sensing and pacing of the heart muscle. Cardiac pacing may be permanent or temporary.

Permanent Pacing Systems

Box 8-7 summarizes indications for permanent cardiac pacing. Most permanent pulse generators are inserted in a subcutaneous pocket in the pectoral region below the clavicle (Fig. 8-22). The pulse generator for a permanent pacemaker is a lithium iodide battery, which lasts for about 6 to 12 years. The permanent pacemaker lead is typically inserted either through a subclavian vein or a cephalic vein through the chest wall (see Fig. 8-22). The lead is then positioned with fluoroscopic guidance and affixed in the right atrial appendage or in the apex of the right ventricle, or in both locations. A third lead may be inserted in a coronary sinus branch to stimulate the left ventricle for biventricular pacing.

TABLE 8-9   Precautions and Relative Contraindications to Cardioversion

Condition	Complications
Digoxin toxicity	Ventricular irritability, asystole
Hypokalemia	Ventricular irritability/fibrillation
Atrial fibrillation with slow ventricular response	Postcardioversion asystole
Atrial fibrillation of unknown duration with inadequate anticoagulation	Thromboembolization
Pacemaker dependency	Rise in thresholds with loss of capture
Low-amplitude R wave	Synchronization on T wave leading to ventricular fibrillation

BOX 8.6   Clinical Terminology Related to Pacemakers

Active fixation lead: A pacing lead with some design at the lead tip (corkscrew, coil) that allows the tip to be embedded in heart tissue, thus decreasing the likelihood of dislodgment

Asynchronous pacing: A pacemaker that fires at a fixed rate regardless of the intrinsic activity of the heart

Bipolar lead: A pacing lead containing two electrodes. One electrode is at the tip of the lead and provides stimulation to the heart. A second electrode is several millimeters proximal to the tip and completes the electrical circuit. Both electrodes provide sensing of the intrinsic cardiac activity.

Capture: The depolarization of a cardiac chamber in response to a pacing stimulus

Chronotropic incompetence: Inability of the sinus node to accelerate in response to exercise

Demand pacing (inhibited pacing): A pacemaker that withholds its pacing stimulus when sensing an adequate intrinsic heart rate

Dual-chamber pacing (physiological pacing): Pacing in both the atria and the ventricles to artificially restore atrioventricular (AV) synchrony

Electromagnetic interference: Electrical or magnetic energy that can interfere with or disrupt the function of the pulse generator

Milliamperage (mA): The unit of measure used for the electrical stimulus (output) generated by the pacemaker

Multisite pacing: The ability to stimulate more than one site in a chamber (eg, right ventricle and left ventricle stimulation in biventricular pacing)

Overdrive pacing: A method of suppressing tachycardia by pacing the heart at a rate faster than the patient's intrinsic rate

Oversensing: Inhibition of the pacemaker by events other than those that the pacemaker was intended to sense (eg, electromagnetic interference, tall T waves)

Pacing threshold: The minimal electrical stimulation required to initiate atrial or ventricular depolarization consistently; expressed as milliamperage (mA) in temporary pacing systems and voltage (V) in permanent pacing systems

Passive fixation lead: A pacing lead that lodges in the trabeculae of the heart without actually penetrating the cardiac wall

Rate-responsive (rate-adaptive, rate-modulated) pacing: A pacemaker that alters pacing rate in response to detected changes in the body's metabolic demand

Sensing: The ability of the pacemaker to detect intrinsic cardiac activity and respond appropriately; how the pacemaker responds depends on the programmed mode of pacing

Sensing threshold: The minimal atrial or ventricular intracardiac signal amplitude required to inhibit or trigger a demand pacemaker

Situational vasovagal syncope: Syncope associated with bradycardia by vagal stimulation during coughing, micturition, or severe pain

Triggered: A response to sensing in which the pacemaker fires a stimulus in response to intrinsic cardiac activity

Undersensing: Failure of the pacemaker to sense the heart's intrinsic activity, resulting in inappropriate firing of the pacemaker

Temporary Pacing Systems

Temporary pacing is used both emergently (eg, to correct life-threatening situations such as asystole, complete heart block, severe bradydysrhythmias, and cardiac arrest) and electively (eg, to evaluate the need for permanent pacing, after cardiac surgery, or for overdrive pacing of tachydysrhythmias). Temporary pacing systems may be transvenous, epicardial, transcutaneous, or transthoracic.

Transvenous Pacing. A transvenous pacing system consists of an external pulse generator and a temporary transvenous pacing lead. The temporary transvenous lead system usually includes a bipolar catheter. The bipolar catheter has a negative distal electrode and a positive proximal electrode that attach to the negative and positive generator terminals, respectively, on the pulse generator. The

BOX 8-7   Indications for Permanent Cardiac Pacing

- Second-degree atrioventricular (AV) block—Mobitz II
- Third-degree (complete) heart block
- Bilateral bundle branch blocks
- Symptomatic bradydysrhythmias
- Asystole
- Sick sinus syndrome
- Prophylaxis during open heart surgery
- Tachydysrhythmias
- Bifascicular LBBB

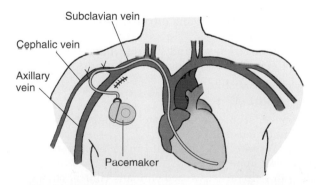

FIGURE 8-22 Transvenous installation of a permanent pacemaker. For dual-chamber pacing, a separate pacing wire would be in the atrium.

catheter is introduced into the brachial, internal or external jugular, subclavian, or femoral vein. The subclavian and internal jugular sites promote catheter stability and allow patient mobility. The catheter is threaded through a sheath in the vein, and the tip is placed in contact with the endocardial surface of the right ventricular apex for stability and reliability.[5] For atrial pacing, an atrial bipolar catheter is placed in the right atrial appendage.

After catheter placement, the sheath is attached to a continuous drip (if it will be used for drawing blood or administering drugs). To maintain sterility, a sterile protective sleeve over the catheter can be used before insertion and then connected to the end of the sheath after satisfactory position is confirmed. The insertion site is covered with a biopatch and a self-adhesive, semipermeable transparent dressing. Nursing care of a patient with a temporary transvenous pacemaker is summarized in Box 8-8.

Epicardial Pacing. In epicardial pacing, the pacing electrodes are placed directly on the outer surface of the heart. Placement of the electrodes can be accomplished by thoracotomy or through a subxiphoid incision. Epicardial pacing is often used as a temporary adjunct during and after open heart surgery. After attaching the pacing wires to the epicardium, the proximal end is brought outside through the chest incision and either connected to a temporary pacemaker generator or capped and then connected if the need for pacing arises. The wires are extracted without reopening the incision, even after scar tissue has formed over the tips.

Transcutaneous Pacing. Transcutaneous pacing involves placing large gelled electrode patches directly on the chest wall, anteriorly to the left of the sternum, and posteriorly on the patient's back (Fig 8-23). It may be used as a "bridge" (temporary measure) until either a transvenous or permanent pacemaker can be placed. Indications for transcutaneous pacing include symptomatic bradycardia (unresponsive to drug therapy), new Mobitz type II heart block, and new third-degree (complete) heart block. Transcutaneous pacing may also be used when transvenous pacing is contradicted or

BOX 8-8 Nursing Responsibilities in Transvenous Pacing

Assessment

During insertion:

- Vital signs, oxygen saturation, peripheral pulses
- Level of sedation/sedative agents used
- Date, time, method, and site of insertion
- Location of wire inserted (atrial, ventricular, atrial and ventricular)
- Measured values: capture threshold (mA) and intrinsic amplitude (mV)
- Patient's tolerance of procedure
- Complications
- Continuous cardiac monitoring and 12-lead electrocardiogram (ECG)
- Final settings: mode, rate, output, and sensitivity

After insertion:

- Rate setting, mV setting, mA setting, mode of operation (demand, asynchronous) and atrioventricular (AV) interval (if appropriate)
- Pacemaker turned off or on
- Rhythm strip, capture and intrinsic (if appropriate); 12-lead ECG
- Status of insertion site and sutures (if present)
- Completion of chest radiograph and results on chart

Every change of shift:

- Pacemaker turned off or on
- Pacemaker secured appropriately to patient
- All connections secured
- Setting for rate, mA, sensitivity, mode of operation AV interval (if appropriate)
- Rhythm strip (also assessed with any clinical change or intervention)
- Sensing and capture thresholds (compare to baseline)

- Presence/absence of hiccupping or muscle twitching
- Status of insertion site and sutures (if present)
- Signs of infection
- Pulse perfusion distal to insertion site (if appropriate)
- Connective ends of pacer wires covered (as appropriate)

Interventions

- Continuous cardiac monitoring
- Verify replacement 9-V battery available.
- Verify connections are intact.
- Label epicardial pacer wires *atrial* or *ventricular*.
- Clean and dress pacer wire insertion site(s) daily with gauze dressing or transparent dressing per institutional protocol. Label time and date of dressing change and initial.
- Observe electrical safety precautions.
  - Keep electrical equipment in the room to a minimum and ensure that it is properly grounded.
  - Avoid simultaneous contact with the patient and any electrical equipment.
  - Cover connective ends of pacer wires to prevent microshock hazard.
  - Wear rubber or latex gloves when handling the connective ends of pacer wires.

Documentation

- Assessments
- Instructions to patient/family
- Pacing wire insertion site care
- Pacing and sensing thresholds (print ECG strips)
- Pacing problems or complications, nursing interventions, and results of interventions

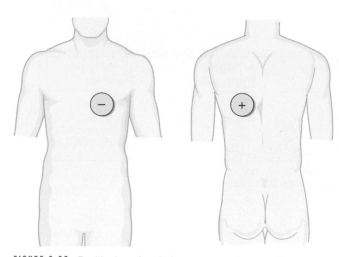

FIGURE 8-23   Positioning of pads for transcutaneous pacing.

not immediately available. The transcutaneous pacemaker is used in a "demand mode" for brady-cardia and asystole; it paces the heart only when needed. This mode is safer because the chance of firing on the T wave (R-on-T phenomenon) is greatly reduced.

The procedure for initiating transcutaneous pacing and monitoring considerations are summarized in Box 8-9. Because transcutaneous pacing can cause significant discomfort, the patient should be made aware of this and adequately sedated. Following initiation of therapy, diligent monitoring is required. A loss of capture can occur if the electrodes fail to maintain good contact with the skin. Inappropriate pacing may result if the pacemaker cannot detect

BOX 8-9   Nursing Responsibilities in Transcutaneous Pacing

1. Explain procedure to patient.
2. Clip excess hair from chest (do not shave skin); ensure skin is dry.
3. Apply anterior electrode to chest at the fourth inter-costal space to the left of the sternum.
4. Apply posterior electrode to patient's back in the area of the left scapula.
5. Connect pacing electrodes to transcutaneous pacemaker.
6. Set pacemaker mode, heart rate, and output.
7. Turn unit on.
8. Assess for effectiveness of pacing:
   • Observe for pacemaker spike with subsequent capture.
   • Assess heart rate and rhythm.
   • Assess blood pressure. (Measure blood pressure in the right arm to avoid interference from the pacemaker.)
   • Check level of consciousness.
   • Observe for patient anxiety/pain and treat accordingly.

the heart's intrinsic rhythm. In either case, the nurse must recognize the problem and reposition either the patient or the electrodes to ensure efficacious transcutaneous pacing.

Transthoracic Pacing. Transthoracic pacing, which involves placing a pacing needle in the ante-rior wall of the heart, is used only as a last resort in emergency situations. It has limited success rates and a high potential for complications.

Functioning of Pacing Systems

The sensing function is the ability of the pacemaker to detect the heart's intrinsic activity. The sensing amplitude is the largest intrinsic signal that is consistently detected by the pacemaker electrode (eg, the R wave is usually the largest signal sensed by the ventricular lead). The smallest number on the sensor control represents the most sensitive set-ting in millivolts (mV), and it indicates the smallest signal the pacemaker will sense.

When the intrinsic heart rate is adequate, the pace-maker responds by inhibiting a pacing stimulus. When the intrinsic heart rate drops below the programmed minimum rate, the pacemaker delivers an electrical stimulus that depolarizes the cardiac chamber con-taining the pacemaker lead. The minimal amount of voltage required from the pacemaker to initiate con-sistent capture is known as the pacing threshold and is measured in milliamps (mA). Many factors affect the pacing threshold, including hypoxia, hyperkale-mia, antidysrhythmic drugs, catecholamines, digoxin toxicity, and corticosteroids. The pacing threshold is determined by establishing successful pacing at higher energy and then gradually decreasing the energy out-put of the generator until capture ceases. The gen crator output is then set at two or three times the threshold level to allow for an adequate safety margin.

A coding system, called the NBG pacemaker code, has been formed to identify the various modes of pacemaker operation (Box 8-10). Knowledge of the three- and five-letter pacemaker code helps the nurse determine the type of implanted device, the intended mode of operation, and the actual mode of operation.

Nursing Care of the Patient Undergoing Cardiac Pacing

Preprocedure

Prior to permanent pacemaker implantation, the nurse assesses the patient's medical and social history. Information gleaned from the medical and social his-tory can influence decisions such as which approach to use during the procedure, and which side is favored for implantation. For example, a subclavian approach may be avoided in a person with a history of a collapsed lung or previous lobectomy, and the right pectoral region may be avoided for pacemaker implantation in a right-handed tennis player. Psychosocial assessment is also important. Patients' psychosocial responses to the need for cardiac pacing may differ. Some may be relieved to have a device that supports the functioning

BOX 8-10 Using the NBG Pacemaker Code

I: Chamber(s) Paced	II: Chamber(s) Sensed	III: Response to Sensing	IV: Rate Modulation	V: Multisite Pacing
O = none A = atrium V = ventricle D = dual (A +V)	O = none A = atrium V = ventricle D = dual (A + V)	O = none T = triggered I = inhibited D = dual (T + I)	O = none R = rate modulation	O = none A = atrium V = ventricle D = dual (A + V)

Adapted from North American Society of Pacing and Electrophysiology/British Pacing and Electrophysiology Group: The revised NASPE/BPEG generic code for antibradycardia, adaptive-rate, and multisite pacing. Pacing Clin Electrophysiol 25(2):260–264, 2002.

- The first position describes the chamber or chambers paced.
- The second position describes the chamber or chambers sensed.
- The third position describes the pacemaker's response to sensed intrinsic cardiac activity.

   The letter "I" means that the pacemaker is inhibited from firing in response to a sensed intrinsic event.

   The letter "T" indicates that the pacemaker triggers pacing stimuli in response to a sensed intrinsic beat.

   The letter "D" designates a dual response (inhibited pacing output and triggered pacing after sensed event).

   The letter "O" designates a mode in which the pacemaker does not respond to sensed intrinsic activity (asynchronous pacing).

- The fourth position describes the presence or absence of rate modulation (variation of the pacing rate in response to a physiological variable).

   The letter "O" denotes no rate modulation.

   The letter "R" means that the rate modulation feature is active. When the rate modulation feature is active, the pacer detects the physiological response in response to patient activity (eg, muscle vibration, increased respiratory rate) and increases the pacing rate to meet increased metabolic demands. The rate modulation feature is not used in temporary pacing.

- The fifth position describes whether multisite pacing is present.

   The absence of a fourth- or fifth-letter designation signifies no rate modulation and no multisite pacing.

of their heart, whereas others may be anxious about the technology and express fears of dying.

Patient and family teaching about cardiac pacing begins at the time the decision for pacemaker insertion is made. After assessing the patient's baseline knowledge about pacemakers and clarifying any misperceptions, the nurse explains the need for pacing, how the pacing system works, the insertion procedure, and the immediate postprocedure care that can be expected. Patient teaching continues during the postprocedure period, when the nurse provides the patient with product specifications for all components of the system (eg, manufacturer, model number, serial number), explains signs and symptoms of pacemaker malfunction and how to report them, explains the importance of keeping follow-up appointments, and explains the general time line and procedure for pulse generator replacement.

Postprocedure

Assessment helps the nurse determine the patient's physiologic response to cardiac pacing. Important parameters to assess include pulse rate; underlying cardiac rhythm; blood pressure; activity tolerance; signs and symptoms such as dizziness, syncope, dyspnea, palpitations, or edema; and the results of

chest radiographs, blood tests, and other relevant laboratory tests. In addition, the nurse monitors for potential complications (Table 8-10).

Electrocardiogram Monitoring. Careful monitoring of the ECG of the patient with a cardiac pacemaker is an essential component of comprehensive patient assessment.

The first step in ECG analysis involves examining the strip for evidence of pacemaker stimulation. When the pacemaker discharges, an artifact called a pacing spike appears on the ECG. If the pacing lead is in the atria, a pacing spike is followed by a P wave. If the pacing wire is in the ventricle, the spike is followed by a wide QRS complex (Fig. 8-24, p. 87). Failure of the pacing stimulus to capture the ventricles or atria is noted by the absence of the QRS or P wave immediately after the pacing spike on the ECG (Fig. 8-25, p. 88).

The sensing function of the pacemaker is evaluated next. If the pacemaker does not sense intrinsic cardiac activity (undersensing), inappropriate pacemaker spikes may appear throughout the underlying rhythm (Fig. 8-26A, p. 88). An oversensing problem can be detected when the pacemaker senses events other than the intrinsic rhythm and is inappropriately inhibited in that chamber or

TABLE 8-10 **Pacemaker Complications**

Complication	Presentation	Confirmation
Pneumothorax	Pleuritic pain; hypotension; respiratory distress or hypoxia	Chest radiograph
Ventricular irritability	Premature ventricular complexes (PVCs) appear similar in configuration to the pacemaker complexes	12-lead electrocardiogram (ECG) or cardiac monitoring
Perforation of ventricular wall or septum	Change in precordial lead waveform morphology or negative QRS complex in lead V_1	12-lead ECG or cardiac monitoring
	Pericardial tamponade (decrease in blood pressure, increase in heart rate)	Two-dimensional echocardiogram
Catheter or lead dislodgement	Failure to capture	12-lead ECG, chest radiograph
Infection and phlebitis or hematoma formation	Swelling, inflammation, drainage, hematoma	Inspection and cultures
Abdominal twitching or hiccups	Twitching, hiccups, discomfort; when associated with perforation, a drop in blood pressure	Observation
Pocket erosion	Swelling, inflammation, drainage	Inspection, culture

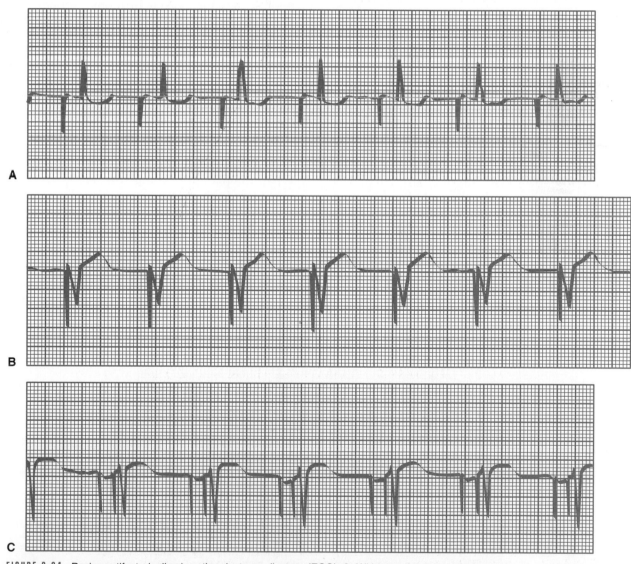

FIGURE 8-24 Pacing artifacts (spikes) on the electrocardiogram (ECG). **A:** With an atrial pacemaker, each pacing spike is followed by a P wave. **B:** With a ventricular pacemaker, each pacing spike is followed by a wide QRS complex. **C:** With a dual-chamber pacemaker, the first pacing spike is followed by a P wave and the second pacing spike is followed by a QRS complex. All strips show 1:1 capture.

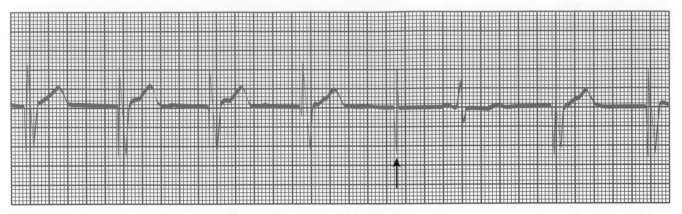

FIGURE 8-25   Failure to capture. The pacing spike is not followed by a QRS complex.

causes a triggered response in the other chamber (see Fig. 8-26B).

The third step in evaluating the ECG is to measure various intervals (Fig. 8-27). The duration of each interval is compared with the programmed setting for that interval.

- The pacing interval (ie, the amount of time between two consecutive pacing spikes in the chamber being paced) is used to determine the pacing rate.
- The AV interval is analogous to the PR interval on the ECG. The AV interval is measured from the beginning of an intrinsic P wave or an atrial pacing spike to the beginning of the intrinsic QRS complex or the ventricular pacing spike (see Fig. 8-27).
- The ventriculoatrial (VA) interval, also called the atrial escape interval, is the amount of time from a ventricular paced or sensed event to the next atrial paced stimulus (see Fig. 8-27).

Troubleshooting Pacing Systems. Malfunction of a pacemaker can be a result of inappropriate programming (pseudomalfunction) or a true component malfunction. A malfunction of the pacemaker is addressed systematically. Immediate action is required to restore pacemaker function when the patient has no underlying rhythm. The following steps are taken:

1. Increase pulse generator output (in mA) to the highest setting, asynchronous mode (VOO, DOO). Asynchronous mode allows assessment for appropriate firing and capture when the patient's rhythm is overridden by the fixed pacing pulse.
2. Check the patient's hemodynamics and simultaneous multiple ECG lead recordings and intervene if appropriate with transcutaneous pacing or atropine sulfate.
3. Check all connections.
4. Replace the pulse generator or battery; be prepared to provide transcutaneous pacing backup during the change.
5. When the patient is stable, proceed with troubleshooting (Table 8-11).

Implantable Cardioverter–Defibrillators

An ICD monitors the patient's rhythm continuously, diagnoses rhythm changes, and treats life-threatening ventricular dysrhythmias. Similar to a pacemaker, the ICD consists of a lead system and a pulse generator. Ideally, the ICD generator is

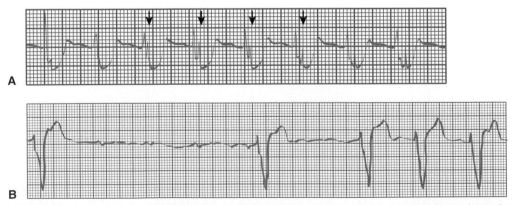

FIGURE 8-26   Undersensing and oversensing. **A:** Failure of the ventricular demand pacemaker to detect the intrinsic rhythm (undersensing) is shown by pacemaker spikes at inappropriate intervals after spontaneous QRS complexes. **B:** Failure of the pacemaker to discharge (oversensing) causing pacing inhibition (noted in the first half of the strip).

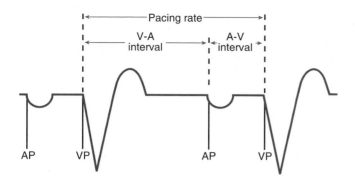

AP = atrial pacing spike
VP = ventricular pacing spike

FIGURE 8-27 The intervals measured on an electrocardiogram (ECG) strip for a patient with a pacemaker.

implanted in the left pectoral area so that the heart is central to the vector of the defibrillation current (Fig. 8-28).

ICDs have been categorized into "generations," based on their functionality.

- The first-generation ICDs were nonprogrammable devices that used a factory-specified rate criterion.
- The second-generation ICDs have programmable features, including bradycardia and antitachycardia pacing and synchronized cardioversion. These features allow the use of tiered therapy (ie, different levels of therapy to treat a dysrhythmia). The first tier of therapy is usually antitachycardia pacing, which involves the carefully timed delivery of pacing stimuli. If antitachycardia pacing is not successful, the second tier of therapy (low-energy synchronized cardioversion) is initiated. Some devices allow multiple attempts at cardioversion. If cardioversion is not successful, the third tier of therapy, defibrillation, is used. The number of defibrillation attempts varies with different devices, but six attempts is usually the maximum. If the patient is successfully converted to a life-compatible rhythm, but the rate is slow, ventricular demand pacing is initiated. Bradycardia pacing is usually intended for brief periods of pacing until normal rhythm resumes.

TABLE 8-11 Troubleshooting a Temporary Pacemaker

Problem	Cause	Intervention
Failure to pace: No evidence of pacing stimulus, patient's heart rate below programmed rate	Battery depletion or pulse generator failure, output or timing circuit failure Loose cable connection	Replace battery or generator. Check all connections for tightness.
Failure to capture: Pacing stimulus not followed by electrocardiogram (ECG) evidence of depolarization	Lead dislodgment	Review chest film, turn patient to left lateral decubitus position until lead can be replaced.
	Broken connector pins or fractured extension connecting cable	Connect wire directly to generator to diagnose cable problem, replace connecting cable.
	Incompatibility of wire pins with cable or to generator	Ascertain a secure fit of the exposed pin to the cable or the generator, adjust connection or replace pulse generator.
	Output setting (mA) too low Perforation	Check capture thresholds and adjust output to a two- to threefold safety margin.
	Lead fracture without insulation break	Review 12-lead ECG, report signs of perforation, stabilize hemodynamics.
	Increase in pacing threshold from medication or metabolic changes	Check intracavitary ECG; if evidence of fracture in one pole, unipolarize lead; if total fracture, replace lead. Check laboratory test results, correct metabolic alterations, review medications and vital signs, increase output.
Oversensing: Device detects noncardiac electrical events and interprets them as depolarization	Oversensitive setting	Reduce sensitivity (value [in millivolts] should be larger to make pacer less sensitive); if patient is pacer dependent (no intrinsic R wave), program to asynchronous mode until problem is corrected.
	Device detecting tall T waves and interpreting them as R waves	Increase ventricular refractory period beyond T wave.

TABLE 8-11   Troubleshooting a Temporary Pacemaker (continued)

Problem	Cause	Intervention
In dual-chamber pacing, cross talk is a form of oversensing: The device detects signals from the other chamber and inhibits; in atrial channel, R waves are detected as P waves.	Atrial lead dislodgment	Recheck atrial capture thresholds; if high, dislodgment is probable.
In ventricular channel, atrial pacing stimulus afterpotential is detected as an R wave, with V pacing inappropriately inhibited	High output from atrial channel	Reduce output from atrial channel, decrease ventricular channel sensitivity (higher millivolt value).
	Electrical interference, improperly grounded electrical devices	Remove nongrounded equipment.
Undersensing: Device fails to detect intrinsic cardiac activity and fires inappropriately	Asynchronous mode setting (VOO, DOO, AOO)	Reprogram to synchronous mode (VVI, DDD, AAI).
	Small intrinsic amplitude	Increase sensitivity (turn sensitivity dial toward lower millivolt value).
	Lead dislodgment	Recheck capture thresholds; if high, lead probably dislodged and needs repositioning.
	Lead insulation break	Check lead with pacing system analyzer, if impedance too low (<200 Ω), insulation break is likely, and lead needs to be replaced or can be temporarily placed in unipolar configuration.

- Third-generation devices have many programmable features that allow the physician to tailor the device to the patient's needs and that provide memory and event retrieval capabilities. Bradycardia pacing therapies with biventricular pacing are common features of current ICDs. To improve discrimination of tachydysrhythmias, the device allows programming of discrimination algorithms, which withhold therapy for ventricular tachycardia when PSVT is confirmed. The availability of an atrial sensing lead allows for a more specific PSVT discrimination algorithm. Some devices also have separate tiers of therapy for atrial tachycardia and atrial fibrillation or flutter. All third-generation ICDs are "noncommitted" (ie, therapy is aborted if the tachycardia terminates even while the ICD is charging).

As with cardiac pacemakers, a coding system, known as the NBD defibrillator code, has been developed to describe modes of ICD function. The first position of the code indicates the shock chamber—none, atrium, ventricle, or dual (O, A, V, or D). The second position indicates the chamber in which antitachycardia pacing is delivered—also coded O, A, V, or D. Position three indicates the means by which tachydysrhythmia is detected, either with the intracardiac electrogram (E) or by hemodynamic means (H). Most current ICDs detect dysrhythmias through intracardiac electrograms. The fourth position of the code is the three- or five-letter code for the pacemaker capability of the device. For example, a ventricular defibrillator that detects tachydysrhythmias using intracardiac electrograms and with adaptive rate ventricular antibradycardia pacing would be labeled VOE-VVIR.

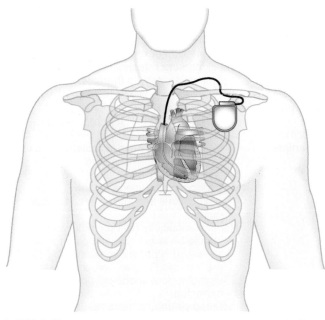

FIGURE 8-28   Positioning of the implantable cardioverter–defibrillator (ICD).

CASE STUDY

Mr. M. is a 64-year-old man admitted to the critical care unit for unstable angina and to rule out non-ST-segment elevation myocardial infarction (NSTEMI). He is placed on a continuous cardiac monitor using a five-lead placement. The monitor is set to read leads II and MCL₁ and display the ECG waveform continuously. A 12-lead ECG is obtained to assess for signs of ischemia, injury, or infarction.

Mr. M is noted initially to be in a sinus tachycardia (rate of 110 beats/min). Two hours later, the high rate alarms sound on the cardiac monitor and he is found to have an irregular rhythm with indiscernible P waves. On further assessment, he is noted to have the following vital signs: BP, 97/64 mm Hg; HR, 140 beats/min; RR, 32 breaths/min, as well as increasing chest pain and shortness of breath. The physician decides to perform synchronized cardioversion. The nurse prepares Mr. M. for the procedure and sedation is administered. The rhythm is converted with 50 J into a sinus tachycardia with a rate of 106 beats/min. On assessment, Mr. M.'s blood pressure is increased to 138/74 mm Hg. An antidysrhythmic is ordered and cardiac monitoring is continued.

1. What are the advantages of monitoring in leads I and MCL₁?

2. What rhythm did Mr. M. develop?

3. What are the immediate nursing priorities for a patient who develops a rhythm change?

4. Why was synchronized cardioversion used for Mr. M.?

References

1. Collins M: Using continuous ST segment monitoring. Nursing 40:11–13, 2010.
2. Pickham D, et al: How many patients need QT interval monitoring in critical care units? J Electrocardiol 43(6):572–576, 2010.
3. Advanced Cardiovascular Life Support (ACLS) for Healthcare Providers. (2010); American Heart Association.
4. Wilber DJ, et al.: Comparison of antiarrhythmic drug therapy and radiofrequency catheter ablation in patients with paroxysmal atrial fibrillation: a randomized controlled trial. JAMA 303(4):333–340, 2010.
5. Wigand, D. (ed): AACN Procedure Manual for Critical Care, 5th ed. Philadelphia: Elsevier, 2011.

Want to know more? A wide variety of resources to enhance your learning and understanding of this chapter are available on **thePoint**. Visit **http://thepoint.lww.com/MortonEss1e** to access chapter review questions and more!

Hemodynamic Monitoring

Based on the content in this chapter, the reader should be able to:

1 Describe the type of information provided by, and common indications for, hemodynamic monitoring.
2 State the basic components of a pressure monitoring system and describe nursing interventions that ensure accuracy of pressure readings and waveforms.
3 Describe nursing interventions associated with arterial pressure monitoring.
4 Interpret data obtained through arterial pressure monitoring.
5 Describe nursing interventions associated with central venous pressure monitoring.
6 Interpret data obtained through central venous pressure monitoring.
7 Describe nursing interventions associated with pulmonary artery pressure monitoring.
8 Interpret data obtained through pulmonary artery pressure monitoring.
9 Describe methods commonly used in the critical care setting to determine cardiac output.
10 List factors that affect oxygen demand and oxygen delivery, and describe methods used to evaluate the balance of oxygen supply, oxygen consumption, and oxygen demand.

Hemodynamic monitoring provides information at the bedside about intracardiac and intravascular pressures and cardiac output. It is used in the critical care setting to assess cardiac function and evaluate the effectiveness of therapy. Because a primary goal of management of critically ill patients is to ensure adequate oxygenation of tissues and organs, hemodynamic monitoring is indicated for patients with conditions that are characterized by insufficient cardiac output due to alterations in intravascular volume (preload), alterations in vascular resistance (afterload), or alterations in myocardial contractility (Box 9-1). Although invasive hemodynamic monitoring technology is used most frequently in the critical care setting, minimally invasive and noninvasive hemodynamic monitoring technologies also exist.

Common Indications for Hemodynamic Monitoring

- Cardiogenic shock
- Severe heart failure
- Sepsis or septic shock
- Multiple organ system dysfunction (MODS)
- Acute respiratory distress syndrome (ARDS)
- Cardiac surgery

Overview of the Pressure Monitoring System

System Components

A pressure monitoring system (Fig. 9-1) transmits pressures from the intravascular space or cardiac chambers through a catheter and fluid-filled noncompliant pressure tubing to a pressure transducer. The transducer converts the physiological signal from the patient into an electrical signal, which the monitor converts to a pressure tracing and digital value. The monitor is able to display several pressure tracings and digital values simultaneously. Controls on the monitor also allow the user to label waveform locations, set or adjust alarms and tracing scale size, and zero the system.

A patent pressure system is maintained by using a continuous flush solution, typically normal saline or dextrose and water (D_5W). The flush solution may also be heparinized. The bag of solution is placed in a continuous pressure infusion device to exert approximately 300 mm Hg of pressure. A continuous flow of approximately 3 to 5 mL/h prevents backflow of blood through the catheter and tubing, thereby maintaining system patency and ensuring accurate transmission of pressures. The system can be flushed manually by activating the flush device.

Ensuring Accuracy

For optimal use of pressure monitoring systems, it is essential to ensure accurate pressure recordings and waveform display. Techniques used to ensure accuracy include the square-wave test (dynamic response testing) and leveling and zeroing the system.

Square-Wave Test (Dynamic Response Testing)

The square-wave test is used to determine the system's ability to accurately measure pressures. Each beat of the heart generates a pressure waveform, which is propagated at a certain frequency (ie, beats per minute) through the systemic circulation. Vascular resistance diminishes (dampens) the waveform's magnitude over time. In a pressure monitoring system, the natural frequency indicates how fast the pressure monitoring system oscillates in response to a signal (eg, the arterial pressure pulse). The

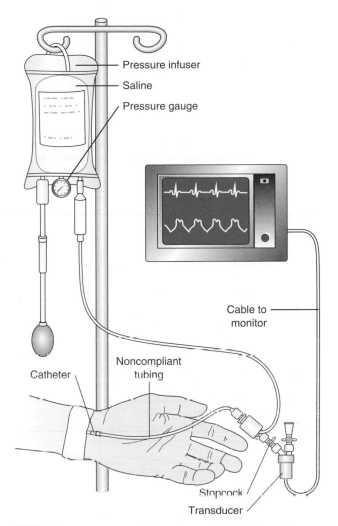

FIGURE 9-1 Pressure monitoring system. An indwelling catheter is attached by noncompliant pressure tubing to a transducer. The transducer is connected to a monitor that displays a waveform and systolic, diastolic, and mean pressure values. The system is composed of a solution under pressure to maintain system patency, a flush device and stopcocks are used for drawing arterial blood samples and zeroing the system.

damping coefficient is a measure of how quickly the oscillations diminish (dampen) and eventually cease. The dynamic response of the system determines the natural frequency and the damping coefficient of the system. Factors that can affect the dynamic response of the system include the system's natural frequency, the quality of the pressure tubing, the number of stopcocks, and the presence of blood sampling systems.

The test done to evaluate dynamic response is commonly known as the "square-wave test."[1] To perform the square-wave test, the flush device is activated and rapidly released. The nurse observes the bedside monitor for the waveform to rise sharply and "square off" at the top of the scale. After the flush device is released, the nurse observes the waveform as it returns to baseline, counts the number of oscillations, and observes the distance between them. In an ideal (optimally damped) system, the square wave has a straight vertical upstroke from the baseline, a

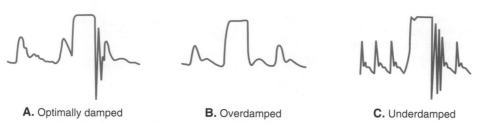

A. Optimally damped   **B.** Overdamped   **C.** Underdamped

FIGURE 9-2 Dynamic response (square-wave) testing. **A:** Optimally damped system. Activation of the flush device generates a sharp vertical upstroke, horizontal line, and straight vertical downstroke ending with 1.5 to 2 oscillations close together before returning to baseline. **B:** Overdamped system. Activation of the flush device generates a slurred upstroke and downstroke with less than 1.5 oscillations above or below the baseline. **C:** Underdamped system. Activation of the flush device generates more than 2 to 3 oscillations above and below the baseline. (Courtesy of Edwards Lifesciences LLC.)

straight horizontal component, and a straight vertical downstroke with approximately 1.5 to 2 sharp oscillations before returning to baseline. The distance between the oscillations is also short. Figure 9-2 depicts the results of dynamic response testing for an optimally damped system, an overdamped system, and an underdamped system. Overdamped systems, which may be caused by system leaks, blood clots, excessively long tubing, or large air bubbles in the tubing or transducer, produce erroneously low systolic pressures. Underdamped systems, which may be caused by small air bubbles in the system or very rigid pressure tubing, produce erroneously high systolic pressures and erroneously low diastolic pressures.

Leveling and Zeroing

To ensure accurate pressure monitoring, the transducer is leveled to an external landmark known as the phlebostatic axis (zero reference point), and then zeroed to atmospheric pressure. The phlebostatic axis is the fourth intercostal space, midaxillary level (Fig. 9-3A). Once the phlebostatic axis is established, the patient's chest wall can be marked to ensure consistent leveling when obtaining subsequent pressure readings. With the patient placed in the supine position, a carpenter-type level or laser-light level is used to align the air–fluid interface

(typically, the stopcock nearest the transducer) with the phlebostatic axis. If the air–fluid interface is raised above the phlebostatic axis, the values displayed will be erroneously low, and if the interface is lowered below the phlebostatic axis, the values displayed will be erroneously high.

Pressure measurements are taken with the patient in the supine position. The head of the bed may be elevated as much as 60 degrees, provided that the air–fluid interface is releveled after any changes in the patient's position (see Fig. 9-3B). The elevation of the head of the bed should be noted to maintain consistency among measurements.

 RED FLAG! Consistency in leveling and measurement techniques is important because small variations in the zero reference point can elicit large and erroneous changes in the pressures observed.

Troubleshooting

Technical or mechanical factors can produce erroneously high or low pressures and altered waveforms. Any impedance between the patient and transducer (eg, air bubbles, blood, additional stopcocks) can alter the signal and consequently, the pressures and waveforms. Less than 300 mmHg in the continuous

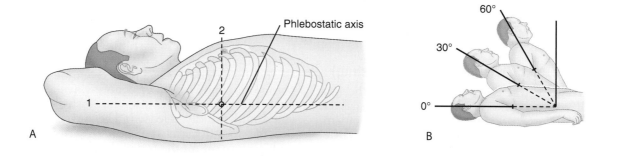

FIGURE 9-3 **A:** The phlebostatic axis is the intersection of the midaxillary line drawn between the anterior and posterior surfaces of the chest (*1*) and the line drawn through the fourth intercostal space at the sternum (*2*). **B:** The position of the phlebostatic axis changes when the head of the bed is raised; therefore, the air–fluid interface must be releveled if the patient's position changes.

pressure device, compliant tubing, or excessive lengths of tubing may also distort the signal to the transducer. The nurse periodically checks the system to ensure patency of the catheter and tubing, sufficient pressure in the pressure bag, and proper positioning of the stopcocks, and to ensure that the alarms are set and functioning properly. Table 9-1 describes causes of technical problems that can affect pressure monitoring systems and troubleshooting techniques to address them.

Arterial Pressure Monitoring

Arterial pressure monitoring allows continuous monitoring of the systemic arterial blood pressure and provides vascular access for obtaining blood samples. Vasoactive IV infusions; cardiovascular instability; fluctuating, unstable blood pressures; and frequent blood draws are indications for arterial pressure monitoring. In addition, when therapeutic decisions depend on obtaining accurate blood pressure values, arterial pressure monitoring is the gold standard.

Equipment and Setup

When selecting the artery for cannulation

- The artery should be large enough to accommodate the catheter without occluding or significantly impeding flow.
- The site should be easily accessible and free from contamination by body secretions.
- There should be adequate collateral blood flow in the event that the cannulated artery becomes occluded.

The radial artery, which usually meets all of these criteria, is the most frequently used site for arterial catheter placement. It is superficially located and therefore easy to palpate. Cannulation of this artery also poses the least limitation on the patient's mobility. Before a catheter is inserted into the radial artery, the presence of adequate collateral circulation to the hand via the ulnar artery is assessed by ultrasound or by performing Allen's test (Fig. 9-4, p. 97). Alternative sites for arterial catheter placement include the femoral and brachial arteries.

After the catheter is inserted, the nurse ensures that the arterial blood pressure alarms on the monitor are properly set and activated. The alarms must be visible and audible to the caregiver. Alarms are set either around specific parameters for the patient, or according to facility protocol. Typically, high and low alarms are set for systolic, diastolic, and mean pressures and for pressures within 10 to 20 mm Hg of the patient's blood pressure.

 RED FLAG! *Although the arterial monitoring system provides vascular access for obtaining blood samples, no IV solution or medication should be administered through the arterial pressure monitoring system at any time.*

Data Interpretation

The normal arterial pressure waveform (Fig. 9-5, p. 97) consists of a rapid upstroke (produced by the rapid ejection of blood from the left ventricle into the aorta), a clear dicrotic notch (which signals closure of the aortic valve and the beginning of diastole), and a definite end point (which reflects the end of diastole). Loss of the dicrotic notch is a sign of overdamping.

The value measured at the peak of the waveform is the systolic pressure, and the value measured at the lowest point of the waveform is the diastolic pressure. The difference between the systolic and diastolic pressure is the pulse pressure. The pulse pressure closely reflects the stroke volume from the ventricle. Bedside monitors do not automatically display the pulse pressure but can be easily calculated and is a value useful in assessing the patient's volume status.

Mean arterial pressure (MAP) is used to evaluate perfusion of vital body organs. Normal MAP is 70 to 105 mm Hg. The formula used to calculate MAP takes into account the fact that diastole is approximately two times longer than systole during a cardiac cycle:

$$\frac{\text{Systolic pressure} + (\text{Diastolic pressure} \times 2)}{3}$$

Most bedside monitors automatically calculate and continuously display the MAP. Algorithms to determine MAP may vary depending on the manufacturer of the equipment.

Blood pressures obtained by an intra-arterial catheter using an optimally damped pressure monitoring system are the most accurate. In normotensive patients, blood pressure measurements obtained through arterial pressure monitoring are very similar to those obtained with a cuff (the intra-arterial systolic pressure is 5 to 10 mm Hg higher). However, comparisons between intra-arterial and cuff pressures may be misleading because the methods of measurement reflect different physiologic events and therefore are not truly comparable. A trend value obtained using one method of measuring blood pressure consistently is often more helpful than comparing values obtained using different methods. Documenting the site of pressure measurements and what method was used to obtain them is important.

Complications
Accidental Blood Loss

Accidental blood loss from an arterial catheter can be catastrophic. Prevention of accidental dislodgement and easy access to the insertion site and connections is imperative. To reduce the risk for accidental blood loss, a Luer-Lok–type connector is used for all connections in the system. The extremity in which the catheter is placed may be immobilized (eg, by placing the wrist on

TABLE 9-1 Troubleshooting Pressure Monitoring Systems

Problem	Cause	Prevention	Intervention
No waveform	Transducer not open to catheter	...	Check and correct stopcock position.
	Settings on bedside monitor incorrect or off	...	Check scale setting and monitor setup.
	Catheter clotted	Maintain continuous flush.	Aspirate blood clot. Do not irrigate with syringe.
	Faulty cable	...	Check function with cable checking device; change cables if necessary.
	Faulty transducer	...	Change transducer if necessary.
Overdamped waveforms	Improper scale selection	...	Change to proper scale.
	Air bubbles in tubing and near transducer	Flush system by gravity. On initial setup, expel all air from flush solution bag.	Flush air from system.
	Blood clot partially occluding catheter tip	Use heparinized solution according to facility protocol.	Aspirate clots with syringe. Use heparinized solution according to facility protocol.
	Forward migration of catheter		Reposition patient.
	Catheter tip occluded by balloon or vessel wall		Reposition catheter by pulling back on it while observing waveforms.
	Leak in pressure system	Tighten all connections and stopcock on set up.	Tighten all connections and stopcocks. Change faulty system components if necessary.
	Pressure bag not inflated at 300 mm Hg	...	Reinflate bag or apply pressure to device to 300 mm Hg. Change device if faulty.
Underdamped waveforms	Excessive movement of catheter	Ensure correct catheter placement. Use appropriate catheter size for vessel.	Try different catheter tip position. Eliminate excessive stopcocks.
	Air bubbles in tubing	Eliminate excessive length of pressure tubing.	Eliminate excessive tubing.
False low readings	Leveling or zero reference (transducer) is too high	Check level periodically. Check monitor settings. Observe waveforms.	Relevel transducer air–fluid interface to phlebostatic axis. Rezero monitor. Optimize length of pressure tubing.
	Improper zeroing	...	
	Overdamped waveforms	Perform square waveform test	
False high readings	Leveling or zero reference (transducer) is too low	Check level periodically. Check monitor settings. Observe waveforms.	Relevel transducer air–fluid interface to phlebostatic axis.
	Improper zeroing	...	Rezero monitor.
	Overdamped waveforms	Perform square waveform test	Remove excessive length of pressure tubing.
Inappropriate pressure waveform	Incorrect catheter position	Establish optimal position carefully during the insertion process.	Reposition patient. Obtain chest x-ray.
	Migration of pulmonary artery catheter (PAC) into mechanical wedge position	Use proper balloon inflation volume (1.25–1.5 mL air) for obtaining a pulmonary artery occlusion pressure (PAOP) tracing.	Reposition catheter.[a] Observe waveforms and confirm with initial insertion tracings. If right ventricular tracing is observed from PAC distal tip, slowly inflate balloon to allow PAC to "float" into pulmonary artery. If PAOP tracing is observed with balloon deflated, withdraw catheter slightly while observing waveforms. Stop withdrawing as soon as a pulmonary artery tracing is observed.
Bleed back into pressure tubing or transducer	Loose connections	...	Tighten connections.
	Stopcocks not returned to proper position	...	Ensure stopcocks are in correct position.
	Pressure bag not at 300 mm Hg	...	Check pressure device.

[a]A physician or advanced practice nurse is usually responsible for repositioning a PAC.

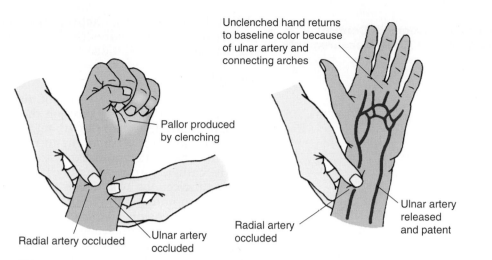

FIGURE 9-4 Modified Allen's test. If color returns in less than 7 seconds, the ulnar circulation to the hand is adequate. If color returns in 7 to 15 seconds, ulnar filling may be impaired. If the hand remains blanched for longer than 15 seconds, ulnar circulation is inadequate and the radial artery should not be cannulated.

an arm board). If a wrist restraint is used, optimally, it should not be placed over the insertion site. Similarly, the extremity should not be covered by bed linens, to facilitate visual checks. Frequent assessments of the site is required if a wrist restraint is present.

Infection

Factors that reduce the risk for infection include proper attention to sterile technique during catheter insertion, care of the insertion site, and blood sampling, and maintenance of a sterile, closed monitoring system. The nurse assesses the insertion site for signs of infection; uses sterile technique when changing dressings, tubing, and flush solution; and maintains the integrity of the system. Applying sterile nonvented ("dead-ender") caps to the stopcock ports helps eliminate contamination. Closed systems for blood sampling help reduce the potential for open stopcock infections and assist with managing potential blood loss.

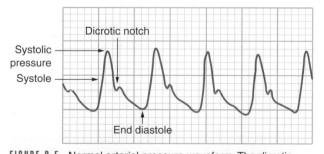

FIGURE 9-5 Normal arterial pressure waveform. The dicrotic notch indicates the end of ventricular systole and the beginning of diastole.

Impaired Circulation

Circulation to the extremity in which the arterial line is placed must be monitored frequently. The nurse assesses the color, sensation, temperature, and movement of the extremity after insertion of the arterial catheter and per facility policy. Any sign or symptom of impaired circulation may be an indication for catheter removal and must be reported immediately.

Central Venous Pressure Monitoring

Central venous pressure (CVP) is typically measured in the superior vena cava near the right atrium via a PICC line or a central line catheter placed in the jugular or subclavian vein. The CVP reflects the pressure of blood in the right atrium and provides information about intravascular blood volume, right ventricular end-diastolic pressure (RVEDP), and right ventricular volume. To a limited degree, in people with normal pulmonary vasculature and left ventricular function, the CVP also indirectly reflects left ventricular end-diastolic pressure (LVEDP) and function, because the left and right sides of the heart are linked by the pulmonary vascular bed.

Data Interpretation

Normal CVP is 2 to 8 mmHg. Abnormally high or low CVP measurements are usually associated with alterations in intravascular volume status or ventricular function (Box 9-2). A CVP value alone is meaningless, but when used in conjunction with other clinical data (eg, breath sounds, heart and respiratory rate, neck vein distention, urine output, electrocardiographic data), it is a valuable aid in managing and predicting the patient's clinical course.

> **BOX 9-2**   **Causes of Alterations in Central Venous Pressure (CVP) Measurements**
>
> **Low CVP Measurements**
> - Hypovolemic state
> - Diuretic therapy
> - Vasodilation (eg, sepsis, vasodilating medications)
>
> **High CVP Measurements**
> - Right ventricular failure
> - Pulmonary embolism
> - Pulmonary hypertension
> - Left ventricular failure
> - Mechanical ventilation
> - Hypervolemic state

Complications

Infection

Infection may occur intravascularly or around the insertion site. Signs and symptoms of central venous catheter–associated infection may include erythema at the insertion site, fever, or an elevated white blood cell (WBC) count. Definitive diagnosis is obtained with blood cultures. Primary measures to prevent infection include routine dressing and IV fluid tubing changes (per Centers for Disease Control and Prevention [CDC] guidelines and facility protocol) and adherence to sterile technique during catheter insertion and dressing changes.

Thrombosis

Thrombi occasionally form and may vary from a thin layer of fibrin over the catheter tip to a large thrombus. Loss of the hemodynamic waveform or the inability to infuse fluid or withdraw blood from the catheter may be indications that the catheter is occluded by a large thrombus. Because a thrombus may embolize (putting the patient at risk for pulmonary embolism) or impair circulation to a limb, it constitutes an emergency and must be reported to the physician immediately. Facility protocol may permit nurses to attempt aspirating the clot. Frequently, facilities also have protocols to administer small doses of thrombolytic agents to dissolve the clot.

Pneumothorax

Anatomical factors can make placement of a central line difficult, particularly if the patient is obese or has torturous subclavian veins. The needle or introducer sheath may pass through the vessel wall and puncture the lung during insertion, causing an apical pneumothorax. A postinsertion chest radiograph is routinely obtained to verify proper catheter placement and assess for pneumothorax. Signs and symptoms of a pneumothorax include pleuritic chest pain, shortness of breath and dyspnea, asymmetrical chest wall movement, diminished or absent breath sounds, tachycardia, and elevated peak inspiratory pressures (if the patient is receiving mechanical ventilation).

Air Embolism

Air embolism occurs as a result of air entering the vasculature and traveling through the vena cava to the right ventricle. When the tubing is disconnected from the catheter, changes in intrathoracic pressure with inspiration and expiration can draw air into the catheter. Approximately 10 to 20 mL of air entering the venous system can cause the patient to become symptomatic. Signs and symptoms include sudden hypotension, confusion, lightheadedness, anxiety, and unresponsiveness. Cardiac arrest may occur if the air bolus is large. If air embolism is suspected, turning the patient on the left side in the Trendelenburg position may allow the air to rise to the wall of the right ventricle and improve blood flow. Supplemental oxygen is started unless contraindicated.

Pulmonary Artery Pressure Monitoring

In pulmonary artery pressure (PAP) monitoring, a catheter is placed through the right side of the heart into the pulmonary artery. By measuring pressures in the right atrium, right ventricle, and pulmonary artery, it is possible to assess right ventricular function, pulmonary vascular status, and, indirectly, left ventricular function. The pulmonary artery catheter (PAC) also allows evaluation of cardiac output.

Equipment and Setup

Pulmonary Artery Catheter

Several types of PACs are available. The type of catheter used is determined by the parameters to be monitored. All PACs have multiple external lumens. A typical PAC (Fig. 9-6) has four lumens:

- The *distal lumen* is located into the pulmonary artery and is attached to the transducer to measure PAPs. Mixed venous blood (used to calculate mixed venous oxygen saturation [SvO_2], oxygen extraction, oxygen consumption, and intrapulmonary shunt measurements) may be withdrawn from the distal lumen. Use of the distal lumen for administering fluid or medication is not recommended.
- The *proximal lumen* terminates in the right atrium or the superior vena cava. The lumen is used for infusing fluids and is often connected to a transducer to provide RAP measurements and display of the RAP waveform. The proximal lumen is also used to inject solution for cardiac output measurement.
- The *thermistor* receives input from a thermistor on the tip of the PAC and measures the patient's core temperature. It detects the blood temperature change when solution is injected through

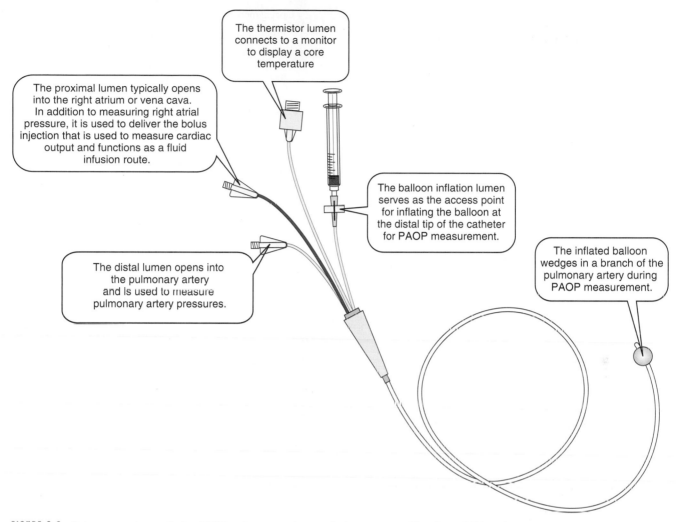

FIGURE 9-6 Pulmonary artery catheter. PAOP, pulmonary artery occlusion pressure. (Courtesy of Edwards Lifesciences, LLC.)

the proximal lumen during cardiac output measurements.

- The *balloon inflation lumen* is used to inflate the balloon near the catheter tip with air. Inflation of the balloon causes the catheter to occlude (or wedge) into a distal artery, allowing measurement of the pulmonary artery occlusion pressure (PAOP), formerly known as the pulmonary artery wedge pressure (PAWP). Fluid is never inserted into the balloon inflation lumen. It is an indirect measurement of LAP.

Specialty PACs have additional lumens and capabilities (Fig. 9-7). For example, a five-lumen catheter has an additional lumen for venous infusion into the right atrium. A seven-lumen catheter includes an additional lumen for venous infusion, as well as an optical module lumen (which connects to a special oximetry monitor for SvO_2 monitoring) and a thermal filament lumen (which allows display of cardiac output on a continuous basis). Another type of specialty PAC determines right ventricular volumes, and then calculates the right ventricular ejection fraction.

Pulmonary Artery Catheter Insertion

The nurse assists with PAC insertion.[2] Strict sterile technique is required. The physician inserts the PAC through a large vein, usually the right internal jugular, the right or left subclavian, or the femoral vein. The physician advances the catheter with the balloon inflated once it is in the right atrium. To determine catheter tip location, the nurse monitors the waveforms and pressures on the bedside monitor as the catheter passes into the right atrium, through the tricuspid valve into the right ventricle, across the pulmonic valve, into the pulmonary artery, and eventually into the wedged position (Fig. 9-8, p. 101). The balloon is allowed to deflate passively after the pulmonary artery wedge is noted on the monitor and the return of the pulmonary artery is confirmed. The amount of air required to 'wedge' the balloon is noted. The PAC is secured, a sterile dressing is placed over the insertion site, and a chest radiograph is obtained to verify catheter position. The distal (pulmonary artery) lumen is connected to pressure tubing, and

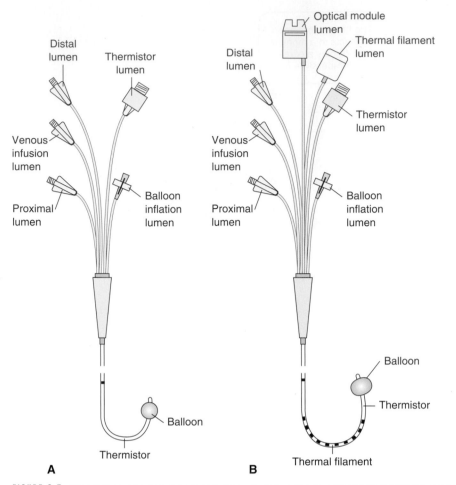

FIGURE 9-7   Specialty pulmonary artery catheters. **A:** A five-lumen catheter that includes an additional venous infusion lumen that is used for infusions into the right atrium. **B:** A seven-lumen catheter that includes a venous infusion lumen, an optical module lumen for continuous mixed venous oxygen saturation (SvO$_2$) monitoring, and a thermal filament lumen for continuous cardiac output monitoring. (Courtesy of Edwards Lifesciences, LLC.)

the other lumens are connected as appropriate, either to the pressure monitoring system or an IV solution.

If the PAC is not properly secured, it may become dislodged and the tip may "fall back" into the right ventricle. The patient may experience dysrhythmias (as a result of endocardial irritation by the catheter tip), and the hemodynamic pressures and waveform will reflect those of the right ventricle instead of the pulmonary artery. Inflating the balloon may cause the catheter to "refloat" into the pulmonary artery. Alternatively, if the catheter is in a sleeve (to protect from contamination), it may be advanced into the proper position in the pulmonary artery.

Data Interpretation

The pressures and waveforms obtained through PAP monitoring are generated by pressure changes in the heart that occur throughout the cardiac cycle. The mechanical activity of the heart (ie, systole and diastole) follows the electrical activity of the heart. Therefore, mechanical activity must be correlated to electrical activity by interpreting the hemodynamic waveforms alongside an electrocardiographic

tracing. Interpretation of pressure measurements obtained through PAP monitoring is summarized in Table 9-2, on page 102.

Measurement of all pressures is most accurate when obtained at the end of expiration. During the end-expiration period, there is minimal airflow and little variation in pleural pressures that influence cardiac pressures. Thus, end expiration provides a standard reference point for obtaining measurements. Spontaneous breathing causes negative intrathoracic pressure during inspiration, which produces a decline in the waveform. The waveform used for measurement is the last clear wave occurring just before the inspiratory dip (Fig. 9-9A), p. 103. Mechanical ventilation causes positive intrathoracic pressure during inspiration, which produces an inspiratory "push," or rise, in the waveform. In mechanically ventilated patients, the waveform used for measurement is the last clear wave occurring just before the inspiratory rise (see Fig. 9-9B).

Right Atrial Pressure

The right atrium is a low-pressure chamber, receiving blood volume passively from the vena cava. The

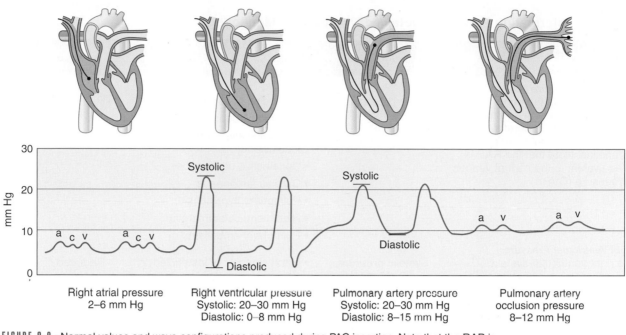

FIGURE 9-8 Normal values and wave configurations produced during PAC insertion. Note that the RAP is equivalent to the RVEDP, the right ventricular systolic pressure is equivalent to the pulmonary artery systolic pressure, and the pulmonary artery diastolic pressure closely approximates the PAOP.

RAP is used to make assumptions about the volume in the right ventricle during end diastole (when the ventricle is the fullest).

Atrial waveforms have three positive waves (Fig. 9-10A, p. 104):

- The *a wave* reflects the increase in atrial pressure during atrial systole (end of ventricular diastole). The tricuspid valve is open at this time, allowing pressures between the atrium and ventricle to equalize. The a wave is used to obtain the RAP (CVP) reading.
- The *c wave* results from a small increase in pressure associated with closure of the tricuspid valve and early atrial diastole (onset of ventricular systole). It may be a distinct wave or a dicrotic notch. It is not present in all waveforms.
- The *v wave* represents atrial diastole (and ventricular systole) and reflects the increase in pressure caused by the filling of the atrium with blood.

Atrial waveforms also have two primary negative waves (descents):

- The *x descent* follows the a wave (or c wave, if present) and represents a decrease in pressure caused by atrial relaxation at the beginning of atrial diastole.
- The *y descent* follows the v wave and represents the initial, passive atrial emptying into the ventricle as the tricuspid valve opens.[1,2]

Accurate identification of the a, c, and v waves requires correlation of the waveform with the electrocardiogram (ECG) (see Fig. 9-10A). On the ECG, the P wave represents atrial depolarization, which causes the right atrium to contract. Therefore, the a wave occurs after the P wave, usually in the PR interval. The mitral and tricuspid values are open, and thus more accurately measures the pressures in the ventricles. The QRS complex represents ventricular depolarization and ventricular contraction. Simultaneously, the atria relax and fill with blood. The v wave generated by these events thus occurs in the T-to-P interval. The mitral and tricuspid valves are closed, and thus do not accurately reflect the pressure (volume) in the ventricles.

Abnormalities of the right atrial waveform include large, elevated a or v waves. Increased resistance to ventricular filling and impaired atrial emptying cause an elevated a wave. Elevated v waves are related to regurgitant flow during ventricular contraction.

Right Ventricular Pressure

Typically, the right ventricular pressure is obtained only on initial PAC insertion. The right ventricle is a low-pressure chamber. When the tricuspid valve is open, the RAP and the RVEDP are similar. During right ventricular systole, the pressure increases to generate enough pressure to open the pulmonic valve and eject blood into the pulmonary artery. Therefore, the right ventricular systolic pressure normally equals the pulmonary artery systolic pressure.

The right ventricular waveform has a distinctive "square root" configuration (see Fig. 9-10B). The initial rapid increase in right ventricular pressure represents right ventricular systole, which follows the QRS complex of the ECG. After ventricular systole, the pulmonic valve closes, and the right ventricular pressure rapidly decreases, creating a diastolic dip. Next in the cardiac cycle, the tricuspid valve opens, allowing the right ventricle to passively fill with blood from the right atrium. Right ventricular diastole occurs within the period from the T wave to the next Q wave on the ECG. The point on the waveform just before the rapid increase in pressures represents the RVEDP.

TABLE 9-2	Interpreting Pressures Obtained Through PAP Monitoring

Pressure and Description	Normal Values	Causes of Increased Pressure	Causes of Decreased Pressure
Right Atrial Pressure (RAP) The RAP reflects the right ventricular end-diastolic pressure (RVEDP) and is therefore an indication of right ventricular function. Note that the RAP is equivalent to the central venous pressure (CVP).	Mean pressure: 2–6 mm Hg	• Right-sided heart failure • Volume overload • Tricuspid valve stenosis or insufficiency • Constrictive pericarditis • Cardiac tamponade • Pulmonary hypertension • Right ventricular infarction • Pulmonary embolism	Reduced circulating blood volume
Right Ventricular Pressure The right ventricular systolic pressure normally equals the pulmonary artery systolic pressure. The right ventricular diastolic pressure is reflected by the RAP.	Systolic pressure: 20–30 mm Hg Diastolic pressure: 0–8 mm Hg	• Mitral stenosis or insufficiency • Pulmonary disease • Hypoxemia • Constrictive pericarditis • Chronic heart failure • Atrial and ventricular septal defects • Patent ductus arteriosus	Reduced circulating blood volume
Pulmonary Artery Systolic Pressure The pulmonary artery systolic pressure results from right ventricular systolic pressure and reflects right ventricular function.	Systolic pressure: 20–30 mm Hg Mean pressure: 8–15 mm Hg	• Left-sided heart failure • Increased pulmonary blood flow (left or right shunting, as in atrial or ventricular septal defects) • Mechanical ventilation • Any condition causing increased pulmonary arteriolar resistance (such as pulmonary hypertension, volume overload, mitral stenosis, or hypoxia)	Reduced circulating blood volume
Pulmonary Artery Diastolic Pressure The pulmonary artery diastolic pressure is an indirect reflection of left ventricular end-diastolic pressure (LVEDP) in a patient without significant pulmonary artery disease.	Diastolic pressure: 8–15 mm Hg Mean pressure: 10–20 mm Hg	• Any condition causing increased pulmonary arteriolar resistance (such as pulmonary hypertension, pulmonary embolism, volume overload, mitral stenosis, or hypoxia)	Reduced circulating blood volume Right ventricular failure
Pulmonary Artery Occlusion Pressure (PAOP) The PAOP indirectly reflects the LAP and the LVEDP, unless the patient has obstructions from the tip of the PAC to the left ventricle. Changes in PAOP reflect changes in left ventricular filling pressure.	Mean pressure: 8–12 mm Hg	• Left-sided heart failure • Mitral stenosis or insufficiency • Pericardial tamponade	Reduced circulating blood volume Right ventricular failure

Modified from Springhouse: Critical Care Nursing Made Incredibly Easy. Philadelphia, PA: Springhouse, 2004, p 170.

Pulmonary Artery Pressure

In healthy people, the pulmonary vasculature is a relatively compliant, low-resistance, low-pressure system. The pulmonary artery systolic pressure is generated by right ventricular systolic ejection. The pulmonary artery diastolic pressure reflects the resistance of the pulmonary vascular bed and, to a limited degree, the LVEDP because the open mitral valve allows equalization of pressure from the left ventricle back to the tip of the PAC. Under normal conditions, with no obstructions or primary pulmonary hypertension, the pulmonary artery diastolic pressure may be used to monitor the LVEDP.

The pulmonary artery waveform characteristics are similar to those of the systemic arterial waveform (see Figs. 9-5 and 9-10C). The dicrotic notch in the downward

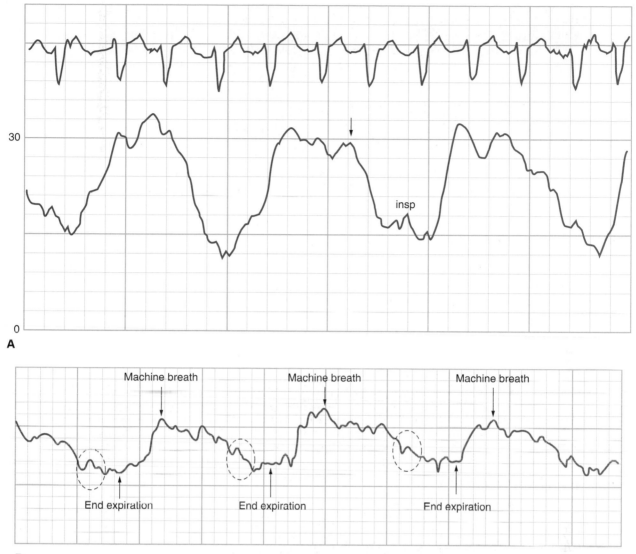

FIGURE 9-9 Measurement of pressures is most accurate when obtained at the end of expiration. **A:** Spontaneous breathing. **B:** Pulmonary artery occlusion pressure (PAOP) tracing with positive pressure mechanical ventilation. Measurement of the PAOP is made at the last clear waveform (*circled areas*) before the inspiratory rise.

slope of the pulmonary artery waveform corresponds with pulmonic valve closure and represents the beginning of the pulmonary artery diastolic phase.

Pulmonary Artery Occlusion Pressure

The PAOP is the measure of the left atrial pressure (LAP) and the LVEDP. The PAOP is obtained by inflating the balloon at the catheter tip. The balloon wedges in a branch of the pulmonary artery, occluding forward flow and creating an unrestricted vascular channel between the tip of the catheter and the left ventricle (Fig. 9-11). In this way, the PAOP reflects the LVEDP when the reading is obtained at end diastole, when the mitral valve is open. (In the presence of mitral valve stenosis, the PAOP does not accurately reflect the LVEDP.)

A PAOP tracing is essentially a LAP tracing; therefore, it has a, c, and v waves and x and y descents just like the RAP tracing (see Fig. 9-10D). The a

wave corresponds to left atrial systole, and is used to obtain the measured pressure in the left atrium. The v wave corresponds to left atrial diastole. The c wave is rarely visible on the PAOP tracing because the slight increase in pressure from backward bulging of the mitral valve is difficult to observe.

The a and v waves on the PAOP tracing are slightly delayed relative to the ECG because of the distance from the left side of the heart over which these pressures are transmitted. The a wave falls more closely in line with the QRS complex, and the v wave correlates with the T wave.

Left ventricular dysfunction and mitral valve disease occur more frequently than right ventricular dysfunction and tricuspid valve disease; therefore abnormal PAOP waveforms are more common than abnormal right atrial waveforms. Left ventricular failure usually causes elevation of both the a and v waves and significantly increases the PAOP (and

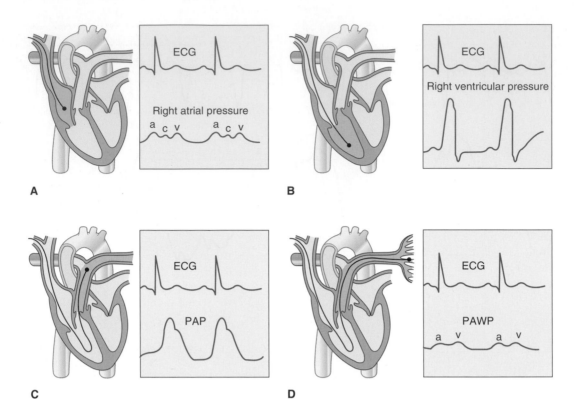

FIGURE 9-10 **A:** Right atrium. A waveform with three small upright waves appears. The a waves represent the right atrial systole; the v waves, right atrial diastole. **B:** Right ventricle. A waveform with sharp systolic upstrokes and lower diastolic dips appears. **C:** Pulmonary artery. A pulmonary artery pressure (PAP) waveform appears. Note that the upstroke is smoother than on the right ventricular waveform. The dicrotic notch indicates pulmonic valve closure. **D:** Distal branch of the pulmonary artery. The balloon wedges where the vessel becomes too narrow for it to pass, and a PAOP waveform, with two small upright waves, appears. The a wave represents left atrial systole; the v wave, left atrial diastole. ECG, electrocardiogram. (Courtesy of Edwards Lifesciences, LLC.)

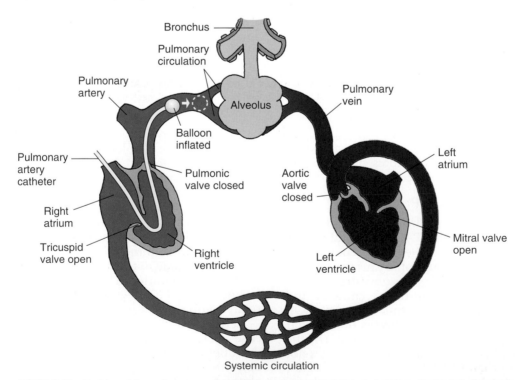

FIGURE 9-11 Position of the pulmonary artery. When the balloon is inflated and the catheter is in the wedge position, there is an unrestricted vascular channel between the tip of the catheter and the left ventricle in diastole. PAOP thus reflects LVEDP, an important indicator of left ventricular function. (Courtesy of Philips.)

the pulmonary artery diastolic pressure) because of reduced contractility and forward blood flow. Normally, the PAOP closely approximates the pulmonary artery diastolic pressure with a gradient of 1 to 4 mm Hg. A widened pressure gradient (greater than 4 mm Hg) is a differential diagnostic sign of primary pulmonary hypertension or increased pulmonary vascular resistance (PVR) (as opposed to left ventricular dysfunction).

Complications

Generally, most complications that occur with PAP monitoring relate to the need for percutaneous central venous access. Complications such as infection, thrombus, pneumothorax, and air embolus were discussed earlier in the chapter. Other complications that may occur with PAP monitoring include ventricular dysrhythmias, pulmonary artery rupture or perforation, and pulmonary infarction.

Ventricular Dysrhythmias

Ventricular dysrhythmias may occur during the insertion of a PAC. As the catheter passes through the right ventricle, it may irritate the endocardium, causing premature ventricular contractions (PVCs) and occasionally ventricular tachycardia. The dysrhythmias typically resolve when the catheter is advanced into the pulmonary artery; however, it is essential to have ready access to emergency medications and equipment in case the ventricular dysrhythmias persist. Migration of the PAC back into the right ventricle may also cause ventricular dysrhythmias.

Pulmonary Artery Rupture or Perforation

Pulmonary artery rupture or perforation is a rare but potentially fatal complication that may occur during insertion or manipulation of the PAC. During insertion of the PAC, proper technique (ie, advancing the catheter with the balloon fully inflated with 1.5 mL of air, avoiding advancing the catheter too far into a small artery) minimizes the chance of rupture or perforation. When obtaining a PAOP tracing, the nurse closely observes the pulmonary artery waveform as the balloon is inflated, and fills the balloon with the proper amount of air (usually 1.25 to 1.5 mL). Overfilling the balloon can cause overdistention of the pulmonary artery, putting the patient at risk for rupture.

Pulmonary Infarction

Pulmonary infarction resulting from loss of blood flow distal to the PAC is typically a result of the PAC migrating distally into a smaller artery (ie, spontaneous wedging). If less than 1.25 to 1.5 mL of air is needed to inflate the balloon and obtain the PAOP waveform, then spontaneous wedging is a higher risk. Changing of the pulmonary artery waveform to a PAOP waveform on the bedside monitor may also indicate spontaneous wedging. (The bedside

---

EVIDENCE-BASED PRACTICE GUIDELINES
Accuracy in Hemodyamic Monitoring

PROBLEM: Technical aspects of monitoring affect the accuracy and reliability of the data obtained through hemodynamic monitoring. Accurate and reliable data are essential to providing optimal patient care.

EVIDENCE-BASED PRACTICE GUIDELINES

1. Verify the accuracy of the invasive pressure monitoring system by performing a square-wave test at the beginning of each shift and any time the system is disturbed (eg, blood draw). (level A)
2. Position the patient in the supine position (head of bed between 0 and 60 degrees), the lateral position (20, 30, or 90 degrees with the head of the bed flat) or prone before obtaining pulmonary artery pressure (PAP), pulmonary artery occlusiive pressure (PAOP), and central venous pressure (CVP) measurements. Allow the patient to stabilize for 5 to 15 minutes after a position change. (level A)
3. With the patient in the supine or prone position, level and reference the transducer air–fluid interface to the phlebostatic axis (4th ICS, ½ AP diameter of the chest) or to the lateral angle-specific reference using a laser or carpenter's level before obtaining PAP, PAOP, and CVP measurements. (level A)
4. Obtain PAP, PAOP, and CVP measurements from a graphic (analog) tracing at end expiration or adjust the measurement point if the patient is receiving airway pressure release ventilation (APRV) or is actively exhaling. (level A)
5. Use a simultaneous electrocardiogram (ECG) tracing to assist with proper PAP, PAOP, and CVP waveform identification. (level A)

KEY

Level A: Meta-analysis of quantitative studies or metasynthesis of qualitative studies with results that consistently support a specific action, intervention, or treatment

Level B: Well-designed, controlled studies with results that consistently support a specific action, intervention, or treatment

Level C: Qualitative studies, descriptive or correlational studies, integrative review, systematic reviews, or randomized controlled trials with inconsistent results

Level D: Peer-reviewed professional organizational standards with clinical studies to support recommendations

Level E: Multiple case reports, theory-based evidence from expert opinions, or peer-reviewed professional organizational standards without clinical studies to support recommendations

Level M: Manufacturer's recommendations only

■ Adapted from American Association of Critical-Care Nurses (AACN) Practice Alert, revised 12/2009.

---

monitor should continuously display the pulmonary artery waveform.) Prompt identification and management (eg, by pulling the catheter back, per facility protocol) can prevent a pulmonary infarction from occurring.

Determination of Cardiac Output

Assessment of cardiac output and its determinants are important adjuncts to the care of critically ill patients. Cardiac output is the volume of blood ejected from the heart per minute. Normally, cardiac output is 4 to 8 L/min at rest. Cardiac output is a function of heart rate and stroke volume (the amount of blood ejected from the left ventricle during systole). Table 9-3 summarizes calculations that are commonly used in evaluating cardiac output.

The cardiac index relates cardiac output to body size. To obtain the cardiac index, the cardiac output is divided by the patient's body surface area (BSA).

Standard bedside monitors and cardiac output computers automatically calculate the cardiac index when the patient's height and weight (needed to calculate the BSA) are entered. Normally, the cardiac index is 2.5 to 4 L/min/m².

An increased or decreased cardiac output provides global information only and needs to be evaluated in light of the factors that affect cardiac output (Fig. 9-12).[5] stroke volume, one of the primary determinants of cardiac output, is influenced by preload, afterload, and contractility.

- **Preload** is the amount of stretch on the myocardial muscle fibers at end diastole. Preload is primarily

TABLE 9-3   Parameters Used in the Evaluation of Cardiac Output

Parameter	Definition	Formula	Normal Values
Cardiac output (CO)	The number of liters pumped by the heart per minute	HR × SV	4–8 L/min
Cardiac index (CI)	CO indexed to the patient's body surface area (BSA)	CO/BSA	2.5–4 L/min/m²
Stroke volume (SV)	The milliliters of blood ejected from the ventricle with each contraction	CO/HR × 1000	60–100 mL/beat
Stroke volume index (SVI)	SV indexed to the patient's BSA	CI/HR	33–47 mL/beat/m²
Mean arterial pressure (MAP)	The calculated average arterial pressure over a full cardiac cycle	[Systolic BP + (diastolic BP × 2)]/3	70–105 mm Hg
Right atrial pressure (RAP)	Pressure created by volume of blood in the right heart	Direct measurement	2–6 mm Hg
Left atrial pressure (LAP)	Pressure created by volume of blood in the left heart	Direct measurement	6–12 mm Hg
Pulmonary artery occlusion pressure (PAOP)	Pressure measured in the pulmonary artery when the PAC's balloon is inflated	Direct measurement	8–15 mm Hg
Right ventricular end-diastolic volume index (RVEDVI)	Amount of volume in the right ventricle at the end of diastole indexed to patient BSA	SVI/RV ejection fraction	60–100 mL/m²
Left ventricular end-diastolic volume index (LVEDVI)	Amount of volume in the left ventricle at the end of diastole indexed to patient BSA	SV/LV ejection fraction	40–80 mL/m²
Systemic vascular resistance (SVR)	The resistance to blood flow offered by the systemic vasculature	[(MAP – RAP) × 80]/CO	800–1200 dyne/s/cm⁻⁵
Systemic vascular resistance index (SVRI)	SVR indexed to patient's BSA	[(MAP – RAP) × 80]/CI	1360–2200 dyne/s/cm⁻⁵
Pulmonary vascular resistance (PVR)	The resistance to blood flow offered by the pulmonary vasculature	(MPAP – PAOP) × 80/CO	<250 dyne/s/cm⁻⁵
Pulmonary vascular resistance index (PVRI)	PVR indexed to patient's BSA	(MPAP – PAOP) × 80/CI	
Left ventricular stroke work index (LVSWI)	A measure of work performed by the left ventricle with each beat	SVI (MAP – PAOP) × 0.0136	40–70 g-m²/beat
Right ventricular stroke work index (RVSWI)	A measure of work performed by the right ventricle with each beat	SVI (MPAP – RAP) × 0.0136	5–10 g-m²/beat
Stroke volume variation (SVV)	Variation in stroke volume over a respiratory cycle	SV maximum – SV minimum/ SV mean	<10%–15%

HR, heart rate.

influenced by total blood volume. The RAP or CVP is used to indirectly assess right ventricular preload, and the PAOP is used to indirectly assess left ventricular preload. Because PAP monitoring measures pressures, not volumes, assumptions are made that equate volume and pressure. However, many factors alter the pressure–volume relationship; therefore, the use of pressures to evaluate preload must be considered in light of these.

- **Afterload** is the resistance to ejection of blood from the ventricles. Primary factors affecting afterload are aortic and pulmonic valve stenosis and vascular resistance. PVR and systemic vascular resistance (SVR) are clinical assessments of right and left ventricular afterload, respectively. PVR and SVR can be indexed to body size using the patient's BSA.
- **Contractility** refers to the ability of the heart to contract independent of preload and afterload. Contractility can be assessed by determining stroke volume and calculating the stroke work index for both the left and right ventricles.

There are several methods of evaluating cardiac output. Methods may use invasive, minimally invasive, or noninvasive technologies. The most commonly used methods in the critical care setting are the thermodilution method, arterial pressure– and waveform-based methods, electrical bioimpedance cardiography, and esophageal Doppler monitoring.

Thermodilution Method

Thermodilution is the most common method used to measure cardiac output and is considered the clinical gold standard. Determination of cardiac output using the thermodilution method may be intermittent or continuous.

- Intermittent determinations require the injection of a known amount of "cooler than blood" indicator solution. The indicator solution is injected into the proximal (right atrial) lumen of the PAC. A thermistor near the end of the catheter continuously measures the temperature of blood flowing past it. The change in blood temperature following injection of the indicator solution generates a thermodilution curve, which the computer uses as a basis for calculating cardiac output.
- Continuous determinations require the use of a specialized PAC, which houses thermal filaments that emit heat as the indicator (see Fig. 9-7B). The "warmer than blood" signal is measured at the thermistor, and thermodilution curves are produced on a 30- to 60-second frequency for continuous cardiac output assessment.

For intermittent thermodilution cardiac output determination, the injectate syringe is usually part of a closed system that remains intact and attached to the proximal (right atrial) lumen by a stopcock

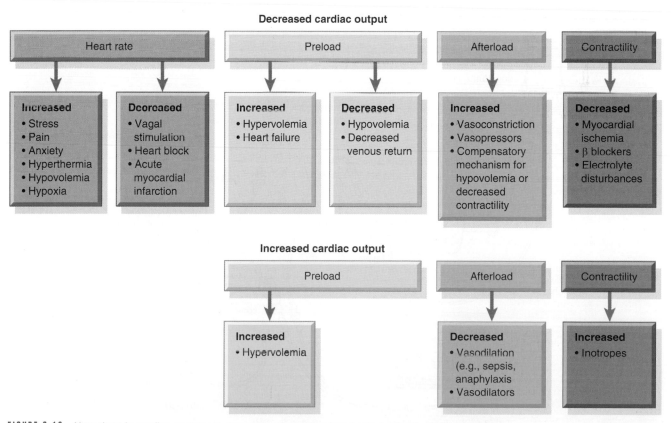

FIGURE 9-12 Alterations in cardiac output are caused by changes in heart rate, preload, afterload, and contractility.

(Fig. 9-13). A computation constant (based on the catheter size, volume and temperature of the injectate, and injection method) is set on the computer or programmed into the bedside cardiac output computer. For most patients, 10 mL of room-temperature injectate (sterile D_5W or normal saline) provides accurate results, although iced (0°C to 4°C) solution may be used for patients with hypothermia or very low cardiac output states to improve the accuracy. A temperature difference between the patient's blood temperature and the injectate of at least 10°C provides a greater signal and improves accuracy. Additional steps to promote accurate measurements include

- Ensuring that the volume of injectate in the syringe is correct
- Injecting the volume smoothly and rapidly, in less than 4 seconds
- Waiting approximately 1 minute between injections to allow the catheter thermistor to return to baseline

The average of several cardiac output determinations is required to obtain a final measurement. Three or more consecutive measurements are usually necessary. Measurements included in the averaging process should be within 10% to 15% of each other and demonstrating acceptable CO curves (Fig. 9-14A). Abnormal curves (see Fig. 9-14B) are eliminated from the cardiac output averaging process.

Arterial Pressure– and Waveform-Based Methods

Another method for determining cardiac output and stroke volume involves using arterial pressures and arterial waveforms. This method is based on the premise that there is a proportional relationship between pulse pressure and stroke volume, and an inverse relationship between pulse pressure and aortic compliance.

An arterial line, a special sensor, and a monitor that uses an algorithm for the stroke volume and cardiac output determinations are required. Although the specific algorithm used to determine the cardiac output value may vary depending on the equipment in use, all of the algorithms rely on the arterial pressure and the arterial waveform shape or size. Therefore, obtaining accurate values and ensuring optimal waveforms are critical.

Other values obtained using arterial pressure– and waveform-based methods include stroke volume variation, pulse pressure variation, and systolic pressure variation. These values reflect the difference between the maximum and minimum values of stroke volume, pulse pressure, and systolic pressure during a respiratory cycle and can be used to identify pulsus paradoxus (ie, an abnormally large decrease in systolic blood pressure during inspiration). These values are used to evaluate a patient's response to fluid administration.

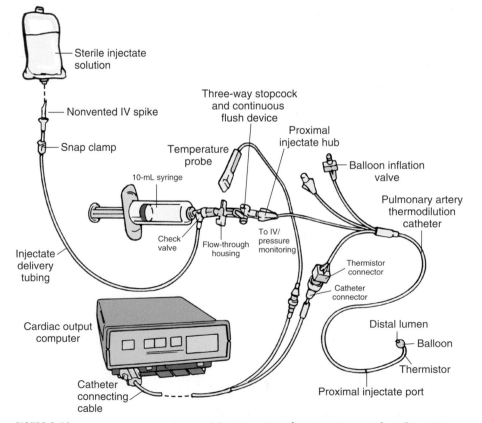

FIGURE 9-13 A closed room-temperature injectate system for measurement of cardiac output.

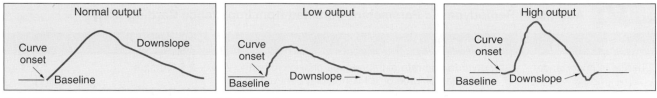

A. Acceptable cardiac output curves (good technique)

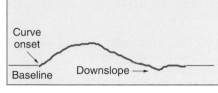

B. Irregular cardiac output curve (poor technique)

FIGURE 9-14 Cardiac output curves obtained using the intermittent thermodilution method. **A:** Acceptable curves representing normal cardiac output, low cardiac output, and high cardiac output. Normal cardiac output curves have a smooth upstroke from the rapid injection followed by a gradual decline. The area under the curve is inversely proportional to the cardiac output. Curves associated with a low cardiac output have a greater area under the curve, with a more sloped upstroke and slower return to baseline. Curves associated with a high cardiac output have a small area under the curve, with a steeper upstroke and a more rapid return to baseline. **B:** An irregular cardiac output curve can result from improper injection technique (eg, irregular or uneven emptying of the injectate syringe) and must be eliminated from the averaging process.

Impedance Cardiography

Impedance cardiography (thoracic electrical bioimpedance) is a noninvasive method for monitoring cardiac output.[3] In impedance cardiography, two sets of electrodes are placed at the base of the neck and the lower thorax (Fig. 9-15). The outer set of electrodes transmits a low-voltage electrical current, which seeks the path of a least resistance (ie, the blood-filled thoracic aorta), while the inner set of electrodes measures the impedance to that current. The impedence changes due to the pulsatile blood flow in the descending aorta during systole and diastole. The change in impedance over time directly reflects left ventricular contractility and is mathematically converted into stroke volume and cardiac output values using an algorithm. Other hemodynamic parameters can also be measured or calculated from the data obtained using impedance cardiography and are provided on a continuous, real-time basis (Table 9-4).

Esophageal Doppler Monitoring

An esophageal Doppler monitor (EDM) incorporates a Doppler transducer into a nasogastric tube. When placed in the esophagus, the EDM allows monitoring of blood flow velocity through the descending aorta (Fig. 9-16). The pulsatile velocity waveform directly reflects left ventricular contractility as well as the patient's intravascular volume status (preload).[4]

Continuous cardiac output and stroke volume determinations are calculated from the Doppler waveform using an algorithm based on the Doppler waveform configuration and the patient's height, weight, and age.

The waveform shape can also be used to determine changes in myocardial contractility and preload. The peak velocity (an indicator of myocardial contractility) is determined from the amplitude of the waveform. The flow time (a reflection of systolic ejection time and thus intravascular volume and changes in preload) is determined by measuring the width of the base of the waveform. As flow from the left ventricle increases, the base widens. Conversely, hypovolemia causes the base of the waveform to narrow.

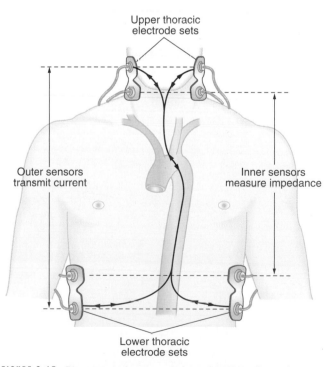

FIGURE 9-15 Placement of sensors in impedance cardiography. (Courtesy of Cardiodynamic International.)

TABLE 9-4 Additional Hemodynamic Parameters Obtained from Impedance Cardiography

Parameter	Clinical Significance	Normal Values
Change in impedance/time (dZ/dt)	Magnitude and rate of impedance change; direct reflection of force of left ventricular contraction	0.8–2.5 Ohms/s
Velocity index (VI)	Peak velocity of blood flow in the aorta; direct reflection of force of left ventricular contraction	33–65/1000 s
Acceleration contractility index (ACI)	Initial acceleration of blood flow in the aorta; direct reflection of myocardial contractility	Males: 70–150/100 s^2 Females: 90–170/100 s^2
Preejection period (PEP)	Systolic time interval, measuring length of time for isovolumetric contraction	0.05–0.12 s
Ventricular ejection time (VET)	Systolic time interval, measuring length of time for left ventricular ejection	0.25–0.35 s (depends on heart rate, preload, and contractility)
Thoracic fluid content status (Zo)	Base thoracic impedance and the electrical conductivity of the chest cavity (primarily determined by the intravascular, intra-alveolar, and interstitial fluids in the thorax) Lower values indicate greater thoracic fluid volume.	Males, 20–30 ohms Females, 25–35 ohms (Normal ranges may vary slightly depending on equipment used.)
Thoracic fluid content (TFC)	The inverse of Zo (1/Zo × 1000) Electrical conductivity of the chest cavity; reflects intravascular, interstitial, alveolar, and intracellular fluid Higher values indicate greater thoracic fluid volume	Males: 30–50/k ohms Females: 21–37/k ohms (Normal ranges may vary slightly depending on equipment used.)

Evaluation of Oxygen Delivery and Demand Balance

When patients are critically ill, careful evaluation of the adequacy of oxygen delivery, oxygen extraction (removal of oxygen from hemoglobin for cellular use), and oxygen consumption with respect to oxygen demand is paramount. If oxygen delivery and consumption are insufficient to meet oxygen demand, the result is hypoxia and the accumulation of an oxygen deficit. Persistent oxygen deficit causes cell and organ dysfunction and eventually leads to cell death and organ failure. Parameters used to evaluate oxygen delivery and demand balance are summarized in Table 9-5.

Arterial oxygen delivery (DaO_2) is the amount of oxygen transported to the tissues. Arterial oxygen delivery depends on cardiac output, hemoglobin levels, and the arterial oxygen saturation (ie, the amount of oxygen bound to hemoglobin). Deficiencies of hemoglobin, arterial saturation, or cardiac output decrease arterial oxygen delivery.

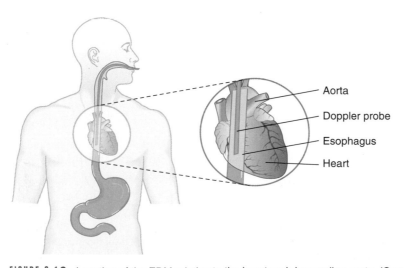

Aorta

Doppler probe

Esophagus

Heart

FIGURE 9-16 Location of the EDM relative to the heart and descending aorta. (Courtesy of Deltex Medical, Inc.)

TABLE 9-5 Oxygen Utilization Variables

Parameter	Definition	Formula	Normal Values
Arterial oxygen content (CaO$_2$)	The amount of oxygen carried by hemoglobin in a deciliter of arterial blood	(Hb × 1.37 × SaO$_2$) + (0.003 × PaO$_2$)	20 mL O$_2$/dL
Venous oxygen content (CvO$_2$)	The amount of oxygen carried by hemoglobin in a deciliter of venous blood	(Hb × 1.37 × SvO$_2$) + (0.003 × PvO$_2$)	15 mL O$_2$/dL
Arterial oxygen delivery index (DaO$_2$I)	The amount of oxygen transported in the blood from the left ventricle through the arteries and capillaries to the tissues in 1 min, indexed to the patient's body surface area (BSA)	CI × CaO$_2$ × 10	500–600 mL O$_2$/min/m²
Venous oxygen delivery index (DvO$_2$I)	The amount of oxygen in the blood returned to the right ventricle from the tissues via the veins in 1 min, indexed to the patient's BSA	CI × CvO$_2$ × 10	375–450 mL O$_2$/min/m²
Mixed venous oxygen saturation (SvO$_2$)	The oxygen saturation of venous blood, measured in the pulmonary artery	Direct measurement	60%–80%
Central venous oxygen saturation (ScvO$_2$)	The oxygen saturation of venous blood, measured in the superior vena cava	Direct measurement	65%–85%
Partial pressure of oxygen, venous blood (PvO$_2$)	The amount of oxygen dissolved in the plasma of venous blood	Direct measurement	35–45 mm Hg
O$_2$ extraction	The amount of oxygen that is removed (extracted) from hemoglobin for use by the cells	CaO$_2$ – CvO$_2$	3–5 mL O$_2$/dL
Oxygen extraction ratio (OER)	The percent of oxygen delivered that is removed (extracted) from hemoglobin for use by the cells	$\dfrac{CaO_2 - CvO_2}{CaO_2}$	22%–30%
Oxygen consumption index (VO$_2$I)	The amount of oxygen used by the cells every minute, indexed to the patient's BSA	(CaO$_2$ – CvO$_2$) × CI × 10	120–170 mL/min/m²
Arterial pH (pHa)	The acidity (pH) of arterial blood	Direct measurement	7.35–7.45
Base excess/base deficit (BE/BD)	The amount of base required to titrate 1 L of arterial blood to a pH of 7.40; decreases with metabolic acidosis	Direct measurement	–2 to +2
Lactate	A metabolic byproduct of the Krebs cycle that increases with anaerobic metabolism	Direct measurement	0.5–2.2 mmol/L

Oxygen consumption (VO$_2$) is the amount of oxygen used by the cells of the body. The primary determinants of oxygen consumption are oxygen demand, oxygen delivery, and oxygen extraction.

- **Oxygen demand** (the cells' requirement for oxygen) is not directly measurable. Stressors (eg, surgery, infection, pain) increase oxygen demand. Factors that decrease the metabolic rate (eg, hypothermia, sedation, pharmacological paralysis) reduce oxygen demand.
- **Oxygen delivery** also influences oxygen consumption (Fig. 9-17). If oxygen delivery is inadequate, as the oxygen delivery decreases, oxygen consumption increases to meet the existing oxygen demand (ie, oxygen consumption becomes supply dependent). When the requirement for oxygen is met, further increases in oxygen delivery do not increase consumption (ie, oxygen consumption is now supply independent). The point of critical oxygen delivery is the point at which oxygen delivery is sufficient to meet the oxygen demand and oxygen consumption does not increase further. The goal in critical care is for the patient to become supply independent, thus ensuring adequate oxygen delivery.
- **Oxygen extraction** is equal to the arterial oxygen content (CaO$_2$) minus the venous oxygen

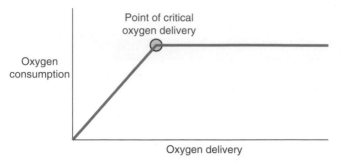

FIGURE 9-17 Delivery-dependent oxygen consumption curve. At the point of critical oxygen delivery, oxygen delivery is sufficient to meet oxygen demand, and oxygen consumption becomes supply independent.

content (CvO_2). Like the arterial oxygen content, the venous oxygen content is determined primarily by the amount of hemoglobin that is saturated with oxygen. Normally, provided that oxygen is supplied in adequate amounts, the cells extract the oxygen they need to support tissue and organ function. Increased demand for oxygen results in a compensatory increase in oxygen extraction, as more oxygen is "unloaded" from the hemoglobin for cellular use. The decreased amount of oxygen in venous blood means that the $CaO_2 - CvO_2$ difference is larger. Conversely, as oxygen demands decrease, less oxygen is required and extracted from the blood, and the $CaO_2 - CvO_2$ difference becomes smaller.

An imbalance of oxygen supply and demand occurs whenever oxygen delivery is inadequate to meet cellular demand or the cells are unable to extract sufficient quantities of oxygen. Threats to the balance of oxygen supply and demand include

- Decreased cardiac output, hemoglobin, or arterial saturation
- Impaired cellular extraction of oxygen
- Oxygen demands so great that they cannot be met by increased oxygen delivery or extraction

Evaluation of Global Tissue Oxygenation Status

Metabolic Indicators

Inadequate oxygen delivery to meet oxygen demands results in anaerobic metabolism and cellular hypoxia. During anaerobic metabolism, lactic acid is produced and begins to accumulate, causing metabolic acidosis. Therefore, laboratory measurement of lactate levels, serum pH, and base excess/base deficit (BE/BD) are means to evaluate oxygen deficit. Elevated lactate levels or metabolic acidosis correlate with oxygen deficit, particularly when the patient has a low or normal level of oxygen delivery and oxygen consumption. Lactate levels, pH, and BE/BD should always be viewed in conjunction with other assessment parameters.

Venous Oxygen Saturation

The venous oxygen saturation is used to evaluate the global balance of oxygen supply and oxygen consumption (oxygen demand). Mixed venous oxygen saturation (SvO_2) is measured using a PAC and reflects the level of saturated hemoglobin in venous blood returning to the right ventricle and pulmonary artery. Alternatively, the venous oxygen saturation ($ScvO_2$) can be measured in the superior vena cava through a central venous catheter. (The values obtained using a central venous catheter are slightly higher than normal because the blood sampled does not represent a "true" mixed venous saturation). Either a decrease in oxygen delivery or an increase in oxygen consumption (oxygen demand) can decrease the amount of oxygen returning to the right side of heart, due to greater tissue extraction of oxygen.

Specialized central venous catheters or PACs containing fiberoptic filaments facilitate continuous measurement of venous oxygen saturation. The fiberoptic filaments emit infrared light that reflects off red blood cells that are saturated with oxygen. The computer calculates the percentage of saturated hemoglobin compared with the total hemoglobin to yield the venous saturation value and updates the information every few seconds.

A low venous oxygen saturation is an early warning that oxygen delivery is inadequate or oxygen demand is high. The nurse assesses the components of oxygen delivery (ie, cardiac output, hemoglobin, and arterial oxygen saturation) and for any increase in oxygen demand (eg, shivering, pain).

A high venous oxygen saturation may be the result of

- Oxygen delivery that is much greater than oxygen demand
- A low metabolic rate and oxygen demand (eg, hypothermia, anesthesia)
- Pathological conditions (eg, sepsis) in which cells cannot extract oxygen from the blood or in which tissue beds are not well perfused with oxygenated blood (ie, oxygen is not extracted from the blood despite the cellular oxygen demand)

Venous oxygen saturation monitoring may be a helpful guide in nursing interventions. For example, endotracheal suctioning may cause a temporary decrease in arterial oxygenation and increase discomfort and anxiety (leading to increased oxygen demand). Monitoring the venous oxygen saturation allows the nurse to judge the impact of this activity on the patient's oxygen supply and demand and take appropriate measures (eg, hyperoxygenating and hyperventilating before suctioning) to mitigate the negative effects of the intervention on oxygen supply and demand.

Evaluation of Regional Tissue Oxygenation Status

Gastric tonometry and sublingual capnometry are used to evaluate perfusion of specific tissue beds that have early susceptibility to hypoperfusion.

- **Gastric tonometry.** In early shock or shock states, a compensatory mechanism occurs in which blood flow is diverted from the nonvital organs (gastrointestinal tract) to vital organs, causing underperfusion of the gastric mucosa and upper gastrointestinal tract. Anaerobic metabolism produces increased amounts of carbon dioxide and lactate; thus, measuring the carbon dioxide level or pH of these tissue beds provides an early indicator of oxygen supply and demand mismatch. In gastric tonometry, a nasogastric tube with a gas-permeable balloon near the distal end is used to measure the partial pressure of carbon dioxide (PCO_2) and calculate the pH of the gastric mucosa. Decreasing gastric mucosal pH or an increasing gastric PCO_2 out of the normal range suggests hypoperfusion and is an indication that oxygen delivery and consumption should be analyzed and optimized.[5]
- *Sublingual capnometry.* In sublingual capnometry, a thermometer-like device is placed under the tongue to measure the PCO_2. Sublingual capnometry is based on the same physiological principles as gastric tonometry. Blood flow to the area under the tongue is reduced in response to shock or hemorrhage.

CASE STUDY

Ms. J., a 68-year-old woman, collapsed in her garden. She was subsequently admitted to the coronary care unit. She has a 10-year history of coronary artery disease and is taking propranolol, digoxin, and nitroglycerin ointment. On admission, she appears pale, diaphoretic, lethargic, and disoriented. Heart sounds S_1, S_2, S_3, and S_4 are audible. Her ECG shows second-degree atrioventricular block (Mobitz type II), premature ventricular contractions (PVCs), and ST segment elevation in leads V_3, V_4, and aVL. Vital signs are HR, 90 beats/min, BP, 90/50 mm Hg; and RR, 24 breaths/min. ABGs are PaO_2, 73 mm Hg; $PaCO_2$, 25 mm Hg; SaO_2, 96%; and pH, 7.35.

Initial interventions include control of anginal pain, supplemental oxygen, and amiodarone infusion. Because of Ms. J.'s age and history, a pulmonary artery catheter (PAC) is inserted. One hour after admission, the following hemodynamic data are obtained: RAP, 10 mm Hg; pulmonary artery systolic/diastolic pressure, 35/20 mm Hg; PAOP, 19 mm Hg; cardiac index (CI), 1.3 L/min/m²; systemic vascular resistance (SVR), 1688 d/s/cm⁻⁵; mixed venous oxygen saturation, 48%.

Interventions to improve Ms. J.'s cardiac function and organ perfusion include amiodarone, nitroglycerin infusion at 10 µg/min, dobutamine infusion at 7 µg/min, morphine for pain, IV, PRN; oxygen, 4 L/min by nasal cannula; intra-aortic balloon counterpulsation, 1:1; and external pacemaker with standby for pacemaker insertion. Therapeutic goals are stabilized cardiac conduction, enhanced myocardial contractility at the least cost to the heart by reducing

preload and afterload, and improved oxygen supply to the myocardium. The combination of drugs and supplemental oxygen serves to achieve these goals. Intra-aortic balloon pumping primarily decreases afterload but also augments coronary perfusion.

Several hours later, assessment shows that Ms. J. is still pale but has improved capillary refill and is oriented to person, place, and time. Audible heart sounds are S_1, S_2, and S_4. The ECG shows rare PVCs with ST elevation and T inversion in leads V_3, V_4, and aVL. Vital signs are HR, 85 beats/min; BP, 100/50 mm Hg; RR, 18 breaths/min. ABGs are PaO_2, 138 mm Hg; $PaCO_2$, 31 mm Hg; SaO_2, 99%; and pH, 7.44. At this time, hemodynamic data are RAP, 9 mm Hg; pulmonary artery systolic/diastolic pressure, 33/17 mm Hg; PAOP, 15 mm Hg; cardiac index, 2.6 L/min/m²; SVR, 1014 d/s/cm⁻⁵; and mixed venous oxygen saturation, 60%.

The results of the interventions are improved left ventricular function, which reduced the backward failure; loss of S_3; and improved arterial oxygenation. The Mobitz II conduction defect resolves as coronary perfusion increases. The metabolic acidosis also appears to be resolving due to improved oxygen delivery to the organs as evidenced by normalization of both the $PaCO_2$ and pH.

1. What are the main concerns associated with the initial assessment findings?
2. What is the significance of the first set of hemodynamic data?
3. How did the interventions affect Ms. J.'s hemodynamic status and oxygen delivery?

References

1. Best Practices: Evidence Based, 2nd ed. Lippincott Williams & Wilkins, 2007, p 201
2. Chapter 73 Pulmonary artery catheter insertion (assist) and pressure monitoring. In: Wiegand D, ed. AACN Procedure Manual, 6th ed. 2011.
3. Kamath SA, Drazner MH, Tasissa G, et al: Correlation of impedance cardiography with invasive hemodynamic measurements in patients with advanced heart failure: the BioImpedance CardioGraphy (BIG) substudy of the Evaluation Study of Congestive Heart Failure and Pulmonary Artery Catheterization Effectiveness (ESCAPE) Trial. Am Heart J 158(2):217–223, 2009
4. Phan T, et al: Improving perioperative outcomes: fluid optimization with esophageal Doppler monitoring: A metaanalysis and review. J Am Coll Surg 207(6):935–941, 2008
5. Palizas F, et al: Gastric tonometry versus cardiac index as resuscitation goals in septic shock: A multicenter randomized controlled rials. Crit Care 13:R44, 2009

Want to know more? A wide variety of resources to enhance your learning and understanding of this chapter are available on thePoint⁂. Visit **http://thepoint.lww.com/MortonEss1e** to access chapter review questions and more!

Airway Management and Ventilatory Support

OBJECTIVES

Based on the content in this chapter, the reader should be able to:

1 Describe nursing care for a patient with an oropharyngeal airway, nasopharyngeal airway, endotracheal tube, or tracheostomy tube.
2 Describe proper suctioning technique and indications for suctioning.
3 Compare and contrast commonly used ventilator modes.
4 Describe nursing care for a patient receiving mechanical ventilation.
5 Describe general principles of weaning.

Airway Management

Artificial Airways

Artificial airways are used to:

• Establish an airway
• Protect the airway
• Facilitate airway clearance
• Facilitate mechanical ventilation

Oropharyngeal Airway

An oropharyngeal airway is a hard plastic device that is inserted through the mouth and extends to the pharynx to prevent the tongue from occluding the airway when muscle tone is decreased.

 RED FLAG! *An oropharyngeal airway is never placed in a conscious patient because it stimulates the gag reflex and can cause vomiting and aspiration.*

The oropharyngeal airway is inserted by holding down the tongue with a depressor and guiding the airway over the back of the tongue. Alternatively, the airway can be inserted with the opening of the curve facing the roof of the mouth, and gently advanced into the correct position by rotating the airway 180 degrees (Fig. 10-1). Following insertion of the oropharyngeal airway, the nurse monitors the patient frequently for airway patency by listening to breath sounds and observing chest wall movement and provides oropharyngeal suction as needed for emesis or oral secretions. To remove an oropharyngeal airway, the oropharynx is suctioned, and the airway is gently removed.

Nasopharyngeal Airway

A nasopharyngeal airway (nasal trumpet) is a flexible tube that is inserted nasally past the base of the tongue to maintain airway patency. Awake patients with an intact gag reflex may tolerate a nasopharyngeal airway better than an oropharyngeal airway.[1] In patients who require frequent nasotracheal suctioning, nasopharyngeal airways are used to prevent the discomfort and airway trauma that can result from repeated introduction of the suction catheter through the nares.

A nasopharyngeal airway that is too long will extend into the patient's trachea. To measure

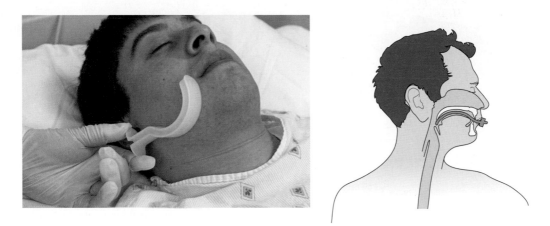

FIGURE 10-1 Sizing and positioning of the oropharyngeal airway.

length, the nurse holds the airway alongside the patient's face. The airway should extend from the tip of the nose to the earlobe (Fig. 10-2). The airway with the largest outer diameter that fits the patient's nostril should be used to facilitate suctioning.

Because the nasopharyngeal airway increases the patient's risk for epistaxis, the patient's history of epistaxis or coagulopathy is carefully reviewed before placing the airway. The nurse explains the procedure to the patient and lubricates the airway with water-soluble jelly or lidocaine jelly to alleviate discomfort. The airway is inserted into the nostril, pointing it down, toward the back of the throat. Once the airway is positioned, the patient is asked to exhale with the mouth closed. If the tube is in the correct position, air will be felt exiting from the tube opening. The proper positioning can also be confirmed visually, by depressing the tongue and looking for the airway's tip just behind the uvula.

During removal, the nasopharyngeal airway may have to be gently rotated to withdraw it from the nares. It is important to be prepared for the possibility of epistaxis following removal.

Endotracheal Tube

An endotracheal tube is a semi-rigid tube that is inserted through the nose or mouth and extends into the trachea (Fig 10-3). Advantages and disadvantages of oral and nasal placement are summarized in Table 10-1. An endotracheal tube is often indicated when it is necessary to obtain an airway or protect the airway from aspiration; endotracheal tubes come with a cuff, which is inflated to secure the airway in place and prevent aspiration. Endotracheal tubes are also frequently used for patients who require mechanical ventilation.

Endotracheal intubation is performed by personnel who have received advanced training in the procedure. Before the procedure, the nurse assembles the necessary equipment (Box 10-1) and confirms that the equipment and suction is working properly. Using a manual resuscitation bag (MRB) and mask, the nurse preoxygenates

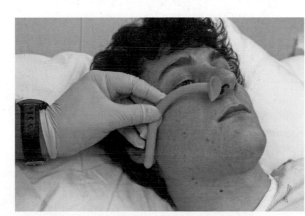

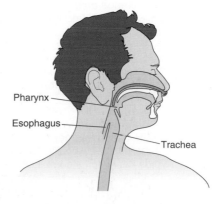

Pharynx

Esophagus

Trachea

FIGURE 10-2 Sizing and positioning of the nasopharyngeal airway.

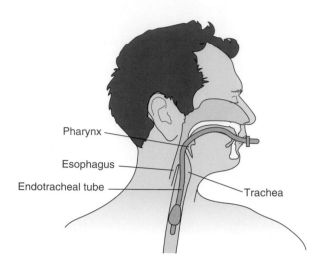

FIGURE 10-3   Positioning of the endotracheal tube.

the patient. The physician may use topical anesthetics, sedatives, short-acting IV anesthetics, or a short-acting neuromuscular blocking (NMB) agent to facilitate rapid and nontraumatic intubation.

The nurse assists during intubation by providing suction as necessary and monitoring the patient's heart rate, blood pressure, and arterial oxygen saturation (SaO_2) using pulse oximetry. Intubation attempts must be held and the patient oxygenated with the MRB if the SaO_2 falls below 90%. Oxygenation and ventilation with the MRB are also performed between intubation attempts. Hypoxemia during intubation may cause bradycardia, hypotension, dysrhythmias, and other complications.

After placement of the endotracheal tube, the cuff is inflated with air to the proper pressure (20 to 25 mm Hg). Underinflation of the cuff puts the patient at risk for aspiration, whereas overinflation can place excess pressure on the tracheal wall mucosa, leading to complications such as tracheal erosion and eventually stenosis. A manometer attached to the endotracheal tube pilot balloon allows measurement of the cuff pressure. Alternatively, the minimal occluding volume can be determined by inflating the cuff slowly while auscultating over the trachea. When the harsh "squeak" of air escaping is no longer audible, the minimal occluding volume has been reached, and the tube cuff is occluding the airway without excessive pressure on the trachea.

To prevent tube movement, tube migration, or inadvertent extubation, the endotracheal tube must be anchored securely with a tube holder. Proper tube placement is determined by auscultation and

TABLE 10-1   Nasal Versus Oral Endotracheal Tube Placement

Placement	Advantages	Disadvantages
Nasal	Patient comfort Prevents tube obstruction from biting Easily anchored and reduced risk for extubation Oral hygiene more effective Appropriate for use in patients with cervical spine injuries Improved ability for communication	Can kink and obstruct airway Predisposes to acute sinusitis, which may result in septic states Epistaxis and pressure necrosis of the nares can develop High risk for shearing off nasal polyps in patients with asthma Tube size usually limited to 6.0–6.5, which increases airway resistance Can penetrate into the brain through the basilar skull fracture
Oral	Less trauma during intubation Permits use of a larger endotracheal tube (less airway resistance) Avoids nasal/sinus complications	Uncomfortable for patient Pressure sores can develop on lips, gums, and tongue Easily obstructed by biting, necessitates a bite block Tube, bite block, and tube-securing devices complicate oral hygiene More difficult to secure, making self-extubation easier Makes communication more difficult

carbon dioxide monitoring and then confirmed with a chest radiograph:

- **Auscultation.** The nurse auscultates the chest bilaterally for equal breath sounds and the abdomen for evidence of esophageal intubation. Unequal breath sounds (greater on the right than on the left) indicate that the tube has been displaced into the right mainstem bronchus. The ability to auscultate air in the abdomen suggests esophageal, rather than tracheal, intubation.
- **Carbon dioxide monitoring.** An absence of carbon dioxide (detected using an end-tidal carbon dioxide monitor or disposable detector) suggests esophageal, rather than tracheal, intubation.
- **Chest radiograph.** A chest radiograph provides definitive confirmation of the tube's position. The endotracheal tube should be 2 to 3 cm above the carina.

 RED FLAG! *Persistent coughing may be a sign of downward displacement of the endotracheal tube.*

Once proper positioning is confirmed and the endotracheal tube is secured, the centimeter mark is noted at the lips or teeth (for an orally placed tube) or nostril (for a nasally placed tube). Noting the level of the tube facilitates ongoing assessment of the tube's position. Displacement of the tube could result in either right mainstem bronchus placement with left lung collapse or self-extubation.

Complications of endotracheal intubation are listed in Box 10-2. The nurse auscultates breath sounds for equality at least once every 4 hours, obtains a chest radiograph to assess tube placement every 24 hours, and monitors the cuff pressure with the manometer or minimal cuff leak technique every 6 to 8 hours. To prevent unintentional extubation,

---

BOX 10-2 Complications of Endotracheal Intubation

- Laryngospasm or bronchospasm
- Hypoxemia or hypercapnia during intubation
- Dysrhythmias, hypertension, or hypotension during intubation
- Laryngeal edema resulting in stridor with extubation
- Trauma to the nasal cavity, oral cavity, esophagus, trachea, or larynx
- Fractured teeth
- Nosocomial infection (pneumonia, sinusitis, abscess)
- Right mainstem bronchus or esophageal intubation
- Aspiration of oral or gastric contents
- Tracheal stenosis or tracheomalacia (collapse of the walls of the trachea)
- Laryngeal stenosis, paralysis, or necrosis
- Tracheoesophageal fistula
- Rupture of the innominate artery
- Vocal cord paralysis

---

the nurse orients the patient to the need for the endotracheal tube and takes measures to ensure the patient's comfort. If these measures are not effective, the physician may order physical or pharmacological restraints.

 RED FLAG! *If a patient is unintentionally extubated for any reason, the airway must be assessed immediately and kept patent. Oxygenation and ventilation may be provided, if required, with an MRB and mask until reintubation can be accomplished.*

Ongoing care of the patient with an endotracheal tube includes replacing the tube holder when it is soiled or becomes insecure. In orally intubated patients, the position of the endotracheal tube is changed from side to side to facilitate oral care and to prevent areas of pressure necrosis on the lips, mouth, and tongue.[2] Before resecuring the tube, the nurse verifies proper positioning by comparing the centimeter markings at the lips, teeth, or nostril with the last radiological documentation of position. Placement of a short oral bite block can prevent biting on the tube, which can cause tube occlusion. Proper oral care and regular inspection of the oral mucosa are of paramount importance when a bite block is used.

Before extubation, the patient must be able to maintain his own airway, as evidenced by an appropriate level of consciousness and the presence of cough and gag reflexes. In all patients, but especially in those with a history of difficult intubation or reactive airway disease, the cuff-leak test should be performed before extubation. After suctioning the oropharynx, the tube cuff is deflated and the endotracheal tube is briefly occluded to demonstrate an air leak around the tube with patient inspiration. Absence of a leak can indicate edema and may predict laryngeal stridor or loss of the airway after extubation. If the cuff-leak test fails, the patient may be given corticosteroids to reduce edema for 24 to 48 hours and then reassessed using the cuff-leak test. In addition, the trachea may be directly visualized with a bronchoscope before extubation to verify that the edema has resolved.

Extubation should never occur unless a qualified person is available to reintubate emergently if the patient does not tolerate extubation. An MRB and mask are kept readily available at the bedside. After explaining the procedure and preparing the patient, the nurse suctions the endotracheal tube and posterior oropharynx, loosens the endotracheal tube holder, and deflates the cuff. The endotracheal tube is removed quickly while having the patient cough. The patient's mouth is suctioned, and humidified oxygen is applied immediately. The patient is evaluated for immediate signs of distress (eg, stridor, dyspnea, a decrease in SaO_2). If signs of distress are present, racemic epinephrine and 100% FiO_2 may be administered. If these interventions fail, immediate reintubation may be necessary.

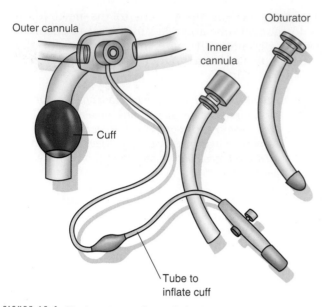

FIGURE 10-4   Tracheostomy tube and obturator.

Tracheostomy

A tracheostomy tube is inserted directly into the trachea through a stoma made in the neck. Advantages of a tracheostomy tube over an endotracheal tube include improved patient comfort, an improved ability to communicate, and the possibility for oral feeding. In patients requiring long-term mechanical ventilation, the tracheostomy tube is the preferred method of airway management to prevent tracheal complications and improve suctioning of secretions (Fig. 10-4). Current practice promotes early tracheostomy (eg, after 7 to 10 days on the ventilator) to facilitate earlier weaning.[3,4] Indications for tracheostomy are summarized in Box 10-3.

A tracheostomy may be performed in the operating room or at the bedside, using a percutaneous progressive dilatation technique. Percutaneous tracheostomy performed at the bedside is associated with less morbidity than the standard procedure performed in the operating room.[4] The equipment used for tracheostomy is summarized in Box 10-4. Complications of tracheostomy are listed in Box 10-5.

Initially, the tracheostomy tube is sutured to the neck in both surgical and percutaneous procedures. The sutures are removed after 48 to 72 hours. The tracheostomy tube is secured at all times with twill tape or a tracheostomy tube holder, even with the sutures in place, to prevent accidental dislodgment (decannulation). If decannulation occurs within the first 7 days of tracheostomy insertion (before a tract is formed in the tissue), the patient may be intubated with an endotracheal tube if emergent tracheostomy tube replacement cannot be done safely. If inadvertent decannulation occurs after a tract has developed, the tracheostomy tube is carefully replaced through the stoma. An obturator and a new, appropriately sized tracheostomy tube are kept at the bedside for this purpose.

The routine care of tracheostomies, which includes cleaning the tracheostomy site every 8 to

12 hours and as needed and cleaning or replacing the inner cannula daily or according to facility policy, is performed as a sterile procedure while in the hospital.[5] The stoma is cleansed with half-strength hydrogen peroxide, followed by rinse with sterile saline, and observed for wound healing, bleeding, and signs of infection. Longer care intervals (eg, daily or as needed) usually are instituted after 7 to 10 days or when secretion and tracheostomy drainage are minimal. Tracheostomy care also includes frequent changing of the tracheal ties and dressing, although initially the ties are not changed until at least 24 to 48 hours after placement to allow for hemostasis of the site. The ties should be tied so that one to two fingers can be inserted between the ties and the skin. This amount of slack minimizes movement of the tracheostomy tube while maintaining the patient's comfort. The midline position of the tracheostomy tube must be maintained to prevent pressure on the surrounding tissue, which can result in erosion.

Prior to removing the tracheostomy tube, the tracheostomy tube may be capped and the cuff deflated for 24 to 48 hours. The patient's ability to breathe and speak around the tracheostomy tube is the final test to ensure airway patency.

Suctioning

Oral Suctioning

Oral suctioning is important when the patient's trachea is intubated because the patient's ability to swallow can be limited. The nurse performs oral suctioning as needed for copious oral secretions and after suctioning the artificial airway. Removal of posterior oropharyngeal secretions with subglottic suctioning minimizes the buildup of oral secretions on top of the endotracheal tube cuff and reduces the risk for aspiration and ventilator-associated pneumonia (VAP).

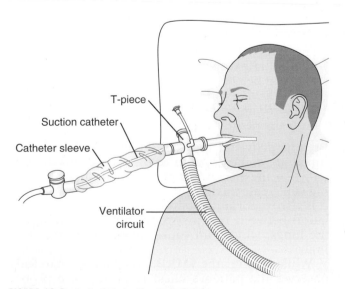

T-piece

Suction catheter

Catheter sleeve

Ventilator circuit

FIGURE 10·5 An in-line suction catheter.

> ### BOX 10·6 Complications of Suctioning
>
> - Hypoxemia
> - Dysrhythmias
> - Vagal stimulation leading to bradycardia and hypotension
> - Bronchospasm
> - Elevated intracranial pressure
> - Atelectasis
> - Tracheal mucosal trauma and bleeding
> - Nosocomial infection
> - Discomfort

Nasotracheal Suctioning

Nasotracheal suctioning is done as a sterile procedure by the nurse or respiratory therapist. A flexible red rubber suction catheter is lubricated and passed through the nostril or nasopharyngeal tube to the back of the nasopharynx. Asking the patient to cough opens the epiglottis, facilitating advancement of the catheter. A change in the sound of the cough and the return of sputum with suctioning indicates passage into the tracheal tree.

Endotracheal and Tracheostomy Suctioning

The presence of the artificial airway prevents glottic closure. As a result, the patient is unable to use the normal clearing mechanism (ie, effective coughing). In addition, the artificial airway is a foreign object, which increases the production of secretions. Suctioning is required to remove secretions and maintain airway patency. In-line suction catheters (Fig. 10-5), which remain connected to the artificial airway and ventilator circuit, are recommended for use in all intubated and ventilated patients. Subglottic suctioning catheters (continuous and intermittent) are also frequently used to prevent the subglottic accumulation of secretions that may lead to aspiration.

Suctioning is not without risks (Box 10-6) and should be done only when needed. Indications for suctioning include visualization of secretions in the artificial airway; the presence of crackles, rhonchi, mucus plugs, or coughing; an increase in the peak airway pressure or a decrease in tidal volume during pressure ventilation; and deterioration of the patient's oxygenation status (ie, decreased SaO_2). The sterile procedure for endotracheal or tracheostomy suctioning (based on the Centers for Disease Control and Prevention recommendations) is given in Box 10-7.

RED FLAG! *The routine instillation of normal saline to facilitate removal of thick secretions is not recommended. Saline instillation causes oxygenation to decrease and may predispose patients to nosocomial infection by transporting bacteria to lower airways.*[6]

BOX 10-7   Endotracheal and Tracheostomy Suctioning

Equipment

Sterile suction catheter sized for either endotracheal tube or tracheostomy

Sterile gloves

Sterile normal saline for irrigation, only when indicated

Sterile disposable container

Technique

1. Prepare for the procedure: Administer medication, assemble equipment, explain the procedure to the patient, adjust the bed to a comfortable working position, prepare suction pressure, wash hands, prepare and open equipment and supplies, and don gloves.
2. Hyperoxygenate the patient with 100% oxygen with the ventilator. Preoxygenate must last at least 2 minutes. Return to the previous oxygen setting after suctioning is completed and an in-line suctioning should be used to avoid loss of PEEP and desaturation.
3. Quickly but gently, insert the catheter as far as possible into the artificial airway without applying suction. For tracheostomy patients, limit the distance to just beyond the end of the tracheostomy device.
4. Withdraw the catheter 1 to 2 cm, and apply intermittent suction while rotating and removing the catheter. Limit suction pressure to 80 to 120 mm Hg. Each suctioning attempt should not exceed 10 to 15 seconds (3 to 5 seconds for patients with a tracheostomy tube). Prolonged suctioning can lead to severe hypoxemia, hemodynamic instability, and cardiac arrest.
5. Monitor the patient's heart rate and rhythm and pulse oximetry values during and after suctioning. Discontinue the procedure if the patient does not tolerate it, as evidenced by dysrhythmias, bradycardia, or a drop in arterial oxygen saturation (SaO_2).
6. Remove equipment.
7. Provide oral hygiene. Cleanse suction tubing with a saline rinse to flush secretions into the suction container.
8. Complete the procedure: Wash your hands and document.

Ventilatory Support

Manual Ventilation

An MRB (Ambu bag, bag-valve-mask device) connected to an oxygen source is typically used in emergencies (eg, unintential extubation, acute respiratory failure). In situations such as cardiopulmonary resuscitation (CPR) where a high concentration of oxygen (eg, 74% to 100%) is required, an MRB with a reservoir must be used.

EVIDENCE-BASED PRACTICE GUIDELINES: Endotracheal Suctioning of Mechanically Ventilated Patients

PROBLEM: Although necessary for patients with artificial airways, endotracheal suctioning is associated with substantial risks. Clinicians must be aware of the risks and take appropriate precautions to ensure patient safety.

EVIDENCE-BASED PRACTICE GUIDELINES

1. Perform endotracheal suctioning only when secretions are present, not routinely. (recommended)
2. Consider pre-oxygenation if the patient has a clinically important reduction in oxygen saturation with suctioning. (suggested)
3. Perform suctioning without disconnecting the patient from the ventilator. (suggested)
4. Use shallow, rather than deep, suction. (suggested)
5. Do not routinely instill normal saline prior to endotracheal suctioning. (suggested)
6. Use closed suction for patients with high FiO_2 or positive end-expiratory pressure (PEEP) and those who are at risk for lung derecruitment. (suggested)
7. If suctioning-induced lung derecruitment occurs in patients with acute lung injury, avoid disconnection and use lung recruitment maneuvers. (suggested)
8. In adults, use a suction catheter that occludes less than 50% the lumen of the endotracheal tube. (suggested)
9. Limit the duration of the suctioning event to less than 15 seconds. (suggested)

■ These clinical practice guidelines, developed by the American Association for Respiratory Care Clinical Practice Guidelines Steering Committee, are based on an electronic literature search between January 1990 and October 2009 and include a review of 114 clinical trials, 62 reviews, and 6 meta-analyses on endotracheal suctioning. Recommendations are graded according to the Grading of Recommendations Assessment, Development, and Evaluation (GRADE) criteria.

■ Published in Respiratory Care 55(6):758–764, 2010.

When operating an MRB:

- The force of squeezing the bag determines the tidal volume delivered to the patient.
- The number of hand squeezes per minute determines the assisted respiratory rate.
- The force and rate that the bag is squeezed determine the peak flow.

Breaths delivered to a conscious patient must be timed to coincide with spontaneous inspiratory effort, or the discomfort of dyssynchronous breathing will create anxiety and resistance to ventilation. It is also important to allow time for complete exhalation between breaths to prevent air trapping in the lungs, which can cause hypotension and lung injury.

While using the MRB, the nurse carefully observes the patient's chest rise to ensure proper ventilation. In addition, the nurse monitors for the development of abdominal distention, which is an indication of esophageal intubation. If a patient becomes progressively more difficult to ventilate using an MRB, conditions associated with decreased lung compliance (eg, an increase in secretions, pneumothorax, worsening bronchospasms) must be considered.

Mechanical Ventilation

When a patient is unable to maintain a patent airway, adequate gas exchange, or both, despite aggressive pulmonary management, more invasive support with intubation and mechanical ventilation must be considered. This step carries its own risks (Box 10-8) and imposes significant physical and psychological burdens on the patient and family. Every effort is made to avoid intubation and mechanical ventilation, but it becomes necessary when respiratory distress becomes respiratory failure. Respiratory failure is defined as the inability to maintain adequate respiration, as measured by an arterial blood pH less than 7.25, an arterial carbon dioxide level ($PaCO_2$) greater than 50 mm Hg, and an arterial oxygen level (PaO_2) less than 50 mm Hg (even with the patient on oxygen).

The goal of mechanical ventilation is to maintain alveolar ventilation appropriate for the patient's metabolic needs and to correct hypoxemia and maximize oxygen transport. Desired clinical outcomes of mechanical ventilation may include:

- Reversal of hypoxemia
- Reversal of acute respiratory acidosis

BOX 10-8 Complications of Mechanical Ventilation

Airway
- Aspiration
- Ventilator-acquired pneumonia (VAP)
- Complications of endotracheal intubation or tracheostomy (see Boxes 10-2 and 10-5)

Mechanical
- Lung injury (eg, barotrauma, volutrauma)
- Atelectasis (resulting from hypoventilation)
- Hypocapnia and respiratory alkalosis (resulting from hyperventilation)
- Hyperthermia (resulting from overheated inspired air)
- Hypercapnia and respiratory acidosis (hypoventilation)

Physiological
- Depressed cardiac function, resulting in hypotension
- Fluid overload
- Respiratory muscle weakness and atrophy
- Complications of immobility
- Gastrointestinal problems (eg, paralytic ileus, stress ulcers, distention)

- Relief of respiratory distress
- Prevention or reversal of atelectasis
- Resting of ventilatory muscles
- Reduction in systemic oxygen consumption, myocardial oxygen consumption, or both
- Stabilization of the chest wall

Overview of Mechanical Ventilation

Ventilators are classified as either negative-pressure or positive-pressure ventilators. Negative-pressure ventilators encase the patient's body and exert negative pressure that pulls the thoracic cage outward to initiate inspiration. In current clinical practice, use of negative-pressure ventilators is limited. Positive-pressure ventilators, which are much more commonly used, deliver air by pumping it into the patient's lungs. With positive-pressure ventilation, the normal relationship between intrapulmonary pressures during inspiration and expiration is reversed (ie, pressures during inspiration are positive and pressures during expiration are negative).

 RED FLAG! *Using positive pressure ventilation, intrathoracic pressures are increased causing venous return to decrease. As a result, patients with conditions associated with decreased sympathetic response (eg, hypovolemia, sepsis, heart disease, advanced age) may develop hypotension during positive pressure ventilation.*

There are three major modes of positive-pressure ventilation:

- **Volume ventilation.** With volume ventilation, a designated volume of air (tidal volume) is delivered with each breath. Volume ventilation is commonly used in critical care settings.
- **Pressure ventilation.** With pressure ventilation, a selected gas pressure is delivered to the patient and sustained throughout the phase of ventilation.
- **High-frequency ventilation.** High-frequency ventilation accomplishes oxygenation by the diffusion of oxygen and carbon dioxide from high to low gradients of concentration. Diffusion is increased when the kinetic energy of the gas molecules is increased. High-frequency ventilation uses small tidal volumes (1–3 mL/kg) at frequencies greater than 100 breaths/minute.[7] The breathing pattern of a person receiving high-frequency ventilation is somewhat analogous to that of panting, which entails moving small volumes of air at a very fast rate (Fig. 10-6). High-frequency ventilation is used to achieve lower peak ventilatory pressures, which reduces the risk for lung injury caused by high pressures. In addition, its different flow delivery characteristics are associated with improved ventilation-perfusion matching. Potential adverse effects associated with high-frequency ventilation include air trapping and necrotizing tracheobronchitis, when used in the absence of adequate humidification.[7]

Various types of lung injury can occur with positive pressure ventilation:

- **Barotrauma** can result from high pressures. With barotrauma, air can leak from the alveoli into the pleural space, resulting in pneumothorax or pneumomediastinum.
- **Volutrauma** is caused by the delivery of large tidal volumes. The alveoli develop fractures that allow fluid and protein to seep into the lungs, resulting in a form of noncardiogenic pulmonary edema.
- **Atelectrauma** is a shear-induced injury resulting from repeated opening and closing of the alveoli.
- **Biotrauma** is damage to the alveoli caused by the release of cytokines and other chemical mediators of the inflammatory response in response to positive-pressure ventilation.
- **Ventilator-associated lung injury (VALI)** and **ventilator-induced lung injury (VILI)** are terms used to describe damage to the lungs resulting from prolonged ventilation. Prolonged high levels of oxygen, high volumes, and pressures may lead to loss of surfactant and increased inflammation of the lung parenchyma and alveoli. The increase in inflammatory mediators damages the alveolar-capillary membrane, resulting in fluid leaking into the lungs and noncardiogenic pulmonary edema.

Mechanical ventilation bypasses the upper airway; therefore, a humidifier with a temperature control is added to the ventilator circuit to humidify and warm the inspired air. The humidity in the air helps to prevent drying of the secretions, which can lead to mucus plugging and make suctioning of secretions more difficult. In most instances, the temperature of the air is about body temperature. Rarely, the air temperatures may be increased (eg, for a patient with severe hypothermia); however, caution is necessary with higher temperatures because they increase the patient's risk for tracheal burns.

Ventilator Settings

Although the respiratory therapist may share or have complete responsibility for managing the ventilator settings, the nurse must still assess and understand the ventilator settings to provide effective nursing care. Common settings include:

- **Fraction of inspired oxygen (FiO$_2$).** The FiO$_2$ is the percentage of oxygen in the air delivered to the patient. Usually, the FiO$_2$ is adjusted to maintain an SaO$_2$ of greater than 90%. Initially, the patient is placed on a high level of FiO$_2$ (60% or higher),

but because oxygen toxicity is a concern when an FiO$_2$ of greater than 60% is required for more than 24 hours, strategies are implemented to maintain the FiO$_2$ at 60% or less after the initial intubation. Subsequent changes in FiO$_2$ are based on arterial blood gases and the SaO$_2$.

- **Tidal volume.** The tidal volume is the amount of air to be delivered with each breath. With volume ventilators, the tidal volume is set by the clinician. Tidal volumes of 5 to 8 mL/kg of body weight are recommended.
- **Respiratory rate.** The respiratory rate (ie, the number of breaths per minute delivered to the patient) is set on most ventilator models. Because minute ventilation, which determines alveolar ventilation, is equal to the respiratory rate multiplied by the tidal volume, adjustments in either of these parameters affect the PaCO$_2$. Increasing the minute ventilation decreases the PaCO$_2$, whereas decreasing it increases the PaCO$_2$. Slowing the respiratory rate may also be necessary to enhance patient comfort or when rapid rates cause air trapping in the lungs (due to decreased exhalation time).
- **Positive end-expiratory pressure (PEEP).** The PEEP control adjusts the pressure that is maintained in the lungs at the end of expiration. PEEP increases the functional residual capacity (FRC) by reinflating collapsed alveoli, maintaining the alveoli in an open position, and improving lung compliance. This decreases shunting and improves oxygenation. It is common practice to use low levels of PEEP (5 cm H$_2$O) in the intubated patient. PEEP is increased in 2- to 5-cm H$_2$O increments when FiO$_2$ levels greater than 50% are required to attain an acceptable SaO$_2$ (greater than 90%) or PaO$_2$ (greater than 60 to 70 mm Hg). High levels of PEEP should rarely be interrupted (eg, by disconnecting the ventilator tubing from the airway) because it may take several hours to recruit alveoli again and restore the FRC.[8] Reduction of PEEP is considered when the patient has a PaO$_2$ of 80 to 100 mm Hg or an FiO$_2$ of 50% or less, is hemodynamically stable, and has stabilization or improvement of the underlying illness.

RED FLAG! *Gas trapped in the lungs at the end of exhalation (eg, due to increased airway resistance or a shortened expiratory time) can result in auto-PEEP and a total PEEP level that is excessive. Excessive PEEP can lead to regional alveolar overdistention and barotrauma.*

- **Peak flow.** Peak flow is the velocity of gas flow per unit of time and is expressed as liters per minute. On many volume ventilators, peak flow can be set directly. Very high peak flow is associated with increased turbulence (reflected by increasing airway pressures), shallow inspirations, and uneven distribution of volume.
- **Peak inspiratory pressure limit (high-pressure alarm).** The peak inspiratory pressure (PIP)

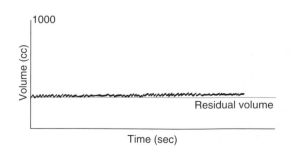

FIGURE 10-6 High-frequency ventilation.

limit is the highest pressure allowed in the ventilator circuit. With volume ventilators, once the high pressure limit is reached, the high-pressure alarm sounds and the inspiration is terminated. If the inspiratory pressure limit is being constantly reached, the patient will not receive the designated tidal volume, and steps must be taken to identify and address the underlying cause (eg, coughing, accumulation of secretions, kinked ventilator tubing, pneumothorax, decreasing compliance, or a high pressure alarm that is set too low).

- **Sensitivity.** The sensitivity function controls the amount of patient effort needed to initiate an inspiration, as measured by negative inspiratory effort. Increasing the sensitivity (requiring less negative force) decreases the amount of work the patient must do to initiate a ventilator breath. Likewise, decreasing the sensitivity increases the amount of negative pressure that the patient needs to initiate inspiration and increases the work of breathing.

- **Inspiratory:expiratory (I:E) ratio.** Most ventilators operate with a short inspiratory time and a long expiratory time (1:2 or 1:3 ratio). This allows time for air to passively exit the lungs, lowering pressures in the thoracic cavity and allowing for increased venous return. However, in conditions of reduced compliance (eg, acute respiratory distress syndrome [ARDS], sarcoidosis), the I:E ratio may be reversed so that the inspiratory time is equal to, or greater than, the expiratory time (eg, 1:1, 2:1, 3:1, 4:1). The inverse I:E ratio improves oxygenation by expanding stiff alveoli using longer inspiratory times, thereby providing more opportunity for gas exchange and preventing alveolar collapse.

Ventilator Modes

The ventilator mode describes how breaths are delivered to the patient. Commonly used modes are summarized in Table 10-2.

Volume Modes

With volume modes of ventilation, a respiratory rate, inspiratory time, and tidal volume are selected for the mechanical breaths. Because the amount of pressure required to deliver the set volume depends on the patient's lung compliance and patient-ventilator resistance factors (Box 10-9, p. 125), the nurse must monitor the PIP to ensure that pressures are within acceptable limits. Common volume modes of ventilation are illustrated in Figure 10-7 on page 125.

- **Assist-control (A/C) mode.** A respiratory rate and tidal volume are preset. If the patient attempts to initiate a breath, the ventilator is triggered and delivers the full preset tidal volume with every breath (see Fig. 10-7A).

- **Synchronized intermittent mandatory ventilation (SIMV) mode.** As with the A/C mode, the respiratory rate and tidal volume are preset. If the patient attempts to initiate a breath above this preset rate, the ventilator allows the patient to take the spontaneous breath. However, unlike the A/C mode, any breaths taken above the preset rate are at the patient's own spontaneous tidal volume. The tidal volume of these breaths is different from the tidal volume set on the ventilator because the tidal volume is determined solely by the patient's spontaneous effort (see Fig. 10-7B).

Pressure Modes

A typical pressure mode of ventilation sets a maximum PIP, not a tidal volume. When the ventilator delivers a breath, it continues delivering the volume until the preset pressure limit is reached, then it stops delivering the breath. The clinician selects the inspiratory pressure limit (which is equal to the PIP), respiratory rate, and I:E ratio, but not the tidal volume. When a pressure mode of ventilation is in use, the tidal volume varies per breath due to lung compliance and airway resistance and must be closely monitored to ensure that the patient is receiving adequate tidal volumes. With some pressure modes, the gas flow rate determines the duration of inspiration. The higher the flow rate, the faster the PIP is reached, and the shorter the inspiration; conversely, the lower the flow rate, the longer the inspiration. If auto-PEEP (due to inadequate expiratory time) is present, peak flow may be increased to shorten inspiratory time so that the patient may exhale completely. Common pressure modes are illustrated in Figure 10-8 on page 126.

- **Pressure-controlled ventilation (PCV) mode.** The PCV mode delivers breaths at a preset pressure limit (see Fig. 10-8A). The "unnatural" feeling of this mode often requires sedation and the use of NMB agents to ensure patient–ventilator synchrony.

> **RED FLAG!** *When the PCV mode is in use, the mean airway and intrathoracic pressures rise, potentially resulting in a decrease in cardiac output. Therefore, it is necessary to monitor the patient's hemodynamic status closely.*

- **Pressure support ventilation (PSV) mode.** PSV mode augments or assists spontaneous breathing efforts by delivering a high flow of gas to a selected pressure level early in inspiration and maintaining that level throughout the inspiratory phase (see Fig. 10-8B). By meeting the patient's inspiratory flow demand throughout the inspiratory phase, patient effort is reduced and comfort is increased. When PSV mode is used as a stand-alone mode of ventilation, the pressure support level is adjusted to achieve the approximate targeted tidal volume and respiratory rate. At high pressure levels, PSV mode provides nearly total ventilatory support. PSV mode is also used with SIMV mode and as a weaning technique. Because the level of pressure support can be gradually decreased, endurance conditioning is enhanced.

TABLE 10-2 Modes of Ventilation

Ventilatory Mode	Common Uses	Advantages	Disadvantages	Nursing Considerations
Volume Modes				
A/C	As an initial mode of ventilation For patients too weak to perform the work of breathing	Ensures ventilator support during every breath Delivers consistent tidal volumes Allows patient to rest	Increased risk for hyperventilation and air trapping May require sedation and paralysis Ventilatory muscle atrophy with longer use	Work of breathing may be increased if sensitivity or flow rate is too low.
SIMV	As a long-term mode of ventilation As a weaning mode	Allows spontaneous breaths (tidal volume determined by patient) between ventilator breaths Allows patient to use own respiratory muscles, preventing muscle atrophy	Patient–ventilator asynchrony possible Work of breathing is increased through artificial airway	…
Pressure Modes				
PCV	For patients with conditions in which compliance is decreased and the risk for barotrauma is high For patients with persistent hypoxemia despite a high FiO_2	Lower peak inspiratory pressures reduce risk for barotraumas Improved oxygenation.	Patient–ventilator asynchrony necessitates sedation/paralysis	Monitor tidal volumes. Monitor for barotrauma and hemodynamic instability.
PSV	As a weaning mode, and in some cases of dyssynchrony Used in combination with SIMV to decrease work of breathing by helping to overcome resistance created by the endotracheal tube	Decreases work of breathing Increases patient comfort	…	Patient must have an intact respiratory drive. PSV mode cannot be used in patients with acute bronchospasm. Monitor respiratory rate and tidal volume at least hourly. Monitor for changes in compliance, which can cause tidal volume to change.
IRV	Used to improve oxygenation in patients with conditions characterized by decreased compliance	Longer inspiratory time provides more opportunity for gas exchange and shorter expiratory times prevent alveolar collapse.	Almost always requires sedation/paralysis Auto-PEEP may develop	Usually used in conjunction with PCV Monitor for auto-PEEP, barotrauma, and hemodynamic instability.
APRV	For patients with high airway pressures to reduce airway pressure and lower minute volume while allowing spontaneous breathing As a weaning mode	Allows lung protective strategies by limiting plateau and peak pressures Allows spontaneous breathing Need for paralysis/sedation is decreased	…	…
VGPO	For acutely ill, unstable patients to provide pressure ventilation while guaranteeing tidal volume and minute ventilation at a set rate For stable, weaning patients as a "safety" when pressure ventilation is desired	Ensures a delivered tidal volume while limiting pressures	Requires sophisticated knowledge of the mode and waveform analysis	Monitor for auto-PEEP, barotrauma, and hemodynamic instability.
PEEP	Used to maintain alveoli inflation at end expiration and decrease the work of breathing For patients on high levels of FiO_2 with refractory hypoxemia	Improves oxygenation Increases FRC, allowing lower FiO_2 levels	High levels of PEEP may cause barotrauma Increases intrathoracic pressures, leading to decreased venous return and cardiac output Increases ICP	Monitor total PEEP (set PEEP and auto-PEEP) and hemodynamics Limit disconnection from ventilator (eg, for suctioning), because of time required to reestablish PEEP.
CPAP	For spontaneously breathing patients to improve oxygenation As a weaning mode For nocturnal ventilation to prevent upper airway obstruction in patients with sleep apnea	May be used in intubated or non-intubated patients	On some systems, no alarm if respiratory rate decreases	Monitor for increased work of breathing.
Noninvasive BiPap	For nocturnal hypoventilation in patients with neuromuscular disease, chest wall deformity, obstructive sleep apnea, and COPD To prevent intubation To prevent reintubation initially after extubation	No need for artificial airway	Patient discomfort or claustrophobia Use of full facemask increases risk for aspiration and rebreathing carbon dioxide.	Thick or copious secretions and poor cough may be relative contraindications for BiPap. Monitor for gastric distention, air leaks from mouth, aspiration risk.

BOX 10-9 Resistance and Compliance

An understanding of how resistance and compliance affect pressures and volumes helps the nurse provide adequate ventilatory support while minimizing adverse effects.

Resistance

Small changes in airway diameter can have enormous effects on airflow resistance. Normally, airway resistance is so small that only small changes in pressure are needed to move large volumes of air into the lungs. But in conditions that decrease airway diameter (eg, pulmonary secretions, the presence of an artifical airway, bronchospasm) marked increases in airway resistance occur. To maintain the same rate of airflow as before the onset of increased airway resistance, the driving pressure (or respiratory effort) must be increased to move air into the lungs.

Compliance

Compliance refers to the ability of the lung to distend. In conditions that reduce the lung's elasticity such as inflammation, fibrotic changes, or edema, the lung requires more force to distend. A patient on a ventilator with normal lungs should have a compliance near 100 mL/cm H_2O (normal). In contrast, a patient on a ventilator with pulmonary disease that causes "stiff" lungs (eg, acute respiratory distress syndrome, sarcoidosis) has a compliance as low as 20 to 30 mL/cm H_2O. Serial measurements of compliance performed by the respiratory therapist can alert the nurse to sudden decreases in compliance, which may be due to pneumothorax, mucus plugging, or pulmonary edema.

Compliance is either static or dynamic:

- **Static compliance** only measures lung compliance. The measurement used to obtain static compliance is the plateau pressure (ie, the pressure applied in positive pressure ventilation to the small airways and alveoli).[17] Plateau pressure is obtained by holding the end-inspiratory time on the ventilator while on a volume mode of ventilation. This holds the volume of delivered air in the patient's chest by preventing exhalation, thus measuring the plateau pressure.

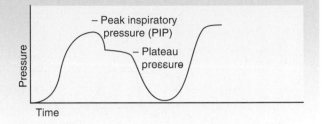

Static compliance is determined by dividing the tidal volume by the plateau pressure and subtracting the positive end-expiratory pressure(PEEP):

Static compliance = V$_T$/ [plateau pressure – PEEP]

- **Dynamic compliance** takes into account airway resistance, thoracic chest wall compliance, and lung compliance. The peak inspiratory pressure (PIP) is the amount of pressure required to deliver the preset tidal volume. The pressure measures the airways' resistance (to flow) as well as by lung and chest wall compliance. Dynamic compliance is obtained by dividing the tidal volume by the PIP and subtracting the PEEP:

Dynamic compliance = V$_T$/PIP – PEEP

To prevent lung injury, it is important to determine lung compliance using airway pressure so that the ventilator can be appropriately adjusted to minimize airway pressures.

- **Inverse ratio ventilation (IRV).** This type of ventilation inverses the I:E ratio so that inspiratory time is equal to, or longer than, expiratory time (eg, 1:1 to 4:1; see Fig. 10-8C). Because the expiratory time is decreased, the nurse must monitor for the development of auto-PEEP.

- **Airway pressure release ventilation (APRV) mode.** This is a time-triggered, pressure-limited, time-cycled mode of ventilation (see Fig. 10-8D). A high-pressure and a low pressure are set. Alveolar recruitment and oxygenation occur during the high-pressure setting (which lasts 5.4

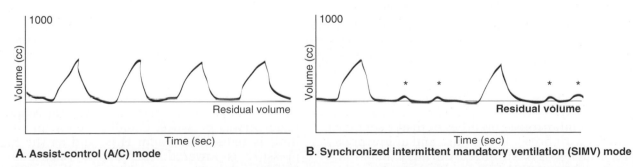

FIGURE 10-7 Volume modes of positive-pressure ventilation. *Asterisks* (*) indicate spontaneous breaths. **A:** Assist-control (A/C) mode. **B:** Synchronized intermittent mandatory ventilation (SIMV) mode.

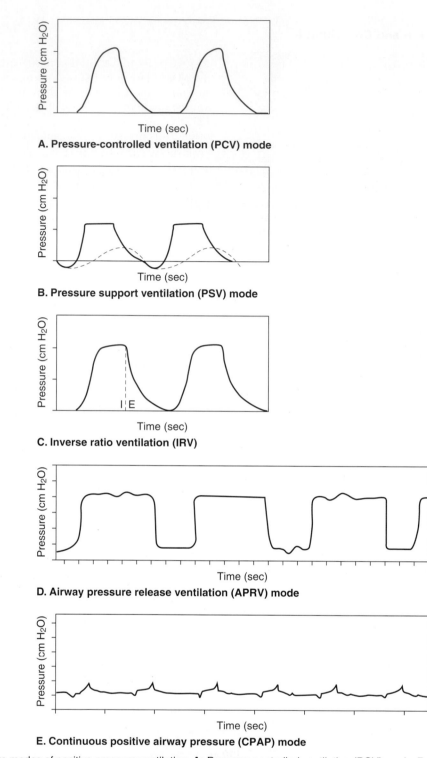

FIGURE 10-8 Pressure modes of positive-pressure ventilation. **A:** Pressure-controlled ventilation (PCV) mode. **B:** Pressure support ventilation (PSV) mode. *Dashed line* indicates spontaneous breathing. **C:** Inverse ratio ventilation (IRV). Inspiration (*I*) is as long, or longer than, expiration (*E*). **D:** Airway pressure release ventilation (APRV) mode. **E:** Continous positive airway pressure (CPAP) mode.

seconds), followed by a brief controlled release (0.6 second) to the low-pressure setting. The patient spontaneously breathes both at a set high pressure with preset brief times and at low pressure, which is synchronized during exhalation. Weaning from APRV is done by decreasing the high-pressure limit while increasing the time at high pressure. At the same time, the low-pressure limit may be dropped, allowing for reduced mean airway pressure. Usually, the low-pressure limit is reduced to 5 cm H_2O, and as the high pressure is lowered, this allows release to a PEEP level that prevents alveolar collapse. When the patient tolerates an FiO_2 of 50% or less, the patient can be switched to PSV mode and further weaning.

- **Volume-guaranteed pressure options (VGPO) mode.** This mode ensures delivery of a prescribed tidal volume while using a pressure control mode of ventilation. In an acutely ill, unstable patient, the VGPO mode may be used to limit the PIP while guaranteeing tidal volume and minute ventilation at a set rate. In a more stable, spontaneously breathing patient, this mode is used as a "safety" when pressure ventilation is desired. The use of a volume guarantee in the spontaneously breathing patient may be especially important at night (when respiratory rates and volumes normally decrease) and in patients for whom secretions are a problem (because secretions increase resistance and result in decreased spontaneous volumes).
- **Continuous positive airway pressure (CPAP) mode.** This mode supplies pressure throughout the respiratory cycle, helping to improve oxygenation in spontaneously breathing patients (see Fig. 10-8E). CPAP can be used for intubated and nonintubated patients. It may be used as a weaning mode from mechanical ventilation and for nocturnal ventilation (nasal or mask CPAP) to splint open the upper airway, preventing upper airway obstruction in patients with obstructive sleep apnea. During expiration, the pressure in the lungs decreases to the "baseline" end-expiratory pressure level and continues to be positive throughout expiration, allowing greater volumes to be generated during inspiration.
- **Noninvasive bilevel positive-pressure (BiPAP) mode.** BiPAP is a noninvasive form of mechanical ventilation provided by means of a nasal mask, nasal prongs, or a full facemask. The system allows the clinician to select two levels of positive-pressure support: an inspiratory pressure referred to as IPAP and an expiratory pressure referred to as EPAP (CPAP/PEEP level). BiPAP may be used in patients with acute, short-term respiratory problems to avoid intubation and mechanical ventilation.

Nursing Care of the Patient Receiving Mechanical Ventilation

A collaborative care guide for the patient receiving mechanical ventilation is given in Box 10-10. Key nursing responsibilities include the following.

Ensuring Adequate Oxygenation and Ventilation

Several important nursing interventions for the patient receiving mechanical ventilation are directed at ensuring that alveolar ventilation appropriate for the patient's needs is maintained. These interventions include:

- Maintaining the airway, as described earlier
- Monitoring the patient's vital signs, arterial oxygen saturation, mental status, respiratory status, and arterial blood gases (Table 10-3, p. 130)

- Monitoring ventilator settings and alarms (Table 10-4, p. 131)

 RED FLAG! *Alarm systems on ventilators warn of developing problems. A nurse or respiratory therapist must respond to every ventilator alarm. Alarms must never be ignored or disarmed.*

Recurrent alarms may indicate an equipment-related issue or a patient complication. When device malfunction or a patient complication is suspected, the patient must be manually ventilated while the nurse or therapist looks for the cause. If the problem is equipment-related and cannot be promptly corrected by ventilator adjustment, a new ventilator must be procured and the malfunctioning ventilator must be taken out of service.

Preventing Aspiration and Ventilator-Associated Pneumonia

Aspiration can occur before, during, or after intubation and greatly increases the patient's risk for developing VAP. VAP (nosocomial pneumonia in a patient who has been mechanically ventilated with an endotracheal tube or tracheostomy for at least 48 hours at the time of diagnosis) is the second most common hospital-acquired pneumonia (HAP) and the leading cause of death from nosocomial infections.[9,11]

 RED FLAG! *Clinical manifestations of VAP include new or progressive and persistent infiltrates on chest radiograph, a temperature higher than 100.4°F (38°C), leukocytosis, new-onset purulent sputum or cough, and worsening gas exchange.*

Because aspiration of oral or gastric secretions is thought to contribute to the development of VAP, strategies that decrease the risk for aspiration will also decrease the risk for VAP. These include:

- Maintaining appropriate cuff inflation
- Evacuating gastric distention with nasogastric suction
- Performing subglottic suctioning to prevent pooling of secretions above the cuff
- Keeping the head of the bed elevated 30 degrees or more at all times unless medically contraindicated
- Providing oral care per unit protocol

Frequent oral care must be performed on all mechanically ventilated patients. Oral care preserves the integrity of the oropharyngeal mucosa, which helps prevent infection and colonization of organisms that has been shown to lead to VAP. General oral care guidelines are not suitable for patients with an endotracheal tube and are not effective for preventing VAP. Current oral care guidelines for the mechanically ventilated patient include:

- Systematic assessment of the oral mucosa daily and with each cleaning
- Handwashing before and after every intervention

BOX 10-10 COLLABORATIVE CARE GUIDE for the Patient on Mechanical Ventilation

OUTCOMES	INTERVENTIONS
Oxygenation/Ventilation A patent airway is maintained. Lungs are clear to auscultation. Patient is without evidence of atelectasis. Peak, mean, and plateau pressures are within normal limits. ABGs are within normal limits.	• Auscultate breath sounds q2–4h and PRN. • Suction as needed for crackles, coughing, or oxygen desaturation. • Hyperoxygenate before and after each suction pass. • Monitor airway pressures q1–2h. • Monitor airway pressures after suctioning. • Administer bronchodilators and mucolytics as ordered. • Perform chest physiotherapy if indicated by clinical examination or chest x-ray. • Turn side to side q2h. • Consider kinetic therapy or prone positioning as indicated by clinical scenario. • Get patient out of bed to chair or standing position when stable. • Monitor pulse oximetry and end-tidal CO_2. • Monitor ABGs as indicated by changes in noninvasive parameters, patient status, or weaning protocol.
Circulation/Perfusion Blood pressure, heart rate, cardiac output, central venous pressure, and pulmonary artery pressure remain stable on mechanical ventilation.	• Assess hemodynamic effects of initiating positive-pressure ventilation (eg, potential for decreased venous return and cardiac output). • Monitor ECG for dysrhythmias related to hypoxemia. • Assess effects of ventilator setting changes (inspiratory pressures, tidal volume, PEEP, and FiO_2) on hemodynamic and oxygenation parameters. • Administer intravascular volume as ordered to maintain preload.
Fluids/Electrolytes I & O measurements are balanced. Electrolyte values are within normal limits.	• Monitor hydration status in relation to clinical examination, auscultation, amount and viscosity of lung secretions. • Assess patient weight, I & O totals, urine specific gravity, or serum osmolality to evaluate fluid balance. • Administer electrolyte replacements (IV or enteral) per physician's order.
Mobility Patient maintains or regains baseline functional status related to mobility and self-care. Joint range of motion is maintained.	• Collaborate with physical/occupational therapy staff to encourage patient effort/participation to increase mobility. • Progress activity to sitting up in chair, standing at bedside, ambulating with assistance as soon as possible. • Assist patient with active or passive range-of-motion exercises of all extremities at least every shift. • Keep extremities in physiologically neutral position using pillows or appropriate splint/support devices as indicated.
Safety Endotracheal tube will remain in proper position. Proper inflation of endotracheal tube cuff is maintained. Ventilator alarm system remains activated.	• Securely stabilize endotracheal tube in position. • Note and record the "cm" line on endotracheal tube position at lip or teeth. • Use restraints or sedation per hospital protocol. • Evaluate endotracheal tube position on chest x-ray daily (by viewing film or by report). • Keep emergency airway equipment and manual resuscitation bag readily available, and check each shift. • Inflate cuff using minimal leak technique, or pressure <25 mm Hg by manometer. • Monitor cuff inflation/leak every shift and PRN. • Protect pilot balloon from damage. • Perform ventilator setting and alarm checks q4h (minimum) or per facility protocol.

BOX 10-10 COLLABORATIVE CARE GUIDE for the Patient on Mechanical Ventilation (continued)

OUTCOMES	INTERVENTIONS
Skin Integrity Patient is without evidence of skin breakdown.	• Assess and document skin integrity at least every shift. • Turn side to side q2h; reassess bony prominences for evidence of pressure injury. • When patient is out of bed to chair, provide pressure relief to sitting surfaces at least q1h. • Remove self-protective devices from wrists, and monitor skin per hospital policy.
Nutrition Nutritional intake meets calculated metabolic need (eg, basal energy expenditure equation). Patient will establish regular bowel elimination pattern.	• Consult dietitian for metabolic needs assessment and recommendations. • Provide early nutritional support by enteral or parenteral feeding, start within 48 hours of intubation. • Monitor actual delivery of nutrition daily with I&O calculations. • Weigh patient daily. • Administer bowel regimen medications as ordered, along with adequate hydration.
Comfort/Pain Control Patients will indicate/exhibit adequate relief of discomfort/pain while on mechanical ventilation.	• Document pain assessment, using numerical pain rating or similar scale when possible. • Provide analgesia as appropriate, document efficacy after each dose. • Prevent pulling and jarring of the ventilator tubing and endotracheal or tracheostomy tube. • Provide meticulous oral care q1–2h with oropharynx suctioning and application of mouth moisturizer as needed; teeth brushing scheduled at least three times daily; antimicrobial rinse twice daily; oral assessment at least daily. • Administer sedation as indicated.
Psychosocial Patient participates in self-care and decision making related to own ADLs (eg, turning, bathing). Patient communicates with healthcare providers and visitors.	• Encourage patient to move in bed and attempt to meet own basic comfort/hygiene needs independently. • Establish a daily schedule for bathing, time out of bed, treatments, and so forth with patient input. • Provide a means for patient to write notes and use visual tools to facilitate communication. • Encourage visitor conversations with patient in normal tone of voice and subject matter. • Teach visitors to assist with range-of-motion and other simple care delivery tasks, to facilitate normal patterns of interaction.
Teaching/Discharge Planning Patient cooperates with and indicates understanding of need for mechanical ventilation. Potential discharge needs are assessed.	• Provide explanations to patient and family regarding: • Rationale for use of mechanical ventilation • Procedures such as suctioning, airway care, chest physiotherapy • Plan for and progress toward weaning and extubation • Initiate early social work to screen for needs, resources, and support systems.

TABLE 10-3 Abnormal Arterial Blood Gases in the Mechanically Ventilated Patient			
Abnormality	**Possible Causes**	**Action**
Hypoxemia	*Patient-related* Secretions Increase in disease pathology Positive fluid balance	Suction. Increase FiO_2. Evaluate patient and chest radiograph. Evaluate intake and output.
Hypocapnia	*Patient-related* Hypoxia Increased lung compliance' Increased minute ventilation *Ventilator-related* Incorrect ventilator settings	Evaluate ABGs and patient. Evaluate for wean potential. Decrease respiratory rate, tidal volume, or minute ventilation.
Hypercapnia	*Patient-related* Sedation Fatigue Decreased minute ventilation *Ventilator-related* Incorrect ventilator settings	Increase respiratory rate or tidal volume settings. Increase respiratory rate, tidal volume, or minute ventilation.

- Routine brushing of the teeth to remove dental plaque (every 8 hours)
- Cleansing of the mouth (every 2 hours and as needed)
- Use of an alcohol-free or antimicrobial (chlorhexidine) oral rinse per unit protocol to reduce oropharyngeal colonization
- Oral and subglottic pharyngeal suctioning with an in-line suction catheter to minimize aspiration risk
- Replacement of the suction set (every 24 hours)
- Application of a water-based mouth moisturizer to prevent mucosal drying and maintain oral mucosa integrity

Providing Nutritional Support

Patients who require long-term mechanical ventilation typically need additional calories per day. Clinical starvation can lead to pulmonary complications and death (Box 10-11). In prolonged starvation, the body cannibalizes the intercostal and diaphragmatic muscles for energy.[12,13] In addition, respiratory muscles, like all other body muscles, need energy to work. If energy needs are not met, muscle fatigue occurs, leading to discoordination of respiratory muscles and a decrease in tidal volume.

Providing Eye Care

Many patients who are receiving mechanical ventilation are comatose, sedated, or chemically paralyzed and therefore have lost the blink reflex or ability to close their eyelids completely. Measures to prevent corneal dryness and ulceration include the instillation of lubricating drops or ointment, taping the eyes, applying eye shields, or applying a moisture chamber. Eye care should be scheduled (as opposed to being provided on an as-needed basis).

Providing Psychosocial Support

A patient on a ventilator is subjected to extreme physical and emotional stress. Psychological distress can be caused by sleep deprivation, sensory overstimulation, sensory deprivation for familiar cues, pain, fear, an inability to communicate, feelings of helplessness and lack of control, and commonly used pharmacological agents. Treatments can often seem dehumanizing. In many cases, the prognosis is poor, and the possibility of death is ever present. General interventions that help to alleviate psychological distress are discussed in Chapter 2.

Weaning From Mechanical Ventilation

The objective of mechanical ventilation is to support the patient through an episode of illness. As soon as mechanical ventilation is started, plans begin for weaning the patient from mechanical support. The patient is evaluated daily for readiness to wean. It is important to perform this assessment and address weaning impediments before initiating weaning trials. Many indices have been developed for use in predicting weaning readiness. Some look exclusively at respiratory factors, whereas others look at a broad range of physiological factors.

The approach to weaning also varies. Some clinicians maintain total ventilatory support up until the time of weaning trials; others use intermittent weaning trials of increasing frequency and duration. Advantages of a gradual approach to weaning may include a reduced risk for complications (because over time the patient on partial rather than full ventilation is exposed to lower levels of pressure and volume) and reduced deconditioning and atrophy of the respiratory muscles (because the patient is required to perform some level of work to breathe during the weaning trials).[14]

Regardless of the approach, certain factors have been found to influence weaning success positively. These include the use of a collaborative, multidisciplinary team to formulate a comprehensive plan of care based on assessment of the

TABLE 10-4 Troubleshooting the Ventilator

Problem	Possible Causes	Action
Volume or low-pressure alarm	*Patient-related*	
	Patient disconnected from ventilator	Reconnect STAT.
	Loss of delivered tidal volume	Auscultate neck for possible leak around endotracheal tube cuff. Review chest film for endotracheal tube placement—may be too high. Check for loss of tidal volume through chest tube.
	Decrease in patient-initiated breaths	Evaluate patient for cause: check respiratory rate, ABGs, last sedation.
	Increased compliance	Evaluate patient for clearing of secretions or relief of bronchospasms.
	Ventilator-related	
	Leaks	Check all tubing for loss of connection, starting at patient and moving toward humidifier. Check for change in ventilator settings. (*Note*: If problem is not corrected STAT, use MRB until ventilator problem is corrected.)
High-pressure or peak-pressure alarm	*Patient-related*	
	Decreased compliance	Suction patient.
	Decreased dynamic compliance	Administer inhaled β-agonists. If sudden, evaluate for pneumothorax. Evaluate chest film for endotracheal tube displacement in right mainstem bronchus. Sedate if patient is bucking the ventilator or biting the endotracheal tube.
	Decreased static compliance	Evaluate ABGs for hypoxia, fluids for overload, chest film for atelectasis. Auscultate breath sounds.
	Ventilator-related	
	Tubing kinked	Check tubing.
	Tubing filled with water	Empty water into a receptacle.
	Patient–ventilator asynchrony	Recheck sensitivity and peak flow settings. Provide sedation/paralysis if indicated.
Heater alarm	Adding cold water to humidifier.	Wait.
	Altered setting	Reset.
	Cold air blowing on humidifier	Redirect airflow.

individual patient, the use of standardized weaning protocols that are assigned to each patient based on individual assessment, and the use of critical pathways.[15]

BOX 10-11 Effects of Clinical Starvation

- Atrophy of respiratory muscles
- Decreased protein (results catabolic state requiring breakdown muscle for calories)
- Decreased albumin (loss oncotic pressure resulting in edema and ascites)
- Decreased cell-mediated immunity
- Decreased surfactant production
- Decreased replication of respiratory epithelium
- Intracellular depletion of adenosine triphosphate (loss of the cellular energy source)
- Impaired cellular oxygenation
- Central respiratory depression

Guidelines for Weaning

Although weaning procedures vary from hospital to hospital, general guidelines remain the same. For instance, weaning is generally initiated in the morning when the patient is rested. The nurse explains the procedure to the patient and administers medications for comfort (eg, bronchodilators, sedatives, pain medication) as indicated. (The use of sedatives and narcotics during weaning is limited to only the level of medication clearly needed to control pain or anxiety.) The nurse raises the head of the bed, ensures a patent airway, and provides suction if necessary. The nurse remains with the patient throughout the weaning trial to provide support and reassurance. At the conclusion of the trial, the nurse also evaluates and documents the patient's response to weaning.

Short-Term Ventilation Weaning

Patients are often intubated electively for surgical or other procedures, or more urgently owing to respiratory distress related to underlying pulmonary disease or traumatic injury. In these situations, ventilation support is usually short-term (ie, less than 3 days). Once the procedure is completed or the patient is stabilized, the goal is extubation as soon as the patient is able to protect the airway. The weaning process in this setting may proceed rapidly, based on individual patient response to reduced ventilatory support. Frequently used predictive criteria for short-term weaning success are a negative inspiratory pressure of less than or equal to –20 cm H_2O, a positive expiratory pressure of greater than or equal to +30 cm H_2O, and a spontaneous minute volume of less than 12 L/min. Guidelines for short-term ventilation weaning are given in Box 10-12.

Long-Term Ventilation Weaning

Patients on mechanical ventilation for longer than 72 hours or those who have failed short-term weaning often have significant deconditioning of the respiratory muscles. These patients usually require a period of "exercising" the respiratory muscles to regain the strength and endurance needed for successful return to spontaneous breathing. During the reconditioning program, goals are to:

- Have the patient tolerate two to three daily weaning trials of reduced ventilatory support without exercising to the point of exhaustion
- Rest the patient between weaning trials and overnight on ventilator settings that provide diaphragmatic rest, with minimal or no work of breathing for the patient

The process of long-term weaning often takes days to weeks, and multiple delays and setbacks are common. Guidelines for long-term ventilation weaning are given in Box 10-13.

Methods of Weaning

Common methods of weaning include the following.
- **T-piece trial (flow-by).** The T-piece (an endotracheal tube adapter that provides oxygen only) is connected to the patient at the desired FiO_2 (usually slightly higher than the previous ventilator setting). In this weaning trial, the patient must breathe through the endotracheal tube without ventilator assistance. Because of the increased resistance caused by the narrowed airway, the patient's work of breathing is increased; therefore, the nurse continuously observes the patient's response and tolerance to the trial. The duration of T-piece trials is not standardized, and some clinicians extubate if an initial trial of 30 minutes ends with acceptable ABG measurements and patient response. Increasing frequency and duration of T-piece trials builds the patient's endurance, with periods of rest on the ventilator between extended trials.
- **SIMV method.** Weaning with the SIMV method entails gradually reducing the number of delivered breaths until a low rate is reached (usually 4 breaths/min). The patient is then extubated if all

---

BOX 10-12 Guidelines for Weaning From Short-Term Ventilation

CRITERIA
Readiness Criteria
- Hemodynamically stable, adequately resuscitated, and not requiring significant vasoactive support
- SaO_2 greater than 90% on FiO_2 less than or equal to 40%; PEEP less than or equal to 5 cm H_2O
- Chest x-ray reviewed for correctable factors; treated as indicated
- Metabolic indicators (serum pH, major electrolytes) within normal range
- Hematocrit greater than 25%
- Core temperature greater than 36°C and less than 39°C
- Adequate management of pain/anxiety/agitation
- No residual neuromuscular blockade (NMB)
- ABGs normalized or at patient's baseline

Tolerance Criteria
If the patient displays any of the following, the weaning trial should be stopped and the patient returned to "rest" settings.
- Sustained respiratory rate greater than 35 breaths/min
- SaO_2 less than 90%
- Tidal volume less than or equal to 5 mL/kg
- Sustained minute ventilation greater than 200 mL/kg/min
- Evidence of respiratory or hemodynamic distress:
Labored respiratory pattern
Increased anxiety, diaphoresis, or both

Sustained heart rate greater than 20% higher or lower than baseline
Systolic blood pressure greater than 180 mm Hg or less than 90 mm Hg

Extubation Criteria
- Mental status: alert and able to respond to commands
- Good cough and gag reflex, able to protect airway and clear secretions
- Able to move air around endotracheal tube with cuff deflated and end of tube occluded

WEANING INTERVENTION
- Reduce ventilator rate, then convert to pressure-support ventilation (PSV) only.
- Wean PSV as tolerated to less than or equal to 10 cm H_2O.
- If patient meets tolerance criteria for at least 2 hours on this level of support *and* meets extubation criteria, may extubate.
- If patient fails tolerance criteria, increase PSV or add ventilator rate as needed to achieve "rest" settings (consistent respiratory rate less than 20 breaths/min) and review weaning criteria for correctable factors.
- Repeat wean attempt on PSV 10 cm H_2O after rest period (minimum, 2 hours). If patient fails second wean trial, return to rest settings and use "long-term" ventilation weaning approach.

Adapted from evidence-based practice guidelines used in the Surgical/Trauma Intensive Care Unit, University of Virginia Health System, Charlottesville, Virginia.

BOX 10-13 Guidelines for Weaning From Long-Term Ventilation

CRITERIA

Readiness Criteria

- Same as for short-term ventilation (see Box 10-12), with emphasis on hemodynamic stability, adequate analgesia/sedation (record scores on flow sheet), and normalizing volume status

WEANING INTERVENTION

- Transfer to pressure-support ventilation (PSV) mode, adjust support level to maintain patient's respiratory rate at less than 35 breaths/min.
- Observe for 30 min for signs of early failure (same tolerance criteria as with short-term ventilation; see Box 10-12).
- If tolerated, continue trial for 2 hours, then return patient to "rest" settings by adding ventilator breaths or increasing PSV to achieve a total respiratory rate of less than 20 breaths/min.
- After at least 2 hours of rest, repeat trial for 2 to 4 hours at same PSV level as previous trial. If the patient exceeds the tolerance criteria (listed in Box 10-12), stop the trial and return to "rest" settings. In this case, the next trial should be performed at a higher support level than the failed trial.
- Record the results of each weaning episode, including specific parameters and the time frame if failure is observed, on the bedside flow sheet.
- The goal is to increase the length of the trials and reduce the PSV level needed on an incremental basis. With each successive trial, the PSV level may be decreased by 2 to 4 cm H_2O, the time interval may be increased by 1 to 2 hours, or both, while keeping the patient within tolerance parameters. The pace of weaning is patient-specific, and tolerance may vary from day to day. Review readiness criteria for correctable factors daily *and* each time the patient fails a weaning trial.
- Ensure nocturnal ventilation at "rest" settings (with a respiratory rate of less than 20 breaths/min) for at least 6 hours each night until the patient's weaning trials demonstrate readiness to discontinue ventilatory support.

DISCONTINUING MECHANICAL VENTILATION

The patient should be weaned until ventilator settings are FiO_2 less than or equal to 40%, PSV less than or equal to 10 cm H_2O, and PEEP less than or equal to 8 cm H_2O. Once these settings are well tolerated, the patient should be placed on continuous positive airway pressure (CPAP) 5 cm H_2O or (if the patient has a tracheostomy) on tracheostomy collar. If the patient meets tolerance criteria over the first 5 minutes, the trial should be continued for 1 to 2 hours. If clinical observation and ABGs indicate that the patient is maintaining adequate ventilation and oxygenation on this "minimal" support, the following options can be considered:

- Extubation can be attempted if the patient meets extubation criteria (see Box 10-12).
- If the patient is on tracheostomy collar, the trials should be continued two to three times per day with daily increases in time on tracheostomy collar by 1 to 2 hours per trial until the total time off the ventilator reaches 18 hours per day. At this point, the patient may be ready to remain on tracheostomy collar for longer than 24 hours unless the tolerance criteria are exceeded.
- Ventilator weaning is considered successful once the patient achieves spontaneous ventilation (extubated or on tracheostomy collar) for at least 24 hours.

Adapted from evidence-based practice guidelines used in the Surgical/Trauma Intensive Care Unit, University of Virginia Health System, Charlottesville, Virginia.

---

other weaning criteria are met. However, low levels of SIMV (fewer than 4 breaths/min) may result in a high level of work and fatigue and may prolong weaning.[16] SIMV plus PSV, called synchronized pressure support ventilation (SPSV), may be used to decrease the work of breathing associated with spontaneous breaths (Fig. 10-9). In SPSV mode, the added pressure overcomes the resistance of the artificial airway. Weaning can be accomplished by lowering the number of breaths or amount of pressure support.

- **CPAP method.** The small amount of positive pressure supplied throughout the inspiratory and expiratory cycles in CPAP mode may decrease the patient's work of breathing. Weaning occurs by decreasing the amount of pressure.
- **PSV method.** Low levels of PSV decrease the work of breathing associated with endotracheal tubes and ventilator circuits. Weaning using the PSV method entails progressively decreasing the inspiratory pressure limit to 8 to 10 cm H_2O

based on the patient maintaining an adequate tidal volume and a respiratory rate of less than 25 breaths/min. The 8-cm H_2O inspiratory pressure limit is thought to overcome the work of breathing through the endotracheal tube and ventilator circuit, so longer weaning trials may be tolerated.

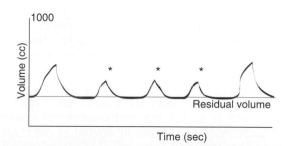

FIGURE 10-9 Pressure support mandatory ventilation (PSMV) mode. *Asterisks* (*) indicate spontaneous breaths.

CASE STUDY

Mrs. Q,. a 74-year-old woman, is admitted with a diagnosis of esophageal cancer. She had an esophagectomy 1 week ago. Following initial extubation, she was reintubated the day of surgery (failed extubation) for respiratory distress, hypercarbia and inability to clear her secretions. Mrs. Q.'s history includes a 13-kg weight loss and limited ADLs while living at home (limited by her dependence on supplemental oxygen and nasojejunal nutrition.) Mrs. Q.'s nutrition status was improved by 6 weeks of home therapy before admission. Her current medications include albuterol, fluticasone, lisinopril, insulin, thyroxine, prednisone, and paroxetine, as well as alprazolam and zolpidem as needed. The current ventilator settings on day 7 of ventilation are: FiO$_2$, 0.40; no rate; PEEP, 5 cm H$_2$O; RR, 20; and tidal volume, 550 mL (current weight 68 kg, a gain of 6 kg from 2 months ago); and minute volume, 10.9 L/min. Mrs. Q.'s vital signs are stable, she is afebrile, and her pain is well controlled with scheduled oral and as-needed IV opioids. Mrs. Q. is generally weak, but able to turn in bed on her own. For 2 days, Mrs. Q. has tolerated sitting up in a chair (three times daily) and she took her first walk today with physical therapy. She is able to cough out secretions from her endotracheal tube. Nutrition and medications are delivered through a percutaneous endoscopic gastrostomy (PEG) tube inserted during surgery. Mrs. Q. tolerates ventilation with resumption of her as-needed alprazolam and is sleeping better with nocturnal zolpidem.

1. Describe appropriate weaning goals for Mrs. Q., based on her status today. What ventilator settings should be used?

2. When would Mrs. Q. be considered ready for extubation? What weaning assessment and laboratory tests, including arterial blood gases and chemistry, should be obtained before a second trial extubation?

3. This is day 7 of ventilation following a failed extubation trial the day of surgery, and Mrs. Q. has progressed physically. What respiratory assessments should the nurse follow while Mrs. Q. is working with physical therapy?

4. The nurse observes Mrs. Q. on continuous positive airway pressure (CPAP) for 1 hour, and she remains stable without changes to her respiratory rate, tidal volume, or minute volume, and her arterial blood gases are within normal limits. Should Mrs. Q. be extubated after this 1-hour CPAP trial if she complained of feeling exhausted (in a written note)? What additional weaning assessments should be done?

5. The medical team decides to wait 1 day longer to allow Mrs. Q. to continue on the ventilator with the reduced inspiratory pressure limit at 10 cm H$_2$O. How does reducing the inspiratory pressure limit affect Mrs. Q.'s work of breathing and the strength and endurance of her respiratory muscles?

References

1. Wiegand D (ed): Section I, Nasopharyngeal airway insertion. AACN Procedure Manual for Critical Care, 6th ed. Philadelphia, PA: Saunders, 2011
2. St. John RE, Seckel MA: Airway management. In Burns SM (ed): AACN Protocols for Practice: Care of the Mechanically Ventilated Patient, 2nd ed. Sudbury, MA: Jones & Bartlett, 2007, pp 1–57
3. Practice Management Guidelines for the Timing of Tracheostomy. AHRQ National Guideline Clearinghouse, 2007
4. Wu Y, Tsai C, Lan C: Prolonged mechanical ventilation in a respiratory care setting: A comparison of outcome between tracheostomized and translaryngeal intubated patients. Crit Care 14(2), 2010
5. Weigand, D (ed): Section IV, Tube care. AACN Procedure Manual for Critical Care, 6th ed. Philadelphia, PA: Saunder, 2011
6. Burns S: AACN Protocols for Practice: Care of Mechanically Ventilated Patients. 2007
7. Fessler H, Derdak S, Ferguson N, et al: A protocol for high frequency oscillatory ventilation in adults. Crit Care Med 35(7):1649–1654, 2007
8. Acosta P, Santisbon E, Varon J: The use of positive end-expiratory pressure in mechanical ventilation. Crit Care Clin 23(2):251–261, 2007
9. Cason CL, Tyner T, Saunders S, et al.: Nurses' implementation of guidelines for ventilator-associated pneumonia from the Centers for Disease Control and Prevention. Am J Crit Care 16(1):28–38, 2007
10. AACN practice alert: Ventilator-associated pneumonia. AACN Clin Issues 16(1):105–109, 2005
11. Chlebicki MP, Safdar N: Topical chlorhexidine for prevention of ventilator-associated pneumonia: A meta-analysis. Crit Care Med 35(2):595–602, 2007
12. Klaude M, Fredriksson K, Tjader I: Protease proteolytic activity in skeletal muscle is increased in patients with sepsis. Clin Sci (112):499–506, 2007
13. Markou NK, Myrianthefs PM, Baltopoulos GJ: Respiratory failure: An overview. Crit Care Nurs Q 27(4):353–379, 2004
14. Schweickert W, Hall J: ICU acquired weakness. Chest 131:1541–1549, 2007
15. Girard T, Wesley E: Weaning from mechanical ventilation. American College of Chest Physicians, 2008
16. Marini J, Wheeler A: Critical Care Medicine: The Essentials. Philadelphia, PA: Lippincott Williams & Wilkins, 2009

Want to know more? A wide variety of resources to enhance your learning and understanding of this chapter are available on **the Point** ✳. Visit **http://thepoint.lww.com/MortonEss1e** to access chapter review questions and more!

Code Management

Based on the content in this chapter, the reader should be able to:

1 Describe measures facilities take to prevent adverse events (eg, cardiopulmonary arrest) and improve patient outcomes.
2 Discuss the roles of code team members and describe the equipment and medications used during a code.
3 Explain basic life support (BLS) measures in cardiopulmonary arrest.
4 Explain the proper implementation of cardiopulmonary resuscitation (CPR).
5 Explain advanced cardiac life support (ACLS) measures.
6 Describe post–cardiac arrest care.

Improving Patient Outcomes

It has been estimated that 15% to 20% of all hospitalized patients develop serious adverse events, including cardiopulmonary arrest (also called sudden cardiac arrest, or SCA).[1] These adverse events are rarely unforeseen. In fact, they are usually preceded by at least one sign or symptom of physiological deterioration that occurs in the hours before the critical change in status (Box 11-1).[1] Many facilities have implemented a rapid response team (RRT) program to facilitate early detection and rapid treatment of unstable patients outside of the critical care unit (Box 11-2). The early intervention of RRTs has been shown to decrease the incidence of cardiac arrest and improve mortality rates.[2]

The causes of cardiopulmonary arrest are myriad (Box 11-3), and patients in the critical care unit are at particularly high risk for experiencing cardiopulmonary arrest during the course of their hospitalization. Early recognition of a patient's deterioration in clinical status and rapid initiation of treatment can prevent some cases of cardiopulmonary arrest

in the critical care unit. If a patient does experience cardiopulmonary arrest, the nurse calls the code and initiates basic life support (BLS) and advanced cardiac life support (ACLS) measures immediately. Other critical care staff members respond to assist with the code; common roles and responsibilities of code team members are given in Box 11-4. The chain of survival (Box 11-5) is completed by providing appropriate post–cardiac arrest care.

BOX 11-1 Signs and Symptoms of Impending Physiologic Deterioration

- Threatened airway
- Respiratory rate less than 8 breaths/min or greater than 28 breaths/min
- SpO_2 less than 90%
- Heart rate less than 40 beats/min or greater than 130 beats/min
- Systolic blood pressure less than 90 mm Hg
- Urine output less than 50 mL in 4 hours
- Acute mental status change

BOX 11-2   Considerations When Implementing a Rapid Response Team (RRT) System

Gaining leadership support. The support of senior leadership is essential for the success of the proposed RRT system. Advantages of an RRT system include

- Marketing advantage in a competitive healthcare environment
- Greater medicolegal protection and decreased liability
- Decreased patient and family complaints
- Avoidance of unnecessary critical care unit admissions
- Decreased number of in-hospital arrests

Determining team structure. The structure of the RRT varies according to facility size, level of patient acuity, availability of resources, and the frequency of adverse events and cardiac arrest. Examples of different models include

- Critical care nurse and respiratory therapist
- Critical care nurse, respiratory therapist, and nurse practitioner or physician assistant
- Critical care nurse, respiratory therapist, and intensivist or hospitalist

Establishing communication tools and protocols. Communication tools provide the RRT leader with a template for gathering pertinent information, facilitating communication with the physician, and facilitating triage decision making.

Training for responders. Members of the RRT must receive the proper training. Areas to be reviewed include

- The benefits of early rescue
- Teamwork with non–critical care staff
- Protocols available to guide RRT therapy

- Triage skills and advanced cardiac life support (ACLS) certification
- What is expected of RRT members when responding to a call
- The use of communication tools
- The chain of command for nurse-led teams

Training for staff. Staff members must be made aware that the RRT exists, educated about the role of the RRT, and taught how to activate the RRT system. Methods of raising staff awareness include the following:

- Formal teaching and in-service training
- Newsletters
- Posters with the RRT calling criteria
- Pocket cards and badge holders with calling criteria
- Brochures with RRT concepts and calling criteria
- Inclusion of RRT education in employee orientation sessions

Calling criteria and the mechanism for activating the RRT system. When considering the RRT calling criteria that will be used, evidence-based data should be considered. The mechanism for activating the RRT system should be clear, quick, and easy so that the staff will use it and the team will respond rapidly.

Evaluation of effectiveness. A means by which to measure the success of the RRT system is imperative. Three key measures that are used include

- Codes per 1000 discharges
- Codes outside the critical care unit
- Utilization of the RRT system

Adapted from 5 Million Lives Campaign. Getting Started Kit. Rapid Response Teams. Cambridge, MA: Institute for Healthcare Improvement, 2008 (Available at www.ihi.org).

RED FLAG! *When a patient is determined to be in cardiopulmonary arrest, seconds matter. Unless definitive action is taken within 4 to 6 minutes, the patient will experience irreversible brain injury. Prompt intervention is necessary if the patient is going to have a chance of survival.*

Equipment and Medications Used During a Code

The equipment and medications used during resuscitative efforts are kept in a central location,

BOX 11-3   Common Causes of Cardiopulmonary Arrest

Cardiac Causes
- Myocardial infarction
- Heart failure
- Dysrhythmia
- Coronary artery spasms
- Cardiac tamponade

Pulmonary Causes
- Respiratory failure secondary to respiratory depression
- Airway obstruction
- Impaired gas exchange, as in acute respiratory distress syndrome (ARDS)

- Impaired ventilation, such as pneumothorax
- Pulmonary embolus

Electrolyte Imbalances
- Hyperkalemia
- Hypomagnesemia
- Hyper- or hypocalcemia

Interventions
- Pulmonary artery catheterization
- Cardiac catheterization
- Surgery
- Medications (drug toxicity, drug side effects)

BOX 11-4 Roles and Responsibilities of Code Team Members

The specific members of the code team will vary depending on the facility.

Code Director (Physician/Nurse Practitioner/ACLS Qualified Personnel)
• Make diagnosis.
• Direct treatment.

Primary Nurse
• Provide information to code director.
• Contact attending physician.

Second Nurse
• Coordinate use of emergency cart.
• Prepare medications.
• Assemble/pass equipment.
• Defibrillate.

Medication Nurse
• Administer medications.

Charge Nurse
• Coordinate personnel performing cardiopulmonary resuscitation (CPR).

Nursing Supervisor
• Control crowd.
• Provide explanations and support to family members who may be present.

Anesthesiologist/Nurse Anesthetist
• Intubate patient.
• Manage airway/oxygenation.

Respiratory Therapist
• Assist with intubation.
• Set up mechanical ventilator.
• Assist with manual ventilation.
• Draw arterial blood gases (ABGs).

Recorder
• Record events, personnel involved.

usually on a rolling cart referred to as a "crash cart" (Table 11-1). Crash carts are stocked in a standard way to assist personnel in locating specific equipment and medications during an emergency. The intubation tray and a cardiac monitor–defibrillator are located on the top of the cart. An oxygen tank, oxygen tubing, a manual resuscitation bag (MRB, Ambu bag), and suctioning equipment are also stowed on the outside of the cart. Labeled drawers hold medications (Table 11-2) and other supplies. The cart must be inventoried daily to ensure that its contents are complete and available in the event of a cardiopulmonary arrest.

Responding to a Code

Basic Life Support Measures (Primary Survey)

BLS measures for a person in cardiopulmonary arrest include cardiopulmonary resuscitation (CPR) and early defibrillation with an automated external

BOX 11-5 The American Heart Association (AHA)/Emergency Cardiac Care (ECC) Chain of Survival

1. Immediate recognition of cardiac arrest and activation of the emergency response system
2. Early cardiopulmonary resuscitation (CPR) with an emphasis on chest compressions
3. Rapid defibrillation
4. Effective advanced cardiac life support (ACLS)
5. Integrated post–cardiac arrest care

defibrillator (AED). In the hospital, the nurse initiating CPR is usually operating as part of a team. One team member starts compressions, one obtains the AED and calls for help, and another opens the airway and initiates ventilation using the MRB.

Cardiopulmonary Resuscitation

In 2010, the American Heart Association (AHA) changed the guidelines for CPR. Whereas previously an "ABC" (airway, breathing, circulation) approach was recommended, the current recommendations are for a "CAB" (circulation, airway, breathing) approach. This change was made in response to studies that showed that the amount of oxygen in a person's blood at the time of collapse is sufficient to sustain basic processes until emergency help arrives, and that better outcomes are achieved by circulating the blood first (as opposed to oxygenating blood that is not being circulated throughout the body). In addition to compressions first, the new AHA guidelines for CPR call for faster and deeper compressions.

Circulation

If a pulse is not detected, then chest compressions are initiated per BLS protocol. To facilitate chest compressions, the patient is placed in a supine position on a firm, flat surface. Many hospital beds have a "CPR" setting that provides a hard, flat surface, or a resuscitation board may be placed under the patient's torso. Hard chest compressions are applied directly downward, with the sternum depressed 2 in and released abruptly (Fig. 11-1). The chest must be allowed to recoil fully between compressions. This rhythm is maintained at a rate of approximately 100 compressions per minute. When working in tandem with other team members (as is the case when CPR

TABLE 11-1 Resuscitation Equipment Cart

Equipment	Purpose

Intubation equipment
  Straight and curved blades
  Endotracheal tubes
  Syringes
  Oropharyngeal airways
  Nasopharyngeal airways
	• Provides adequate, patent airway, thus ensuring oxygenation of the lungs during resuscitation
	• Allows the patient to be placed on mechanical ventilation
	• Reduces chances for gastric distention, aspiration, or vomiting
	• Allows for the administration of oxygen in high concentrations
	• Provides route for NAVEL medications (ie, those that can be administered via endotracheal tube): **n**aloxone, **a**tropine, **v**alium, **e**pinephrine, **l**idocaine

Oxygen tank
Manual resuscitation bag (MRB)
Suctioning equipment
  Suction source
  Suction catheters
  Suction tubing
	• Ensures that oxygen is available if wall oxygen is unavailable
	• Permits delivery of breaths manually
	• Clears oropharyngeal (nasopharyngeal) airway before intubation
	• Ensures that suctioning is available if wall suction is unavailable

IV fluids and tubing
Nitroglycerin tubing
Medications (advanced cardiac life support [ACLS] drugs as a minimum)
  Amiodarone
  Lidocaine
  Atropine
  Epinephrine
  Sodium bicarbonate
  Calcium chloride
  D_{50}
  Adenosine
  Magnesium
  Premixed dopamine infusion
	• Improves hypotension
	• Prevents precipitation of IV nitroglycerin
	• Used to support circulation, correct underlying dysrhythmias or electrolyte imbalances

Drip chart	• Allows for rapid titration of ACLS/critical care drugs during and after resuscitation without having to perform complex calculations

Blood tubes
  Red—chemistries
  Blue—coagulation studies
  Purple—hematology (complete blood count)
  Green—troponin
	• Allows for the rapid drawing and sending of blood for analysis

Arterial blood gas (ABG) kits Peripheral IV supplies Prefilled flush syringes (normal saline) Needles Decompression (cardiac) needles Clipboard with paper and pen; code sheets Pressure bags Manual blood pressure cuff Gloves (latex, nonlatex, sterile) Defibrillator/transcutaneous pacemaker Resuscitation board	• Allows for rapid drawing and sending of ABGs • Ensures access for fluid and IV drug administration • Allows for faster flushing of IV lines • Allows for drawing up of medications • Used in cardiac tamponade • Used to document the arrest • Used for rapid infusion of fluid boluses • Used to monitor effectiveness of resuscitation • Used for infection control • Used for defibrillation, cardioversion, and temporary transcutaneous pacing • Used to create a flat, hard surface to improve chest compressions

is being performed in the critical care unit), there is no pause for the breath; one team member provides uninterrupted chest compressions, while the other administers the breaths using the MRB. A third team member checks the patient's carotid or femoral pulses at regular intervals to determine the adequacy of compressions. If no third team member is present, CPR should not be interrupted for a pulse check.[3]

Airway
The nurse assesses for an adequate airway. In an unintubated patient, the airway is opened using the head tilt–chin lift method or the jaw thrust maneuver (Fig. 11-2). If the patient is intubated, the nurse suctions the artificial airway and attempts to ventilate the patient with the MRB. If spontaneous respirations do not return once a patent airway is established, then the patient must be assisted with breathing and an artificial airway secured if not already present.

Breathing
Oxygen is delivered as rescue breaths using an MRB. The MRB is connected to 100% high-flow oxygen, and either the mask portion is placed over the patient's mouth and nose or the adapter is connected directly to the endotracheal or tracheostomy

TABLE 11-2 Medications Used to Treat a Patient in Cardiopulmonary Arrest

Drug	Class	Uses	Dosages
Adenosine	Antidysrhythmic	Supraventricular tachycardia, atrial fibrillation	6 mg rapid IV followed by 10 mL NS flush Repeat twice with 12 mg Max. dose: 30 mg
Amiodarone	Antidysrhythmic	Ventricular tachycardia, supraventricular tachycardia, atrial fibrillation, ventricular fibrillation	150–300 mg bolus, 1 mg/min for 6 h, then 0.5 mg/min for 18 h
Atropine	Anticholinergic	Bradycardia	0.5–1.0 mg IV Max. dose: 3 mg
Calcium chloride	Electrolyte	Hyperkalemia, hypocalcemia, calcium channel blocker toxicity	Syringe 10 mL of 10% solution (100 mg/mL), 2–4 mg/kg
Dobutamine	Inotrope; β_1 agonist	Decreased cardiac output	5–20 µg/kg/min
Dopamine	Inotrope; β_1 agonist	Hypotension	5–20 µg/kg/min
Epinephrine	Catecholamine	Ventricular fibrillation Pulseless ventricular tachycardia, pulseless electrical activity	Syringe 1:10,000, 1-mg bolus IV Repeat q 3–5 min
Isoproterenol	Catecholamine; β agonist	Ventricular tachycardia, ventricular fibrillation	Drip 0.5–5 µg/min
Lidocaine	Antidysrhythmic	Ventricular tachycardia, ventricular fibrillation	Bolus 1–1.5 mg/kg Drip 20–50 µg/kg/min
Magnesium sulfate	Electrolyte	Torsades de pointes	Drip 1–2 g/50 mL Normal saline
Nitroglycerin	Coronary vasodilator	Myocardial infarction, angina	5–100 µg/min
Procainamide	Antidysrhythmic	Ventricular tachycardia, ventricular fibrillation	Bolus 5–10 mg/kg over 8–10 min Drip 20–30 mg/min
Sodium bicarbonate	Alkalinizer	Acidosis	50 mEq syringe Normal dose is 1 mEq/kg
Vasopressin	Nonadrenergic, endogenous antidiuretic hormone; vasoconstrictor	Ventricular fibrillation Pulseless ventricular tachycardia	40 U to be substituted for the first of second dose of epinephrine
Verapamil	Calcium channel blocker	Supraventricular tachycardia	2.5–5 mg IV over 2 min Repeat 5–10 mg in 15–30 min

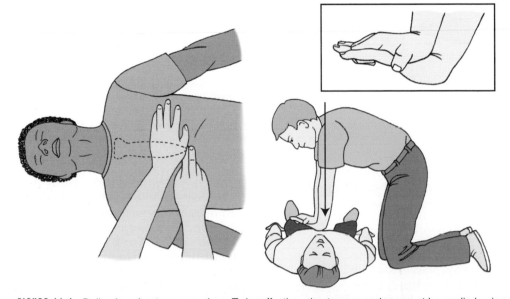

FIGURE 11-1 Delivering chest compressions. To be effective, chest compressions must be applied using proper technique.

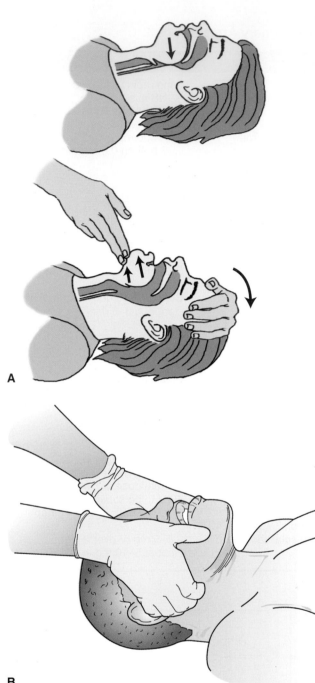

A

B

FIGURE 11-2   A: The head tilt–chin lift maneuver is used to open the airway in an unintubated patient. **B:** The jaw thrust maneuver is used without head extension if cervical spine trauma is suspected.

tube. The bag reservoir is squeezed to deliver breaths while observing the rise and fall of the chest wall to verify that the breaths are actually ventilating the lungs. Another team member can auscultate the patient's lung fields to confirm that the delivered breaths are reaching the lungs.

RED FLAG! Chest compressions should not be interrupted to deliver the breaths. The AHA recommends asynchronous breathing with chest compressions.

Automated External Defibrillation

AEDs are frequently used in the hospital setting, including critical care units. Once the AED is placed on the patient, chest compressions are stopped so that the AED can read the rhythm and deliver a countershock.

RED FLAG! When an AED is being used and is reading the rhythm, all personnel must avoid touching the patient, the bed, or any of the equipment attached to the patient.

Advanced Cardiac Life Support Measures (Secondary Survey)

ACLS assessments and interventions are more in-depth and sophisticated than those used during the BLS primary survey. While the ACLS steps are being carried out, chest compressions continue with minimal interruptions. The "ABCDs" of ACLS are

- **Airway.** If needed, definitive airway management (eg, endotracheal intubation) takes place now.
- **Breathing.** Proper placement of the endotracheal tube is verified using end-tidal carbon dioxide ($ETCO_2$) monitoring. Oxygen is administered, and oxygenation is evaluated using pulse oximetry.
- **Circulation.** If not already present, an IV line may be inserted. Medications (eg, antidysrhythmics, inotropes, vasoconstrictors, electrolyte replacements) and electrical therapies (eg, defibrillation, transcutaneous pacing) may be used to correct dysrhythmias and support circulation.
- **Differential diagnosis.** The underlying cause of the cardiopulmonary arrest is explored in more depth so that measures to treat it can be initiated.

The nurse assesses the electrocardiogram (ECG) rhythms on the monitor throughout the resuscitation effort. If the patient is in ventricular fibrillation or pulseless ventricular tachycardia, preparations for defibrillation need to be started immediately while continuing to provide chest compressions and ventilation. The defibrillator paddles are positioned so that the heart is in the current pathway (Fig. 11-3). The procedure for defibrillation is given in Box 11-6. Current recommendations are to attempt defibrillation using one shock, with immediate resumption of CPR. Following this first shock, five cycles of CPR are performed. If the patient remains in a shockable rhythm, then a second shock is delivered. After each subsequent shock, five more cycles of CPR are performed before determining whether the patient is in a shockable rhythm.[3]

If the patient has bradycardia that is unresponsive to drug therapy, Mobitz type II heart block, or third-degree (complete) heart block, transcutaneous pacing may be used to try and correct the dysrhythmia (see Chapter 8). On most defibrillators, the large pacing electrodes ("combination pads") can be used to pace a patient transcutaneously. In patients with profound asystolic arrest, transcutaneous pacing should not be relied on indefinitely.

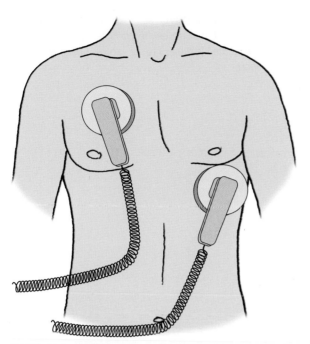

FIGURE 11-3 Standard positioning of defibrillator paddles (sternum–apex position). The anterior paddle is placed firmly on the patient's upper right chest below the clavicle and to the right of the sternum. The apex paddle is positioned firmly on the patient's lower left chest in a midaxillary line.

Post–Cardiac Arrest Care

Following successful conversion to a perfusing rhythm, the patient may be hemodynamically unstable and require continuous intensive monitoring. Vasoconstrictors may be administered to maintain an adequate blood pressure. If the patient was placed on a transcutaneous pacemaker during the cardiopulmonary arrest, then a transvenous pacemaker may need to be inserted until a permanent pacemaker can be placed.

Induced therapeutic hypothermia (32° to 34° Celsuis) may benefit unconscious adult patients who experience out-of-hospital cardiac arrest due to ventricular fibrillation and who are resuscitated in the field. In addition, there is evidence that supports

hypothermic therapy for cardiac arrest caused by other dysrhythmias.[4] During cardiac arrest, blood flow to the brain is compromised, and even prompt interventions may not counteract the deleterious effects of this hemodynamic compromise. Studies have shown that cooling the patient after cardiac arrest may preserve neurological function by reducing the cerebral metabolic rate for oxygen ($CMRO_2$).

CASE STUDY

Mr. B. was being cared for in the critical care unit following an acute myocardial infarction. He presented to the emergency department complaining of "heaviness" in his chest. He was diaphoretic and dyspneic. The initial 12-lead ECG revealed ST-segment elevation in leads I, aVL, and V_1 through V_5, with significant Q waves in V_1 through V_4.

Mr. B. is admitted to the critical care unit following cardiac catheterization for angioplasty and placement of drug-eluting stents. He is kept in a supine position with his leg straight. Initial assessment of the groin access site reveals an intact, dry dressing, and no swelling or hematoma. Mr. B. is awake, oriented, and cooperative.

Three hours following the cardiac catheterization procedure, Mr. B. develops some swelling at the groin site and pressure is applied. At this time, Mr. B. is awake, alert, and cooperative, but an hour later, he becomes restless and agitated and complains of low back pain. He is thrashing around in the bed and will not remain supine. The nurse pages the physician and requests that he come to the bedside urgently. Mr. B. is becoming progressively more combative, and suddenly he loses consciousness. A code is called and the code team responds with the crash cart to the bedside.

The nurse quickly assesses Mr. B. and finds that he is not breathing. A manual resuscitation bag (MRB) is used to ventilate Mr. B after opening the airway with a head tilt. The cardiac monitor shows a rhythm, but no pulse is palpable. Chest compressions are started immediately. Another nurse assesses pulses during chest compressions to assure adequate compressions. A nurse anesthetist intubates Mr. B., and a respiratory therapist maintains ventilation.

The responding physician orders laboratory studies and the administration of IV fluid boluses and ACLS medications. Mr. B. is noted to have pulseless electrical activity and potential underlying causes are managed. Mr. B. dies following multiple attempts to reestablish a perfusing rhythm.

1. Why did the nurse call the physician to the bedside when Mr. B. became agitated?

2. How should the nurse performing cardiopulmonary resuscitation (CPR) deliver chest compressions?

BOX 11-6 **Procedure for Defibrillation**

1. Apply defibrillator pads to the patient.
2. Turn on defibrillator.
3. Set the number of joules (J):
   Monophasic device: 360 J
   Biphasic device: 120 or 200 J, depending on device
4. Ensure that personnel are not touching the patient or bed.
5. Deliver shock.
6. Continue cardiopulmonary resuscitation (CPR).
7. Prepare to deliver subsequent shocks per advanced cardiac life support (ACLS) protocol.

References

1. Jones D, Bellomo R, Goldsmith D: General principles of medical emergency teams. In DeVita MA, Hillman K, Bellomo R (eds): Medical Emergency Teams: Implementation and Outcome Measurement. New York, NY: Springer Press, 2006, pp 80–90
2. Butner S: Rapid response team effectiveness. Dimens Crit Care Nurs 30(4):201–205, 2011
3. American Heart Association: 2010 American Heart Association guidelines for cardiopulmonary resuscitation and emergency cardiovascular care. Circulation 122(18), 2010
4. Holzer M, et al: Targeted temperature management of cardiac arrest. N Engl J Med 363:1256–1264, 2010

Want to know more? A wide variety of resources to enhance your learning and understanding of this chapter are available on the**Point**. Visit **http://thepoint.lww.com/MortonEss1e** to access chapter review questions and more!

Cardiovascular System

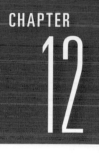

THREE

Patient Assessment: Cardiovascular System

OBJECTIVES

Based on the content in this chapter, the reader should be able to:

1 Describe the components of the history for cardiovascular assessment.
2 Explain the use of inspection, palpation, percussion, and auscultation for cardiovascular assessment.
3 Discuss the mechanisms responsible for the production of the first, second, third, and fourth heart sounds and their timing in the cardiac cycle.
4 Describe the attributes of common systolic and diastolic murmurs.
5 Discuss the use of routine blood tests, serum lipid levels, and biochemical markers in the diagnosis and monitoring of cardiovascular disease.
6 Discuss the purpose of cardiovascular diagnostic studies and associated nursing implications.

Although advanced and complex technologies are being used with increasing frequency to assess and manage cardiovascular conditions, a comprehensive history and physical examination is also an integral part of care for critically ill patients with cardiovascular conditions.

History

The cardiovascular history provides information that guides the physical assessment, the selection of diagnostic tests, and the choice of treatment options.

Elements of the cardiovascular history are summarized in Box 12-1.

The nurse begins the history by investigating the patient's chief complaint. Obtaining answers to the questions posed in Box 12-2 helps the nurse to better understand the nature of the patient's signs and symptoms, and may provide clues to the underlying cause. Chest pain, one of the most common symptoms of cardiovascular disease, is commonly caused by coronary artery disease (CAD). Chest pain may also be secondary to cardiovascular problems that are unrelated to CAD (eg, pericarditis). Differential diagnoses of chest pain are summarized in Table 12-1.

BOX 12-1 Cardiovascular Health History

History Of The Present Illness

Complete analysis of the following signs and symptoms (using the NOPQRST format; see Box 12-2 below):

- Chest pain
- Nausea or vomiting
- Dyspnea
- Edema
- Palpitations
- Syncope/dizziness
- Cough and hemoptysis
- Nocturia
- Cyanosis
- Extremity pain or paresthesias

Past Health History

- **Relevant childhood illnesses and immunizations:** rheumatic fever, murmurs, congenital anomalies, streptococcal infections
- **Past acute and chronic medical problems, including treatments and hospitalizations:** heart failure, hypertension, coronary artery disease, myocardial infarction, hyperlipidemia, valve disease, cardiac dysrhythmias, diabetes mellitus, endocarditis, thrombophlebitis, DVT, peripheral vascular disease, chest injury, pneumonia, pulmonary embolism, thyroid disease, tuberculosis
- **Risk factors:** age, heredity, gender, race, tobacco use, elevated cholesterol, hypertension, physical inactivity, obesity, diabetes mellitus (see Box 12-3)
- **Past surgeries:** coronary artery bypass grafting (CABG), valvular surgery, peripheral vascular surgeries
- **Past diagnostic tests and interventions:** ECG, electrocardiogram, echocardiogram, stress test, electrophysiology studies, myocardial imaging studies, thrombolytic therapy, cardiac catheterization, percutaneous transluminal cardiac angioplasty, stent placement, atherectomy, pacemaker or implantable cardioverter defibrillator implantation, valvuloplasty

- **Medications, including prescription drugs, over-the-counter drugs, vitamins, herbs, and supplements:** angiotensin-converting enzyme (ACE) inhibitors, anticoagulants, antihypertensives, antiplatelets, antiarrhythmics, angiotensin II receptor blockers (ARBs), β-blockers, calcium channel blockers, antihyperlipidemics, diuretics, electrolyte replacements, nitrates, inotropes, hormone replacement therapies, oral contraceptives, use of agents for erectile dysfunction
- **Allergies and reactions to medications, foods, contrast dye, latex or other materials**
- **Transfusions, including type and date**

Family History

- **Health status or cause of death of parents and siblings:** CAD, hypertension, diabetes mellitus, sudden cardiac death, stroke, peripheral vascular disease, lipid disorders

Personal and Social History

- Tobacco, alcohol, and substance use
- Environment
- Diet: restrictions, supplements, caffeine intake
- Sleep patterns: number of pillows used
- Exercise

Review of Other Systems

- **HEENT:** retinal problems, visual changes, headaches, carotid artery disease
- **Respiratory:** shortness of breath, dyspnea, cough, lung disease, recurrent infections, pneumonia, tuberculosis
- **Gastrointestinal:** nausea, vomiting, weight loss, change in bowel habits
- **Genitourinary:** incontinence, erectile dysfunction
- **Musculoskeletal:** pain, weakness, varicose veins, change in sensation, peripheral edema
- **Neurological:** transient ischemic attacks, stroke, change in level of consciousness, changes in sensations
- **Endocrine:** thyroid disease, diabetes mellitus

BOX 12-2 Assessment Parameters: Questions to Ask in a Symptom Assessment

N—Normal: Describe your normal baseline. What was it like before this symptom developed?

O—Onset: When did the symptom start? What day? What time? Did it start suddenly or gradually?

P—Precipitating and palliative factors: What brought on the symptom? What seems to trigger it—factors such as stress, position change, or exertion? What were you doing when you first noticed the symptom? What makes the symptom worse? What measures have helped relieve the symptom? What have you tried so far? What measures did not relieve the symptom?

Q—Quality and quantity: How does it feel? How would you describe it? How much are you

experiencing now? Is it more or less than you experienced at any other time?

R—Region and radiation: Where does the symptom occur? Can you show me? In the case of pain, does it travel anywhere such as down your arm or in your back?

S—Severity: On a scale of 0 to 10, with 0 being the absence of pain and 10 being the worst ever experienced, rate your symptom. How bad is the symptom at its worst? Does it force you to stop your activity and sit down, lie down, or slow down? Is the symptom getting better or worse, or staying about the same?

T—Time: How long does the symptom last? How often do you get the symptom? Does it occur in association with anything, such as before, during, or after meals?

TABLE 12-1 Differential Diagnosis of Chest Pain

Diagnosis	Onset of Pain	Quality of Pain	Relieved By
Angina pectoris	Sudden, after heavy meal or exertion; may also occur at rest (unstable angina)	Heavy, crushing, squeezing, choking	Rest, nitroglycerin
Acute myocardial infarction	Varies, may be associated with feeling of doom	Similar to angina, but more severe	No relief with rest or nitroglycerin
Pericarditis	Varies, may be preceded by "flu-like" symptoms for several days to weeks; onset usually accompanied by fever and chills	Pleuritic Sharp, stabbing, worsens with inspiration and coughing	Sitting up, leaning forward, breathing shallowly, decreasing movement of chest and arms, nonsteroidal anti-inflammatory drugs (NSAIDs)
Acute aortic dissection	Sudden, may be associated with syncope; intense from the onset	Ripping, tearing sensation; may be followed by a period of minimal pain (latency period) before severe, unrelenting pain often described as the worst pain the patient has ever experienced	No relief

The patient's past health history, family history, and personal and social history can provide important information about the patient's risk factors for cardiovascular disease (Box 12-3). The history concludes with a review of relevant systems. The information obtained during the review of systems provides insight into the patient's overall health status and helps determine the impact of cardiovascular disease on the functioning of other body systems.

BOX 12-3 Risk Factors for Cardiovascular Disease

Major Uncontrollable Risk Factors
- **Age:** Incidence of all types of atherosclerotic disease increases with aging.
- **Heredity:** Even when other risk factors are controlled, the chance for development of coronary artery disease (CAD) increases when there is a familial tendency
- **Gender:** Men have a greater risk for developing CAD than do women at earlier ages. After menopause, women's death rate from myocardial infarction increases but is not as great as men's.
- **Race:** Rates of cardiovascular disease are higher for African Americans, Mexican Americans, Native Americans, Native Hawaiians, and some Asian Americans.

Risk Factors That Can Be Modified, Treated, or Controlled
- **Tobacco smoking:** A smoker's risk for a myocardial infarction is more than twice that of a nonsmoker.
- **High blood cholesterol:** The risk for CAD increases as the blood cholesterol level rises. When other risk factors are present, this risk increases even more.
- **Hypertension:** Hypertension increases the risk for stroke, myocardial infarction, kidney failure, and heart failure.
- **Physical inactivity:** Moderate to vigorous regular exercise plays a significant role in preventing heart disease and CAD, and in controlling cholesterol, diabetes, obesity, and hypertension.
- **Obesity:** Excess body fat, especially at the waist, increases a person's risk for developing heart disease and stroke, even in the absence of other risk factors. Excess weight raises blood pressure, blood cholesterol, and blood triglyceride levels; lowers high-density lipoproteins; and promotes the development of diabetes.
- **Diabetes mellitus:** Even when blood glucose levels are under control, diabetes greatly increases the risk for heart disease and stroke.

Contributing Risk Factors
- **Stress:** A person's response to stress may be a contributing factor to heart disease.
- **Excessive alcohol intake:** Drinking too much alcohol can raise blood pressure, cause heart failure, lead to stroke, contribute to high triglycerides and obesity, and produce arrhythmias.

Metabolic Syndrome
A group of risk factors associated with an increased risk for developing cardiovascular disease and type 2 diabetes, metabolic syndrome is diagnosed when three or more of the following risk factors are present:

- Fasting blood glucose of 100 mg/dL or higher
- HDL cholesterol below 40 mg/dL in men or below 50 mg/dL in women
- Triglycerides of 150 mg/dL or higher
- Waist circumference of 40 in (102 cm) or higher in men or 35 in (88 cm) or higher in women
- Systolic blood pressure of 130 mm Hg or higher, diastolic blood pressure of 85 mm Hg or higher, or drug treatment for hypertension

Physical Examination

Inspection

Inspection encompasses several points:

- **General appearance and presentation.** The patient's general appearance and presentation are key elements of the initial inspection. The nurse notes first impressions of the patient's age, nutritional status, self-care ability, alertness, overall physical health, and ability to move and speak with or without distress. The patient's posture, gait, and musculoskeletal coordination are also considered.
- **Jugular venous distention.** Evaluation of jugular venous distention provides insight into hemodynamics and cardiac function. The height of the level of blood in the right internal jugular vein is an indication of right atrial pressure (RAP) because there are no valves or obstructions between the vein and the right atrium. Jugular venous distention is assessed by measuring the highest point of visible pulsation as the vertical distance above the sternal angle (Fig. 12-1). A level more than 3 cm above the sternal angle indicates an abnormally high volume in the venous system (eg, as a result of right-sided heart failure, obstruction of the superior vena cava, or pericardial effusion). An increase in the jugular venous pressure of more than 1 cm while pressure is applied to the abdomen for 60 seconds (hepatojugular or abdominojugular test) indicates the heart's inability to accommodate the increased venous return.
- **Chest.** Inspection of the chest may reveal the location of the point of maximal impulse (PMI). Usually, the PMI is located at the fifth intercostal space (ICS) on the midclavicular line; however, in some pathological conditions, it may be displaced. (For example, left ventricular hypertrophy displaces the PMI laterally.) The nurse also notes abnormally strong precordial pulsations (thrusts),

asymmetry, any depression or bulging of the precordium, and any signs of trauma or injury.
- **Extremities.** The nurse examines the extremities for lesions, ulcerations, unhealed sores, varicose veins, and hair distribution. A lack of normal hair distribution on the extremities may indicate diminished arterial blood flow to the area.
- **Skin.** The nurse evaluates the skin for moistness or dryness, color, elasticity, edema, thickness, lesions, ulcerations, and vascular changes. Cyanosis and clubbing of the nailbeds may indicate chronic cardiac or pulmonary abnormalities. General differences in color and temperature between body parts may provide perfusion clues.

Palpation

Pulses

The nurse palpates the brachial, radial, femoral, popliteal, posterior tibial, and dorsalis pedis pulses bilaterally to determine symmetry and strength (rated on a scale of 0 to +4). The nurse also compares the warmth of the palpated areas to monitor perfusion.

> **RED FLAG!** *The carotid pulses are never assessed simultaneously, because doing so can obstruct blood flow to the brain.*

Abnormal pulses include the following.

- **Pulses tardus** (a prolonged pulse with a weak, slow upstroke) is often associated with aortic stenosis.
- **Pulsus alternans** (a pulse that alternates in strength with every other beat) is often found in patients with left ventricular failure.
- **Pulsus paradoxus,** often seen in hypovolemic patients, is a pulse that decreases during inspiration but returns to normal during expiration. To measure pulsus paradoxus, the sphygmomanometer is deflated until the pulse is heard only during expiration, and the corresponding systolic pressure is noted. As the cuff continues to deflate, the point at which the pulse is heard throughout the inspiratory and expiratory cycle is noted. The second systolic pressure reading is subtracted from the first; if the difference is greater than 10 mm Hg during normal respirations, the pulsus paradoxus is considered pathological.
- **Pulsus bisferiens** is an arterial pulse with two systolic peaks.

Precordium

The chest wall is palpated to assess for the PMI, thrills (palpable vibrations that usually represent a disruption in blood flow related to a defect in one of the semilunar valves), and abnormal pulsations. The nurse follows a systematic palpation sequence with the patient in a supine position. The PMI is palpated, and its location, diameter, amplitude, and duration are noted. If the PMI is difficult to palpate, assisting the patient into the left lateral decubitus position may facilitate palpation. Next,

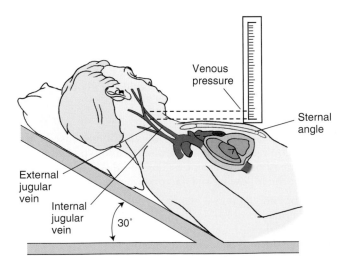

FIGURE 12-1 To assess jugular venous pressure, place the patient supine in bed and gradually raise the head of the bed to 30, 45, 60, and 90 degrees. Using tangential lighting, note the highest level of venous pulsation. Measure the vertical distance between this point and the sternal angle. Record this distance in centimeters and the angle of the head of the bed.

the lower and upper left sternal border areas, the sternoclavicular area, the upper and lower right sternal border areas, the lower right sternal border area, and the epigastric area are palpated to assess for thrills.

Percussion

Although radiologic methods give more precise data about heart size, a gross estimation of heart size can be made by percussing for the dullness that reflects the cardiac borders.

Auscultation

The precordium is auscultated systematically (Fig. 12-2). In each area auscultated, the nurse identifies the first (S_1) and second (S_2) heart sound noting the intensity of the sound, respiratory variation, and splitting. After S_1 and S_2 are identified, the nurse notes the presence of extra heart sounds (S_3 and S_4). Finally, each area is auscultated for the presence of murmurs and friction rubs.

Heart Sounds

First Heart Sound

S_1 is produced by the closure of the atrioventricular (mitral and tricuspid) valves and correlates with the beginning of ventricular systole (Fig. 12-3A). Because the mitral valve closes first, and thus is responsible for most of the sound heard, S_1 is heard best in the mitral (apical) area. The intensity (loudness) of S_1 varies with the length of time the valve is open and the structure of the leaflets (thickened or normal):

• A loud S_1 is produced when the valve leaflets are wide open at the onset of ventricular systole, and it corresponds to a short PR interval on the electrocardiogram (ECG) tracing. Mitral stenosis also

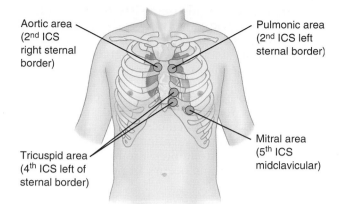

Aortic area (2nd ICS right sternal border)

Pulmonic area (2nd ICS left sternal border)

Tricuspid area (4th ICS left of sternal border)

Mitral area (5th ICS midclavicular)

FIGURE 12-2   Areas of auscultation.

increases the intensity of S_1 because of a thickening of the valvular structures.

• A soft S_1 is produced when the valve leaflets have had time to float partially closed before ventricular systole, and it corresponds to a lengthening of the PR interval on the ECG.

S_1 is made of two component sounds: the closing of the mitral valve (left side), followed by the closing of the tricuspid valve (right side). Usually, S_1 is heard as a single sound. However, if right ventricular systole is delayed, S_1 may be heard as a split sound. The most common cause of this splitting is delay in the conduction of impulses through the right bundle branch; the splitting correlates with a right bundle branch block pattern on the ECG. Splitting of S_1 is heard best over the tricuspid area.

Second Heart Sound

S_2 is produced by the closure of the semilunar (aortic and pulmonic) valves and is heard best over the aortic area. S_2, which represents the beginning of

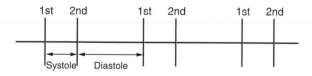

A. First (S_1) and second (S_2) heart sound.

Normal: S_1 is produced by the closure of the AV valves and correlates with the beginning of ventricular systole. It is heard best in the apical or mitral area.

Normal: S_2 is produced by the closure of aorta and plumonic valves and correlates with the beginning of ventricular diastole

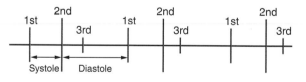

B. Third heart sound (S_3) Occurs during the early, rapid filling phase of ventricular diastole; heard best at apex

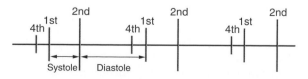

C. Fourth heart sound (S_4) Occurs during the late diastolic phase during the atrial contraction; heard best at apex

FIGURE 12-3   Graphic depiction of heart sounds.

ventricular diastole, also consists of two separate components: aortic valve closure followed by pulmonic valve closure. With inspiration, right ventricular systole is prolonged slightly because of increased filling of the right ventricle. This causes the pulmonic valve to close later than the aortic valve and S_2 to be heard as a split sound. This normal finding is termed physiological splitting. The intensity of S_2 may be increased in the presence of aortic or pulmonic valvular stenosis or when an increase in the diastolic pressure forces the semilunar valves to close, as occurs in pulmonary or systemic hypertension.

Third Heart Sound

An S_3 is a low-frequency sound that occurs during the early, rapid-filling phase of ventricular diastole (see Fig. 12-3B). A physiological S_3 is a normal finding in children and healthy young adults; it usually disappears after 25 to 35 years of age. A pathological S_3 is produced when a noncompliant or failing ventricle cannot distend to accept the rapid inflow of blood.

This causes turbulent flow, resulting in the vibration of the atrioventricular valves or the ventricles themselves, producing a low-frequency sound. An S_3, most commonly associated with left ventricular failure, is heard best at the apex with the stethoscope bell. The sound may be accentuated by having the patient turn slightly to the left side. A right ventricular S_3 is heard best at the lower left sternal border and varies in intensity with respiration, becoming louder on inspiration.

Fourth Heart Sound

An S_4 (atrial gallop) is a low-frequency sound heard late in diastole just before S_1 (see Fig. 12-3C). It is rarely heard in healthy patients. The sound is produced when atrial contraction forces blood into a noncompliant ventricle. Systemic hypertension, myocardial infarction, angina, cardiomyopathy, and aortic stenosis all may produce a decrease in left ventricular compliance and an S_4. A left ventricular S_4 is auscultated at the apex with the bell of the stethoscope. Conditions affecting right ventricular compliance, such as pulmonary hypertension or pulmonic stenosis, may produce a right ventricular S_4 heard best at the fourth ICS at the left sternal border; it increases in intensity during inspiration.

Summation Gallop

With rapid heart rates that shorten ventricular diastole, if an S_3 and S_4 are both present, they may fuse together and become audible as a single diastolic sound. This is called a summation gallop. This sound is loudest at the apex and is heard best with the stethoscope bell while the patient lies turned slightly to the left side.

Heart Murmurs

Murmurs are sounds produced either by the forward flow of blood through a stenotic valve or by the backward flow of blood through an incompetent valve or septal defect. Murmur classification is based on several attributes (Box 12-4).

BOX 12-4 Attributes of Heart Murmurs

Timing
Systolic murmurs:
- *Midsystolic* murmur begins after S_1 and stops before S_2.
- *Pansystolic (holosystolic)* murmur starts with S_1 and stops with S_2 without a gap between the murmur and the heart sound.
- *Late systolic* murmur starts in mid to late systole and continues up to S_2.

Diastolic murmurs:
- *Early diastolic* murmur starts right after S_2 and fades before the next S_1.
- *Middiastolic* murmur starts a short time after S_2 and fades away or merges into a late diastolic murmur.
- *Late diastolic* murmur starts late in diastole and continues up to S_1.

Location of maximal intensity. This is the anatomical location where the murmur is heard best, identified based on ICS and its relation to the sternum, the apex, the midclavicular line, or one of the axillary lines.

Radiation. This is the site farthest from the location of the greatest intensity at which the sound is still heard, identified using the anatomical landmarks described previously.

Pitch. The terms *high, medium,* and *low* are used to describe the pitch of the murmur.

Shape. The shape of a murmur is determined by its intensity over time.

- A *crescendo murmur* grows louder.
- A *decrescendo murmur* grows softer.
- A *crescendo-decrescendo murmur* first rises in intensity, then falls.
- A *plateau murmur* has the same intensity throughout.

Intensity. A grading system is used to describe the intensity of the murmur (scales 1 through 4, 1 through 5, and 1 through 6 are used).

- Grade 1: barely audible in a quiet room, very faint; may not be heard in all positions
- Grade 2: quiet, but clearly audible
- Grade 3: moderately loud
- Grade 4: loud with palpable thrill
- Grade 5: very loud with an easily palpable thrill; may be heard when the stethoscope is partly off the chest.
- Grade 6: very loud with an easily palpable thrill; may be heard with stethoscope entirely off the chest.

Quality. The terms such as *harsh, rumbling, vibratory, blowing,* and *musical* are used to describe the quality of the sound.

Ventilation and position. The murmur may be affected by inspiration, expiration, or a change in body position.

Systolic Murmurs

Systolic murmurs occur after S_1 and before S_2. During ventricular systole, the aortic and pulmonic valves are open. If either of these valves is stenotic, a mid-systolic murmur is heard. The murmurs associated with aortic stenosis and pulmonic stenosis are described as crescendo–decrescendo (diamond) shaped (Table 12-2), meaning that the sound increases and then decreases in intensity.

Mitral or tricuspid valvular insufficiency or a defect in the ventricular septum causes the backward flow of blood from an area of higher pressure to an area of lower pressure. This produces a systolic regurgitant murmur. Systolic regurgitant murmurs are pansystolic and plateau-shaped (see Table 12-2).

Diastolic Murmurs

Diastolic murmurs occur after S_2 and before the next S_1. During diastole, the aortic and pulmonic valves are closed while the mitral and tricuspid valves are open to allow filling of the ventricles. Aortic or pulmonic valvular insufficiency produces an early diastolic murmur that begins immediately after S_2 and decreases in intensity as regurgitant flow decreases through diastole, producing a decrescendo shape (see Table 12-2).

Mitral or tricuspid valve stenosis produces a mid-diastolic murmur. Because the mitral and tricuspid valves open shortly after the aortic and pulmonic valves close, there is a delay between S_2 and the start of the murmur. The murmur decreases in

TABLE 12-2 Common Systolic and Diastolic Murmurs

Type	Where to Auscultate	Radiation	Pitch	Shape	Quality	Ventilation and Position
Systolic murmurs						
Aortic stenosis	Aortic area, right second ICS	Neck, upper back, right carotid, down the left sterna border to the apex	Medium	Crescendo–decrescendo S_1 S_2 S_1	Harsh, may be musical at the apex	Heard best with the patient sitting and leaning forward, loudest during expiration
Pulmonic stenosis	Pulmonic area, left, second ICS	Left side of neck, toward left shoulder	Medium	Crescendo–decrescendo S_1 S_2 S_1	Often harsh	Loudest during inspiration
Mitral regurgitation	Mitral area, apex, mid-clavicular Fifth ICS	Left axilla, left sterna border (less often)	Medium to high	Plateau S_1 S_2 S_1	Blowing, harsh	Heard best with patient in the left lateral decubitus position, does not become louder with inspiration
Tricuspid regurgitation	Tricuspid area, left sternal border, fourth ICS	Right sternal border, to the xiphoid area, and perhaps to the left mid-clavicular line, but not to the axilla	Medium	Plateau S_1 S_2 S_1	Blowing, harsh	May increase slightly with inspiration
Diastolic murmurs						
Aortic regurgitation	Aortic area, right second ICS	Sternal border, apex	High	Decrescendo S_1 S_2 S_1	Blowing	Heard best with the patient sitting, leaning forward, with breath held after exhalation
Mitral stenosis	Mitral area, apex, mid-clavicular, fourth ICS	Usually none	Low	Decrescendo–crescendo Loud S_1 S_2 S_1	Rumbling	Best heard with the patient in a left lateral position Mild exercise and listening during exhalation also make the murmur easier to hear

intensity from its onset and then increases again as ventricular filling increases because of atrial contraction; this is termed decrescendo–crescendo (see Table 12-2).

Friction Rubs

A high-pitched, rasping, scratchy sound that varies with the cardiac cycle is called a pericardial friction rub. A pericardial friction rub is produced when inflamed pericardial layers rub together. The rub may be heard anywhere over the pericardium with the diaphragm of the stethoscope, and is accentuated by having the patient lean forward and exhale. A pericardial friction rub, unlike a pleural friction rub (see Chapter 15), does not vary in intensity with respiration.

Cardiac Laboratory Studies

Routine Blood Tests

Routine blood tests (eg, hematological studies, coagulation studies, and blood chemistries) provide valuable information about the health and functioning of the cardiovascular system. Normal reference ranges for hematologic studies, coagulation studies, and blood chemistries are given in Table 12-3.

Serum Lipid Levels

Serum lipid levels are used to assess risk for developing CAD. Standard elements of a lipid profile are:

- Total cholesterol
- Low-density lipoprotein (LDL) cholesterol

TABLE 12-3   Normal Reference Ranges for Laboratory Blood Tests

Blood Test	Reference Range	Blood Test	Reference Range
Hematological Studies		Blood gases	
Red blood cell count		pH	7.35–7.45
Men	$4.6–6.2 \times 10^6$	PaO_2	80–105 mm Hg
Women	$4.2–5.4 \times 10^6$	$PaCO_2$	35–45 mm Hg
Hematocrit		Bicarbonate	22–29 mEq/L
Men	40%–50%	Base excess, deficit	0 ± 2.3 mEq/L
Women	38%–47%	SaO_2	98%
Hemoglobin		$Sv–CO_2$	75%
Men	13.5–18.0 g/100 mL	**Bilirubin**	
Women	12.0–16.0 g/100 mL	Total	0.2–1.3 mg/dL
Corpuscle indices		Direct	0–20 mg/dL
Mean corpuscular volume	82–98 FL	**Calcium**	
Mean corpuscular hemoglobin	27–31 pg	Total	8.9–10.3 mg/dL
Mean corpuscular hemoglobin concentration	32%–36%	Free (ionized)	4.6–5.1 mg/dL
White blood cell count		**Creatinine**	
Total	4,500–11,000/mm³	Men	0.9–1.4 mg/dL
Differential (in number of cells/mm³ blood)		Women	0.8–1.3 mg/dL
Total leukocytes	5,000–10,000 (100%)	**Electrolytes**	
Total neutrophils	3,000–7,000 (60%–70%)	Glucose (fasting)	65–110 mg/dL
Lymphocytes	1,500–3,000 (20%–30%)	Magnesium	1.3–2.2 mEq/L
Monocytes	375–500 (2%–6%)	Phosphorus	2.5–4.5 mg/dL
Eosinophils	50–400 (1%–4%)	Phosphatase, alkaline	35–148 U
Basophils	0–50 (0.1%)	Protein (total)	6.5–8.5 g/dL
Sedimentation rate	0–30 mm/h	Urea nitrogen	8–26 mg/dL
*Coagulation Studies**		**Uric acid**	65–110 mg/dL
Platelet count	250,000–500,000/mm³	Men	4.0–8.5 mg/dL
Prothrombin time	12–15 s	Women	2.8–7.5 mg/dL
Partial thromboplastin time	60–70 s		
Activated partial thromboplastin time	35–45 s		
Activated clotting time	75–105 s		
Fibrinogen level	160–300 mg/dL		
Thrombin time	11.3–18.5 s		
Blood Chemistries			
Serum electrolytes			
Sodium	135–145 mEq/L		
Potassium	3.3–4.9 mEq/L		
Chloride	97–110 mEq/L		
Carbon dioxide	22–31 mEq/L		

* Example only; regional laboratory techniques and methods may result in variations.

TABLE 12-4 Serum Cholesterol Levels

Cholesterol Level (mg/dL)	Description
LDL	
Less than 100 (less than 70 in very high risk patients)	Optimal
100–129	Near or above optimal
130–159	Borderline high
160–189	High
Greater than or equal to 190	Very High
Total Cholesterol	
Less than 200	Desirable
200–239	Borderline high
Greater than or equal to 240 mg/dL	High
High-Density Lipoprotein	
Less than 40	Low
Greater than 60	High (desirable)
Serum Triglycerides	
Less than 150	Normal
150–199	Borderline high
240–499	High
Greater than or equal to 500	Very high

From the Third Report of the NCEP on detection, evaluation and treatment of high blood cholesterol in adults (ATP III). Circulation 106:3143–3421, 2002.

- Very–low-density lipoprotein (VLDL) cholesterol
- High-density lipoprotein (HDL) cholesterol
- Triglycerides

Because HDL cholesterol has a protective effect, higher levels of HDL cholesterol lower risk for CAD. However, the risk for CAD increases as the ratio of total cholesterol to HDL cholesterol increases, or as the ratio of LDL cholesterol to HDL cholesterol increases. Interpretation of serum cholesterol levels is summarized in Table 12-4.

RED FLAG! Patients who present with a suspected or confirmed acute cardiovascular or coronary event should have a lipid panel sent to a laboratory within 24 hours of presentation.

Biochemical Markers

Cardiac Enzymes

Cardiac enzymes, normally found in cardiac tissue, are released into the serum after cardiac injury. Elevation of one or more of these enzymes is not a specific indicator of cardiac injury. However, because cardiac damage does result in above-normal serum concentrations of these enzymes, quantification of cardiac enzyme levels, along with other diagnostic tests and the patient's clinical presentation, is routinely used for diagnosing cardiac disease, particularly acute myocardial infarction.

Creatine kinase (CK) is an enzyme found in heart muscle, skeletal muscle, and brain tissue. Myocardial infarction can cause elevations of serum CK levels, as can many other cardiac and noncardiac causes (Box 12-5). When assessing CK values, it is important to remember that they vary depending on the patient's muscle mass. Patients with low muscle mass have less ability to release CK into the bloodstream than do patients with high muscle mass.

Serum CK values begin rising 4 to 6 hours after the onset of myocardial necrosis, typically peak at 18 to 24 hours, and return to baseline at 36 to 40 hours. To rule out myocardial infarction, samples are commonly drawn every 8 hours for 24 hours. The noncardiac release of CK generally produces elevations that appear and disappear more slowly than those seen with myocardial necrosis.

Currently, obtaining serial measurements of total CK as an isolated marker is not recommended to diagnose acute myocardial infarction.[1,2] However, total CK remains a relevant test because it provides the basis for calculating levels of more specific CK isoenzymes: CK-MB (heart muscle), CK-MM (skeletal muscle), and CK-BB (brain). Total CK usually consists entirely of CK-MM, and neither CK-BB nor CK-MB is present. An increase in the total CK level and a percentage of CK-MB greater than 5% is generally considered diagnostic for myocardial damage.

BOX 12-5 Cardiac and Noncardiac Causes of Elevated Serum Creatine Kinase (CK)

Cardiac Causes
- Myocardial infarction
- Pericarditis
- Myocarditis
- Cardioversion
- Defibrillation
- Prolonged supraventricular tachycardia (SVT)
- Myositis
- Reperfusion therapy with thrombolytics
- Coronary angioplasty
- Cardiac surgery

Noncardiac Causes
- Musculoskeletal disorders (eg, polymyositis, muscular dystrophy)
- Trauma
- Surgery
- Strenuous exercise
- Seizure activity
- Cerebrovascular insults
- Heavy alcohol intake
- Intramuscular injections
- Acute cholecystitis
- Gastrointestinal or urological insults
- Hypothyroidism
- Collagen disorders

BOX 12-6 Cardiac and Noncardiac Causes of Elevated Troponin Levels

Cardiac Causes
- Myocardial infarction
- Myocardial ischemia
- Heart failure
- Myocarditis
- Myocardial contusion
- Supraventricular tachycardias (SVTs)
- Left ventricular hypertrophy

Noncardiac Causes
- Sepsis and systemic inflammatory response syndrome (SIRS)
- Hypovolemia
- Pulmonary embolism
- Acute stroke
- Renal failure
- Chronic obstructive pulmonary disease (COPD)
- Pulmonary hypertension

Myocardial Proteins

Myoglobin and troponin are proteins that are bound within cardiac muscle. Myoglobin appears in the serum less than 1 hour after the onset of symptoms of myocardial infarction, making it ideal for early detection of myocardial necrosis. An elevated serum myoglobin level 4 to 8 hours after the onset of symptoms in the absence of ECG changes consistent with myocardial infarction is not reliable for diagnosing myocardial infarction because other disorders can also increase myoglobin levels. However, because of the high sensitivity of myoglobin, a negative test in the first 4 to 8 hours after the onset of symptoms is useful for ruling out myocardial necrosis.

Troponins are released into the circulation after necrosis and rupture of myocardial cells. An increase in troponin levels is detected within 4 to 6 hours of myocardial necrosis. Levels generally peak 24 hours after the onset of symptoms and remain elevated for up to 10 days after the cardiac event. In addition to myocardial infarction, other cardiac and noncardiac conditions can be associated with elevated troponin levels (Box 12-6). In critical care patients, elevated troponin levels signify a worse overall outcome.

Three troponin subforms have been identified:

- Cardiac troponin-I (cTnI)
- Cardiac troponin-T (cTnT)
- Cardiac troponin-C (cTnC)

Both cTnI and cTnT are highly specific to cardiac tissue and have equal sensitivity and specificity in detecting myocardial necrosis. As a result, the use of cTnI or cTnT is recommended for the diagnosis of myocardial infarction.[1,2] Because a quantitative relationship exists between the level of cTnI or cTnT detected and the risk for death in patients with myocardial infarction, troponin elevations are also important prognostic indicators that may guide treatment and follow-up.

Brain-Type Natriuretic Peptide

Natriuretic peptides are neurohumoral hormones released by the heart when the cardiac muscle decompensates. Atrial natriuretic peptides are secreted as a result of atrial myocardial distention, but only minute amounts are released in response to ventricular distention. Brain-type natriuretic peptide (BNP) is released primarily from the cardiac ventricles, in response to ventricular dilation and increased intraventricular pressures. As a result, BNP levels are helpful in diagnosing ventricular dysfunction caused by heart failure, particularly in emergency department settings. BNP levels also provide important prognostic information for patients with acute coronary syndromes (eg, myocardial infarction, unstable angina) and patients with heart failure. In these patients, elevated BNP levels are predictive of a greater risk for death, postinfarction heart failure, or reinfarction.[3]

C-Reactive Protein

C-reactive protein (CRP), a marker for inflammation and necrosis, has been shown to be elevated in patients with acute coronary syndromes. A blood test called highly sensitive C-reactive protein (hs-CRP) can be used to determine the risk for heart disease:

• Less than 1.0 mg/dL, low risk
• 1.0 to 3.0 mg/dL, moderate risk
• Greater than 3.0 mg/dL, high risk

Patients with acute coronary syndromes and serum values greater than 3 mg/dL (or greater than 5 mg/dL after a coronary interventional procedure) are at higher risk and merit closer monitoring or more thorough evaluation.[4]

D-Dimer

D-Dimer represents the end product of fibrin dissolution that occurs at the site of a thrombus. Although D-dimer can be elevated in myocardial infarction and heart failure, it is being used more commonly to detect thromboembolic events such as deep venous thrombosis (DVT) and pulmonary embolism.[5]

Cardiac Diagnostic Studies

The number of cardiovascular diagnostic techniques continues to increase, especially in the area of non-invasive testing. Diagnostic studies are used to:

• Obtain a functional assessment of the patient's cardiac status so that the best treatment option can be selected
• Screen before high-risk procedures
• Monitor disease progression and response to treatment

Table 12-5 summarizes information about some of the most commonly used tests. Patients undergoing invasive cardiac studies (eg, cardiac catheterization and related procedures) require careful preprocedure evaluation and postprocedure care and monitoring. Box 12-7 on page 156 presents nursing considerations for the patient undergoing cardiac catheterization.

TABLE 12-5   Cardiac Diagnostic Studies

Test and Purpose	Method of Testing	Nursing Implications
Standard 12-lead electocardiogram (ECG)		
Used to assess dysrhythmias and myocardial ischemia or infarction	Electrodes applied to the patient's chest and limbs record electrical impulses as they travel through heart, producing 12 different views of the heart's electrical activity	• Optimal skin preparation and electrode placement are critical to obtaining high-quality readings • Important patient remains still to prevent artifact
Holter (24-hour) monitoring		
Used to quantify frequency and complexity of cardiac ectopic activity during patient's usual activities	Electrodes applied to the patient's chest are connected to a portable recording device that records the electrical activity of the heart continuously for 24 to 48 h	• The nurse instructs the patient to maintain normal activities and keep a diary to record medications, activities, and symptoms during the monitoring period • Bathing is prohibited while the electrodes are in place
Chest radiography		
Used to evaluate heart size, pulmonary congestion, effusions, and position of medical devices (eg, transvenous pacemaker electrodes, pulmonary artery catheters)	X-rays pass through the chest wall making it possible to visualize structures	• May be performed at the bedside • Patient may be asked to take a deep breath and hold it while the radiograph is taken to displace the diaphragm downward
Transthoracic echocardiography		
Used to assess ejection fraction, wall motion and thickness, valve function and disease, and blood flow through the chambers and valves of the heart	A transducer emits ultrasound waves and receives a signal from the reflected sound waves to produce an image	• Patient must be able to tolerate lying flat or nearly flat and must be able to turn onto the left side for several minutes at a time

(continued on page 154)

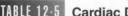 **Cardiac Diagnostic Studies** (continued)

Test and Purpose	Method of Testing	Nursing Implications
Transesophageal echocardiography (TEE)		
Used to obtain high-quality images of cardiac structures	A 2D transducer on the end of a flexible endoscope is passed through the esophagus	• Patient must be NPO for 6 h prior to study and until gag reflex returns after the study • Administer IV sedation as necessary • Monitor for risks include esophageal perforation; dyspnea, hemoptysis, or severe pain which must be reported immediately
Stress testing		
Used to assess prognosis and determine functional capacity in patients with ischemic heart disease	Physiologic parameters (eg, heart rate and ECG) are monitored while the heart is in a resting state and then again when the heart is stressed either by exercise or by a pharmacological agent that simulates exercise	• Caffeine, β-blockers, and digoxin are withheld on day of test • The nurse advises patient that when pharmacologic agents are used in place of exercise, side effects such as flushing, headache, and nausea may occur
Radionuclide cardiac imaging (positron emission tomography [PET], single-photon emission computed tomography [SPECT])		
Often used in conjunction with stress testing to evaluate myocardial perfusion and viability	Cameras capture the photons emitted by infused radiotracers to provide information on the magnitude and location of uptake	• Patient must be NPO for 6 h prior to study • Caffeine must be restricted for 24 h prior to the procedure • Serious side effects from the radiotracer are rare but medications to counteract these side effects should be readily available
Computed tomography (CT)		
Used to obtain detailed two- or three-dimensional views of the heart and surrounding structures	X-rays pass through the body while a detector gathers and records images generated by the beams	• Assess for history of allergies to IV contrast dye (if contrast is to be given)
Magnetic resonance imaging (MRI)		
Used for high-resolution assessment of cardiovascular anatomy, function, blood flow, metabolism, and perfusion	A magnetic field is used to obtain images	• The patient must be able to lie flat, hold his breath for periods of time, and tolerate confinement in the scanner • Metal in the body (eg, non-MRI-compatible aneurysm clips, implanted pacemakers and defibrillators) is a contraindication to MRI
Cardiac catheterization		
Used to evaluate the structure and fuction of the aorta, coronary arteries, valves, and chambers of the heart, and to measure pressures within the chambers and vessels of the heart	A catheter is introduced through the femoral or brachial artery and threaded into the chambers and vessels of the heart to facilitate various diagnostic procedures	• Preprocedure evaluation includes screening for contrast media allergy and obtaining laboratory studies, including complete blood count, prothrombin and partial thromboplastin time, International Normalized Ratio (INR), and chemistry panel • Patient must be NPO for 6 h prior to study

TABLE 12-5 **Cardiac Diagnostic Studies** (continued)

Test and Purpose	Method of Testing	Nursing Implications
Cardiac catheterization		• Risks include bleeding at the entry site, dissection of any of the vessels traversed during the procedure, perforation of peripheral or coronary arteries, irritation of cardiac tissue, plaque embolization leading to myocardial infarction or stroke, and allergic reactions or renal compromise resulting from the use of contrast media • Check distal extremity for pulse, capillary refill and sensorium • Remind patient to lie flat for 4-6 h per institutional protocol • Check site frequently for hematoma or bleeding
Left heart catheterization Used to delineate baseline coronary anatomy and identify abnormalities of the coronary vessels, great vessels, and cardiac chambers; also used to obtain the left ventricular ejection fraction and information regarding wall motion abnormalities and left ventricular size	A catheter is introduced through the brachial or femoral artery and passed through the aorta and aortic valve into the left ventricle	• Same as for cardiac catheterization
Right heart catheterization Used to sample oxygen saturations and pressures in the right atrium and ventricle, pulmonary capillary bed, and pulmonary artery	A catheter is introduced through the inferior jugular vein to the superior vena cava	• Postprocedure restrictions are minimal because a vein is accessed and the risk for bleeding is low • Self-limiting dysrhythmias may occur as a result of stimulation of the myocardium
Electrophysiology study Used during cardiac catheterization to evaluate a broad spectrum of cardiac dysrhythmias	Electrode catheters are introduced into the chambers of the heart, where they are used to record the electrical activity of the heart and also to induce dysrhythmias for study	• Same as for cardiac catheterization
Coronary angiography Used during cardiac catheterization to obtain information regarding the lumen and wall structure of the coronary arteries	Radiographic contrast is injected into the chambers of the heart and the coronary arteries under fluoroscopic guidance and x-ray images are obtained	• Same as for cardiac catheterization
Intravascular ultrasound Used during cardiac catheterization to visualize the inside of the coronary arteries	An ultrasound probe is attached to the end of the cardiac catheterization catheter	• Same as for cardiac catheterization

BOX 12-7 Nursing Interventions for the Patient Undergoing Cardiac Catheterization

Preprocedure
- Explain the procedure to the patient and family.
- Verify that the patient has taken nothing by mouth for at least 6 hours before the procedure except prescribed medications as advised by the physician.
- Ensure that ordered preoperative laboratory studies have been completed and results are available.
- Verify the patient's identity and identify allergy information; alert physician if patient is allergic to radiographic dye, medications, or specific foods.
- Ensure that informed consent has been obtained.
- Establish IV access per facility protocol or physician order.
- Place the patient on cardiac monitoring system with blood pressure and pulse oximetry monitoring.
- Provide supplemental oxygen as ordered or indicated.
- Premedicate the patient per physician order.
- Obtain vital signs before transfer to catheterization laboratory.

During Procedure
- Continually assess the patient's vital signs, oxygenation, level of consciousness, and cardiac rhythm per institutional protocol, and alert the physician of any significant changes or the development of malignant cardiac dysrhythmias (eg, premature ventricular contractions, ventricular tachycardia, ventricular fibrillation).
- Be prepared to initiate cardiac resuscitation with emergency equipment and medications.

Postprocedure
- Ensure that the patient's vital signs are stable before transfer.
- Check catheterization site dressing for bleeding and integrity.
- Check distal pulses below catheterization site; if femoral site was used, check distal pulse, extremity color, capillary refill, and neurosensory status.
- Keep extremity straight and instruct the patient not to bend the leg or arm.
- Maintain IV infusion per physician order or facility protocol.
- Maintain supplemental oxygenation support as ordered or indicated.
- Encourage oral fluids as ordered.
- Check the patient's coagulation status per facility protocol before sheath removal.
- When catheter is removed:
  o Apply direct pressure over site for 20 to 30 minutes to prevent bleeding, or apply commercial hemostatic compression device per facility protocol.
  o Check distal extremity for pulse, color, capillary refill, and sensorium.
  o Remind the patient to lie flat for 4 to 6 hours per facility protocol.
  o Check the site dressing every 4 to 6 hours for bleeding and integrity.

CASE STUDY

Ms. K., a 68-year-old woman, is admitted to the critical care unit following an acute syncopal episode. In the ED, she reported "heaviness" in her chest and was observed to be dyspneic. Auscultation revealed an S_4. Nonspecific changes were noted on ECG, and serial cardiac enzymes remained normal. Mrs. K. was placed on supplemental oxygen with ongoing monitoring of her oxygenation status. Ms. K. has a history of tobacco smoking for 20 years (2 packs/d), but has not smoked in the last 5 years. She also has a history of hypertension and has been taking a calcium channel blocker for the last 2 years.

On the basis of Ms. K.'s symptoms and history, the physician orders a cardiac catheter procedure to assess Ms. K.'s cardiac function and the patency of her coronary arteries. During the procedure, the interventional cardiologist notes an 85% obstruction of the left anterior descending coronary artery and performs angioplasty (balloon inflation) and stent placement. The femoral catheter is removed and pressure is held according to facility protocol. Ms. K. is then transferred back to the critical care unit.

1. What are the nursing interventions to prepare Ms. K. for cardiac catheterization?

2. What nursing care will Ms. K. require following the procedure?

References

1. Antman EM, Anbe DT, Armstrong PW, et al.: ACC/AHA guidelines for the management of patients with ST-elevation myocardial infarction. Update 2007
2. ACC/AHA Guidelines for the Management of Patients with Unstable Angina/non-ST Segment Myocardial Infarction: A report of the ACC/AHA Task Force on Practice Guidelines. Circulation 116:803–807, 2007
3. Pfisterer M: BNP-guided vs symptom guided heart failure therapy. JAMA 301(4):383–392, 2009
4. Sabatine MS, Morrow DA, Jablonski KA, et al.: Prognostic significance of the Centers for Disease Control/American Heart Association high-sensitivity C-reactive protein cut points for cardiovascular and other outcomes in patients with stable coronary artery disease. Circulation 115:1528, 2007
5. Qaseem A, et al.: Diagnosis of venous thromboembolism: Guidelines from ACP-AAFP test characteristics of D-dimer assays alone diagnosis of VTE. Ann Fam Med 5(1):57–62, 2007

Want to know more? A wide variety of resources to enhance your learning and understanding of this chapter are available on thePoint. Visit http://thepoint.lww.com/MortonEss1e to access chapter review questions and more!

Patient Management: Cardiovascular System

OBJECTIVES

Based on the content in this chapter, the reader should be able to:

1 Describe nursing considerations specific to the major classes of drugs used to treat cardiovascular disorders.
2 Describe various surgical interventions for cardiac disease and the critical care nurse's role in caring for a patient undergoing cardiac surgery.
3 Describe various percutaneous coronary intervention (PCI) techniques and the critical care nurse's role in caring for a patient undergoing PCI.
4 Describe nursing interventions for a patient receiving intraaortic balloon pump (IABP) therapy or ventricular circulatory assistance.

Pharmacotherapy

Many medications, alone and in combination, are commonly used in critical care settings to treat cardiovascular disease. Critical care nurses are responsible for preparing and administering these medications, as well as evaluating their effects and using detailed patient assessment data to guide titration of doses. Many patients require treatment with multiple cardiovascular medications, so the nurse must also consider potential drug interactions.

Fibrinolytics, Anticoagulants, and Platelet Inhibitors

An arterial thrombus may transiently or persistently occlude coronary artery blood flow, causing acute coronary syndrome (ACS). Fibrinolytic, anticoagulant, and platelet inhibitor drugs affect different phases of the thrombotic process.

Fibrinolytics

Fibrinolytics either directly or indirectly convert plasminogen to plasmin, which causes the degradation of fibrin and fibrinogen, resulting in clot lysis. In patients with myocardial infarction, early fibrinolytic therapy has been shown to dissolve the thrombus, reestablish coronary blood flow, minimize infarct size, preserve left ventricular function, and reduce morbidity and mortality. Researchers continue to evaluate the efficacy of fibrinolytic agents in conjunction with other medications such as glycoprotein (GP) IIb/IIIa inhibitors, direct thrombin inhibitors, and low-molecular-weight heparins (LMWHs). Because patients are at risk for recurrent thromboembolism, aspirin and heparin are given to most patients who receive fibrinolytic therapy. The most common adverse effects of fibrinolytic therapy are bleeding, intracranial hemorrhage, and reperfusion dysrhythmias. Contraindications to fibrinolytic therapy are given in Box 13-1.

- Active internal bleeding
- History of recent intracranial hemorrhage
- Ischemic stroke within 3 months (except current ischemic stroke)
- Intracranial neoplasm, arteriovenous malformation (AVM), or aneurysm
- Recent intracranial or intraspinal surgery
- Closed-head or facial trauma within 3 months
- Suspected aortic dissection
- Severe uncontrolled hypertension
- A predisposition to abnormal hemostasis and hemorrhage (ie, bleeding diathesis)
- Abnormal coagulation studies

Anticoagulants

Anticoagulants such as unfractionated heparin, LMWHs (fractionated heparins), direct thrombin inhibitors, and warfarin prevent thrombus formation. These agents do not lyse existing thrombi; rather, they prevent additional thrombi from forming.

Unfractionated Heparin

Unfractionated heparin prevents clot formation by combining with antithrombin III (a naturally occurring anticoagulant in the blood) and inhibiting the conversion of prothrombin to thrombin. Unfractionated heparin is commonly used for acute conditions (eg, ACS) and for patients undergoing percutaneous coronary intervention (PCI) procedures or surgical revascularization. However, several factors limit the clinical utility of unfractionated heparin:

- It has a narrow therapeutic range, low bioavailability, and variable anticoagulant response.
- It must be administered parenterally.
- Activated partial thromboplastin time (APTT) monitoring is required.
- Associated risks include bleeding, heparin-induced thrombocytopenia (HIT), and hypersensitivity reactions.

Protamine sulfate reverses the effects of heparin; however, protamine may cause a life-threatening anaphylactic reaction.

Low-Molecular-Weight Heparins

LMWHs are small fragments derived from unfractionated heparin. These drugs inhibit clot formation by blocking factor Xa (which converts prothrombin to thrombin). Advantages of LMWHs over unfractionated heparin include their longer half-life, more predictable anticoagulation effect, greater bioavailability, cost-effectiveness, and lower bleeding risk. In addition, LMWHs are administered subcutaneously once to twice daily and do not require anticoagulation monitoring. The most common adverse effects of LMWHs include bleeding, thrombocytopenia,

elevated aminotransferase levels, and pain, erythema, ecchymosis, or hematoma at the injection site. LMWHs may be used instead of heparin for patients with unstable angina, acute non–ST-segment elevation myocardial infarction (NSTEMI), or deep venous thrombosis (DVT).

Direct Thrombin Inhibitors

Direct thrombin inhibitors interact directly with thrombin, preventing thrombin from converting fibrinogen to fibrin. Like LMWHs, these agents are administered by injection. However, therapeutic drug monitoring is difficult and there is no antidote available. Direct thrombin inhibitors may be administered as alternatives to unfractionated heparin in low-risk patients who undergo PCI procedures or patients with HIT.[1]

Warfarin

Warfarin, an oral drug used for chronic anticoagulation therapy, interferes with the synthesis of vitamin K–dependent clotting factors such as factors II, VII, IX, and X. The most common cardiovascular indications for warfarin include dilated cardiomyopathy, atrial fibrillation, heart failure, venous thromboembolism, valve replacement with a prosthetic heart valve, and post–acute myocardial infarction anticoagulation for high-risk patients. The dose is titrated according to the patient's international normalized ratio (INR). Because warfarin levels do not peak for 3 to 4 days, acute anticoagulant therapy is continued until the INR reaches the desired level for the patient's condition (usually 2.5 to 3.5). The INR is evaluated daily until the therapeutic level is achieved. Elevated INR levels predispose the patient to bleeding, warfarin's most common adverse effect. Contraindications to warfarin are given in Box 13-2.

 RED FLAG! *Warfarin doses are decreased for elderly patients and patients with liver or renal impairment and heart failure.*

- Uncontrolled hypertension
- Severe hepatic or renal disease
- A predisposition to abnormal hemostasis and hemorrhage (ie, bleeding diathesis)
- Gastrointestinal or genitourinary bleeding
- Cerebral or dissecting aortic aneurysm
- Recent central nervous system, eye, or other major surgery
- Recent trauma
- Pregnancy (first and third trimesters)
- Pericarditis
- Pericardial effusion
- Spinal puncture
- Recent diagnostic procedures with the potential for uncontrolled bleeding

Platelet Inhibitors

Aspirin

Aspirin, the most widely used platelet inhibitor, inhibits thromboxane A_2 (a platelet agonist) to prevent platelet aggregation, thrombus formation and arterial vasoconstriction. Aspirin is used to decrease mortality for patients with acute myocardial infarction; to reduce the incidence of nonfatal acute myocardial infarction and mortality for patients with stable angina, unstable angina, or previous myocardial infarction; to prevent graft closure after coronary artery bypass graft (CABG) surgery; and to prevent coronary artery thrombus after PCI. Adverse effects of aspirin include stomach pain, nausea, vomiting, gastrointestinal bleeding, subdural or intracranial hemorrhage, thrombocytopenia, coagulopathy, and a prolonged prothrombin time (PT). Patients with a history of aspirin intolerance, gastrointestinal or genitourinary bleeding, peptic ulcers, severe renal or hepatic insufficiency, or bleeding disorders should not take aspirin.

Adenosine Diphosphate Receptor Antagonists

Adenosine diphosphate receptor antagonists, such as clopidogrel (Plavix), prevent adenosine diphosphate–induced platelet activation and platelet aggregation, resulting in an irreversible inhibition of platelet function. The effects of clopidogrel begin within 2 to 3 hours, steady-state platelet inhibition is achieved after 3 to 7 days of therapy. Once clopidogrel is discontinued, bleeding times and platelet function normalize within 3 to 7 days. Major adverse effects include bleeding disorders, gastrointestinal upset, thrombotic thrombocytopenic purpura (TTP), and neutropenia.

Glycoprotein (GP) IIb/IIIa Inhibitors

GP IIb/IIIa inhibitors inhibit the GP IIb/IIIa receptor (the final common pathway for platelet aggregation) thus preventing platelet aggregation which inhibits thrombus formation. GP IIb/IIIa inhibitors are recommended for patients with ACS or NSTEMI who undergo PCI procedures, and prior to PCI for patients with ST-segment elevation myocardial infarction (STEMI).[2] These agents are administered in conjunction with either an LMWH or unfractionated heparin. Adverse effects include bleeding, thrombocytopenia, stroke, and allergic reactions.

Inotropes

Inotropes increase the force of myocardial contraction by acting on adrenergic receptors in the sympathetic nervous system (Table 13-1). This, in turn, increases stroke volume, cardiac output, blood pressure, and coronary artery perfusion. These drugs are commonly given to patients with ventricular dysfunction or cardiogenic shock. However, as contractility and heart rate increase, myocardial oxygen demand also increases, and myocardial ischemia can worsen. The nurse must closely monitor the patient for evidence of ischemia, angina, and dysrhythmias. Commonly used inotropes are summarized in Table 13-2.

Antidysrhythmics

Antidysrythmics (also discussed in Chapter 8) include class I sodium channel blockers, class II β-adrenergic blockers, class III potassium channel blockers, class IV calcium channel blockers, adenosine, magnesium sulfate, atropine, and digoxin. These agents are used to restore the heart to a regular rhythm. The action of these drugs is complex; drugs within the same class can work differently, and actions of those in different classes may overlap. The therapeutic window is small, and caution must be used to prevent complications.

β-Adrenergic Blockers

β-Adrenergic blockers interfere with sympathetic nervous system stimulation, contributing to decreased heart rate, depressed atrioventricular (AV) node conduction, decreased contractility, and decreased myocardial oxygen demand. β-Adrenergic agents are used in the treatment of dysrhythmias, heart failure, and hypertension.

These agents may be classified as cardioselective (inhibiting β_1 receptors) or nonselective (inhibiting β_1 and β_2 receptors). Nonselective agents affect bronchial and vascular smooth muscle, leading to bronchoconstriction and vasoconstriction. Although cardioselective β-adrenergic agents are sometimes used with caution in patients with pulmonary disease, in general, severe asthma, bronchospasm, and severe

TABLE 13-1 Adrenergic Receptors Affecting Cardiovascular Function

Receptor	Location	Effects of Stimulation
β_1	Heart	Positive inotropic (increased contractility) and chronotropic action (increases rate)
β_2	Bronchial smooth muscle	Bronchodilation
	Vascular smooth muscle	Vasodilation
	AV node	Positive dromotropic action (increased conduction velocity)
α_1	Vascular smooth muscle	Vasoconstriction
	Heart	Weak positive inotropic and chronotropic actions
α_2	Presynaptic sympathetic nerve endings	Inhibition of norepinephrine release
Dopaminergic	Kidney and splanchnic vessels	Renal and splanchnic vessel vasodilation

TABLE 13-2 **Commonly Used Inotropes**

Drug	Indications	Mechanism of Action	Adverse Effects
Dopamine	Conditions characterized by hypotension, decreased cardiac output, and oliguria	Stimulates dopaminergic, β-adrenergic, and α-adrenergic receptors • Low doses (eg, 3–10 µg/kg/min) increase myocardial contractility • Higher doses cause vasoconstriction and increased blood pressure	Tachycardia, palpitations, and dysrhythmias Headache Nausea and vomiting Hypertension
Dobutamine	Conditions that cause poor cardiac contractility or low cardiac output (eg, heart failure, shock)	Stimulates β_1 receptors to increase myocardial contractility	Tachycardia and dysrhythmias Headache Nausea Blood pressure fluctuations
Epinephrine	Cardiac arrest; symptomatic bradycardia; severe hypotension; anaphylaxis; shock	Stimulates α_1, β_1, and β_2 receptors • Low doses (eg, 1–2 µg/min) act on the β receptors to increase cardiac output by increasing heart rate and myocardial contractility • Higher doses act on the α_1 receptors to cause profound vasoconstriction, increased blood pressure and SVR, and decreased renal and spanchic perfusion	Tachycardia and dysrhythmias Cerebral hemorrhage Pulmonary edema Myocardial ischemia and angina Headache, dizziness, and nervousness
Vasopressin	Ventricular fibrillation; asystole; pulseless electrical activity	Promotes smooth muscle contraction to increase peripheral vascular resistance	Dysrhythmias Myocardial ischemia or infarction and angina Tremors and vertigo Water intoxication Sweating
Isoproterenol	Conditions characterized by a decreased heart rate (eg, cardiac transplantation; refractory torsades de pointes; β-blocker overdose; symptomatic bradycardia in absence of external pacemaker)	Stimulates β_1 and β_2 receptors to increase myocardial activity, cardiac output, heart rate, blood pressure	Tachycardia, palpitations, and dysrhythmias Myocardial ischemia Pulmonary edema and bronchospasm Hypotension Vomiting Sweating
Norepinephrine	Cardiogenic shock; significant hypotension with low SVR (eg, septic shock)	Stimulates α receptors to cause peripheral vasoconstriction and increase blood pressure and SVR	Tachycardia, bradycardia, and dysrhythmias Hypertension Tissue necrosis from extravasation Headache

chronic obstructive pulmonary disease (COPD) are contraindications for the use of β-adrenergic blockers. Other contraindications include cardiogenic shock, severe left ventricular failure, bradycardia, and second- or third-degree heart block.

 RED FLAG! *Cardioselective β-adrenergic blockers lose their selectivity at higher doses.*

Calcium Channel Blockers

Calcium channel blockers prevent the movement of calcium into cells, slowing conduction through the sinoatrial (SA) and AV nodes in the myocardium. These agents also have anticoagulant, negative inotropic, and peripheral vasodilation effects. In addition to dysrhythmias, calcium channel blockers are used to treat diastolic dysfunction heart failure and hypertension. Adverse effects include hypotension, systolic heart failure, and AV block, bradycardia, headache, dizziness, peripheral edema, nausea, constipation, and flushing. Contraindications include hypotension, heart failure, and severe aortic stenosis.

Digoxin

Digoxin, a mild positive inotrope frequently used in the treatment of heart failure, works by inhibiting the sodium–potassium pump, causing intracellular sodium levels to increase. This promotes calcium influx and enhanced myocardial contractility. Digoxin also activates the parasympathetic system, decreasing heart rate and increasing AV node inhibition.

Most patients benefit from a low dose, which also reduces the incidence of toxicity. Toxicity is common and is frequently associated with severe dysrhythmias. It is no longer common practice to administer loading doses. Routine doses are individualized based on the patient's diagnosis, symptoms, underlying disease processes, age, response to therapy, and blood levels. Blood levels of 0.5 to 1.0 ng/mL are recommended for patients with heart failure, and levels of 0.8 to 2 ng/mL for those with dysrhythmias. Electrolyte imbalances (eg, hypokalemia, hypomagnesemia) and concurrent therapy with other medications used to treat cardiovascular disorders (eg, β-adrenergic blockers, calcium channel blockers) can increase the risk for digitalis toxicity.

 RED FLAG! *Signs and symptoms of digitalis toxicity include palpitations, dysrhythmias, gastrointestinal upset (eg, anorexia, nausea, vomiting, diarrhea), fatigue, insomnia, confusion, headache, depression, vertigo, syncope, facial pain, and visual disturbances.*

Phosphodiesterase III Inhibitors

Phosphodiesterase III inhibitors are used in the treatment of severe heart failure that is refractory to other drugs, and for short-term treatment of acute heart failure. These agents increase contractility, venous vasodilation, and peripheral arterial vasodilation by inhibiting an enzyme that breaks down cyclic adenosine monophosphate (cAMP). Phosphodiesterase III inhibitors reduce ventricular filling pressures and tend to decrease arterial pressure; however, they minimally affect heart rate. Typically, an IV bolus dose is administered, followed by an IV maintenance infusion that is titrated to effect. Adverse effects include hypotension, dysrhythmias, and thrombocytopenia.

Vasodilators

Vasodilators decrease preload, afterload, or both.

Nitrates

Nitrates have several actions. They

- Cause venous dilation, which decreases venous return to the heart and reduces preload
- Cause arterial vasodilation (at high doses), which reduces afterload
- Promote coronary artery vasodilation, improve collateral blood flow, and reduce platelet aggregation, enhancing myocardial perfusion, and decreasing myocardial oxygen demand
- Reduce blood pressure and elevated pulmonary vascular resistance, systemic vascular resistance (SVR), central venous pressure (CVP), and pulmonary artery occlusion pressure (PAOP)

Nitrates are used to treat acute angina, and angina that is unresponsive to other therapies. They are also indicated for the treatment of large anterior acute myocardial infarction and myocardial infarction associated with acute or chronic heart failure, acute pulmonary edema, persistent ischemia, or hypertension.

Nitrates may be administered intravenously, sublingually, or topically. Contraindications to IV nitrates include hypotension, uncorrected hypovolemia, hypertrophic obstructive cardiomyopathy, and pericardial tamponade.

Adverse effects of nitrates include headache, hypotension, syncope, and tachycardia. Tolerance may develop to the antianginal, hemodynamic, and antiplatelet effects of nitrates, especially with continuous or high-dose therapy; however, dosing regimens that allow for nitrate-free intervals may prevent this occurrence.

Nitroprusside Sodium

Nitroprusside (Nitropress) is a potent arterial and venous vasodilator that decreases SVR and increases cardiac output. Uses include the treatment of severe left ventricular heart failure, hypertension after CABG surgery, hypertensive crisis, and dissecting aneurysm. Adverse effects include hypotension, myocardial ischemia, nausea, vomiting, abdominal pain, and cyanide toxicity.

 RED FLAG! *The usual IV infusion dosage is 0.5 to 10 µg/kg/min; to prevent cyanide toxicity, the maximal dose should not be given for longer than 10 minutes. The dose is titrated to effect; if blood pressure does not respond after 10 minutes, the drug is discontinued.*

Because nitroprusside is sensitive to light, the infusion bag is covered with an opaque material to prevent degradation.

Nesiritide

Nesiritide (Natrecor), a recombinant form of human brain-type natriuretic peptide (BNP), is identical to the hormone produced by the left ventricle in response to volume overload and increased wall stress. A venous and arterial vasodilator, nesiritide reduces preload and afterload and increases cardiac output without increasing heart rate. Adverse effects include hypotension, bradycardia, ventricular dysrhythmias, angina, dizziness, and apnea. As a result of concerns about renal toxicity and increased mortality, clinical trials are being conducted to assess nesiritide's efficacy and safety.

Angiotensin-Converting Enzyme Inhibitors

Angiotensin-converting enzyme (ACE) inhibitors are used to treat heart failure, hypertension, acute myocardial infarction with or without left ventricular dysfunction or failure, and asymptomatic left ventricular dysfunction. They are also used to decrease morbidity and mortality for patients at high risk for acute myocardial infarction, stroke, or cardiovascular death. Unless contraindicated, patients with anterior acute myocardial infarction, pulmonary congestion, or a left ventricular ejection fraction of less than 40% should receive an ACE inhibitor within 24 hours.

ACE inhibitors block the conversion of angiotensin I to the potent vasoconstrictor angiotensin II, reduce aldosterone synthesis, and may promote fibrinolysis. As a result, these agents mitigate left ventricular remodeling, increase cardiac output, and decrease sodium retention, blood pressure, CVP, PAOP, SVR, and pulmonary vascular resistance.

Adverse effects of ACE inhibitors include hypotension, dizziness, angioedema, cough, headache, fatigue, nausea, vomiting, diarrhea, hyperkalemia, and renal function impairment. All ACE inhibitors are contraindicated in pregnant patients, and for those with angioedema, bilateral renal artery stenosis, or preexisting hypotension. In the presence of impaired renal function, hyperkalemia, or concurrent diuretic use, these agents must be used with caution; a lower dosage is required.

Antihyperlipidemics

The pharmacological management of hyperlipidemia decreases morbidity and mortality from coronary artery disease (CAD).[8,9] Desirable lipid levels are as follows:

- Total cholesterol less than 200 mg/dL
- Low-density lipoprotein (LDL) cholesterol less than 100 mg/dL (less than 70 mg/dL in very high-risk patients)
- High-density lipoprotein (HDL) cholesterol greater than 60 mg/dL
- Triglycerides less than 150 mg/dL

The primary target of antihyperlipidemic therapy is LDL cholesterol. Drug therapy with LDL-lowering drugs is recommended for patients who meet the following criteria:

- 0 to 1 risk factors for CAD (see Chapter 12, Box 12-3) and an LDL cholesterol level greater than or equal to 190 mg/dL
- 2 or more risk factors for CAD and an LDL cholesterol level greater than or equal to 130 mg/dL
- Documented CAD or CAD risk equivalents (eg, stroke, diabetes, peripheral artery disease) and an LDL cholesterol level greater than or equal to 100 mg/dL

Drug therapy may also be indicated when the triglyceride level is 200 mg/dL or greater, and for patients with borderline-high triglycerides (150 to 199 mg/dL) and CAD or CAD risk equivalents. For these patients, drugs to increase HDL cholesterol levels may be given.

There are five major classes of antihyperlipidemic drugs:

- Hydroxymethylglutaryl coenzyme-A (HMG-CoA) reductase inhibitors (statins) decrease total and LDL cholesterol, decrease triglycerides, and increase HDL cholesterol by inhibiting the rate-limiting enzyme that promotes cholesterol biosynthesis.
- Nicotinic acid inhibits lipolysis in adipose tissue and inhibits hepatic production of very-low-density lipoprotein (VLDL) cholesterol, thus decreasing total cholesterol, triglycerides, VLDL cholesterol, and LDL cholesterol, as well as increasing HDL cholesterol.
- The bile acid sequestrants bind bile acids in the intestine and form an insoluble complex that is excreted in the feces. Because bile acids are not absorbed, the liver is stimulated to manufacture more bile acids from cholesterol. This promotes movement of cholesterol out of the serum and into the liver, lowering serum total cholesterol and LDL cholesterol levels.
- The fibrates inhibit peripheral lipolysis and decrease the hepatic extraction of free fatty acids, which reduces triglyceride production. These agents decrease total cholesterol, triglycerides, and VLDL cholesterol, and they increase HDL cholesterol.
- Cholesterol absorption inhibitors selectively inhibit the intestinal absorption of cholesterol. They are used more effectively when combined with a statin to further reduce LDL cholesterol.

Cardiac Surgery

Surgical Interventions

Coronary Artery Bypass Graft Surgery

In coronary artery bypass graft (CABG) surgery, native vessels (conduits) are "harvested" and grafted into place to reroute blood flow past diseased areas of the coronary arteries. CABG surgery has proved effective in relieving symptoms and prolonging life in patients with left main CAD and three-vessel disease with poor left ventricular function.[2] Increased use of PCI techniques has decreased the need for CABG surgery in many cases. Patients selected for CABG surgery today are older; have more advanced coronary disease; have more impaired left ventricular function; and, in many cases, have had previous CABG surgery.

Commonly used grafts include saphenous vein grafts, internal mammary artery grafts, and radial artery grafts (Table 13-3).

- **Saphenous vein grafts.** Saphenous vein grafts are used to bypass the obstruction in the coronary artery by anastomosing one end of the vein to the aorta (proximal anastomosis) and the other end to the coronary artery just past the obstruction (distal anastomosis). Although the saphenous vein can be taken from above or below the knee, a vein from below the knee is preferred because it is close in diameter to the size of the coronary artery. To remove the vein, an incision is made along the inner aspect of the leg. Alternatively, small incisions can

TABLE 13-3   Common Conduits Used for Coronary Artery Bypass Grafting

Type of Graft	Advantages	Disadvantages
Saphenous vein	• Technically easier to harvest • Longer length may allow for several grafts	• Less long-term patency compared with internal mammary artery graft • Leg incision has tendency toward edema and infection; less common with fiberoptic approach
Internal mammary artery	• Vascular endothelium adapted to arterial pressure and high flow, resulting in decreased intimal hyperplasia and atherosclerosis • Improved long-term patency • Retains nerve innervation and therefore its ability to adapt diameter to blood flow • No leg incision • Diameter closer to coronary artery	• Dissection off the chest wall takes more time; long dissection time may increase risk for postoperative bleeding • Pleural chest tube needed because pleural space violated • Increased postoperative pain • Use of bilateral internal mammary arteries may increase risk for infection and sternal infection, especially in patients with diabetes
Radial artery	• Technically easier to harvest • Better patency rate compared with saphenous vein graft • Vascular endothelium adapted to arterial pressure and high flow, resulting in decreased intimal hyperplasia and atherosclerosis	• Tendency to spasm, although this can be treated medically • Preoperative assessment of ulnar artery's ability to supply alternative blood flow is important

be made in the area of the vein, and a flexible fiberoptic scope is inserted to visualize the vessel and remove it. The fiberoptic method of vein removal is associated with improved wound healing and reduced complications involving the incision site. Only 50% of saphenous vein grafts are patent after 10 years. Three main processes account for saphenous vein failure: thrombosis, fibrointimal hyperplasia, and atherosclerosis. Aspirin is recommended postoperatively and should be continued indefinitely to prevent early saphenous vein graft closure.[2]

• **Internal mammary artery grafts.** The internal mammary artery, the second branch of the subclavian artery, is used as a pedicle graft (ie, the proximal end remains attached to the subclavian artery). Both the left and the right internal mammary artery can be used. The internal mammary artery descends the anterior chest wall just lateral to the sternum behind the costal cartilage. To isolate the internal mammary artery, the pleural space is entered and the internal mammary artery is dissected free from the chest wall. Ninety percent of internal mammary artery grafts are patent 10 years after surgery. As compared with saphenous artery grafts, internal mammary artery grafts exhibit less atherosclerosis over time and are associated with lower long-term morbidity and improved long-term survival.[2]

• **Radial artery grafts.** The radial artery, a thick, muscular artery, is prone to spasm with mechanical stimulation. To prevent spasm, the artery is perfused with a calcium channel blocker solution during surgery and minimally stimulated.

Administration of nitroglycerin followed by oral nitrates postoperatively helps decrease the occurrence of spasm following grafting of the artery. Patency rates of 89% for 1 year have been reported.[3]

CABG surgery typically requires a midline sternotomy. In some cases, surgeons may use less invasive "mini" left or right thoracotomy approaches, known as minimally invasive direct coronary artery bypass grafting (MIDCABG). With MIDCABG, the number of grafts that can be performed is restricted because the small incision does not allow access to the entire heart surface. MIDCABG is most frequently used for grafts to the left anterior descending artery; grafts to the right coronary artery and the posterior descending artery can also be made.

CABG surgery is usually performed with the patient on cardiopulmonary bypass. The cardiopulmonary bypass machine (also called a pump oxygenator) assumes the job of oxygenating the patient's blood and circulating it throughout the body (Box 13-3). However, it is also possible to perform CABG surgery "off pump" (OPCABG). Available data comparing CABG and OPCABG indicates that length of stay in patients after OPCABG surgery is decreased, and patients seem to have fewer neurological complications. The stroke rate is similar in both groups of patients; however, in patients undergoing CABG, the symptoms of stroke occur immediately after surgery, and in patients undergoing OPCABG, the symptoms of stroke appear later, 48 to 72 hours after surgery.[4] The explanation for this finding is that systemic inflammatory response syndrome (SIRS) causes diffuse microembolic

BOX 13-3 Cardiopulmonary Bypass

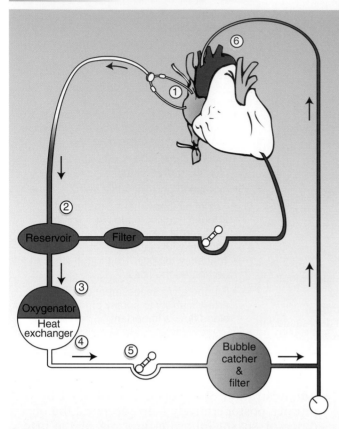

A cardiopulmonary bypass machine is used for cardiac surgeries that require the heart to be still and empty. Before the bypass is implemented, the tubing of the machine is primed with a balanced electrolyte solution or blood. The patient's deoxygenated blood enters the bypass circuit either through one cannula placed in the right atrium or through two cannulae placed in the superior and inferior vena cavae (1), respectively. The blood is temporarily held in the reservoir (2), before moving into the oxygenator (3), which also removes carbon dioxide from the blood. The heat exchanger (4)

cools the blood and then rewarms the blood, and then a series of roller-type pumps (5) pump the blood through the circuit and back to the patient. Oxygenated blood is returned to the ascending aorta (6) by way of a cannula. The flow through the bypass pump is nonpulsatile.

During cardiopulmonary bypass, the patient's core body temperature is lowered to between 82°F and 89°F to reduce the body's metabolic demands and help protect major organ systems from ischemic injury. Heparin is administered to prevent massive extravascular coagulation as the blood circulates through the mechanical parts of the bypass system. Once extracorporeal circulation is established and systemic hypothermia is achieved, the aorta is cross-clamped and a cold (39.2°F) cardioplegia solution that is high in potassium is infused into the aortic root. As it circulates through the coronary arteries, the cold cardioplegia solution induces asystole and hypothermia to decrease the metabolic demands of the myocardium. Topical hypothermia is also created by pouring iced normal saline slush over the heart. Because cold cardioplegia can be associated with postoperative complications (eg, ventricular dysrhythmias, decreased cerebral blood flow, reperfusion injury), some surgeons use a normothermic (98.6°F) cardioplegia solution instead.

Following completion of the surgery, the heat exchanger rewarms the blood (if hypothermic techniques were used). The aortic cross-clamp is removed so that blood again perfuses the coronary arteries. During perfusion and rewarming, a spontaneous cardiac rhythm may resume, ventricular fibrillation may develop (necessitating internal defibrillation), or pacing may be used to initiate a rhythm. After a reliable rhythm and rate are established, total bypass may be reduced to partial bypass (ie, some of the patient's blood is circulated through the heart and lungs, while some continues to circulate through the pump). After the heart can maintain adequate cardiac output on its own, the cannulae are removed and the heparinization is reversed.

events that take time to develop. Following OPCABG surgery, anticoagulation interventions are aggressively implemented to suppress activation of the coagulation cascade. Ongoing nursing assessment of a patient who has undergone OPCABG surgery focuses on detecting embolic events and monitoring for side effects of anticoagulation (eg, gastrointestinal bleeding, HIT).

Transmyocardial Revascularization

Transmyocardial revascularization may be an option for patients who continue to have unstable angina that is refractory to interventions. Eligible patients usually have had prior CABG surgery, multiple cardiac interventions with maximal medication manipulation, or both. A laser probe is used to

create channels in the left ventricle wall that encourage revascularization. The location and number of channels created depend on the patient's preoperative cardiac performance. Revascularization, which takes many months to develop, is thought to involve angiogenesis (ie, the formation of new blood vessels or the modeling of existing blood vessels), which increases collateral flow to the dysfunctional areas.

Nursing Care of the Patient Undergoing Cardiac Surgery

Preoperative Care

The postoperative course depends on the patient's preoperative condition; therefore, history, physical

BOX 13-4 Preoperative Teaching for the Patient Undergoing Cardiac Surgery

Equipment
- Cardiac monitor
- Arterial line
- Pulmonary artery catheter (PAC)
- IV lines and IV infusion pumps
- Endotracheal tube and ventilator: suctioning, how to communicate when intubated, anticipated removal
- Foley catheter: the patient may experience an increased sensation to urinate
- Chest tubes: anticipated removal
- Pacing wires
- Nasogastric tube
- Soft hand restraints

Incisions and Dressings to Expect
- Median sternotomy or other incision
- Leg incision (if saphenous vein is used)

The Patient's Immediate Postoperative Appearance
- Skin yellow owing to use of Betadine solution in operating room
- Skin pale and cool to touch because of hypothermia during surgery
- Generalized "puffiness," especially noticeable in neck, face, and hands, because of third spacing of fluid given during cardiopulmonary bypass

Awakening From Anesthesia
- The patient recovers in the critical care unit; does not go to the postanesthesia care unit

- Each patient recovers from anesthesia differently
- The patient may feel certain sensations
- The patient may hear certain noises
- The patient may be aware or able to hear but unable to respond

Discomfort
- Amount of discomfort to be expected
- When pain might be expected
- Relief mechanisms: positioning/splinting, medications, patient-controlled analgesia (PCA), and the importance of early administration of pain medication

Postoperative Respiratory Care
- Turning
- Use of pillow to splint median sternotomy incision
- Effective coughing and deep breathing after extubation; have the patient practice exercises before surgery
- Incentive spirometry
- Early mobilization

Miscellaneous
- Presence and purpose of postoperative invasive lines and tubes
- Postoperative activity progression
- Visiting policy in critical care unit
- Avoiding use of arms to protect stability of sternotomy

examination, chest radiography, electrocardiography, and laboratory test results are obtained and evaluated preoperatively. Factors that may increase mortality include age; gender; previous similar surgery (resurgery); preoperative occurrence of acute myocardial infarction; and concomitant conditions such as diabetes mellitus, peripheral vascular disease, renal insufficiency, and COPD.[2] Whether the surgery is elective or emergent may also influence outcome. Effective preoperative teaching (Box 13-4) can help improve outcomes and alleviate anxiety and stress for both the patient and the family.

Postoperative Care

Patients are transported directly to the critical care unit, where they recover from anesthesia and usually remain for 24 hours after surgery. Patients arrive in the critical care unit with numerous lines and tubes in place. Some patients will have had temporary pacing electrodes placed on the epicardial surface of the heart during surgery and brought out through the chest wall on either side of the median sternotomy incision (Fig. 13-1). Chest tubes placed in the mediastinum and pericardial space for drainage are

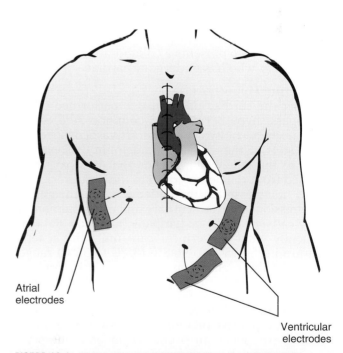

Atrial electrodes

Ventricular electrodes

FIGURE 13-1 Placement of temporary epicardial pacing wires. Ventricular pacing electrodes are typically located to the left and atrial wires to the right of the sternum.

BOX 13-5 Nursing Responsibilities in Caring for the Cardiac Surgery the Patient in the Immediate Postoperative Period

Priority Interventions Performed by the Critical Care Team on Arrival

- Attach the patient to bedside cardiac monitor and note rhythm.
- Attach pressure lines to bedside monitor (arterial and pulmonary artery); level and zero transducers and note pressure values and waveforms.
- Obtain cardiac output/index and note existing inotropic or vasoactive drips.
- After ventilator is connected to endotracheal tube, auscultate breath sounds bilaterally.
- Apply end-tidal carbon dioxide monitor to ventilator circuit and note waveform and value (best indicator of endotracheal tube placement).
- Apply pulse oximetry device to the patient and note the arterial oxygen saturation (SpO_2) and waveform.
- Check peripheral pulses and perfusion signs.

- Monitor chest tubes and character of drainage: amount, color, flow. Check for air leaks.
- Measure body temperature and initiate rewarming if temperature less than 96.8°F (36°C).

Once the Patient Is Determined to Be Hemodynamically Stable

- Measure urine output and note characteristics.
- Obtain clinical data (within 30 minutes of arrival).
- Obtain chest radiograph.
- Obtain 12-lead electrocardiogram (ECG).
- Obtain routine bloodwork within 15 minutes of arrival; tests may include arterial blood gases (ABGs), potassium, glucose, partial thromboplastin time (PTT), hemoglobin (varies with facility).
- Assess neurological status.
- Test pacemaker function by assessing capture and sensing.

---

brought out through stab wounds just below the median sternotomy. If the pleural space has been entered, pleural tubes will also be present.

Immediate postoperative care involves cardiac monitoring and maintenance of oxygenation and hemodynamic stability, as described in Box 13-5. Because cardiopulmonary bypass produces abnormal blood interface and altered blood flow patterns, it has profound physiological effects (Table 13-4).

Ongoing care entails preventing hypothermia, managing pain, and monitoring for and preventing complications. Accurate assessments, vigilant monitoring, and proper interventions are critical in stabilizing patients who have just undergone cardiac surgery. Box 13-6 presents a collaborative care guide for a patient who has undergone cardiac surgery.

Preventing Hypothermia

Whether the cardiac procedure is performed on or off bypass, hypothermia is a common side effect. Hypothermia causes peripheral vasoconstriction and a shift of the oxygen–hemoglobin dissociation curve to the left, which means that less oxygen is released from the hemoglobin to the tissues.

The nurse assesses the patient's core temperature on admission to the critical care unit using pulmonary artery catheter (PAC) or tympanic methods. Patients frequently enter the critical care unit with a temperature in the 95°F to 96.8°F (35°C to 36°C) range. Increasing the room temperature and using radiant heat, blankets, or a warming blanket are effective techniques for increasing core temperature. Rewarming should occur slowly to prevent hemodynamic instability due to rapid vasodilation. After rewarming, many patients experience an overshoot in body temperature, so ongoing temperature assessment is necessary.

Shivering, which occurs most often 1½ to 3 hours after critical care unit admission, increases metabolic rate, oxygen consumption, carbon dioxide production, and myocardial workload. If the patient is hemodynamically compromised, shivering can be managed with sedation, meperidine (Demerol), or a combination of neuromuscular blockade and sedation if the shivering is severe.

Managing Pain

After cardiac surgery, the patient may experience pain resulting from the chest or leg incision, the chest tubes, rib spreading during surgery, and care activities. Pain can result in altered hemodynamics (eg, tachycardia, hypertension) diminished chest expansion, increased atelectasis, and retention of secretions.

Although pain perception varies from person to person, a median sternotomy incision is usually less painful than a lateral thoracotomy incision, and most patients report that the pain is most severe the first 3 to 4 days after surgery. Discomfort from the leg incision often worsens after the patient is ambulatory, especially if leg swelling occurs.

Pain control, often with patient-controlled analgesia (PCA), is aggressively pursued to ensure comfort and rapid mobilization, which can lessen complications. Intercostal nerve blocks and spinal analgesia are less commonly used.

 RED FLAG! *It is important to differentiate angina from incisional pain because angina after CABG surgery may indicate graft failure. Typical median sternotomy pain is localized; does not radiate; is often worse with deep breathing, coughing, or movement; and is often described as sharp, dull, aching, or burning. Angina is usually precordial or substernal; not well localized; frequently radiates to the arms, neck, or jaw; is not affected by respiration or movement; and is often described as a pressure sensation.*

(*text continues on page 169*)

TABLE 13-4 Effects of Cardiopulmonary Bypass

Effects	Clinical Implications
Increased Capillary Permeability Interface between blood and nonphysiological surfaces or bypass circuit leads to • Complement activation that increases capillary permeability • Platelet activation—platelets secrete vasoactive substances that increase capillary permeability • Release of other vasoactive substances that increase capillary permeability	Large amounts of fluid move from the intravascular to the interstitial space during and up to 6 h after cardiopulmonary bypass. Patient becomes edematous.
Hemodilution Solution used to prime extracorporeal circuit dilutes the patient's blood. Secretion of vasopressin (antidiuretic hormone [ADH]) is increased. Levels of renin–angiotensin–aldosterone are increased because of nonpulsatile renal perfusion. Total body water is increased.	Decreased blood viscosity improves capillary perfusion during nonpulsatile flow and hypothermia. Hgb and Hct decrease. Levels of coagulation factors are decreased because of dilution. Intravascular colloid osmotic pressure is decreased, contributing to movement of fluid from intravascular to interstitial spaces. Water is retained at collecting tubule of kidney. Aldosterone causes retention of sodium and water at renal tubule. Weight gain occurs.
Altered Coagulation Procoagulant effects: • Interface between blood and nonendothelial surfaces of bypass circuit activates intrinsic coagulation cascade. • Platelet damage activates intrinsic pathway. Anticoagulant effects: • Interface between blood and nonendothelial surfaces of bypass circuit causes platelets to adhere to tubing and to clump; abnormal platelet function; activation of coagulation cascade, which depletes clotting factors; denaturization of plasma proteins, including coagulation factors. • Coagulation factors are decreased as a result of hemodilution.	Risk for microemboli is increased. Platelet count decreases by 50%–70% of baseline. Abnormal postoperative bleeding occurs. Possibility of bleeding diathesis exists.
Damage to Blood Cells Exposure of blood to nonendothelial surfaces causes mechanical trauma and shear stress. • Platelet damage occurs. • Red blood cell hemolysis occurs. • Leukocytes are damaged.	Platelet count is decreased. Free hemoglobin and hemoglobinuria are increased. Hct is decreased. Immune response is diminished.
Microembolization Emboli form from tissue debris, air bubbles, platelet aggregation.	Microemboli to body organs (brain, lungs, kidneys) are possible.
Increased Systemic Vascular Resistance (SVR) Catecholamine secretion is increased when cardiopulmonary bypass is initiated. Renin secretion is due to nonpulsatile flow to kidney. Hypothermia develops.	Hypertension is possible. Increased SVR may decrease cardiac output.

BOX 13-6 COLLABORATIVE CARE GUIDE for the Patient After Cardiac Surgery

OUTCOMES	INTERVENTIONS
Oxygenation/Ventilation ABGs are within normal limits and pulse oximeter value is >92%. Pulmonary edema is minimized on chest x-ray and demonstrated by improved breath sounds. Atelectasis is improved. Chest tubes remain patent.	• Obtain ABGs per protocol. • Correlate pulse oximeter and end-tidal CO_2 with ABG results. • Adjust ventilator settings after consulting with the respiratory therapist and physician. • Wean from mechanical ventilation per protocol using the expertise of respiratory therapy. • Extubate when the patient is hemodynamically stable; able to protect airway. • Provide supplemental oxygen after extubation. • Encourage use of incentive spirometer, cough and deep breathing q2–4h after extubation. • Milk chest tubes if necessary to facilitate forward drainage movement.
Circulation/Perfusion The patient maintains adequate clinical perfusion. Vital signs will be within normal limits, including MAP > 70 mm Hg; cardiac index will be in a suitable range for the patient's left ventricular function. Heart failure due to decreased cardiac output or perioperative myocardial infarction is minimized. The patient is euthermic.	• Monitor pulmonary artery pressure and PAOP, central venous pressure (CVP) or right atrial pressure (RAP), cardiac output, systemic vascular resistance (SVR), and pulmonary vascular resistance per protocol if pulmonary artery catheter is in place. • Monitor ECG, ST segments, and arterial blood pressure continuously. • Administer positive inotropic agents and reduce afterload with vasodilating agents guided by hemodynamic parameters and physician orders. • Regulate volume administration as indicated by PAOP or CVP values. • Evaluate effect of medications on BP, HR, and hemodynamic parameters. • Monitor and treat dysrhythmias per protocol and physician orders. • Anticipate need for temporary cardiac pacing; isolate wires for electrical safety. • Prepare the patient for IABP assist if necessary. • Assess for neck vein distention, pulmonary crackles, S_3 or S_4, peripheral edema, increased preload parameters, elevated "a" wave of CVP or PAOP waveform. • Monitor 12-lead ECG if ECG changes observed. • Assess temperature q1h. • Warm the patient 1°C/h by using warming blankets, lights, and fluid warmer.
Hematological Issues The patient has minimal bleeding and avoids cardiac tamponade. Chest tube drainage is <200 mL/h.	• Monitor for signs of cardiac tamponade (hypotension, pulsus paradoxus, tachycardia, cardiac pressure equalization). • Evaluate chest x-ray for widened mediastinum, consulting with a physician as needed. • Monitor prothrombin time (PT), partial thromboplastin time (PTT), complete blood count (CBC), and anticoagulant therapy per protocol. • Administer protamine, blood products, and other procoagulants per order or protocol. • Monitor vasoactive drug need and report marked increase of drugs to physician (marked increase may indicate possible tamponade).

BOX 13-6 COLLABORATIVE CARE GUIDE (continued)

OUTCOMES	INTERVENTIONS
Fluids/Electrolytes	
The patient maintains or improves preoperative renal function, as evidenced by urine output of approximately 0.5 mL/kg/h.	• Replace K^+ to maintain level >4.0 mEq/L. • Monitor intake and output q1–2h. • Monitor BUN, creatinine, electrolytes, Mg^+, PO_4^+. • Record daily weights. • Administer fluid volume or diuretics as ordered.
Mobility/Skin Integrity	
The patient maintains range of motion, muscle strength, and skin integrity.	• Turn the patient side to side q2h while on bedrest and evaluate skin closely. • Mobilize out of bed after extubation. • Progress activity to chair for meals, bathroom privileges, increased distance walking, delegating to assistive personnel as indicated. • Monitor vital signs, respiratory effort during activity.
Incisions heal without evidence of infection.	• Check stability of sternotomy incision daily, especially with diabetic patients. • Assess sternotomy and leg incision for redness, swelling, drainage. • Apply compression hose and elevate legs to reduce edema. • Provide caloric and nutrient intake to meet metabolic requirements per calculation for long-term patients. • Monitor prealbumin for trends on long-term patients.
Comfort and Pain Control	
The patient has relief of surgical pain. The patient demonstrates no evidence of pain or anxiety such as increased HR, BP, RR, or agitation during activity or procedures. Timely administration of pain medication is a priority.	• Assess quality, duration, location of pain. Use visual analog scale to assess pain quantity. • Provide a calm environment. Provide for adequate periods of rest and sleep.
Teaching/Discharge Planning	

The patient and family understand:
  Tests, procedures, treatments
  Need for restraints as indicated and per facility policy
  Activity levels, dietary restrictions, medication regimen, and incision care.
	• Consult nutritional support services.
	• Make appropriate social work referrals early during hospitalization.
	• Initiate education regarding heart-healthy diet, physical activity limitations (eg, lifting over 10–15 lb, driving restrictions), stress-reduction strategies, management of pain, incision care.

Supporting Cardiac Output

To maintain optimal cardiac performance and blood pressure, proper volume resuscitation is imperative. A variety of fluids may be used, including normal saline, hetastarch, hyperosmolar fluids (eg, 3% saline), and blood products (if the patient is bleeding). Hemodynamic parameters, including a low CVP (less than 8 to 10 mm Hg), low pulmonary artery diastolic pressure, and low PAOP (less than 14 to 18 mm Hg), in combination with a low cardiac index (less than 2.5 L/min/m²), help guide interventions.

Sympathomimetic drugs or intraaortic balloon pump (IABP) counterpulsation (described later in this chapter) may be used to improve cardiac contractility. Potential underlying causes of myocardial dysfunction include myocardial ischemia and infarction, stunned myocardium (ie, the transient depression of left ventricular function due to a temporary reduction of myocardial blood flow), hibernating myocardium (ie, chronically impaired yet viable myocardial tissue), and cardiac tamponade. Whatever the cause, time and support of function are usually the major factors that improve cardiac performance. Protracted periods of time with mechanical or pharmacological support may indicate the need for a ventricular assist device (VAD), usually as a bridge to heart transplantation.

Reducing SVR can also increase cardiac performance. If the patient has an adequate blood pressure (mean arterial pressure [MAP] greater than 70 mm Hg or systolic blood pressure greater than

120 mm Hg) without pharmacological support, afterload reduction with arterial vasodilators can be started with or without inotropic support. The necessary speed of response dictates the choice of drug.

Monitoring for Dysrhythmias

Dysrhythmias frequently occur after CABG surgery. The hemodynamic response to a change in cardiac rhythm dictates the speed of the intervention in patients. Knowledge of the patient's baseline rhythm is important. The types of dysrhythmias that may occur range from premature atrial contractions to ventricular fibrillation and asystole.

- Sinus tachycardia is very common and can be detrimental because prolonged periods of tachycardia decrease diastolic filling time and coronary artery perfusion.
- Premature atrial contractions that occur frequently may be a precursor to atrial fibrillation. Maintenance of adequate potassium levels (ie, 4 to 4.5 mEq/L) and IV infusion of magnesium may minimize premature atrial contractions.
- Atrial fibrillation can lead to cardiac decompensation and cardioembolic stroke. For new-onset atrial fibrillation, the goals are conversion to sinus rhythm using antidysrythmics or control of the ventricular response rate. If atrial fibrillation persists or reoccurs for more than 24 hours, warfarin anticoagulation may be needed.[1]
- Heart block dysrhythmias occur secondary to edema at the surgical site near the conduction system and are seen most often in patients who have undergone valve surgery. This rhythm usually resolves 48 to 72 hours after surgery, once the edema has decreased.
- Premature ventricular contractions (PVCs) can deteriorate to ventricular tachycardia, ventricular fibrillation, or asystole. If there is no pulse, cardiopulmonary resuscitation (CPR) is started immediately and advanced cardiac life support (ACLS) guidelines are followed.

Preventing Pulmonary Complications

Pulmonary complications after cardiac surgery can be attributed to the inflammatory response and the development of atelectasis and pneumonia. Mechanical ventilation is required to achieve adequate oxygenation and ventilation. Positive end-expiratory pressure (PEEP) is frequently used to help keep the alveoli open and improve oxygenation. The goal for CABG patients is quick weaning from mechanical ventilation. Once the patient has displayed the ability to follow commands and the strength to protect the airway, a short contiuous positive airway pressure (CPAP) trial is instituted. The patient can be extubated when cardiac performance is good (cardiac index greater than 2.2 L/min/m²), adequate oxygenation and ventilation are achieved without acidosis, and chest tube bleeding is minimal. Following extubation, aggressive use of incentive spirometry and physical mobility ensures proper pulmonary function.

Protracted poor cardiac or respiratory function requires continued mechanical ventilation. A tracheostomy should be considered in patients with compromised respiratory function because it can enhance the ventilator weaning process and promote patient comfort.

Preventing Neurological Complications

Once the patient is awake from the anesthesia, frequent evaluation of level of consciousness and motor and sensory ability is mandatory. Postoperative neurological deficits are divided into two categories: (1) major focal deficits (stroke), stupor, or coma and (2) deterioration in intellectual function. Causes of stroke include emboli, hypoxia, hypoperfusion, hemorrhage, and metabolic abnormalities. Cognitive changes (eg, deficits in memory, language, or psychomotor function) are most noticeable immediately after surgery but may still be present 12 to 36 months after the procedure.[5]

Monitoring Postoperative Bleeding

Drainage and decompression of the pericardial and pleural spaces is required after cardiac surgery. Small, flexible chest tubes with bulb suction decrease discomfort, increase early ambulation, and decrease the accumulation of pleural effusions. Vigilant monitoring of chest tube drainage is imperative. The usual mediastinal chest tube output ranges from 100 to 200 mL/h, with periods of increased drainage caused by changes in position or temperature. Measurement of drainage may be required hourly or at more frequent intervals (every 15 or 30 minutes) if drainage is copious.

 RED FLAG! Chest tube bleeding that exceeds 500 mL/h is considered surgical bleeding and mandates surgical reexploration.

If the chest tube output is greater than 200 mL/h, then intervention is necessary. Protamine is given first to reverse the effects of heparin. Aggressive rewarming is very important in a patient who has increased bleeding because of the increased risk of bleeding if hypothermic. However, as the patient's temperature rises, heparin is reactivated, causing increased bleeding. Platelet infusions are also used to decrease bleeding.

Follow-up coagulation studies act as a guide to the need for further infusions and assist with monitoring blood loss. If bleeding is increasing, an elevated PT (greater than 15 seconds) may indicate that bleeding is due to a lack of factors (eg, fibrinogen) that can be replaced using fresh frozen plasma. Coagulation factors such as cryoprecipitate (factors I and VIII) and factor VII are indicated in severe bleeding. Medications such as aminocaproic acid (a potent fibrinolysis inhibitor), aprotinin (a serine–protease inhibitor that blocks kallikrein at the beginning of the coagulation cascade), and desmopressin acetate (which influences factor VIII and enhances platelet adhesion) can be administered to promote coagulation.

RED FLAG! *Cardiac tamponade is a serious complication of increased postoperative bleeding that occurs when excessive fluid or blood accumulates in the pericardial space, resulting in increasing pressure on the ventricle. Tamponade may develop rapidly or slowly, depending on how fast blood accumulates in the pericardial sac. It is important to monitor the chest tube drainage closely and maintain patency. Decreasing cardiac output, blood pressure, and chest tube drainage along with a significant increase in pharmacological support despite volume resuscitation are important warning signs.*

Preventing Renal Complications

Decreasing urine output (less than 0.5 mL/kg/h) is usually caused by decreased renal perfusion due to depressed cardiac function. Mechanical problems (eg, catheter obstruction or malposition) are often overlooked and should be ruled out first. Hypovolemia is a very common problem that can be addressed with fluid administration. For some patients, diuresis with a loop diuretic may be necessary. Urine output, creatinine levels, and blood urea nitrogen (BUN) levels are closely monitored. If acute renal failure develops, dialysis is necessary.

Preventing Endocrine Complications

In the initial postoperative period, maintaining a blood glucose level of less than 200 mg/dL is particularly important in managing wound healing. Use of an insulin drip initially has been shown to reduce the incidence of deep sternal wound infections by 50%.[6] Once good glucose control is achieved, insulin is given subcutaneously, and glucose levels are followed closely.

Adrenal insufficiency may occur, especially in patients who were receiving steroids at regular intervals before surgery. If the patient is taking vasoactive drugs and cannot be weaned from them without becoming hemodynamically unstable, adrenal insufficiency is considered.

Monitoring for Infection

In the early postoperative period, febrile reactions are usually attributed to SIRS and to overshoot from rewarming. If the fever (temperature greater than 100.4°F [38°C]) persists for more than 48 to 72 hours, infection should be considered.

Mediastinitis is the major infection in patients who have undergone CABG surgery and may be a devastating complication that increases the length of hospital stay and mortality. Risk factors associated with mediastinitis are obesity; prior cardiac surgery; preexisting type 1 diabetes mellitus; and perioperative factors such as excessive electrocautery use and use of both internal mammary arteries, resulting in compromised blood flow to the chest wall. Immediate intervention is an extended antibiotic course. Long-term management may include plastic surgery of the thoracic wall. Because sternal instability is thought to contribute to the development of mediastinitis, the nurse teaches the patient measures to maintain the stability of the sternum (eg, avoiding excessive arm movement, placing a small pillow on the sternal incision and squeezing when coughing, and sleeping on the back).

Percutaneous Coronary Intervention Techniques

PCI techniques are less invasive procedures for the treatment of CAD. PCI techniques compare favorably with CABG in terms of risk, success rate, the patient's physical capacity after the procedure, length of hospital stay, and cost.[7] Successful PCI, which is defined as a significant reduction of the luminal diameter stenosis (40% to 50%) without significant in-hospital complications (eg, death, myocardial infarction, abrupt closure necessitating CABG or repeat PCI) ranges from 80% to 100%, depending on the patient's clinical presentation (ie, stable or unstable angina) and angiographic characteristics (ie, subtotal or total occlusion). Long-term survival rates are high, although repeat PCI may be necessary for recurrent or progressive disease.

Commonly used PCI techniques include percutaneous transluminal coronary angioplasty (PTCA) and stent placement.

- **PTCA.** During PTCA, a catheter is introduced into an area of coronary artery stenosis. A balloon attached to the catheter is then inflated, increasing the luminal diameter and improving blood flow through the dilated segment (Fig. 13-2). The process that leads to successful dilation is complex, but it is thought that PTCA stretches the vessel wall, leading to fracture of the inelastic atherosclerotic plaque and to tearing or cracking within the intima and media of the vessel. This cracking or slight dissection of the inner lumen of the vessel may be necessary for successful dilation.
- **Stent placement.** Intracoronary stents are hollow stainless steel tubes that act as "scaffolding" in the coronary artery. The artery is dilated using a PTCA balloon catheter, and then a stent that is premounted on a balloon catheter is inserted through the guide catheter along a guide wire to the lesion site. Once placed across the stenotic lesion, the balloon is inflated, and the stent is expanded and left in the coronary artery. Success of the stenting procedure depends on endothelialization of the stent to provide a smooth flow of blood in the coronary artery and through the stent. Drug-eluting stents are coated with drugs such as heparin, paclitaxel, or rapamycin. It is believed that the gradual release of these drugs at the site of the atherosclerotic plaque inhibits restenosis by limiting smooth muscle cell proliferation and inflammation while allowing reendothelialization to proceed normally. The use of drug-eluting stents has dramatically decreased the need for repeat PCI procedures. Stent thrombosis is a major short- and long-term complication of stent placement, especially with

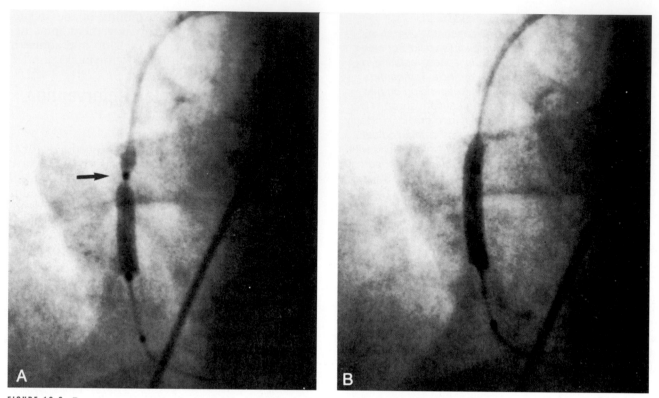

FIGURE 13-2 Percutaneous transluminal coronary angioplasty (PTCA). **A:** Many PTCA balloons expand at both ends and not in the center, where they are pinched by the stenosis. **B:** The central indentation usually disappears as the stenosis is dilated. (Courtesy of John B. Simpson, MD, Palo Alto, CA.)

older bare metal stents, which act as thrombogenic prostheses. Anticoagulation and antiplatelet medication regimens are crucial to successful stenting and long-term prognosis.

PCI is used to alleviate angina pectoris unrelieved by medical treatment and to reduce the risk for myocardial infarction in symptomatic patients and asymptomatic patients with significant stenosis. It is only indicated for coronary arteries that have at least a 70% narrowing. Patients with surgical risk factors (eg, severe underlying noncardiac diseases, advanced age, poor left ventricular function) are particularly suited for PCI because successful dilation obviates the need for an operation that would be poorly tolerated. It is also often appropriate for patients who have undergone CABG surgery previously, but are now experiencing recurrent symptoms because of stenosis and graft closure or progression of coronary disease.

If thrombus and underlying stenosis are causing an infarction, thrombolytic therapy, PCI, or both may be used. If a blood clot has impeded flow to the distal myocardium and precipitates an ischemic episode, a thrombolytic agent can be administered intravenously or directly into the coronary artery. On successful lysis of the thrombus, dilation of the underlying stenosis often further enhances blood flow to the reperfused myocardium. Primary PCI is dilation of an infarct-related coronary artery during the acute phase of myocardial infarction without prior administration of a thrombolytic agent. Primary PCI may benefit patients deemed ineligible for traditional medical therapy (eg, those in cardiogenic shock, those believed to be at high risk for bleeding complications, and those older than 75 years).

Nursing Care of the Patient Undergoing PCI

Preprocedure

The nurse monitors all preliminary laboratory tests, including cardiac enzymes; coagulation studies (PT and partial thromboplastin time [PTT]); and serum electrolytes, creatinine, and BUN levels. Potassium levels must be within normal limits because low levels result in increased sensitivity and excitability of the myocardium, potentially giving rise to life-threatening ventricular dysrhythmias, especially with ischemic myocardium. Evaluation of kidney function is important because PCI entails the use of radiopaque contrast material. Contrast-induced renal failure occurs more frequently in patients with higher baseline creatinine levels.[8] In addition to evaluating kidney function, the nurse ensures that the patient is adequately hydrated to promote excretion of the contrast material.

 The Older Patient. *Elderly patients may be sensitive to small amounts of contrast material; therefore, it is especially important to monitor kidney function in elderly patients, both before and after PCI.*

Twenty-four hours before the procedure, aspirin (325 mg once a day) is administered for its antiplatelet effect. Studies have also shown that administration of an antiplatelet drug before and after a PCI decreases adverse events such as acute closure and subacute thrombosis.[9] Diabetic patients taking metformin are advised to discontinue this medication before their procedure because it is contraindicated with intravascular contrast agents. Anticoagulants such as warfarin are also often withheld for a number of days before the PCI procedure.

Postprocedure

Following PCI, the nurse monitors for complications (Box 13-7). Initial post-PCI laboratory tests may include coagulation studies, cardiac enzymes, and serum electrolytes. Elevation of the cardiac enzymes can indicate that a silent myocardial infarction has occurred and must be reported to the physician immediately. Chest pain may indicate a transient vasospastic episode, which can be resolved with vasodilation therapy, or an acute occlusion, which requires emergent repeat PCI or CABG surgery. At the first sign of vasospasm, the nurse administers oxygen by mask or nasal cannula and obtains a 12-lead electrocardiogram (ECG) to document any acute changes indicative of injury to the myocardium (eg, ST-segment elevation). For fast, temporary (and possibly permanent) relief, nitrates and calcium channel blockers may be administered. In addition, the IV drip of nitroglycerin is titrated to maintain a blood pressure adequate to ensure coronary artery perfusion and to alleviate chest pain. Emergent CABG surgery may be necessary when the vasoconstriction cannot be reversed through the administration of nitrates.

BOX 13-7 **Complications of Percutaneous Coronary Intervention (PCI)**

- Myocardial infarction
- Coronary artery spasm
- Abrupt closure of a dilated segment
- Coronary artery dissection or intimal tear
- Restenosis
- Coronary perforation
- Bradycardia
- Ventricular tachycardia or ventricular fibrillation
- Transient or persistent neurological deficit
- Contrast sensitivity reactions (eg, urticaria, flushing, laryngospasm, nausea, anxiety)
- Retroperitoneal hemorrhage
- Peripheral vascular complications occurring primarily at the catheter site
  - Arterial thrombosis
  - Excessive bleeding/ hematoma formation
  - Pseudoaneurysm
  - Femoral arteriovenous fistula
  - Arterial laceration

Because the femoral approach is used most often in PCI to access the vasculature, most patients have an entry port in either the right or the left groin through which sheaths have been placed percutaneously in a vein and an artery. Many times, the sheaths are removed before the patient leaves the cardiac catheterization laboratory, and a hemostasis device, collagen plug, or surgical suture around the opening of the blood vessel is used to facilitate hemostasis. The nurse instructs the patient on the importance of keeping the involved leg straight and the head of the bed angled at 45 degrees or less.

If the sheath remains in place after the procedure, an IV infusion is attached to the venous sheath and a pressurized arterial flush is attached to the arterial line to prevent clotting in the lumens. This arrangement ensures patency should an immediate return to the cardiac catheterization laboratory be necessary because of a complication. Otherwise, if the post-PCI course is uncomplicated, the sheaths are removed after 2 to 4 hours, and pressure is applied to the site. The patient must remain on complete bedrest for 4 to 6 hours after the sheaths are removed. Bleeding at the sheath site may result in a major hematoma that can require surgical evacuation or compromise distal blood flow to the lower extremity. After sheath removal, the nurse pays careful attention to the area of the puncture site, checking distal pulses frequently and reporting immediately to the physician any changes that may indicate bleeding. To prevent excessive bleeding and to aid hemostasis, the physician may order that a 5-lb sandbag be placed over the puncture site.

After PCI, aspirin is continued indefinitely for its antiplatelet effect. Patients who have had a drug-eluting stent placed are administered clopidogrel for 12 months postprocedure, and possibly indefinitely, unless CABG is planned. Often, long-acting nitrates, calcium channel blockers, ACE inhibitors, and lipid-lowering agents are added to the medical regimen.

Intraaortic Balloon Pump Counterpulsation

In intraaortic balloon pump (IABP) counterpulsation, inflation and deflation of a balloon in the thoracic aorta is used to increase oxygen supply to the myocardium, decrease left ventricular work, and improve cardiac output. Major uses of IABP counterpulsation include the treatment of acute left ventricular failure after cardiac surgery, the treatment of cardiogenic shock after myocardial infarction, and as short-term "bridge" therapy prior to cardiac transplantation. The desired results of IABP therapy are increased coronary artery perfusion and decreased afterload with a subsequent increase in cardiac output. Contradictions to IABP counterpulsation include aortic insufficiency, severe peripheral vascular occlusive disease, and aortic aneurysm.

IABP counterpulsation is usually an unplanned, emergent intervention for a deteriorating condition. Preparing family members prior to their first visit with the patient following device insertion and providing ongoing explanations of the patient's status and care can help to alleviate anxiety. Honest communication helps family members recognize changes in the patient's condition and make informed, realistic decisions regarding the patient's care.

Insertion and Operation

The balloon used in IABP counterpulsation is positioned in the thoracic aorta via the femoral artery. It is positioned just distal to the great vessels and proximal to the renal artery (Fig. 13-3). Once in place,

the balloon catheter is attached to a console that displays the patient's ECG and an arterial waveform for timing of the balloon inflation and deflation. The console also displays a balloon waveform that illustrates the inflation and deflation of the balloon itself. The balloon is inflated and deflated in accordance with the cardiac cycle:

- Inflation occurs during diastole, increasing aortic pressure and retrograde blood flow back toward the aortic valve (Fig. 13-4). This increases coronary artery perfusion pressure and blood flow, thus improving oxygen supply.
- Deflation occurs just before systole (ie, just before blood is ejected from the left ventricle). This decreases the impedance to ejection (ie, afterload), the left ventricle's workload, and myocardial oxygen demand.

Timing of inflation and deflation must coincide with the cardiac cycle to ensure effectiveness of IABP therapy. Two primary methods of timing can be used with IABP therapy:

- **Conventional timing** uses the arterial waveform as the triggering mechanism to determine both inflation and deflation of the balloon. Balloon inflation occurs at the dicrotic notch (which signals the closure of the aortic valve and the beginning of diastole on the arterial waveform). Deflation is timed to occur at end diastole, just before the next sharp systolic upstroke on the arterial waveform.
- **Real timing** uses the same point of reference on the arterial waveform for balloon inflation but uses the ECG signal as the trigger for balloon deflation. The QRS complex is recognized as the onset of ventricular systole. Triggering off the R wave allows for balloon deflation to occur at the time of systolic ejection. Real timing is more effective

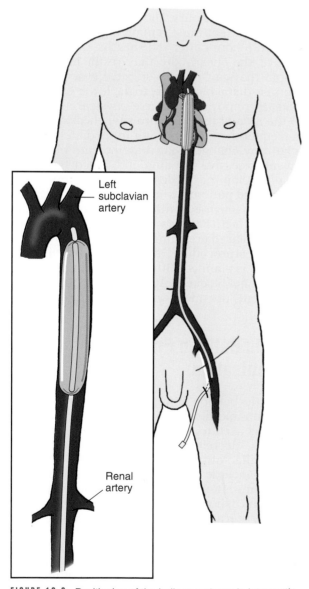

FIGURE 13-3 Positioning of the balloon catheter in intraaortic balloon pump (IABP) counterpulsation.

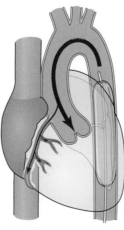 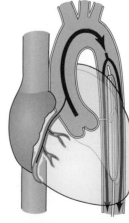

A. Inflation   B. Deflation

FIGURE 13-4 Intraaortic balloon pump (IABP) counterpulsation. A: Inflation of the balloon increases aortic pressure and retrograde blood flow back toward the aortic valve. B: Deflation of the balloon decreases the impedance to ejection, reducing ventricular workload and increasing cardiac output.

in patients with irregular heart rhythms because balloon deflation occurs on recognition of the R wave. Real timing can also be achieved with a special IABP catheter that has a fiberoptic pressure sensor in the tip. The pressure sensor determines the precise time when the aortic valve closes with each contraction of the heart, regardless of the patient's heart rhythm.

Improper timing reduces the effectiveness of therapy and can be detrimental to the patient. For example

- Early inflation shortens systole abruptly and increases ventricular workload as ejection is suddenly interrupted.
- Late inflation does not increase the coronary artery perfusion pressure sufficiently.
- Early deflation allows pressure to rise to normal end-diastolic levels preceding systole, resulting in no decrease in afterload.
- Late deflation encroaches on the next systole and increases afterload because of the presence of the still-inflated balloon during early systolic ejection.

Nurses must be able to recognize and correct problems in balloon pump timing. To do this, analysis of the arterial pressure waveform is necessary. To evaluate the waveform effectively, the patient's unassisted pressure tracing is viewed alongside the assisted pressure tracing. This can be accomplished by adjusting the console so that the balloon inflates and deflates on every other beat (ie, a 1:2 assist ratio). Alternatively, a strip recording of the 1:2 assistance can be obtained for analysis. Box 13-8 summarizes how to evaluate the effectiveness of IABP therapy using the arterial pressure waveform.

Cardiovascular monitoring is also important in determining the effectiveness of IABP therapy. Effective IABP therapy causes a decrease in heart rate, MAP, and PAOP. Heart rhythm and regularity must also be considered. Irregular dysrhythmias may inhibit efficient IABP therapy with some types of consoles because timing is set by the regular R–R interval on the ECG. Urine output, skin perfusion, and mentation are important assessment parameters for determining the adequacy of cardiac output.

Complications

Complications associated with IABP counterpulsation include mechanical problems with the balloon, impaired circulation, bleeding at the insertion site, and infection.

- **Mechanical problems.** The nurse frequently assesses the left radial pulse and urine output to detect problems with balloon placement. A decrease, absence, or change in character of the left radial pulse may indicate that the balloon has advanced up the aorta and is causing either a complete or partial obstruction of the left subclavian artery. An acute, dramatic drop in urine output

---

BOX 13-8 **Assessing the Effectiveness of Intraaortic Balloon Pump (IABP) Therapy Using the Arterial Pressure Waveform**

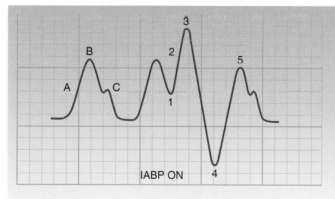

Five Criteria for Assessing the Effectiveness of IABP Using the Arterial Pressure Waveform
- Inflation occurs at the dicrotic notch (1 is equal to C).
- Inflation slope is parallel to the systolic upstroke and is a straight line (2 is parallel to A).
- Diastolic augmentation peak is greater than or equal to the preceding systolic peak (3 greater than or equal to B).
- An end-diastolic dip in pressure is created with balloon deflation (4). The deeper the diastolic dip created by the balloon deflation, the better the afterload reduction.
- The following systolic peak (assisted systole) is lower than the preceding systole (unassisted systole) (5 is less than B).

Unassisted Waveform

A: Systolic upstroke
B: Systolic peak
C: Dicrotic notch

Assisted Waveform

1: Inflation point
2: Inflation slope
3: Diastolic augmentation peak (diastolic peak pressure)
4: End-diastolic dip
5: Next systolic peak

This tracing shows an unassisted arterial waveform, followed by an assisted arterial waveform.

TABLE 13-5 Injuries Secondary to Balloons

Injury	Assessment Findings	Intervention
Balloon entrapment	Balloon pressure waveform indicates leaks Small amounts of blood in tubing or flecks of dried blood in tubing	Surgical removal is usually indicated
Balloon rupture	Presence of bright red blood or flecks of dried blood in the catheter or gas delivery line Gas alarm sounds Decreased augmentation Signs of embolic event Entrapment (may be the first indication)	Immediate removal of the catheter by the appropriate personnel Before removal: Turn pump off Clamp the line Place the patient on left side in Trendelenburg position

may be an indication that the catheter has slipped down the aorta and is obstructing the renal arteries. Although the incidence of injury secondary to balloon rupture or entrapment (ie, formation of a blood clot in the balloon) is low, the nurse also monitors for these complications (Table 13-5).

- **Impaired circulation.** The presence of the balloon catheter in the femoral or iliac artery predisposes the patient to impaired circulation of the involved extremity and development of compartment syndrome. The nurse documents the quality of peripheral pulses and neurological status before IABP insertion. Following insertion, the nurse assesses and documents the quality of pulses, skin perfusion, and neurological status per protocol, and notifies the physician of any changes.

 RED FLAG! Avoid hip flexion, which may obstruct flow to the affected extremity, by keeping the cannulated leg straight and the head of the bed at an angle less than 30 degrees.

- **Bleeding.** Continuous anticoagulation with a heparin infusion is required during IABP therapy to prevent thrombus formation around the catheter. Bleeding related to use of continuous anticoagulation or the development of coagulopathies commonly occurs at the insertion site of the balloon catheter. The nurse maintains anticoagulation therapy as ordered and monitors for bleeding.
- **Infection.** Patients are at increased risk for infection secondary to surgery, the presence of invasive devices, and compromised pulmonary or nutritional status. Early recognition of signs and symptoms of infection and early intervention can prevent the development of sepsis.

Weaning

Weaning patients from balloon assistance usually can begin 24 to 72 hours after insertion; some patients require longer periods of support because of hemodynamic instability. Indications for weaning from IABP therapy are given in Box 13-9. Weaning is commonly achieved by decreasing the assist ratio from 1:1 to 1:2 and so on until the minimal assist ratio is achieved. A patient may be assisted at the first decrease for up to 4 to 6 hours. The minimal amount of time is 30 minutes. During this time, the nurse assesses the patient for any change in hemodynamic status.

Ventricular Assist Devices

When there is profound myocardial injury, the augmentation of systemic blood pressure by IABP counterpulsation may not be adequate because IABP augments cardiac output only by 8% to 10%. A VAD may be used for patients with cardiac failure that is refractory to IABP counterpulsation, pharmacological therapies, and revascularization procedures. These devices, which may be placed internally or externally, support circulation until the heart recovers or a donor heart is obtained for transplantation. Restoration of adequate blood flow and preservation of end-organ function are the fundamental goals of short- or long-term VAD use. Complications associated with VAD use are summarized in Box 13-10.

BOX 13-9 Indications for Weaning From Intraaortic Balloon Pump (IABP) Therapy

Hemodynamic stability
  Cardiac index greater than 2 L/min/m²
  Pulmonary artery occlusion pressure (PAOP) less than 20 mm Hg
  Systolic blood pressure greater than 100 mm Hg
Minimal requirements for vasopressor support
Evidence of adequate cardiac function
  Good peripheral pulses
  Adequate urine output
  Absence of pulmonary edema
  Improved mentation
Evidence of good coronary perfusion
  Absence of ventricular ectopy
  Absence of ischemia on the ECG
  Severe vascular insufficiency
Deteriorating, irreversible condition

BOX 13-10 Complications Associated With Ventricular Assist Devices (VADs)

- Bleeding
- Cardiac tamponade
- Embolic events
- Right ventricular failure (when a left VAD is in use)
- Infection
- Dysrhythmias

The VAD relieves the workload of one or both ventricles by acting as the primary pump supporting systemic circulation, pulmonary circulation, or both. Left ventricular support usually requires cannulation of the left ventricle with a conduit that leads to the device. The ascending aorta, which receives the output from the device, is also cannulated with a conduit. Circulation in the patient supported by a left VAD is similar to the normal circulatory process. Blood passes from the left atrium through the left ventricle and into the device, which then ejects blood into the ascending aorta during pump systole.

In biventricular support, one pump supports right heart circulation while the other supports left heart circulation (Fig. 13-5). The addition of right ventricular assistance requires cannulation of the right atrium (for inflow to the device) and the pulmonary artery (for outflow from the device).

CASE STUDY

Mr. M. is a 63-year-old man who has had CABG surgery with three grafts: an internal mammary artery graft to the left anterior descending coronary artery and a saphenous vein graft to the right coronary artery and diagonal artery. Prior to surgery, Mr. M. had moderate left ventricular dysfunction (ejection fraction 35%). His past medical history is significant for poorly controlled diabetes mellitus, treatment for tuberculosis 20 years ago, and renal insufficiency. After 8 hours in surgery (during which cardiopulmonary bypass was used), Mr. M. has been transferred to the critical care unit from the operating room. He is receiving dobutamine (5 µg/kg/min) to improve cardiac performance. On postoperative day 2, he is still intubated, on dobutamine at 7 µg/kg/min, with a cardiac index of 2.0 L/min/m^2 and a PAOP of 22 mm Hg. His urine output is marginal at 25 mL/h (preoperative weight is 80 kg). Attempts at weaning Mr. M. from the dobutamine have failed.

1. What is occurring in this situation?
2. What are immediate nursing interventions?
3. What interventions would be the most important to make the physician aware of?

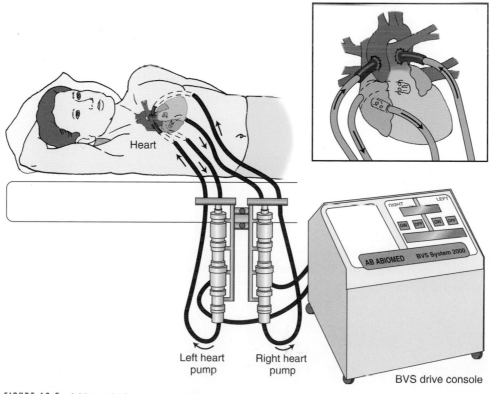

Left heart pump   Right heart pump   BVS drive console

FIGURE 13-5 A biventricular support system.

References

1. Lewis BE, Hursting MJ: Direct thrombin inhibitor during percutaneous coronary intervention in patients with heparin induced thrombocytopenia. Expert Rev Cardiovasc Ther 5(1):57–68, 2007
2. Eagle K, Guyton R, Davidoff R, et al.: ACC/AHA 2004 guideline update for coronary bypass graft surgery. J Am Coll Cardiol 110:e340–431, 2004
3. Goldman S, et al.: Radial artery grafts versus saphenous vein grafts in coronary artery bypass graft. JAMA 305 (2):167–174, 2011
4. ACC/AHA 2011 update to the 2004 guideline for coronary artery bypass graft surgery
5. Selnes O: Etiology of cognitive change after coronary artery bypass graft surgery: More than just a pump? Nat Clin Pract Cardiovasc Med 5:314–315, 2008
6. Lazar H, et al.: The Society of Thoracic Surgeons Practice Guidelines Series: Blood glucose measurement during adult cardiac surgery. Ann Thorac Surg 87:663–669, 2009
7. Serruys P, et al.: Percutaneous coronary intervention versus coronary artery bypass graft for severe coronary artery disease. NEJM 360:961–972, 2009
8. Katzberg R: Cotrast-induced nephropathy. Appl Radiol 39:9, 2010
9. Mahta SR, Yusuf S, Peters RJ, et al.: Effects of pretreatment with clopidogrel and aspirin followed by long term therapy in patients undergoing percutaneous coronary intervention: The PCI-CURE Study. Lancet 358:527–533, 2001

Want to know more? A wide variety of resources to enhance your learning and understanding of this chapter are available on the **Point** ✳. Visit **http://thepoint.lww.com/MortonEss1e** to access chapter review questions and more!

Common Cardiovascular Disorders

OBJECTIVES

Based on the content in this chapter, the reader should be able to:

1 Describe the pathophysiology, assessment, and management of acute coronary syndromes in the critically ill patient.
2 Describe the pathophysiology, assessment, and management of heart failure in the critically ill patient.
3 Describe the assessment and management of hypertensive crisis.
4 Describe the assessment and management of aortic aneurysm and aortic dissection.
5 Describe the assessment and management of cardiomyopathy in the critically ill patient.
6 Describe the pathophysiology, assessment, and management of valvular disease.
7 Describe the pathophysiology, assessment, and management of infectious and inflammatory cardiac disorders.

Acute Coronary Syndromes

Acute coronary syndromes include acute myocardial infarction and unstable angina pectoris (ie, chest pain or discomfort that usually occurs while at rest). The most common cause of the reduced oxygen supply that precipitates acute coronary syndromes is coronary artery disease (CAD; Box 14-1).

 The Older Patient. *CAD is more common and more severe in older patients, and they may have numerous comorbidities (eg, diminished β-sympathetic response, decreased arterial compliance and arterial hypertension leading to increased cardiac afterload, cardiac hypertrophy, ventricular diastolic dysfunction) that complicate management and prognosis.*

A 12-lead electrocardiogram (ECG) can be used to detect patterns of myocardial ischemia, injury, and infarction. When the heart muscle becomes ischemic, injured, or infarcted, depolarization and repolarization of the cardiac cells are altered, causing changes in the QRS complex, ST segment, and T wave in the ECG leads overlying the affected area of the heart:

• **Ischemia.** The ECG may show T-wave inversions and ST-segment depressions of 1 to 2 mm or more for a duration of 0.08 second in the ECG leads associated with the anatomical region of myocardial ischemia (Fig. 14-1). The inverted T-wave representative of ischemia is symmetrical, relatively narrow, and somewhat pointed. Ischemia is also suspected when a flat or depressed ST segment makes a sharp angle when joining an upright

BOX 14·1   Pathophysiology of Coronary Artery Disease (CAD)

Although the atherosclerotic process is not completely understood, evidence suggests that it begins when the endothelium is damaged by elevated levels of cholesterol and triglycerides in the blood, hypertension, or cigarette smoking. Gradually, as fatty substances, cholesterol, cellular waste products, calcium, and fibrin pass through the vessel, they are deposited in the inner lining of an artery. Deposition of these materials leads to the formation of an atheroma (ie, a lipid plaque with a fibrous covering), and blood flow in the artery becomes partially or completely blocked. White blood cells, smooth muscle cells, and platelets aggregate at the site of the atheroma, promoting the formation of a collagen and elastic fiber matrix and causing the endothelium to become much thicker. The inflammatory process is meant to be protective, but in atherosclerosis,

the process has been found to be destructive. The atheroma continues to develop, and a fibrous cap forms over the lipid core. As the cap matures, inflammatory substances weaken the cap and cause it to rupture. Once the cap is ruptured, the coagulation cascade is initiated, and a clot (thrombus) is formed, obstructing blood flow in the vessel.

Symptoms often do not occur until 70% or more of the blood supply to the area is occluded. When an artery becomes about 70% occluded and oxygen demand exceeds oxygen supply, myocardial ischemia may result. If the ischemic state is not corrected, injury to the myocardium may occur. Eventually, if adequate blood flow to the myocardium is not restored, myocardial infarction may result. Ischemia and injury are reversible processes; infarction is not.

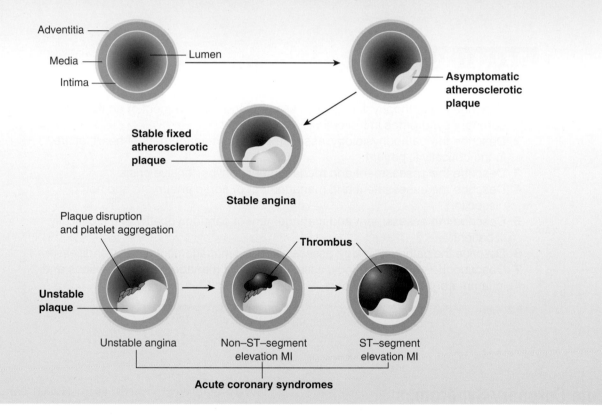

T wave rather than merging smoothly and imperceptibly with the T wave.

- **Injury.** The hallmark of acute myocardial injury is the presence of ST-segment elevations greater than 1 mm in the leads facing the injured area. The elevated ST segments have a downward concave (coved) shape and merge unnoticed with the T wave (Fig. 14-2). Patients without ST-segment elevation either have unstable angina or non–ST-segment elevation myocardial infarction (NSTEMI). Patients with ST-segment elevation have ST-segment elevation myocardial infarction

(STEMI). The pattern on the ECG indicative of STEMI is seen in stages in the leads overlying the infarcted area (Fig. 14-3).

- **Infarction.** Patients with infarction may or may not have ST-segment elevation on the ECG. In most patients with STEMI or NSTEMI, a Q wave ultimately develops on the ECG. The term Q-wave myocardial infarction (QMI) is used to describe this type of infarction. In a much smaller number of patients who present with STEMI, a Q wave does not develop. The term non–Q-wave myocardial infarction (NQMI) is used to classify these patients.

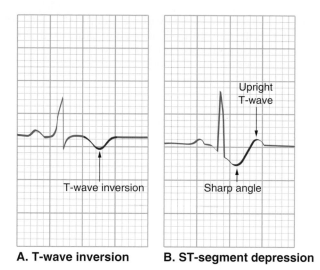

A. T-wave inversion   **B. ST-segment depression**

FIGURE 14-1 12-Lead electrocardiogram (ECG) patterns consistent with myocardial ischemia. **A:** T-wave inversion. **B:** ST-segment depression. Note how the ST segment forms a sharp angle when joining an upright T wave, rather than merging smoothly with it.

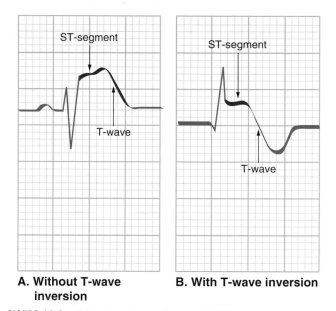

A. Without T-wave inversion   **B. With T-wave inversion**

FIGURE 14-2 12-Lead electrocardiogram (ECG) patterns consistent with acute myocardial injury. The elevated ST segments have a downward concave (coved) shape and merge unnoticed with the T wave. **A:** ST-segment elevation without T-wave inversion. **B:** ST-segment elevation with T-wave inversion.

Unstable Angina Pectoris

Angina pectoris is caused by transient, reversible myocardial ischemia precipitated by an imbalance between myocardial oxygen demand and myocardial oxygen supply. The most common cause of reduced oxygen supply is CAD. A nonocclusive thrombus develops on a disrupted atheroma, resulting in reduced myocardial perfusion. Other, less common, causes of angina include intense focal spasm of a coronary artery, arterial inflammation, or a marked increase in oxygen demand (eg, as a result of fever, tachycardia, or thyrotoxicosis).

There are different types of angina:

- **Stable angina** (chronic stable angina, classic angina, exertional angina) is paroxysmal substernal pain that is usually predictable. The pain occurs with physical exertion or emotional stress and is relieved by rest or nitroglycerin.
- **Unstable angina** (preinfarction angina, crescendo angina) is cardiac chest pain that usually occurs while at rest. The pain of unstable angina is usually more prolonged and severe than that of stable angina.

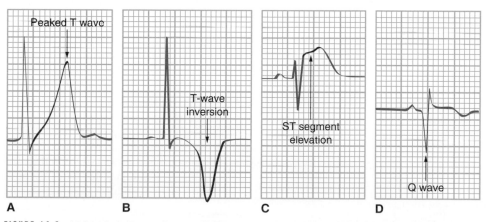

FIGURE 14-3 12-Lead electrocardiogram (ECG) patterns consistent with ST-segment elevation myocardial infarction (STEMI). **A:** During the earliest stage of infarction (the hyperacute phase), the T waves become tall and peaked. **B:** Within a few hours, the hyperacute T waves invert. **C:** Next, the ST segments elevate, a pattern that usually lasts from several hours to several days. Reciprocal ST-segment changes (ie, ST-segment depression in the leads facing away from the injured area) may be seen. **D:** Q waves indicative of infarction usually develop within several hours of the onset of the infarction, but in some patients, they may not appear until 24 to 48 hours after the infarction. Q waves consistent with myocardial infarction are usually 0.04 second or more in width or one-fourth to one-third the height of the R wave in depth.

• **Variant angina** (Prinzmetal's angina, vasospastic angina) is a form of unstable angina caused by coronary artery spasm. The pain usually occurs at rest, most often between midnight and 8:00 AM.

Assessment

The nurse uses the NOPQRST framework to gain more detail about the patient's chest pain (Box 14-2). Based on the information obtained, the angina may be classified as one of three principal presentations: rest angina, new-onset severe angina (onset within the past 2 months), or increasing angina (in intensity, duration, or frequency). Physical examination helps determine the cause of the angina, detect comorbid conditions, and assess any hemodynamic consequences of the angina. If the physical examination is performed during an anginal episode, tachycardia, a fourth heart sound (S_4), and pulsus alternans may be noted, and the patient may be hypertensive. Patients with diabetes mellitus may present with a "silent" myocardial infarction. Women may have an atypical presentation (eg, shortness of breath, GI disturbances).

The Older Patient. *Older patients are more likely to present with atypical angina symptoms (eg, dyspnea, confusion, weakness, fainting) rather than with typical substernal chest pain, pressure, squeezing, fullness, or heaviness. Also, because of differences in the amount and distribution of subcutaneous fat, an older patient may develop anginal symptoms more quickly when exposed to cold.*

A 12-lead ECG is a standard diagnostic test for patients with angina. The newly obtained ECG is compared with previous ECGs. In addition to T-wave inversion or ST-segment elevation, ectopic beats may also be present during an anginal episode. Between anginal episodes, the ECG may appear normal. Transient ST-segment changes (greater than or equal to 0.05 mV) that occur during a symptomatic episode while at rest and that resolve when the patient is asymptomatic are highly suggestive of severe CAD.[1] Other diagnostic studies used in the assessment of angina pectoris include biochemical cardiac markers, exercise stress testing, cardiac imaging studies, and coronary angiography.

Management

The goal of therapy for the patient with angina pectoris is to restore the balance between oxygen supply and oxygen demand. The patient is placed on bedrest until stabilized to minimize oxygen demand, and supplemental oxygen may be given to increase oxygen supply. The nurse assesses the patient's vital signs and mental status frequently and uses pulse oximetry and arterial blood gases (ABGs) to evaluate oxygenation status. The patient is placed on a cardiac monitor for ischemia and dysrhythmia detection.

Pharmacotherapy

Nitroglycerin is a mainstay of therapy and is used sublingually or as a spray for acute anginal attacks. If three sublingual tablets (0.4 mg) or three sprays taken 5 minutes apart do not relieve the pain of

---

BOX 14-2   The NOPQRST Characteristics of Chest Pain Due to Myocardial Ischemia

N—Normal
• The patient's baseline before the onset of the pain

O—Onset
• The time when the pain/discomfort started

P—Precipitating and Palliative Factors

Precipitating
• Exercise
• Exercise after a large meal
• Exertion
• Walking on a cold or windy day
• Cold weather
• Stress or anxiety
• Anger
• Fear

Palliative
• Rest/termination of activity
• Sublingual nitroglycerin

Q—Quality
• Heaviness
• Tightness
• Squeezing
• Choking

• Suffocating
• Viselike

If the patient reports the pain as superficial, knifelike, or throbbing, it is not likely to be anginal.

R—Region and Radiation
• Substernal with radiation to the back, left arm, neck, or jaw
• Upper chest
• Epigastric
• Left shoulder
• Intrascapular

When the patient is asked to point to the painful area, the painful area is typically identified by the hand or clenched fist. It is unusual for true anginal pain to be localized to an area smaller than a fingertip.

S—Severity
• Pain often rated as 5 or above (on a scale of 0 to 10, with 10 being the worst pain ever experienced).

T—Time
• Pain lasts from 30 seconds to 30 minutes.
• Pain can last longer than 30 minutes for unstable angina or myocardial infarction.

angina, an IV nitroglycerin drip is initiated at 5 to 20 µg/min. The dosage is increased every 5 to 15 minutes, up to 200 µg/min, until a blood pressure response is noted or signs and symptoms are relieved. Once a patient has been pain free and has no other indications of ischemia for 12 to 24 hours, the IV nitroglycerin is discontinued and replaced with oral or topical nitrates.

Morphine sulfate is indicated for patients whose symptoms are not relieved after three serial sublingual nitroglycerin tablets or whose symptoms recur with adequate anti-ischemic therapy. A dose of 1 to 5 mg IV is recommended to relieve symptoms and maintain comfort. The nurse carefully monitors the patient's respiratory rate and blood pressure, especially if the patient continues to receive IV nitroglycerin.

β-Adrenergic blockers are started orally within the first 24 hours for patients with unstable angina.[1] These agents decrease myocardial oxygen consumption (by reducing myocardial contractility) and increase blood flow to the coronary arteries (by slowing the heart rate and prolonging diastolic filling). Calcium channel blockers, which also decrease myocardial oxygen demand, may be used for patients with ischemia-related symptoms that do not respond to nitrates and β-adrenergic blockers.[1]

The combination of aspirin, an anticoagulant, and an additional antiplatelet drug (ie, clopidogrel or ticlopidine) is recommended for patients with unstable angina. Aspirin is administered as soon as the diagnosis of unstable angina is made or suspected, unless contraindicated.[1]

Invasive Therapy

Patients with unstable angina may require percutaneous transluminal coronary angioplasty (PTCA) and stent placement or coronary artery bypass grafting (CABG). Intraaortic balloon pump (IABP) support may be used in critically ill patients to provide increased coronary artery perfusion and to decrease afterload.

Myocardial Infarction

Pathophysiology

Prolonged ischemia due to an imbalance between oxygen supply and oxygen demand causes irreversible cell damage and muscle death. Although multiple factors can contribute to the imbalance between oxygen supply and oxygen demand, coronary artery thrombosis characterizes most infarctions. Plaque rupture is believed to trigger the development of the thrombus in most patients with myocardial infarction (see Box 14-1, p. 180).

Irreversible damage to the myocardium can begin as early as 20 to 40 minutes after interruption of blood flow. However, the dynamic process of infarction may not be completed for several hours. Necrosis of tissue appears to occur sequentially (ie, cellular death first occurs in the subendocardial layer and then spreads throughout the thickness of the heart wall). Transmural infarction is an infarction that produces necrosis that extends through all the layers of the myocardium. If the area of the transmural infarction is small, the damaged myocardium may become dyskinetic (ie, unable to contract in a coordinated fashion). If the area of infarction is more extensive, the damaged myocardium may become akinetic (ie, unable to contract at all). As a result, cardiac output is compromised.

Most myocardial infarctions affect the left ventricle, although infarctions can also occur in the right ventricle or in both ventricles (Box 14-3). The larger the area of infarction, the greater the impact on ventricular function. Several factors determine the size of the infarction, including

- The extent, severity, and duration of the ischemic episode
- The metabolic demands of the myocardium at the time of the event
- The size of the occluded vessel
- The amount of collateral circulation (ie, smaller arteries that under normal conditions carry very little of the blood flow but, in the presence of an occlusion, enlarge and dilate over time, creating an alternate route for blood flow)
- Vascular tone
- The status of the intrinsic fibrinolytic system

Several complications can develop following an acute myocardial infarction (Box 14-4). Some of the most life-threatening include cardiogenic shock, ventricular septal rupture, left ventricular free wall rupture, thromboembolism, and dysrhythmias.

- **Cardiogenic shock** (discussed in Chapter 33) occurs when loss of contractile forces results in left ventricular dysfunction. Clinical manifestations of cardiogenic shock include a rapid, thready pulse; a narrow pulse pressure; dyspnea; tachypnea; inspiratory crackles; distended neck veins; chest pain; cool, moist skin; oliguria; and decreased mentation. ABGs reveal a decreased arterial oxygen tension (PaO_2) and respiratory alkalosis. Hemodynamic findings include a systolic blood pressure less than 85 mm Hg, a mean arterial pressure (MAP) less than 65 mm Hg, a cardiac index less than 2.2 L/min/m², and a pulmonary artery occlusive pressure (PAOP) greater than 18 mm Hg. Cardiac enzymes may show an additional rise or a delay in reaching peak values.
- **Ventricular septal rupture** occurs in about 1% of patients with myocardial infarction and accounts for approximately 11% of all in-hospital deaths.[2,3] The greatest risk for ventricular septal rupture is within the first 24 hours and continues for up to 5 days. The patient presents with a new, loud, holosystolic murmur associated with a thrill felt in the parasternal area. In addition, the patient has progressive dyspnea, tachycardia, and pulmonary congestion. Oxygen samples taken from the right atrium, right ventricle, and pulmonary artery catheter (distal lumen) show a higher PaO_2 in the right ventricle than in the right atrium because the

BOX 14-3 Infarction Location

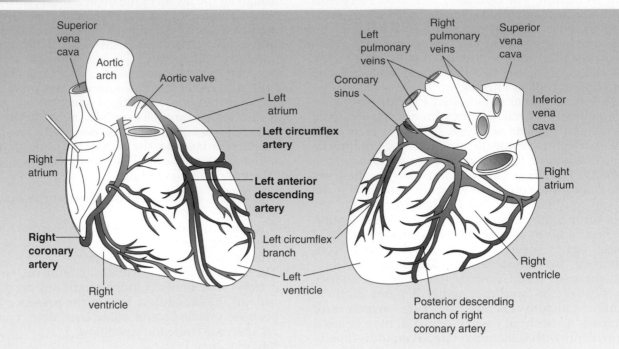

Affected Area of Heart	Occluded Coronary Artery	Structures Supplied	Potential Consequences
Anterior left ventricle, interventricular septum (anteroseptal)	Left anterior descending artery	Anterior wall of left ventricle, interventricular septum, ventricular conducting tissue	• Heart failure, pulmonary edema, cardiogenic shock, and death (due to impaired left ventricular function) • Intraventricular conduction disturbances (eg, bundle branch blocks, fascicular blocks)
Lateral and posterior left ventricle	Left circumflex artery	Lateral and posterior walls of the left ventricle, sinoatrial (SA) node (50% of patients), atrioventricular (AV) node (10% of patients)	• Impaired left ventricular function (although less than with anteroseptal infarctions) • Dysrhythmias associated with dysfunction of the SA or AV nodes (eg, sinus arrest, wandering atrial pacemaker, sinus pause, junction rhythm)
Inferior left ventricle, right ventricle	Right coronary artery	Inferior wall of the left ventricle, right ventricle, SA node (50% of patients), AV node (90% of patients)	• Dysrhythmias associated with dysfunction of the SA and AV nodes (eg, bradycardia, heart blocks) • Concomitant inferior ventricular wall and right ventricular infarction • Significant hemodynamic compromise (due to biventricular dysfunction)

oxygenated left ventricular blood is shunted to the right ventricle. Urgent cardiac catheterization and surgical correction are needed. The patient is supported with fluid administration, inotropic agents (dopamine and dobutamine), afterload reduction (nitroprusside), and IABP counterpulsation until emergency surgery is possible.

• **Left ventricular free wall rupture** occurs in about 1% to 2% of patients with myocardial infarction and accounts for approximately 10%

of in-hospital deaths.[2] Left ventricular free wall rupture is more likely to occur either within the first 24 hours after myocardial infarction or 3 to 5 days after myocardial infarction. Clinical findings include prolonged chest pain, dyspnea, sudden hypotension, jugular venous distention, tamponade, and pulseless electrical activity. Left ventricular free wall rupture occurs so suddenly and with such severity that lifesaving efforts are often futile.

BOX 14-4 Complications of Acute Myocardial Infarction

Vascular Complications
- Recurrent ischemia
- Recurrent infarction

Myocardial Complications
- Diastolic dysfunction
- Systolic dysfunction
- Heart failure
- Cardiogenic shock/hypotension
- Right ventricular infarction
- Ventricular cavity dilation
- Aneurysm formation (true, false)

Mechanical Complications
- Left ventricular free wall rupture
- Ventricular septal rupture
- Papillary muscle rupture with acute mitral regurgitation

Pericardial Complications
- Pericarditis
- Dressler's syndrome
- Pericardial effusion

Thromboembolic Complications
- Mural thrombosis
- Systemic thromboembolism
- Deep venous thrombosis (DVT)
- Pulmonary embolism

Electrical Complications
- Ventricular tachycardia
- Ventricular fibrillation
- Supraventricular tachydysrhythmias
- Bradydysrhythmias
- Atrioventricular (AV) block (first, second, or third degree)

From Becker RC: Complicated myocardial infarction. Crit Pathways Cardiol 2(2):125 152, 2003.

- **Thromboembolism** occurs in about 5% to 10% of patients with myocardial infarction. Patients are often predisposed to deep venous thrombosis (DVT) because of the systemic inflammatory response associated with infarction, immobility, venous stasis, and reduced cardiac output. Pulmonary embolism develops in about 10% to 15% of patients with DVT. After myocardial infarction, patients are also at risk for systemic emboli that usually originate in the wall of the left ventricle. These emboli can occlude the cerebral, renal, mesenteric, or iliofemoral artery. Patients are systemically anticoagulated with unfractionated heparin or low-molecular-weight heparin (LMWH), followed by warfarin for 6 to 12 months.

- **Dysrhythmias** often accompany acute infarctions. Because ischemic myocardium has a lower fibrillatory threshold, few ventricular dysrhythmias are considered benign after an infarct. Supraventricular dysrhythmias (eg, atrial fibrillation, atrial flutter) may be the result of high left atrial pressures caused by left ventricular failure. Conduction defects may also occur. Prophylactic antidysrhythmics during the first 24 hours of hospitalization are not recommended. However, easy access to atropine, lidocaine, amiodarone, transcutaneous pacing patches, transvenous pacing wires, a defibrillator, and epinephrine is essential. Cardioversion may be used to treat patients with new onset atrial fibrillation. Transcutaneous pacing may be indicated in an emergent situation for heart block dysrhythmias until a transvenous temporary pacemaker or permanent pacemaker can be placed. Some patients with ventricular dysrhythmias may require an implantable cardioverter–defibrillator (ICD).

Assessment

History and Physical Examination

The most common presenting complaint of a patient with myocardial infarction is chest discomfort or pain. Unlike the pain of angina, the pain of myocardial infarction is often more prolonged and unrelieved by rest or sublingual nitroglycerin. Additional symptoms include diaphoresis, dyspnea, weakness, fatigue, anxiety, restlessness, confusion, shortness of breath, or a sense of impending death. Some patients (especially those with inferior wall infarction) experience nausea and vomiting (believed to be related to the severity of the pain and vagal stimulation).

On physical examination, the patient may be restless, agitated, and in distress. The skin is cool and moist. Vital signs may show a low-grade fever, hypertension, and tachycardia from increased sympathetic tone or hypotension and bradycardia from increased vagal tone. The pulse may be irregular and faint. Auscultation of the heart may reveal a diminished S_1 due to decreased contractility, an S_4 (due to decreased left ventricular compliance), or an S_3 (due to ventricular dysfunction and heart failure). Transient systolic murmurs may be heard because of papillary muscle dysfunction. After about 48 to 72 hours, many patients develop a pericardial friction rub. Additional findings on physical examination, such as jugular venous distention; labored, rapid breathing; or fine crackles, coarse crackles, or rhonchi on auscultation of the lungs may indicate the development of complications such as heart failure or pulmonary edema. Patients with right ventricular infarcts may present with jugular venous distention as well as peripheral edema and elevated central venous pressure (CVP).

TABLE 14-1 Electrocardiographic (ECG) Findings in Different Types of Myocardial Infarctions

Anatomical Location	ECG Evidence
Anteroseptal wall	V_1 through V_4: Q waves and ST-segment elevations
Lateral wall	I, aVL, V_5, and V_6: Q waves and ST-segment elevations
Posterior wall	V_1 and V_2: tall upright R waves with ST-segment depression
	V_7 through V_9: Q waves and ST-segment elevation
Inferior wall	II, III, aVF: Q waves and ST-segment elevation
Right ventricular wall	RV_1 through RV_6 (right precordial chest leads): Q waves and ST-segment elevations.

Electrocardiography

Myocardial infarction is characterized by changes in the T wave, the ST segment, and the Q wave that evolve over time (see Fig. 14-3). Within a few days after the infarction, the elevated ST segments return to baseline. Persistent elevation of the ST segment may indicate the presence of a ventricular aneurysm. The T waves may remain inverted for several weeks, indicating areas of ischemia near the infarct region. Eventually, the T waves should return to their upright configuration. The Q waves do not disappear and therefore always provide electrocardiographic evidence of a previous infarction. Abnormal Q waves accompanied by ST-segment elevations indicate an acute infarction, whereas abnormal Q waves accompanied by a normal ST segment indicate a previous infarction.

A routine 12-lead ECG does not provide an adequate view of the right ventricle or of the posterior wall of the left ventricle; therefore, additional leads are needed to view these areas. To attain an accurate view of the right ventricle, right-sided chest leads are recorded by placing the six chest electrodes on the right side of the chest using landmarks analogous to those used on the left side. These six right-sided views are examined for patterns of ischemia, injury, and infarction in the same way left-sided chest leads are evaluated. To detect posterior wall abnormalities, the leads anatomically opposite the posterior wall (ie, V_1 and V_2) are examined and the principle of reciprocal change is used. If tall R waves with ST-segment depressions are noted in V_1 and V_2, the pattern is consistent with a posterior wall infarction. Electrocardiographic findings for patients with various types of myocardial infarctions are summarized in Table 14-1.

Laboratory Tests

When myocardial cells are damaged by an infarction, biochemical markers are released into the bloodstream and can be detected by laboratory tests (Fig. 14-4):

- Within 1 to 4 hours of infarction, myoglobin appears in the serum; the peak occurs at 6 to 7 hours.
- Within 4 to 6 hours, the MB isoform of creatinine kinase (CK-MB) begins to appear in serum, and it peaks after approximately 18 to 24 hours. However, the appearance and peak of CK-MB may occur significantly earlier in patients who have a non–Q-wave infarction or who have undergone successful reperfusion therapy (eg, angioplasty or thrombolysis). Because elevated CK-MB values return to baseline 36 to 40 hours after infarction in patients who do not have ongoing necrosis, resampling can be used to detect reinfarction.

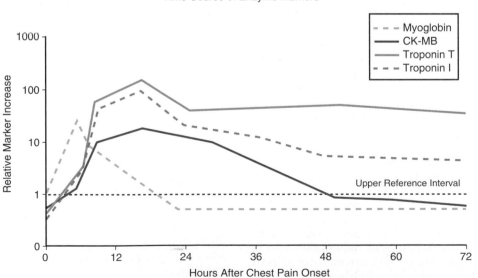

Time Course of Enzyme Markers

FIGURE 14-4 Peak elevation and duration of serum enzymes after acute myocardial infarction.

- Within 4 to 6 hours, an increase in troponin levels is detected, with levels generally peaking 24 hours after the onset of symptoms. As with CK-MB, serial testing is required and reperfusion strategies change the timing of the peak troponin value. Troponins remain elevated for up to 10 days after the cardiac event, facilitating diagnosis of patients who delay seeking treatment.

Diagnostic Studies

A chest radiograph and echocardiogram, obtained as soon as possible, are useful in ruling out an aortic dissection and acute pericarditis and detecting structural abnormalities (eg, valve defects). Other diagnostic studies that may be ordered during the course of the patient's hospitalization or shortly after discharge may include

- Radionuclide studies, to provide information about the presence of CAD as well as the location and quantity of ischemic and infracted myocardium
- Magnetic resonance imaging (MRI), to reveal structural and functional abnormalities of the heart and aorta
- Coronary magnetic resonance angiography (MRA), which uses the principles of MRI in combination with a contrast medium to create images of vessel walls and plaques

- Computed tomography (CT) and CT angiography, to obtain information about the circulation of blood in the heart and coronary arteries
- Coronary angiography, to help the physician determine whether PTCA or stent placement is indicated, or if the patient is a candidate for CABG
- Stress testing, to assess the patient's functional capacity and ability to perform activities of daily living (ADLs), to evaluate the efficacy of the patient's medical therapy, and to risk-stratify the patient based on the likelihood of a subsequent cardiac event

Management

Early Management

Early management entails confirming the diagnosis of myocardial infarction and initiating reperfusion therapy. Diagnosis and initial management must be rapid because the benefit of reperfusion therapy is greatest if therapy is initiated quickly. The initial diagnosis of myocardial infarction is based primarily on the patient's symptoms, the 12 lead ECG, and the serial cardiac enzymes. If the initial screening suggests infarction, the interventions listed in Table 14-2 are initiated. The nurse also checks the vital signs frequently, establishes IV access, and continuously assesses the patient's cardiac rhythm. Blood

TABLE 14-2 Initial Management of the Patient With a Suspected Myocardial Infarction

Action	Rationale
Administer aspirin, 160–325 mg chewed.	Platelets are one of the main components in thrombus formation when a coronary plaque is disrupted, and aspirin diminishes platelet aggregation.
After recording the initial 12-lead ECG, place the patient on a cardiac monitor and obtain serial ECGs.	The 12-lead ECG is central in the decision pathway for the diagnosis and treatment of the patient. Continuous cardiac monitoring is used to detect dysrhythmias and to monitor ST-segment changes.
Give oxygen by nasal cannula and apply a pulse oximeter. If severe pulmonary edema is present and the patient is in respiratory distress, intubation may be necessary.	Pulmonary edema often causes hypoxemia in patients with myocardial infarction.
Administer sublingual nitroglycerin (unless the systolic blood pressure is less than 90 mm Hg or the heart rate is less than 50 or greater than 100 beats/min). Give 0.4 mg every 5 min for a total of three doses. IV nitroglycerin is recommended for patients with acute myocardial infarction with persistent pain, for control of hypertension, or for management of pulmonary congestion.	Sublingual nitroglycerin helps to promote vasodilation (but is relatively ineffective in relieving pain in the early stages of a myocardial infarction).
Provide adequate analgesia with morphine sulfate (2–4 mg IV; doses can be repeated every 5 min until the pain is relieved).	Morphine is the drug of choice to relieve the pain of a myocardial infarction.
Administer β-adrenergic blocker.	During the first few hours after the onset of ST-segment elevation myocardial infarction (STEMI), β-adrenergic blockers may diminish myocardial oxygen demand by reducing heart rate, systemic arterial pressure, and myocardial contractility.

From Antman EM, Anbe DT, Armstrong PW, et al.: ACC/AHA guidelines for the management of patients with ST-elevation myocardial infarction. A report of the American College of Cardiology/American Heart Association Task Force on Practice Guidelines (Committee to revise the 1999 guidelines for the management of patients with acute myocardial infarction). Circulation 110:e82–e293, 2004.

is drawn for serum cardiac markers, hematology, chemistry, and a lipid profile. During the initial evaluation, the patient and family may be anxious. To help alleviate anxiety, the nurse provides reassurance, support, and brief and clear explanations of interventions.

Fibrinolytic Therapy. Fibrinolytic agents may be used in the treatment of patients with acute STEMI, and for those with ST-segment depression if a posterior myocardial infarction is suspected.[4] Fibrinolytic therapy provides maximum benefit if given within 4 hours of the onset of symptoms, and there is a time-dependent decrease in efficacy.[4] These drugs are not effective or appropriate for patients without ST-segment elevation or with nonspecific ECG changes. Unless contraindicated (see Chapter 13, Box 13-1), fibrinolytics may be given to patients with STEMI who meet either of the following criteria:

- Onset of symptoms within the previous 12 hours and ST-segment elevation greater than 0.1 mV in two or more contiguous precordial leads or in two or more adjacent limb leads, or
- New-onset left bundle branch block

The patient is closely monitored during and after the infusion of a fibrinolytic agent. The nurse assesses the patient for signs of reperfusion, which include resolution of chest pain, normalization of elevated ST segments, and the development of reperfusion dysrhythmias (eg, accelerated idioventricular rhythm, ventricular tachycardia, atrioventricular (AV) block). In addition, the nurse assesses for complications from the drug therapy (eg, allergic reactions, bleeding, hypotension), and for reocclusion of the coronary artery. Indicators of reocclusion include new onset of chest pain, return of ST-segment elevation, and hemodynamic instability.

Percutaneous Transluminal Coronary Angioplasty. PTCA may be used instead of fibrinolytic therapy for patients with STEMI who present within 12 hours of the onset of symptoms, for patients with NSTEMI, and for patients with persistent ischemic symptoms. The nurse carefully monitors the patient after a PTCA for retroperitoneal or vascular hemorrhage, other evidence of bleeding, early acute reocclusion, and late restenosis. If PTCA is not successful, the patient may be evaluated for emergent CABG surgery.

Ongoing Management

As the patient progresses out of the immediate crisis stage, the goal of management continues to be maximizing cardiac output while minimizing cardiac workload. Monitoring includes frequent vital sign assessment, continuous cardiac monitoring with ST-segment monitoring, and serial 12- lead ECGs and serum cardiac marker testing. Prompt recognition and management of complications (see Box 14-4) is essential in reducing mortality and morbidity. For the first 12 hours of hospitalization, patients who are hemodynamically stable and free of ischemic chest discomfort remain on bedrest with bedside commode

privileges, and then their activity level is gradually increased. When the oxygen saturation level is stable for more than 6 hours, the need for continuous oxygen therapy is reassessed and the fraction of inspired oxygen (FiO_2) may be weaned down.

The patient is often not given anything by mouth until the pain has resolved. After the pain has resolved, the patient is given clear liquids and progressed to a heart-healthy diet as tolerated. Daily weights are recorded, and intake and output are measured to detect fluid retention. Stool softeners are administered to prevent straining, which can cause sudden and significant changes in systolic blood pressure and heart rate (Valsalva maneuver), placing the patient at risk for ventricular dysrhythmias. A collaborative care guide for patients with acute myocardial infarction is given in Box 14-5.

Pharmacotherapy. Medications administered to patients with myocardial infarction may include the following:

- Daily aspirin is administered indefinitely.
- IV unfractionated heparin or LMWH is used in patients after STEMI who are at high risk for systemic emboli. The risk is highest in patients with an anterior myocardial infarction, atrial fibrillation, cardiogenic shock, or a previous embolus.[4]
- Angiotensin-converting enzyme (ACE) inhibitors are administered orally within the first 24 hours to patients with anterior wall myocardial infarction, pulmonary congestion, or a left ventricular ejection fraction less than 40%, in the absence of hypotension. ACE inhibitors help prevent ventricular remodeling and preserve ejection fraction.[4]
- An insulin infusion may be required to normalize the patient's blood glucose levels during the first several days following STEMI.
- Magnesium is indicated for patients with a documented magnesium deficit and for those with torsades de pointes ventricular tachycardias due to prolonged QT intervals.
- β-Adrenergic blockers are administered intravenously during the initial hours of the evolving infarction, followed by oral therapy provided there are no contraindications. Calcium channel blockers may be given to patients in whom β-adrenergic blocker therapy is ineffective or contraindicated.
- Nitrate therapy may be continued beyond the first 24 to 48 hours for patients with recurrent angina or persistent heart failure.
- Statins are given within the first 24 hours and may be continued for 6 months or indefinitely.
- Antiplatelet (eg, Clopedigrel (Plavix)) is administered for a minimum of 3 months following the placement of a bare metal stent and up to 12 months following a drug–eluting stent placement.

Hemodynamic Monitoring. Pulmonary artery pressure monitoring is indicated in patients with myocardial infarction who have severe or progressive heart failure, pulmonary edema, cardiogenic shock, progressive hypotension, or suspected mechanical

BOX 14-5 COLLABORATIVE CARE GUIDE for the Patient With Myocardial Infarction

OUTCOMES	INTERVENTIONS
Oxygenation/Ventilation	
ABGs are within normal limits and pulse oximeter value is >90%.	• Assess respiratory rate, effort, and breath sounds q2–4h. • Obtain ABGs per order or signs of respiratory distress. • Monitor arterial saturation by pulse oximeter. • Provide supplemental oxygen by nasal cannula or face mask for the first 6 h then as needed. • Provide intubation and mechanical ventilation as necessary.
Pulmonary edema is minimized on chest x-ray and demonstrated by improved breath sounds.	• Obtain chest x-ray daily. • Administer diuretics per order. • Monitor signs of fluid overload.
The patient is without evidence of atelectasis.	• Encourage nonintubated patients to use incentive spirometer and perform coughing and deep breathing q4h and PRN. • While on bedrest, turn side to side q2h.
Circulation/Perfusion	
Vital signs are within normal limits, including MAP >70 mm Hg and cardiac index >2.2 L/min/m².	• Monitor HR and BP q1–2h and PRN during acute failure phase. • Assist with pulmonary artery catheter insertion. • Monitor pulmonary artery pressures and PAOP, CVP, or RAP q1h and cardiac output, systemic vascular resistance, and pulmonary vascular resistance q2–4h (may also use a continuous CO monitor) if pulmonary artery catheter is in place. • Maintain patent IV access. • Administer positive inotropic agents, and reduce afterload with vasodilating agents guided by hemodynamic parameters and physician orders. • Evaluate effect of medications on BP, HR, and hemodynamic parameters. • Prepare the patient for IABP assist if necessary.
The patient has no evidence of heart failure due to decreased cardiac output.	• Restrict volume administration as indicated by PAOP or CVP values. • Assess for neck vein distention, pulmonary crackles, S_3 or S_4, peripheral edema, increased preload parameters, elevated "a" wave of CVP or PAOP waveform. • Monitor 12-lead ECG qd and PRN.
The patient has no evidence of further myocardial dysfunction, such as altered ECG or cardiac enzymes.	• Monitor cardiac markers, Mg, PO_4, Ca^{2+}, and K^+ as ordered. • Monitor ECG for changes consistent with evolving myocardial infarction. • Consider obtaining right sided 12 lead ECG if an inferior wall MI to determine RV involvement. • Report and treat abnormalities per protocols or orders.
Dysrhythmias are controlled.	• Provide continuous ECG monitoring in the appropriate lead. • Document rhythm strips every shift. • Anticipate need for/administer pharmacological agents to control dysrhythmias.
After fibrinolytic therapy, the patient has relief of pain; no evidence of bleeding; no evidence of allergic reaction.	• Assess, monitor, and treat pain. • Monitor for signs of reperfusion, such as dysrhythmias, ST-segment return to baseline, early rise and peak in CK. • Monitor for signs of bleeding, including neurological, gastrointestinal, and genitourinary assessment. • Monitor prothrombin time (PT), activated partial thromboplastin time (aPTT), anticoagulation therapy per protocol. • Have anticoagulant antidotes available, if the drug has an antidote. • Assess for itching, hives, sudden onset of hypotension or tachycardia. • Administer hydrocortisone or diphenhydramine per protocol.
There is no evidence of cardiogenic shock, cardiac valve dysfunction, or ventricular septal defect.	• Monitor ECG, heart sounds, hemodynamic parameters, level of consciousness, and breath sounds for changes. • Report and treat deleterious changes as indicated.

(continued on page 190)

BOX 14-5 COLLABORATIVE CARE GUIDE for the Patient With Myocardial Infarction (continued)

OUTCOMES	INTERVENTIONS
Fluids/Electrolytes Renal function is maintained as evidenced by urine output >30 mL/h, normal laboratory values.	• Monitor intake and output q1–2h. • Monitor BUN, creatinine, electrolytes qd and PRN. Take daily weights. • Administer fluid volume and diuretics as ordered.
Mobility/Safety The patient complies with ADL limitations. The patient does not fall or accidentally harm himself or herself.	• Provide clear explanation of limitations. • Provide bedrest with bedside commode privileges first 12 h. • Progress to chair for meals, bathing self, bathroom privileges. Continually assess patient response to all activities. • Provide environmental modifications to prevent falls, bruising, or injury. • Use restraints as indicated and per facility policy.
Skin Integrity The patient has no evidence of skin breakdown.	• Turn side to side q2h while the patient is on bedrest. • Evaluate skin for signs of pressure areas when turning. • Consider pressure relief/reduction mattress for high-risk patients. • Use Braden scale to monitor risk for skin breakdown.
Nutrition Caloric and nutrient intake meet metabolic requirements per calculation (eg, basal energy expenditure). The patient has normal laboratory values reflective of nutritional status.	• Provide appropriate diet: oral, parenteral, or enteral feeding. • Provide clear or full liquids the first 24 h. • Restrict sodium, fat, cholesterol, fluid, and calories if indicated. • Consult dietitian or nutritional support services. • Monitor albumin, prealbumin, transferrin, cholesterol, triglycerides, total protein.
Comfort/Pain Control The patient has relief of chest pain. There is no evidence of pain, such as increased HR, BP, RR, or agitation during activity or procedures.	• Use visual analog scale to assess pain quantity. • Assess quality, duration, location of pain. • Administer IV morphine sulfate, and monitor pain and hemodynamic response. • Administer analgesics appropriately for chest pain and assess response. • Monitor physiological response to pain during procedures or after administration of pain medication. • Provide a calm, quiet environment.
Psychosocial The patient demonstrates decreased anxiety by calm demeanor and vital signs during, for example, procedures, discussions. The patient and family demonstrate understanding of myocardial infarction and treatment plan by asking questions and participating in care.	• Assess vital signs during treatments, discussions, and so forth. • Provide explanations and stable reassurance in calm and caring manner. • Cautiously administer sedatives and monitor response. • Consult social services and clergy as appropriate. • Assess coping mechanism history. • Allow free expression of feelings. • Encourage patient and family participation in care as soon as feasible. • Provide blocks of time for adequate rest and sleep.

BOX 14-5 COLLABORATIVE CARE GUIDE for the Patient With Myocardial Infarction (continued)

OUTCOMES	INTERVENTIONS
Teaching/Discharge Planning	
The patient reports occurrence of chest pain or discomfort.	• Explain importance of reporting all episodes of chest pain.
	• Provide frequent explanations and information to the patient and family.
Family demonstrates appropriate coping during the critical phase of an acute myocardial infarction.	• Encourage family to ask questions regarding treatment plan, patient response to therapy, prognosis, and so forth.
In preparation for discharge to home, the patient and family understand activity levels, dietary restrictions, medication regimen, what to do if pain recurs.	• Make appropriate referrals and consults early during hospitalization.
	• Initiate education regarding heart-healthy diet, cardiac rehabilitation program, stress-reduction strategies, management of chest pain.

complications. The PAOP is closely followed for assessment of left ventricular filling pressures. A PAOP below 18 mm Hg may indicate volume depletion, whereas a PAOP greater than 18 mm Hg indicates pulmonary congestion or cardiogenic shock. Continuous cardiac output monitoring is used to evaluate the cardiac output and cardiac index. In some situations, monitoring venous oxygen saturation may also be useful. Invasive arterial monitoring is indicated for patients with myocardial infarction who have severe hypotension or for those receiving vasopressor or vasodilator drugs.

Heart Failure

Heart failure is a clinical syndrome characterized by shortness of breath, dyspnea on exertion, paroxysmal nocturnal dyspnea, orthopnea, and peripheral or pulmonary edema. It has many causes, related either to impaired cardiac function or excessive work demands (Box 14-6).

BOX 14-6 Causes of Heart Failure

Impaired Cardiac Function
• Myocardial disease (eg, cardiomyopathies, myocarditis, coronary insufficiency, myocardial infarction)
• Valvular heart disease (stenotic or regurgitant)
• Congenital heart defects
• Constrictive pericarditis

Excess Work Demands
• Increased pressure work (eg, systemic hypertension, pulmonary hypertension, coarctation of the aorta)
• Increased volume work (eg, arteriovenous shunt, fluid overload)
• Increased perfusion work (eg, thyrotoxicosis, anemia)

Heart failure may be acute or chronic. Acute heart failure is the sudden appearance of symptoms, usually over days or hours. Immediate intervention is necessary to save the patient's life. Chronic heart failure is the development of symptoms over months to years. Patients with chronic heart failure may live with minimal or well-controlled symptoms. However, chronic heart failure may become acutely worse. Any factor that increases oxygen demand (eg, hypoxemia, ischemia, hypertension, tachycardia, anemia, exercise), and therefore demand for increased cardiac output beyond the ability of the ventricle to function, can cause an acute exacerbation. Similarly, any factor that depresses the function of the already compromised ventricle (eg, alcohol, drugs that exert a negative inotropic effect such as calcium channel blockers and β-adrenergic blockers) can lead to an exacerbation. Many patients with heart failure have comorbid conditions, such as CAD, hypertension, diabetes mellitus, chronic obstructive pulmonary disease (COPD), and chronic renal insufficiency. Worsening of a comorbid condition may also lead to an acute exacerbation of stable chronic heart failure. Potentially, acute decompensation is reversible if treated quickly and aggressively.

Pathophysiology

The end result of all types of heart failure is insufficient cardiac output. The loss of forward flow (cardiac output) causes a decrease in perfusion to the kidneys and the release of renin. Renin converts angiotensin I to angiotensin II, a potent vasoconstrictor. The vasoconstriction increases the resistance (afterload) that the heart must pump against. Angiotensin II also stimulates the release of aldosterone, which causes the kidneys to retain sodium and water. This increases the circulating volume (preload) and contributes to volume overload. The combination of increased afterload and preload worsens the cardiac output, thus increasing the release of renin from the kidneys and continuing the cycle of heart failure.

Right-Sided Heart Failure

Right-sided heart failure (cor pulmonale) refers to failure of the right ventricle to pump adequately. The most common cause of right-sided heart failure is left-sided heart failure, but right-sided heart failure can also result from pulmonary disease and primary pulmonary artery hypertension. Acute onset of right-sided heart failure is often caused by pulmonary embolus.

Left-Sided Heart Failure

Left-sided heart failure refers to failure of the left ventricle to fill or empty properly. This leads to increased pressures inside the ventricle and congestion in the pulmonary vascular system. The increased pulmonary artery pressures, in turn, lead to orthopnea, possibly pulmonary edema, elevated venous pressures, liver congestion, lower extremity edema, and paroxysmal nocturnal dyspnea. Patients may also present with hypotension, tachycardias, and prerenal azotemia. Heart failure may be classified as systolic and diastolic dysfunction.

Systolic Dysfunction

Systolic dysfunction is usually estimated by ejection fraction, or the percentage of the ventricular end-diastolic volume (VEDV) that is ejected from the ventricle in one cycle. Normal ejection fraction is 50% to 70%. Systolic dysfunction is defined as an ejection fraction of less than 40% and is caused by a decrease in contractility. The ventricle is not emptied adequately because of poor pumping, and the end result is decreased cardiac output.

Diastolic Dysfunction

Diastolic dysfunction is less well defined and more difficult to measure, and it is often referred to as heart failure with preserved left ventricular function. Pumping is normal or even increased, with an ejection fraction as high as 80% at times. Diastolic dysfunction is characterized by impaired relaxation and filling. Ventricular filling is a combination of passive filling and atrial contraction. If the ventricle is stiff and poorly compliant (due to aging, uncontrolled hypertension, hypertrophy, or volume overload), relaxation is slow or incomplete. If the heart rate is fast, diastole is short, or if the patient has atrial fibrillation, there is no organized atrial contraction. These mechanisms all reduce filling of the ventricle and contribute to diastolic dysfunction, therefore decreasing cardiac output.

Assessment

History

The symptoms of heart failure are nonspecific. The history is used to put the symptoms into a context

---

BOX 14-7 **New York Heart Association (NYHA) Functional Classification of Heart Failure**

Class I: No limitation of physical activity. Ordinary physical activity does not cause undue fatigue or dyspnea.

Class II: Slight limitation of physical activity. Comfortable at rest, but ordinary physical activity results in fatigue or dyspnea.

Class III: Marked limitation of physical activity without symptoms. Symptoms are present even at rest. If any physical activity is undertaken, symptoms are increased.

Class IV: Unable to carry on any physical activity without symptoms. Symptoms are present even at rest. If any physical activity is undertaken, symptoms are increased.

---

and differentiate heart failure from other conditions that produce shortness of breath, dyspnea on exertion, coughing, and fatigue (eg, pulmonary disease, deconditioning). Heart failure symptoms typically worsen with activity and improve with rest. Cough and shortness of breath may increase when lying down and improve with sitting up. Determining the severity of symptoms (Table 14-3) aids in establishing functional class (Box 14-7) and evaluating the success of therapy.

The nurse asks the patient about medications (prescription and nonprescription) and herbal supplements because a complete medication history may provide clues to the underlying cause. For example, patients taking nonsteroidal anti-inflammatory drugs (NSAIDs) may present with worsening heart failure and renal function because of the effect of the NSAIDs on renal blood flow.

When the pathophysiological changes of heart failure occur over a long period, the body adapts and compensates. In acute heart failure, there is no time for compensation or adaptation, and the clinical manifestations are severe. Symptoms in patients with an acute exacerbation of heart failure may include

- Increased dyspnea on exertion or rest, decreased exercise tolerance, and increased orthopnea, paroxysmal nocturnal dyspnea, or both
- Weight gain of 5 to 50 lb resulting from fluid retention
- Renal insufficiency with elevated blood urea nitrogen (BUN) and creatinine levels

Physical Examination

The physical findings in heart failure differ depending on whether the patient has acute or chronic heart failure, right and/or left ventricular involvement and whether the dysfunction is systolic or

TABLE 14-3 Assessment of Severity of Heart Failure

Symptom	Measure(s)	Questions
Orthopnea	Number of pillows the patient sleeps on regularly	How many pillows do you sleep on at night? If more than one, is it for comfort or because you cannot breathe with one or two?
Dyspnea on exertion	Number of blocks the patient can walk without stopping to rest or catch breath Number of flights of stairs the patient can climb without stopping to rest or catch breath Number of times the patient must rest while doing ADLs such as toileting or minor housework	How many blocks and flights of stairs can you walk without stopping to rest or catch your breath? Do you stop because you cannot go further or because you want to avoid getting short of breath? For patients who are limited by peripheral vascular disease or orthopedic problems: Do you stop because you cannot breathe or because of pain? Which comes first?
Paroxysmal nocturnal dyspnea	Average number of occurrences per night or week	After you go to bed, do you ever have to sit up suddenly to catch your breath? How much time passes before you can breathe normally? Do you need to do anything besides sit up to relieve the shortness of breath?
Dizziness or light-headedness	Presence or absence (of real concern when symptom occurs when the patient is standing and persists or occurs with activity)	Do you ever become dizzy or light-headed? What are you doing when this occurs?
Chest pain or pressure	Presence or absence	Do you have chest pain or pressure? Do you become short of breath with the chest pain or pressure? Which comes first, the pain or the shortness of breath? (Chest pain that comes after shortness of breath is often caused by the heart failure.)

diastolic. Common physical examination findings are summarized in Box 14-8.

Laboratory Studies

Many laboratory studies are ordered in the initial and ongoing evaluation of a patient with heart failure (Table 14-4). Brain-type natriuretic peptide (BNP) is a naturally occurring substance secreted by the ventricles when overstretched. BNP levels may be used to distinguish between pulmonary and heart failure–related causes of dyspnea (particularly in the emergency department).[5] In addition, BNP is used as a marker for evaluating adequacy of treatment and acute progression of heart failure, but the reliability of BNP for this use has not been established.

Diagnostic Studies

Diagnostic studies include electrocardiography, echocardiography, chest radiography, and exercise testing.

Management

Chronic Heart Failure

A major goal of therapy is symptomatic improvement or, if possible, elimination of symptoms. The underlying cause of the heart failure is identified and treated. If an etiologic factor cannot be identified or cannot be treated, then its manifestations

BOX 14-8 Physical Examination Findings in Heart Failure

General
- Anxiety
- Forward-leaning posture
- Cachexia (chronic)

Cardiovascular
- Hypotension or hypertension
- Tachycardia
- Elevated jugular venous pressure
- Elevated right atrial pressure (RAP)
- Elevated pulmonary artery pressure
- Displaced point of maximal impulse (PMI) (to the left)
- Third heart sound (S_3)
- Murmur (valvular cause)

Respiratory
- Cheyne–Stokes breathing (NYHA class IV)
- Bibasilar crackles
- Wheezing

Abdomen
- Ascites
- Hepatomegaly
- Splenomegaly
- Hepatojugular reflux

Extremities
- Peripheral edema

TABLE 14-4 Laboratory Studies Used in the Evaluation of Heart Failure

Laboratory Study	Purpose	When Performed
Complete blood count	Used to identify any anemia or infection	Yearly if no specific indication With any exacerbation
Iron studies, anemia work-up	Used to rule out hemochromatosis	As needed to evaluate any treatment for iron-deficiency anemia
Thyroid function tests	Used to rule out hyperthyroidism or hypothyroidism as a cause of heart failure	No follow-up unless indicated before initiation of amiodarone
Electrolytes	Used to assess the effects of diuresis on potassium and sodium levels	With changes in diuretic dose, aggressive diuresis, and titration of drugs that affect potassium (ACE inhibitors, angiotensin II receptor blockers [ARBs], spironolactone)
Blood urea nitrogen (BUN) and creatinine	Used to assess renal function; BUN: creatinine ratio distinguishes between prerenal azotemia and kidney disease	With increased edema or an exacerbation With titration of ACE inhibitors
Liver function tests	Used to evaluate bilirubin and alkaline phosphatase (AP) levels, which are often elevated in liver congestion caused by heart failure Used to evaluate albumin levels (low albumin makes peripheral edema more difficult to reduce)	With any exacerbation Before initiation of lipid-lowering drugs or amiodarone
HIV	Used to rule out HIV/AIDS as etiologic factor	As indicated by history or change in status
Lipid panel	Used to assess risk for coronary artery disease (CAD) and nutritional status	Yearly or more often as indicated to evaluate treatment

are treated. Strategies such as sodium restriction, alcohol avoidance, regular exercise, adherence to the medication regimen, and daily weight measurements are very effective for managing symptoms and preventing hospitalizations for acute exacerbations. Several medications are used in the management of chronic heart failure:

- ACE inhibitors are the mainstay of therapy for heart failure. ACE inhibitors work by blocking the renin–angiotensin–aldosterone system, resulting in vasodilation and blocking sodium and water reabsorption. Blockage of the long-term effects of myocardial cell exposure to the renin–angiotensin–aldosterone system is hypothesized to be the mechanism by which ACE inhibitors decrease mortality and limit the progression of remodeling.[6] ACE inhibitors are typically started at low doses and titrated to target doses to avoid hypotension. Angiotensin II receptor blockers (ARBs) may be used for patients who cannot tolerate ACE inhibitors.
- Digoxin is used to manage symptoms and increase exercise tolerance. It is a weak inotrope that also blocks neurohormones such as norepinephrine. Long-term exposure to neurohormones is believed to contribute to the progression of heart failure.
- Loop diuretics are standard therapy for diuresis in patients with heart failure. When patients are receiving large doses yet continue to have edema or have increased edema, diuretic resistance must

be considered. A brief course of an IV diuretic or the addition of a thiazide diuretic until the edema is controlled may be required. The combination of loop and thiazide diuretics works for refractory edema more efficiently than either type of diuretic alone. The resolution of edema should be followed by a return to a loop diuretic alone.
- Spironolactone is a weak diuretic with potassium-sparing properties. It is used in the treatment of heart failure to block the effects of aldosterone.
- β-Adrenergic blockers are used to improve symptoms and increase exercise tolerance.

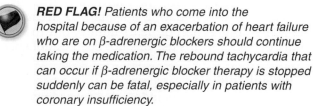

RED FLAG! Patients who come into the hospital because of an exacerbation of heart failure who are on β-adrenergic blockers should continue taking the medication. The rebound tachycardia that can occur if β-adrenergic blocker therapy is stopped suddenly can be fatal, especially in patients with coronary insufficiency.

- Calcium channel blockers are used primarily for patients with diastolic dysfunction. Calcium channel blockers should be avoided in systolic dysfunction because they exert a strong negative inotropic effect but lack the long-term benefits of β-adrenergic blockers.
- Nitrates are venodilators, and their primary effect is to decrease preload. Nitrates are used in heart failure to help alleviate the symptoms of orthopnea and dyspnea on exertion.

Acute Exacerbations of Heart Failure

The main concerns for the care of a patient with an acute exacerbation of chronic heart failure are the same as for any patient with a life-threatening condition. Once the basic priorities (airway, breathing, and circulation) are addressed, etiologic factors and long-term strategies can become the focus of care. Hemodynamic monitoring may be indicated under the following circumstances:

- The patient does not respond to empirical therapy (ie, inotropes and intravenous diuretics) for heart failure.
- The patient has a concomitant respiratory disorder (eg, COPD), and it is necessary to differentiate between pulmonary and cardiac causes of respiratory distress.
- The patient has complex fluid status needs to be evaluated (eg, the patient continues to have peripheral edema or ascites and has renal function parameters indicating worsening prerenal azotemia).

Intubation

The indications for endotracheal intubation in patients with heart failure are the same as for patients in respiratory distress. If the increased work of breathing is leading to fatigue of the respiratory muscles and the arterial carbon dioxide tension ($PaCO_2$) is rising in association with a falling pH, intubation is indicated even if the patient is able to breathe unaided. Noninvasive positive pressure ventilation with bilevel positive pressure (BiPAP) may be used in the acute management of pulmonary edema to avoid more invasive intubation.

Diuresis

Once the airway is protected, attention is directed toward reducing the pulmonary edema. In most cases, aggressive IV diuresis is indicated to facilitate the excretion of excess fluid rapidly and quickly make the patient feel better. If the IV loop diuretic is not sufficient to produce this level of diuresis, a thiazide may be given orally along with the loop diuretic.

Cardiac Output Optimization

The following measures are used to increase cardiac output by optimizing preload, reducing afterload, and increasing contractility.

Fluids

Decreased preload is usually related to iatrogenic overdiuresis. However, patients who are on stable doses of diuretics may become dehydrated if they become hyperglycemic or experience vomiting and diarrhea while continuing to take the prescribed diuretic dose. Careful fluid repletion usually corrects this problem. The symptomatic hypotension and increased BUN and creatinine that are the hallmarks of decreased preload should quickly return to baseline levels.

Inotropes and Inodilators

To increase cardiac output, it is necessary to increase contractility and decrease afterload. Inotropes improve contractility but they also increase myocardial oxygen consumption. To be useful in patients with heart failure, there must be greater improvement in oxygen delivery than in oxygen consumption. The following are indications for the use of inotropes:

- Low cardiac output and high PAOP, especially with symptomatic hypotension
- High PAOP with poor response to diuretics in volume-overloaded patients
- Severe right-sided heart failure that is the result of left ventricular failure
- Symptoms of heart failure at rest despite excellent maintenance therapy

Dopamine is an excellent inotrope at mid-level doses. However, because dopamine is also a vasoconstrictor, especially at higher doses, it increases afterload in patients with heart failure and can decrease stroke volume. Although there are no data to support its use, renal-dose dopamine has been used frequently in patients with heart failure.[7] At low doses of 1 to 3 µg/kg/min, the hypothesized main effect of dopamine is stimulation of dopaminergic receptors that dilate renal and splanchnic circulations.

Inodilators are used to stimulate β-adrenergic receptors in the heart and blood vessels to increase contractility and cause vasodilation. The two inodilators most commonly used in critical care units are dobutamine and milrinone. Because these drugs increase stimulation of β-adrenergic receptors, they are also chronotropic (ie, they increase heart rate), and they must be used carefully and titrated slowly in patients with tachycardia or ventricular dysrhythmia.

The effect of inotropes and inodilators can be measured when a pulmonary artery catheter is in place. As the drugs are titrated to optimum doses, cardiac output increases, and the PAOP decreases. Any organ function that was compromised because of inadequate perfusion should improve (eg, urine output should increase, and BUN and creatinine should return to baseline levels).

Vasodilators

In patients with cardiogenic shock or patients who have an exacerbation related to hypertensive emergency, the afterload is the primary limiting factor. Immediate treatment with parenteral vasodilators is necessary to decrease and control the blood pressure or decrease the workload of the damaged myocardium in order to maintain life or limit end-organ damage. Nitroprusside has the most rapid onset with the shortest half-life of any of these medications. It provides for a rapid decrease in blood pressure, and the effect is limited to minutes if the medication must be stopped because of an exaggerated response. It must be given as a continuous drip and requires reliable monitoring of blood pressure in a setting where emergency resuscitation is available.

Nesiritide, a BNP that is an approved vasodilator for treatment of acute decompensation of chronic heart failure, has had mixed results in studies on clinical efficacy and safety. The ASCEND-HF trial, with over 7000 patients, has shown no significant difference in outcomes when compared to placebo.[8] The study did, however, reinforce the drug's safety, revealing no excess adverse effects although it did not show any improvement over standard care.

Measures to Optimize Heart Rate

Heart rate and rhythm must be optimized for adequate cardiac output. A heart rate that is too fast can compromise filling and, in patients with ischemia, can contribute directly to decreased contractility and increased myocardial oxygenation. A heart rate that is too slow can decrease cardiac output.

If the patient is experiencing bradycardia, the underlying cause must be identified and treated. Bradycardia resulting from ischemic damage to the conduction system is treated with a permanent pacemaker. If the bradycardia is the result of ongoing ischemia, a temporary pacemaker along with treatment of the ischemia is indicated. If the bradycardia is the result of medication, the medication should be held or discontinued until the indication for the medication can be reevaluated. In this situation, β-adrenergic blockers may be held for 24 to 36 hours but should not be discontinued suddenly. If the bradycardia is the result of β-adrenergic blockers, temporary pacing may be required while the drug is titrated down.

In many cases, tachycardia is associated with ischemia or hypertensive crisis, and treatment of the underlying problem also treats the tachycardia. Sinus tachycardia is usually the result of decreased stroke volume and can be resolved by treating the underlying cause of the decreased stroke volume. Treatment of the tachycardia without increasing stroke volume leads to worsening end-organ perfusion. Tachycardia caused by atrial flutter or atrial fibrillation with rapid ventricular response necessitates treatment of the dysrhythmia. If the patient is unstable, direct-current countershock cardioversion is indicated. Otherwise, mechanical methods such as the Valsalva maneuver or carotid massage may be helpful. If medication is required to slow the rhythm, amiodarone is the least dangerous medication to use in systolic dysfunction.

Hypertensive Crisis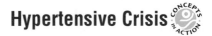

Hypertensive crisis is an acute elevation of blood pressure (greater than 180/120 mm Hg) that is associated with acute or imminent target organ damage.[9] Common causes include exacerbations of chronic hypertension, the sudden withdrawal of antihypertensive medications, and acute or chronic renal disease. Other causes include postsurgical status, pheochromocytoma, eclampsia, and extensive burns. The marked, rapid increase in blood pressure initially leads to intense vasoconstriction as the body attempts to protect itself from the elevated pressure. If the blood pressure remains critically high, compensatory vasoconstriction fails, resulting in increased pressure and blood flow throughout the vascular system. Potential consequences include acute cerebrovascular syndromes (eg, hypertensive encephalopathy, acute stroke), acute cardiovascular syndromes (eg, myocardial infarction, aortic dissection, pulmonary edema), and acute renal damage.

Clinical findings depend on the degree of vascular injury and the type of end-organ damage. Signs of encephalopathy include headache, visual disturbances, confusion, nausea and vomiting, retinal exudates and hemorrhages, and papilledema. Chest pain may be a manifestation of an acute coronary syndrome or aortic dissection. Oliguria or azotemia may be seen in patients with kidney damage.

Most patients who present with hypertensive crisis are critically ill and in need of immediate treatment. The goal is to reduce the mean blood pressure by no more than 25% (to avoid hypoperfusion) within 1 hour of starting treatment, and to prevent or reverse target organ damage.[9] The goal of managing a hypertension encephalopathy is to decrease the MAP by 25% over 8 hours.[10] Several IV medications are used in the treatment of hypertensive crises; the choice depends on availability and the clinical situation (Table 14-5). Constant monitoring with an intra-arterial catheter is necessary to avoid lowering the blood pressure too quickly.

Aortic Disease

Aortic Aneurysm

Aortic aneurysm is a localized dilation of the aorta to a size greater than 1.5 times its normal diameter. True aneurysms involve the entire vessel wall and are classified according to their morphology and location (Fig. 14-5). Fusiform aneurysms, the more common type, are diffuse dilations of the entire circumference of the artery. Saccular aneurysms are localized balloon-shaped outpouchings. False aneurysms (which are not actually aneurysms) are formed when blood leaks through the wall of the aorta and is contained by the surrounding tissues. Aortic aneurysms may be abdominal, thoracic, or both.

- **Abdominal aortic aneurysm** occurs more frequently in men. Smoking is the leading risk factor, followed closely by atherosclerosis, age, hypertension, and lipid disorders.[11] Most patients are asymptomatic. Abdominal or back pain is the most common symptom; worsening of the pain is usually related to expansion or rupture of the aneurysm. Detection of abdominal aortic

TABLE 14-5 IV Medications Used in the Treatment of Hypertensive Emergencies

Drug	Class	Onset of Action
Nitroprusside sodium	Vasodilator	Immediate
Nitroglycerin	Vasodilator	1–2 min
Fenoldopam	Vasodilator	less than 5 min
Hydralazine	Vasodilator	15–30 min
Labetalol	Adrenergic blocker	less than 5 min
Esmolol	Adrenergic blocker	Immediate
Nicardipine	Calcium channel blocker	5–6 min
Enalaprilat	Angiotensin-converting enzyme (ACE) inhibitor	10–15 min

Adapted from Mansoor GA, Frishman WH: Comprehensive management of hypertensive emergencies and urgencies. Heart Dis 4:358, 2002; Tuncel M, Ram VCS: Hypertensive emergencies: Etiology and management. Am J Cardiovasc Drugs 3(1):21–31, 2003.

aneurysm by physical examination is difficult, especially in obese patients. The abdomen is examined for the presence of bruits or masses, and peripheral pulses are carefully evaluated. Abdominal ultrasonography or abdominal CT angiography is the most practical method of confirming the diagnosis.

- **Thoracic aortic aneurysm** is classified by the involved segment of the aorta (root, ascending, arch, or descending). Symptoms, when present, are related to the size and location of the aneurysm and include aortic insufficiency and signs of pericardial tamponade or aortic insufficiency if the aneurysm involves the aortic root.

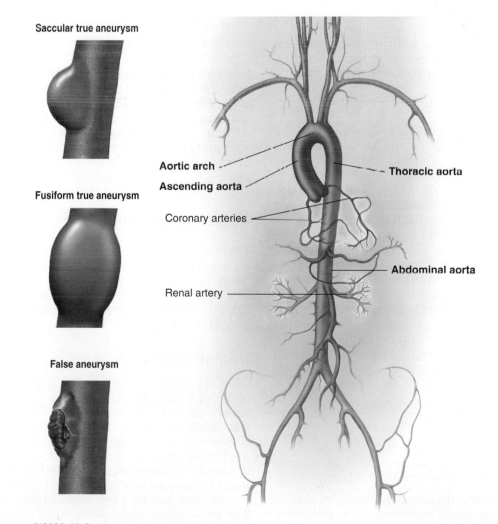

Saccular true aneurysm

Fusiform true aneurysm

False aneurysm

Aortic arch

Ascending aorta

Coronary arteries

Renal artery

Thoracic aorta

Abdominal aorta

FIGURE 14-5 Types of aortic aneurysms.

BOX 14-9 General Indications for Surgical Repair of Aortic Aneurysms

Abdominal
- Diameter greater than or equal to 5.5 cm in men (4.5 to 5.0 cm in women)
- Diameter 4.5 to 5.5 cm; clinical setting, patient preference

Thoracic
- Ascending aorta: diameter greater than or equal to 5.5 cm (5 cm in patients with Marfan syndrome)
- Descending aorta: diameter greater than or equal to 6.0 cm
- Symptoms suggesting expansion or compression of surrounding structures

Other
- Rapidly expanding aneurysms (growth rate greater than 0.5 cm over a 6-month period)
- Symptomatic aneurysm regardless of size

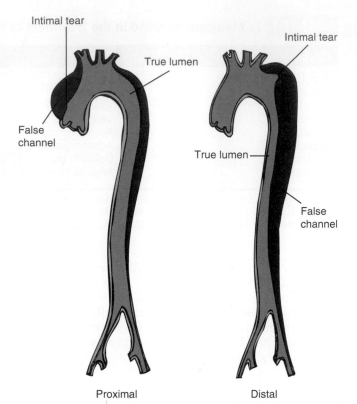

FIGURE 14-6 Two major patterns of aortic dissection.

Serial noninvasive tests (eg, ultrasonography) are used to monitor progression of the aneurysm. Indications for surgical repair are given in Box 14-9. Endovascular repair, a minimally invasive approach to aortic aneurysm repair, is the treatment of choice for high-risk patients.[12] The graft is placed through the femoral artery and anchored to the wall of the aorta with self-expanding or balloon-expanded stents.

Aortic Dissection

Acute aortic dissection is the most common and the most lethal process involving the aorta. Dissection involves a longitudinal separation of the medial layers of the aorta by a column of blood. The dissection begins at a tear in the aortic wall, usually at the proximal end of the dissection. Blood pumped through this tear creates a false channel (lumen) that rapidly becomes larger than the true aortic lumen (Fig. 14-6). The incidence is highest in men older than 60 years with a history of hypertension. Other risk factors include cystic medial degeneration, pregnancy, and trauma.[11]

More than 90% of patients present with sudden, intense chest pain that is frequently described as "ripping" or "tearing." The chest pain may be accompanied by syncope or a latency period of less pain. Additional clinical manifestations depend on the location of the dissection:

- Coronary arteries: cardiac ischemia
- Aortic root: cardiac tamponade and aortic insufficiency
- Aortic arch: neurological deficits
- Renal arteries: elevated serum creatinine, decreased urine output, and severe hypertension

In most patients, the diagnosis is made by detecting the murmur of aortic regurgitation or alteration of the peripheral pulses in patients with known risk factors, such as hypertension. The chest radiograph may show a widened mediastinum. Transesophageal echocardiography (TEE) or contrast medium–enhanced CT may be used to confirm the diagnosis.[11]

Management focuses on controlling blood pressure and pain. Surgery is necessary when the aortic dissection is greater than 4.5 cm in length or rapidly expanding.

Cardiomyopathies

The cardiomyopathies are diseases of the heart muscle that cause cardiac dysfunction resulting in heart failure, dysrhythmias, or sudden death.[21–23] The most common types of primary cardiomyopathies in Western countries are dilated and hypertrophic (Table 14-6).

Dilated Cardiomyopathy

Dilated cardiomyopathy is the third most common cause of heart failure, the most common cause of heart failure in the young, and the most common indication for heart transplantation.[21]

Some patients remain asymptomatic or have minimal clinical findings. Symptoms usually develop gradually and are typically related to left ventricular heart failure. Asymptomatic ventricular tachycardia is common, but its prognostic impact is unknown. The presence of right-sided heart failure is associated with poor prognosis.[22,24]

TABLE 14-6 **Primary Cardiomyopathies**

Cardiomyopathy	Etiology	Pathology	Clinical Manifestations	Management
Dilated	Idiopathic Genetic factors Viral infection Immunodeficiency (eg, HIV) Exposure to toxins (eg, alcohol)	Systolic dysfunction Chamber dilation with normal or reduced left ventricular wall thickness	• Heart failure • Fatigue, weakness • Dysrhythmias • Systemic or pulmonary emboli	• Identify and eliminate potential causes • Manage heart failure, dysrhythmias • Heart transplant • Genetic testing and family screening to identify asymptomatic family members
Hypertrophic	Genetic factors	Diastolic dysfunction Marked hypertrophy of left ventricle, occasionally also of right ventricle, and usually (but not always) disproportionate hypertrophy of septum	• Dyspnea • Angina • Fatigue • Syncope • Palpitations • Dysrhythmias • Heart failure • Sudden death	• Symptomatic treatment • Septal wall ablation or surgery in select patients • Volume reduction surgery • Genetic testing and family screening to identify asymptomatic family members

Dilated figure labels: Increased atrial chamber size; Increased ventricular chamber size; Decreased muscle size

Hypertrophic figure labels: Thickened interventricular septum; Left ventricular hypertrophy

Figures courtesy of the Anatomical Chart Company.

Laboratory tests include screening for potentially reversible causes (see Table 14-6). Echocardiography is used to identify the primary abnormality and determine the ejection fraction. Cardiac catheterization may be needed to exclude CAD.[22,24,25]

Treatment goals include identifying and eliminating potential causes and controlling heart failure, dysrhythmias, and other problems such as intracoronary thrombus. In patients with dilated cardiomyopathy, the incidence of sudden cardiac death from ventricular tachycardia or ventricular fibrillation is very high. For patients who have syncopal episodes or survive sudden death, an ICD is usually indicated. If this device fires frequently or symptomatic nonsustained ventricular tachycardia occurs, amiodarone may be added to the regimen for rhythm control.

Hypertrophic Cardiomyopathy

Hypertrophic cardiomyopathy is probably the most frequently occurring cardiomyopathy in the United States. Sudden death (usually from a ventricular dysrhythmia) is a catastrophic outcome in asymptomatic or mildly symptomatic people of any age group. Early identification of patients at risk for hypertrophic cardiomyopathy (and therefore, sudden death) is imperative. Mortality is higher in younger patients.[24]

Many patients with hypertrophic cardiomyopathy are asymptomatic or have only mild symptoms.[22,24,25] Hypertrophic cardiomyopathy is often found unexpectedly during investigation of heart murmurs or family screening. The most common symptom is dyspnea, which may be exacerbated with exertion. Presyncope and syncope also frequently occur. Left ventricular hypertrophy on the echocardiogram confirms the diagnosis.

Management includes controlling symptoms, preventing complications, and reducing the risk for sudden death through screening.[22,24,26]

Valvular Disease

Cardiac valves maintain the unidirectional flow of blood. If structural changes occur as a result of disease, this function is disrupted. Disease causes either valvular stenosis or insufficiency (regurgitation). The stenotic valve has a narrowed orifice that creates a partial obstruction to blood flow, resulting in increasing pressure behind the valve and decreasing forward blood flow. The insufficient valve is incompetent or leaky; blood flows backward, increasing the pressure and volume behind the valve. Stenosis and insufficiency can occur alone or in combination, in the same valve, or in more than one valve.

Although abnormalities can affect any of the four valves, Table 14-7 focuses on mitral and aortic abnormalities, which are more common and produce profound hemodynamic changes.

Assessment

The diagnosis of valvular disease is suggested by the history, clinical signs and symptoms, physical

TABLE 14-7 Mitral and Aortic Valve Disorders

Disorder	Causes	Pathophysiology	Clinical Manifestations
Mitral stenosis	Rheumatic heart disease	As forward flow from the left atrium to the left ventricle decreases, cardiac output decreases. Blood backed up behind the stenotic valve causes left atrial dilation and increased left atrial pressure, which is reflected backward into the pulmonary circulation. With prolonged high pressures, fluid moves from the pulmonary capillaries into the interstitial space and alveoli. Pulmonary hypertension develops, which can lead to right-sided heart failure.	Fatigue, exertional dyspnea, orthopnea, pulmonary edema, atrial fibrillation
Mitral insufficiency	**Chronic:** Rheumatic heart disease, myxomatous degeneration of the mitral valve, degenerative changes associated with aging, left ventricular dilation	During ventricular systole, some of the ventricular blood regurgitates into the atrium rather than being ejected through the aortic valve, decreasing forward cardiac output. Left ventricular hypertrophy occurs as a compensatory measure, but ultimately worsens the regurgitation. Left ventricular overload causes left ventricular dilation. Regurgitant flow into the left atrium causes increased left atrial pressure and dilatation; volume overload may be reflected backward to the pulmonary circulation.	Fatigue, palpitations, shortness of breath, pulmonary and right-sided heart symptoms (late in the disease process)
	Acute: Endocarditis, chest trauma, myocardial infarction	Cardiac output decreases dramatically. Because of the acute nature, dilation and hypertrophy do not occur.	Pulmonary edema and shock
Aortic stenosis	Rheumatic heart disease, calcification of a congenital bicuspid valve, calcific degeneration (especially in elderly patients)	Obstructed left ventricular outflow leads to diminished cardiac output. The left ventricle hypertrophies to maintain cardiac output. Extreme left ventricular hypertrophy increases myocardial oxygen demand at the same time that cardiac output and coronary artery perfusion are decreased. As the stenosis worsens, compensation fails and volume and pressure overload in the left ventricle causes left ventricular dilation. Increased left ventricular pressures are reflected backward through the left atrium and pulmonary vasculature.	Angina, syncope, exertional dyspnea, orthopnea, and paroxysmal nocturnal dyspnea
Aortic insufficiency	**Chronic:** Rheumatic heart disease, ascending aortic aneurysm	Blood flows backward from the aorta into the left ventricle during ventricular diastole. Forward cardiac output decreases, and left ventricular volume and pressure increase, leading to left ventricular hypertrophy. Eventually, the increase in left ventricular pressure is reflected backward into the left atrium and pulmonary circulation.	Fatigue, low diastolic blood pressure, widened pulse pressure, water-hammer (Corrigan's) pulse, angina
	Acute: Blunt chest trauma, ruptured ascending aortic aneurysm, infective endocarditis	Left-sided heart failure and pulmonary edema develop rapidly because compensatory left ventricular hypertrophy does not have time to develop. In response to the diminished cardiac output, systemic vascular resistance increases to maintain the blood pressure. The increased systemic vascular resistance increases the regurgitation and worsens the situation.	Left-sided heart failure, pulmonary edema

examination, and auscultation of the characteristic murmur (see Chapter 12, Table 12-2). Diagnosis is confirmed by echocardiography and catheterization of both sides of the heart. On the echocardiogram, valvular insufficiency is recognized by regurgitation of the contrast medium backward through the incompetent valve. Stenosis is diagnosed by measuring valvular gradients and calculating the valve area.

- To determine the gradient across the mitral valve, left atrial and left ventricular pressures are measured during diastole. A left atrial diastolic pressure that is 15 to 20 mm Hg higher than left ventricular diastolic pressure means that severe mitral stenosis exists. The normal mitral valve area is 4 to 6 cm^2. An area less than 1.5 cm^2 signifies critical mitral stenosis, and surgery is indicated.
- To determine the gradient across the aortic valve, the left ventricular and aortic root pressures are measured during systole. A gradient of more than 50 mm Hg is associated with clinically significant aortic stenosis. Normal aortic valve area is 2.6 to 3.5 cm^2. Hemodynamically significant aortic stenosis occurs if the valve area is less than 1 cm^2.

Management

Surgery is indicated before left ventricular function deteriorates significantly and the patient's activity becomes severely limited, or before severe signs and symptoms develop. The goals of valvular surgery are to relieve symptoms and restore normal hemodynamics. Surgical intervention consists of either valve reconstruction or valve replacement. Valve reconstruction is associated with decreased operative mortality and fewer thromboembolic and anticoagulation-related complications than valve replacement. Percutaneous balloon valvuloplasty may be used for patients considered too high risk for surgery.

Valve Reconstruction

Reconstruction procedures are more likely to be successful if performed early in the course of disease, before left ventricular function deteriorates and irreparable damage occurs. Most valve reconstruction procedures are performed on the mitral valve. Compared with mitral valve replacement, reconstruction eliminates the need for long-term anticoagulation, decreases the risks for thromboembolism and endocarditis, decreases the need for reoperation, and increases survival. However, for aortic valve disorders, most attempts at reconstruction have not been successful.

Although not indicated for patients with severe mitral stenosis, commissurotomy may be effective for patients with moderate stenosis with minimal calcification. During commissurotomy, the fused commissures are surgically divided. This procedure improves leaflet mobility and increases the mitral valve area, decreasing the degree of stenosis.

BOX 14-10 **Advantages and Disadvantages of Prosthetic Cardiac Valves**

Mechanical Valves
- Good long-term durability
- Adequate hemodynamics
- High risk for thromboembolism requires long-term anticoagulation
- Increased risk for bleeding complications

Biological Valves
- Poor long-term durability
- Better hemodynamics than mechanical valves (except in small sizes)
- No hemolysis
- Low incidence of thromboembolism; possibly no need for anticoagulation
- Fewer bleeding complications

Mitral insufficiency may be treated with annuloplasty if annular dilation is responsible for the regurgitation. Annuloplasty is performed using sutures or a prosthetic ring. The ring is sewn around the mitral annulus so that excess annular tissue is drawn up, reducing the circumference. When an annuloplasty ring is used, anticoagulation is required for 3 months until the ring is endothelialized. If the chordae tendineae are stretched or ruptured, surgical shortening or surgical repair of ruptured chordae can be effective.

Valve Replacement

Valve replacement surgery is done through a median sternotomy incision, and cardiopulmonary bypass and myocardial preservation techniques are used.

Prosthetic valves may be mechanical or biological. Advantages and disadvantages of each type are summarized in Box 14-10.

Infectious and Inflammatory Cardiac Disorders

Infectious and inflammatory diseases of the heart have multiple etiologies, making diagnosis and treatment a clinical challenge. Patients may present with acute pain mimicking myocardial infarction, or may seek medical attention because of fatigue and vague flu-like symptoms. Because of the permanent damage these diseases can cause to structures of the heart, patients often face serious long-term cardiac disability.

Pericarditis

Pericarditis is inflammation of the pericardium. Acute pericarditis is pericarditis that lasts no longer than 1 or 2 weeks.[27,28] Inflammation often involves the adjoining diaphragm. The causes of pericarditis are listed in Box 14-11. Pericarditis can be a primary

BOX 14-11 Causes of Pericarditis

- Idiopathic (90% of patients, usually presumed to be viral)
- Infectious (bacterial, tubercular)
- Autoimmune or inflammatory (eg, systemic lupus erythematosus, Dressler's syndrome)
- Drugs
- Vaccinations
- Neoplasms
- Radiation therapy
- Device implantation (eg, implantable defibrillator)
- Acute myocardial infarction
- Trauma to the chest wall or myocardium, including cardiopulmonary surgery
- Chronic renal failure requiring dialysis

disease or occur secondary to another disorder, such as acute myocardial infarction or renal failure.[28,29] Dressler's syndrome (ie, the development of pericarditis, malaise, fever, and elevated white blood cell count weeks to months after a myocardial infarction) is believed to be the result of an autoimmune reaction that occurs after the myocardial infarct.[24] Infectious pericarditis is common in immunocompromised patients.[30]

Repeated episodes of pericarditis can lead to the formation of adhesions between the layers of the pericardium or between the pericardium and adjacent structures, resulting in constrictive pericarditis.[31] In constrictive pericarditis, diastolic filling is impaired because of the ventricle's inability to expand, eventually leading to a decrease in cardiac output and systemic signs of heart failure. Even with successful surgical removal of the diseased pericardium, the long-term survival rate is poor.[27,31]

Assessment

The primary symptom in acute pericarditis is chest pain.[27,29] The pain tends to be pleuritic and is made worse by breathing deeply or lying supine. Because of the pain associated with breathing, patients frequently complain of dyspnea. Relief is often obtained by sitting up, leaning forward, and taking shallow breaths. The chest pain of pericarditis can be distinguished from ischemic chest pain by its quality (sharp, as opposed to a feeling of heaviness) and the fact that it can be relieved by changing position.

The patient may have general symptoms of an infection (eg, low-grade fever, chills, tachycardia, malaise). The presence of a pericardial friction rub confirms the diagnosis; however, absence of a rub does not rule out pericarditis. The rub may wax and wane and may even transiently disappear during the course of the illness.

The 12 lead ECG is the most important test in establishing acute pericarditis.[27] It shows diffuse ST-segment elevation with an upward concavity and PR-segment depression in all leads (Fig. 14-7). This contrasts with the ECG seen in acute myocardial injury, which typically shows upward convexity (as opposed to concavity) in only the leads facing the injured area (Fig. 14-8).[27–29] Laboratory tests include complete blood count, cardiac enzymes (which may be elevated if the inflammation extends to the myocardium), rheumatoid factors, and antinuclear antibody titers. Blood cultures may be indicated if there is evidence of infection. Viral studies may be obtained if the rest of the diagnostic work-up is negative.

Management

Treatment goals for the patient with pericarditis are to relieve symptoms, eliminate any possible causative agents, and monitor for complications such as constrictive pericarditis or pericardial effusions that could lead to cardiac tamponade.[24,29] Symptom relief includes the use of NSAIDs. Steroids may be indicated in resistant cases in which infectious causes have been excluded. Anticoagulants should be avoided in the patient recovering from myocardial infarction. Most episodes of pericarditis abate over 2 to 6 weeks. Rarely do patients experience recurrent episodes.

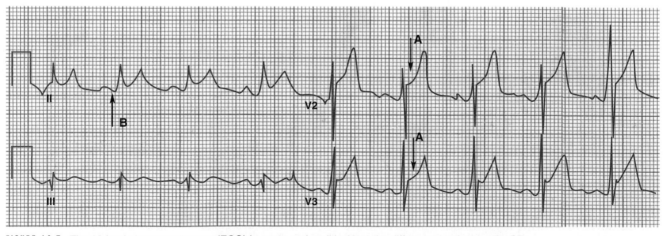

FIGURE 14-7 The 12-lead electrocardiogram (ECG) in acute pericarditis. Note the diffuse upward concavity ST changes (**A**) and the PR-segment depression (**B**).

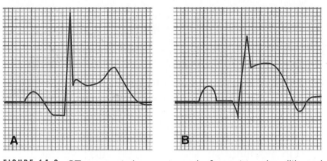

FIGURE 14-8 ST-segment changes seen in **A:** acute pericarditis and **B:** myocardial infarction.

Myocarditis

Myocarditis is an inflammation of the myocardium.[24,32] Some episodes of myocarditis resolve without further sequelae. However, myocarditis can also evolve into a chronic, progressive disease with a poor prognosis. The disorder may result in dysrhythmias or heart failure, and is recognized as a cause of sudden death in young athletes.[33] Myocarditis is believed to be related to an acute infection or an autoimmune response to the infection. Potential causes, which can occur in any age group, are listed in Box 14-12.

Assessment

The clinical presentation of myocarditis is variable. With viral myocarditis, there is typically a delay before the onset of cardiac manifestations (eg, heart failure, dysrhythmias).[24,32] The presence of vague symptoms, such as fatigue, dyspnea, palpitations, and precordial discomfort, accompanied by a slight rise in serum enzymes and nonspecific ST–T-wave changes on the ECG, may point to the diagnosis of myocarditis. Definitive diagnosis requires a positive endomyocardial biopsy.[32,34] However, lack of a positive biopsy does not rule out myocarditis.

Management

Myocarditis is a potentially lethal disease that often has no cure and may require heart transplantation. Although myocarditis evokes a severe inflammatory response, treatment with corticosteroids or immunosuppressive agents has not been shown to be effective in changing the clinical course.[32,34] Treatment is largely supportive, and many of the skills needed by the nurse to care for a patient with myocarditis are similar to those needed to care for a patient with heart failure.

Endocarditis

Endocarditis is an infection of the endocardial surface of the heart, including the valves, caused by bacterial, viral, or fungal agents.[35,36] Infectious endocarditis is a serious illness associated with considerable morbidity and mortality. Common causative organisms include streptococci, enterococci, and *Staphylococcus aureus*. Risk factors are summarized in Box 14-13.[24,35-37]

The development of infectious endocarditis is a complex process.[24,35,37] First, there must be endothelial damage that exposes the basement membrane of the valve to turbulent blood flow. Next, this exposure, especially in patients in a hypercoagulable state, must lead to the development of a platelet and fibrin clot (vegetation) on the valve leaflet. These vegetations must be exposed to bacteria by way of the bloodstream, such as occurs after dental or urological procedures. Finally, bacterial proliferation must take place. The infected vegetation interferes with normal valve function and eventually damages the valve structure, leading to severe heart failure.

BOX 14-12 Potential Causes of Myocarditis

Viruses
- Coxsackie virus
- Adenovirus
- HIV
- Influenza virus

Bacteria
- *Clostridium* species
- *Corynebacterium diphtheriae*
- Streptococci
- Spirochetes (Lyme disease)

Fungi
- *Aspergillus* species
- *Candida* species

Toxins
- Tricyclic antidepressants
- Phenothiazines

BOX 14-13 Risk Factors for Endocarditis

Native Valve Endocarditis
- Mitral valve prolapse
- Congenital heart disease
- Rheumatic heart disease
- Degenerative valve disease (such as aortic stenosis)
- Age greater than 60 years
- IV drug abuse

Prosthetic Valve Endocarditis

Early (Within 60 Days of Surgery)
- Nosocomial infections
- Indwelling catheters
- Endotracheal tubes

Late (After 60 Days)
- Dental, genitourinary, or gastrointestinal manipulations

BOX 14-14 Clinical Features of Endocarditis

- Fever
- Heart murmurs
- Splenomegaly
- Petechiae
    Splinter hemorrhages
    Osler's nodes (small, raised, tender nodules that occur on the fingers or toes)
    Janeway lesions (small erythematous or hemorrhagic lesions on the palms or soles)
- Musculoskeletal complaints
- Systemic or pulmonary emboli
- Neurological manifestations
    Headache
    Mycotic aneurysms

Particles from the infected vegetation or severely damaged valve can break loose and cause peripheral or cerebral emboli.[24,35–37]

Assessment

Clinical manifestations of endocarditis usually occur within 2 weeks of the precipitating infection and are related to four underlying processes: bacteremia or fungemia, valvulitis, immunologic response, and peripheral emboli (Box 14-14).[35,38] Fever and a new or changed heart murmur are present in almost all patients.[35] Nonspecific symptoms (eg, general malaise, anorexia, fatigue, weight loss, night sweats) are common. A careful history focusing on risk factors for infectious endocarditis and a physical examination are needed to alert the nurse to the potential diagnosis of endocarditis.[24]

Definitive diagnosis of infectious endocarditis includes persistent bacteremia caused by pathogens typically responsible for causing infectious endocarditis and evidence of myocardial involvement (eg, echocardiographic visualization of a vegetation or a new or worsening murmur).[39,40]

Management

Rapid diagnosis of infectious endocarditis, initiation of appropriate treatment, and early identification of complications are the keys to good patient outcomes.[24,38] Antibiotic therapy is based on the results of the cultures, the type of heart valve (ie, native or prosthetic), and the prevalence of drug-resistant bacteria.[38] Treatment is usually with a prolonged course of antibiotics and should begin as soon as blood cultures are drawn, without waiting for identification of the specific organism. Immediate surgical intervention is indicated in the presence of severe heart failure secondary to valve dysfunction, uncontrolled infections, and prosthetic valve dysfunction or dehiscence.

CASE STUDY

Mrs. K., a 68-year-old white woman, has been admitted to the critical care unit with shortness of breath at rest. Vital signs are BP, 218/100 mm Hg; HR, 110 beats/min; and RR, 38 breaths/min. She has run out of her antihypertensive medication for the fourth time this year and only came to the hospital because of her breathing difficulties.

On examination, Mrs. K. is pale and clammy sitting upright in a chair. She has bibasilar crackles to her scapulae, and her heart rhythm is irregularly irregular. She has pitting edema bilaterally to her thighs, jugular venous pulsation to the earlobe, and hepatojugular reflux. A chest radiograph shows bilateral infiltrates. An ECG shows a left ventricular ejection fraction of 78% with estimated pulmonary artery pressures of 50 to 55 mm Hg. Laboratory values are unremarkable.

On admission, Mrs. K. is started on lisinopril, 5 mg orally once per day, and given 20 mg of IV furosemide. She is also given 5 mg of IV metoprolol × 3 over the first 24 hours, which results in worsened shortness of breath and frothy sputum. Blood gases show hypoxemia and hypercarbia. She is intubated and placed on a ventilator. Because of her worsening condition, a pulmonary catheter is inserted. Readings are right atrial pressure (RAP) 26 mm Hg; pulmonary artery pressure 68/54 mm Hg; PAOP 36 mm Hg; and cardiac index 1.1 L/min/m². Shortly after the readings are taken, Mrs. K. has a cardiac arrest, from which she cannot be resuscitated.

1. Mrs. K. experienced fluid overload and a hypertensive emergency. What could the healthcare team have done differently in managing her hypertension and fluid overload?

2. Based upon her presentation, physical assessment and hemodynamic numbers, was Mrs. K. experiencing left- or right-sided failure, or both?

3. What role did atrial fibrillation play in Mrs. K.'s heart failure?

References

1. Anderson JL, Adams CD, Antman EM, et al.: ACC/AHA 2007 guidelines for the management of patients with unstable angina/non-ST-segment elevation myocardial infarction: Executive summary. A Report of the American College of Cardiology/American Heart Association Task Force on Practice Guidelines (Writing Committee to Revise the 2002 Guidelines for the Management of Patients With Unstable Angina/Non-ST-Elevation Myocardial Infarction). Circulation 116:803–877, 2007
2. Bhimji S, et al.: Ventricular septal rupture following myocardial infarction, 2008. Retrieved from emedicine.medscape.com
3. Shamshod F, et al.: Fatal myocardial rupture after acute myocardial infarction complicated by heart failure, left ventricular dysfunction or both. Am Heart J 160(1):145–151, 2010

4. Antman EM, Anbe DT, Armstrong PW, et al.: ACC/AHA guidelines for the management of patients with ST-elevation myocardial infarction. A report of the American College of Cardiology/American Heart Association Task Force on Practice Guidelines (Committee to revise the 1999 guidelines for the management of patients with acute myocardial infarction). Circulation 110:e82–e293, 2004

5. 2009 Focused Update ACCF/AHA guidelines for diagnosis and management of heart failure in adults. Circulation 119:1977–2016, 2009

6. Stoller J, Michotery F, Mandell B: Chapter 65: Heart failure. In The Cleveland Clinic Intensive Review of Internal Medicine. Philadelphia, PA: Lippincott Williams & Wilkins, 2009

7. Mehra MR: Optimizing outcomes in the patient with acute decompensated heart failure. Am Heart J 151(3):571–579, 2006

8. O'Conner CM, Staling RC, Hernandez AF: Effect of Nesiritide in patients with acute decompensation heart failure. N Engl J Med 365:32–43, 2011

9. Seventh Report of the Joint National Committee on the Prevention, Detection, Evaluation, and Treatment of High Blood Pressure (JNC 7). Retrieved July 30, 2006, from http://www.nhlbi.nih.gov/guidelines/hypertension

10. Panciolo A: Hypertension management in acute neurological emergencies. Ann Emerg Med 51:524–527, 2008

11. Aortic diseases. In Zipes DP, Libby P, Bonow RO, et al.: (eds): Braunwald's Heart Disease, 9th ed. Philadelphia, PA: Elsevier Saunders, 2011, chapter 60

12. DeBruin JL, et al.: DREAM study group: Long term outcome of open or endovascular repair of abdominal aortic aneurysm. N Engl J Med 362:1863–1871, 2010

13. Isselbacher EM: Thoracic and abdominal aortic aneurysms. Circulation 111:816–828, 2005

14. Katzen BT, Dake MD, MacLean AA, et al.: Endovascular repair of abdominal and thoracic aortic aneurysms. Circulation 112:1663–1675, 2005

15. Maron BJ, Towbin JA, Thiene G, et al.: Contemporary definitions and classification of the cardiomyopathies: An American Heart Association scientific statement from the Council on Clinical Cardiology, Heart Failure and Transplantation Committee; Quality of Care and Outcomes Research and Functional Genomics and Translational Biology Interdisciplinary Working Groups; and Council on Epidemiology and Prevention. Circulation 113:1807–1816, 2006

16. Wynne J, Braunwald E: The cardiomyopathies. In Zipes DP, Libby P, Bonow RO, Braunwald E (eds): Braunwald's Heart Disease, 7th ed. Philadelphia, PA: Elsevier Saunders, 2005, pp 1659–1696

17. Hughes SE, McKenna WJ: New insights into the pathology of inherited cardiomyopathy. Heart 91:257–264, 2005

18. McNeill MM: Pericardial, myocardial, and endocardial disease. In Woods SL, Sivarajan Froelicher ES, Motzer SA, et al.: (eds): Cardiac Nursing, 5th ed. Philadelphia, PA: Lippincott Williams & Wilkins, 2005, pp 776–793

19. Tarolli KA: Left ventricular systolic dysfunction and non-ischemic cardiomyopathy. Crit Care Nurs Q 26:3–15, 2003

20. Ho CY, Seidman CE: A contemporary approach to hypertrophic cardiomyopathy. Circulation 113:858–862, 2006

21. LeWinter MM, Kabbani S: Pericardial diseases. In Zipes DP, Libby P, Bonow RO, et al.: (eds): Braunwald's Heart Disease, 7th ed. Philadelphia, PA: Elsevier Saunders, 2005, pp 1757–1780

22. Lange RA, Hillis LD: Acute pericarditis. N Engl J Med 351(21):2195–2202, 2004

23. Carter T, Brooks CA: Pericarditis: Inflammation or infarction? J Cardiovasc Nurs 20(4):239–244, 2005

24. Maisch B, Ristic AD: Practical aspects of the management of pericardial disease. Heart 89:1096–1103, 2003

25. Wang A, Bashore TM: Undercover and overlooked. N Engl J Med 351(10):1014–1019, 2004

26. Baughman KL, Wynne J: Myocarditis. In Zipes DP, Libby P, Bonow RO, et al.: (eds): Braunwald's Heart Disease, 7th ed. Philadelphia, PA: Elsevier Saunders, 2005, pp 1697–1717

27. Maron BJ, Ackerman MJ, Nishimura RA, et al.: Task Force 4: HCM and other cardiomyopathies, mitral valve prolapse, myocarditis, and Marfan syndrome. J Am Coll Cardiol 45:1340–1345, 2005. Retrieved July 18, 2006, from http://content.onlinejacc.org/ cgi/content/full/45/8/1318

28. Baughman KL: Diagnosis of myocarditis: Death of Dallas criteria. Circulation 113:593–595, 2006

29. Karchmer AW: Infective endocarditis. In Zipes DP, Libby P, Bonow RO, et al.: (eds): Braunwald's Heart Disease, 7th ed. Philadelphia, PA: Elsevier Saunders, 2005, pp 1633–1658

30. Fink AM: Endocarditis after valve replacement surgery. Am J Nurs 106:40–51, 2006

31. Moreillon P, Que Y: Infective endocarditis. Lancet 363:139–149, 2004

32. Baddour LM, Wilson WR, Bayer AS, et al.: Infective endocarditis: Diagnosis, antimicrobial therapy, and management of complications. A statement for health care professionals from the Committee on Rheumatic Fever, Endocarditis, and Kawasaki Disease, Council on Cardiovascular Disease in the Young, and the Councils on Clinical Cardiology, Stroke, and Cardiovascular Surgery and Anesthesia, American Heart Association: Endorsed by the Infectious Diseases Society of America. Circulation 111:e394–e434, 2005

33. Durak DT, Lukes AS, Bright DK, for the Duke Endocarditis Service: New criteria for diagnosis of infective endocarditis: Utilization of specific echocardiographic findings. Am J Med 96:200–209, 1994

34. Li JS, Sexton DJ, Mick N, et al.: Proposed modifications to the Duke criteria for the diagnosis of infective endocarditis. Clin Infect Dis 30:633–638, 2000

Want to know more? A wide variety of resources to enhance your learning and understanding of this chapter are available on **thePoint** ⁂. Visit **http://thepoint.lww.com/MortonEss1e** to access chapter review questions and more!

Respiratory System

Patient Assessment: Respiratory System

OBJECTIVES

Based on the content in this chapter, the reader should be able to:

1 Describe the components of the history for respiratory assessment.
2 Explain the use of inspection, palpation, percussion, and auscultation for respiratory assessment.
3 Explain the components of an arterial blood gas and the normal values for each component.
4 Compare and contrast the arterial oxygen saturation and the partial pressure of oxygen dissolved in arterial blood.
5 Compare and contrast the causes, signs, and symptoms of respiratory acidosis, respiratory alkalosis, metabolic acidosis, and metabolic alkalosis.
6 Analyze examples of an arterial blood gas result.
7 Discuss the purpose of pulse oximetry, end-tidal carbon dioxide monitoring, and mixed venous oxygen saturation monitoring.
8 Discuss the purpose of respiratory diagnostic studies and associated nursing implications.

TABLE 15-1 Sputum Assessment

Sputum Appearance	Significance
Yellow, green, brown	Bacterial infection
Clear, white	Absence of infection
Yellow	Possible allergies
Rust colored (yellow mixed with blood)	Possible tuberculosis
Mucoid, viscid, blood streaked	Viral infection
Persistent, slightly blood streaked	Carcinoma
Clotted blood present	Pulmonary infarct

A comprehensive pulmonary assessment allows the nurse to establish the patient's baseline status and provides a framework for rapidly detecting changes in the patient's condition.

History

Principal symptoms to investigate in more detail commonly include dyspnea, chest pain, sputum production (Table 15-1), and cough. Because smoking has a significant impact on the patient's respiratory health, the patient's use of tobacco should be quantified by amount and how long the patient has smoked. Elements of the respiratory history are summarized in Box 15-1. A pulmonary illness often results in the production (or a change in the production) of sputum.

Physical Examination

High-quality physical assessments often provide information that can lead to the detection of complications or changes in the patient's condition before information from laboratory and diagnostic studies is available.

BOX 15-1 Respiratory Health History

History of the Present Illness

Complete analysis of the following signs and symptoms (using the NOPQRST format; see Chapter 12, Box 12-1):

- Dyspnea, dyspnea on exertion
- Shortness of breath
- Chest pain
- Cough
- Sputum production and appearance
- Hemoptysis
- Wheezing
- Orthopnea
- Clubbing
- Cyanosis

Past Health History

- **Relevant childhood illnesses and immunizations:** whooping cough (pertussis), mumps, cystic fibrosis
- **Past acute and chronic medical problems, including treatments and hospitalizations:** streptococcal infection of the throat, upper respiratory infections, tonsillitis, bronchitis, sinus infection, emphysema, asthma, bronchiectasis, tuberculosis, cancer, pulmonary hypertension, heart failure, musculoskeletal and neurological diseases affecting the respiratory system
- **Risk factors:** age, obesity, smoking, allergens
- **Past surgeries:** tonsillectomy, thoracic surgery, coronary artery bypass grafting (CABG), cardiac valve surgery, aortic aneurysm surgery, trauma surgery, tracheostomy
- **Past diagnostic tests and interventions:** tuberculin skin test, allergy tests, pulmonary function tests, chest radiograph, computed tomography (CT) scan, magnetic resonance imaging (MRI), bronchoscopy, cardiac

stress test, ventilation–perfusion scanning, pulmonary angiography, thoracentesis, sputum culture
- **Medications, including prescription drugs, over-the-counter drugs, vitamins, herbs, and supplements:** oxygen, bronchodilators, antitussives, expectorants, mucolytics, anti-infectives, antihistamines, methylxanthine agents, anti-inflammatory agents
- **Allergies and reactions to medications, foods, contrast dye, latex, or other materials**
- **Transfusions, including type and date**

Family History

- **Health status or cause of death of parents and siblings:** tuberculosis, cystic fibrosis, emphysema, asthma, malignancy

Personal and Social History

- Tobacco, alcohol, and substance use
- Environment: exposure to asbestos, chemicals, coal dust, allergens; type of heating and ventilation system
- Diet
- Sleep patterns: use of pillows
- Exercise

Review of Other Systems

- **HEENT:** strep throat, sinus infections, ear infection, deviated nasal septum, tonsillitis
- **Cardiac:** heart failure, dysrhythmias, coronary artery disease (CAD), valvular disease, hypertension
- **Gastrointestinal:** weight loss, nausea, vomiting
- **Neuromuscular:** Guillain–Barré syndrome, myasthenia gravis, amyotrophic lateral sclerosis, weakness
- **Musculoskeletal:** scoliosis, kyphosis

Inspection

Inspection of the patient involves checking for the presence or absence of several factors (Box 15-2).

- **Central cyanosis** (blueness of the tongue or lips) usually means the patient has low oxygen tension. The presence of cyanosis is a late and often ominous sign. Cyanosis is difficult to detect in a patient with anemia. A patient with polycythemia may have cyanosis even if oxygen tension is normal.
- **Labored breathing** is an important marker of respiratory distress. As part of the inspection, the nurse determines whether the patient is using the accessory muscles of respiration (the scalene and sternocleidomastoid muscles). Intercostal retractions (inward movement of the muscles between the ribs) suggest that the patient is making a larger effort at inspiration than normal. The nurse also observes the patient for use of the abdominal muscles during the usually passive expiratory phase. Sometimes, the number of words a patient can say before having to gasp for another breath is a good measure of the degree of labored breathing.
- **Respiratory rate, depth, and pattern.** These are important parameters to follow and may be indicators of the underlying disease process (Table 15-2).
- **Anterior–posterior diameter of the chest.** The size of the chest from front to back may be increased in patients with obstructive pulmonary disease (due to overexpansion of the lungs) and in patients with kyphosis.
- **Chest deformities and scars** (eg, kyphoscoliosis or flail chest from trauma) are important in helping to determine the reason for respiratory distress.
- **Chest expansion** is important to note. Causes of abnormal chest expansion are listed in Box 15-3. Asynchronous respiratory effort often precedes the need for ventilatory support.

- **Clubbing** of the fingers (see Chapter 30, Fig. 30-2) is seen in many patients with respiratory and cardiovascular diseases, especially chronic hypoxia.

Palpation

In addition to observing expansion of the chest wall, the nurse palpates chest expansion by positioning the thumbs on the patient's back, at the level of the 10th rib, and observing the divergence of the thumbs caused by the patient's breathing. Expansion of the chest wall should be symmetrical (see Box 15-3).

To assess tactile fremitus (the ability to feel sound on the chest wall), the nurse asks the patient to say "ninety-nine" while palpating the posterior surfaces of the chest wall. Tactile fremitus is slightly increased by the presence of solid substances, such as the consolidation of a lung due to pneumonia, pulmonary edema, or pulmonary hemorrhage. Conditions that result in greater air volume in the lung (eg, emphysema) are associated with decreased or absent tactile fremitus, because air does not conduct sound well.

The nurse palpates for subcutaneous emphysema by moving the fingers in a gentle rolling motion across the chest and neck to feel pockets of air underneath the skin. Subcutaneous emphysema may result from a pneumothorax or small pockets of alveoli that have burst with increased pulmonary pressure, (eg, PEEP). In severe cases, the subcutaneous emphysema may spread throughout the body.

Finally, the nurse palpates the position of the trachea. Pleural effusion, hemothorax, pneumothorax, or a tension pneumothorax can cause the trachea to move away from the affected side. Atelectasis, fibrosis, tumors, and phrenic nerve paralysis often pull the trachea toward the affected side.

BOX 15-2 **Components of the Inspection Process in the Physical Assessment of the Respiratory System**

General
- Mentation
- Anxiety level
- Speech
- Skin color (pallor, cyanosis)
- Weight (obese, malnourished)
- Body position (leaning forward, arms elevated)

Thorax
- Symmetry of thorax
- Anterior–posterior diameter (should be less than transverse by at least half)
- Rate, pattern, rhythm, and duration of breathing
- Use of accessory muscles

- Synchrony of chest and abdomen movement
- Alignment of spine

Head and Neck
- Nasal flaring
- Pursed-lip breathing
- Mouth breathing versus nasal breathing
- Use of neck and shoulders
- Tracheal position
- Central cyanosis

Extremities
- Clubbing
- Edema
- Peripheral cyanosis

TABLE 15-2 Respiration Patterns

Type	Description	Pattern	Clinical Significance
Normal	12–20 breaths/min and regular		Normal breathing pattern
Tachypnea	Greater than 24 breaths/min and shallow		May be a normal response to fever, anxiety, or exercise Can occur with respiratory insufficiency, alkalosis, pneumonia, or pleurisy
Bradypnea	Less than 10 breaths/min and regular		May be normal in well-conditioned athletes Can occur with medication-induced depression of the respiratory center, diabetic coma, neurologic damage
Hyperventilation	Increased rate and increased depth		Extreme exercise, fear, or anxiety; central nervous system (CNS) disorders; compensation for acidosis (eg, salicylate overdose)
Kussmaul's respiration	Rapid, deep, labored		Associated with diabetic ketoacidosis
Hypoventilation	Decreased rate, decreased depth, irregular pattern		Usually associated with overdose of narcotics or anesthetics
Cheyne–Stokes respiration	Regular pattern characterized by alternating periods of deep, rapid breathing followed by periods of apnea		May result from severe heart failure, drug overdose, increased intracranial pressure (ICP) stroke, or renal failure May be noted in elderly people during sleep, not related to any disease process
Biot's respiration	Irregular pattern characterized by varying depth and rate of respirations followed by periods of apnea		May be seen with meningitis or severe brain damage
Ataxic	Significant disorganization with irregular and varying depths of respiration		A more extreme expression of Biot's respirations; indicates respiratory compromise and elevated ICP
Air trapping	Increasing difficulty in getting breath out		Seen in chronic obstructive pulmonary disease (COPD) when air is trapped in the lungs during forced expiration

BOX 15-3 Abnormal Chest Expansion

Unilateral diminished expansion
- Atelectasis
- Endotracheal or nasotracheal tube positioned in right mainstream bronchi
- Collapsed lung
- Pulmonary embolus
- Lobar pneumonia
- Pleural effusion
- Pneumothorax
- Rib fracture

Asynchronous expansion
- Flail chest

Percussion

Percussion of the chest normally produces a resonant or hollow note. In diseases in which there is increased air in the chest or lungs (eg, pneumothorax, emphysema), percussion notes may be hyperresonant. A flat percussion note is more likely to be heard if a large pleural effusion is present in the lung beneath the examining hand. A dull percussion note is heard if atelectasis or consolidation is present. Asthma or a large pneumothorax can result in a tympanic drum-like sound.

Auscultation

In general, four types of breath sounds are heard in the normal chest (Table 15-3). Bronchial breath

TABLE 15-3	Characteristics of Breath Sounds			
	Duration of Sounds	**Intensity of Expiratory Sound**	**Pitch of Expiratory Sound**	**Locations Where Heard Normally**
Vesicular[a]	Inspiratory sounds last longer than expiratory ones.	Soft	Relatively low	Over most of both lungs
Bronchovesicular	Inspiratory and expiratory sounds are about equal.	Intermediate	Intermediate	Often in the first and second interspaces anteriorly and between the scapulae
Bronchial	Expiratory sounds last longer than inspiratory ones.	Loud	Relatively high	Over the manubrium, if heard at all
Tracheal	Inspiratory and expiratory sounds are about equal.	Very loud	Relatively high	Over the trachea in the neck

[a]The thickness of the bars indicates intensity; the steeper their incline, the higher the pitch. From Bickley LS: Bates' Guide to Physical Examination and History Taking, 10th ed. Philadelphia, PA: Lippincott Williams & Wilkins, 2009, p 303.

sounds are abnormal when heard over lung tissue and indicate fluid accumulation or consolidation of the lung (eg, as a result of pneumonia or pleural effusion). Bronchial breath sounds are associated with egophony and whispered pectoriloquy:

- **Egophony** (distorted voice sounds) occurs in the presence of consolidation and is detected by asking the patient to say "E" while the nurse listens with a stethoscope. In egophony, the nurse will hear an "A" sound rather than an "E" sound.
- **Whispered pectoriloquy** is the presence of loud, clear sounds heard through the stethoscope when the patient whispers. Normally, the whispered voice is heard faintly and indistinctly through the stethoscope. The increased transmission of voice sounds indicates the presence of fluid in the lungs.

Adventitious sounds are additional breath sounds heard with auscultation and include discontinuous sounds, continuous sounds, and friction rubs:

- **Discontinuous sounds** are brief, nonmusical, intermittent sounds and include fine and coarse crackles. When assessing crackles, the nurse notes their loudness, pitch, duration, amount, location, and timing in the respiratory cycle. Fine crackles are soft, high-pitched, very brief popping sounds that occur most commonly during inspiration. These result from fluid in the airways or alveoli, or from the opening of collapsed alveoli. Restrictive pulmonary disease results in fine crackles during late inspiration, whereas obstructive pulmonary disease results in fine crackles during early inspiration. Crackles become coarser as the air moves through larger fluid accumulations, such as in bronchitis or pneumonia. Crackles that clear with coughing are not associated with significant pulmonary disease.
- **Continuous sounds** include wheezes and rhonchi. Wheezes are high-pitched musical sounds

that have a shrill quality. They are caused by the movement of air through a narrowed or partially obstructed airway, such as in asthma, chronic obstructive pulmonary disease (COPD), or bronchitis. Rhonchi are deep, low-pitched rumbling noises. The presence of rhonchi indicates the presence of secretions in the large airways, such as occurs with acute respiratory distress syndrome (ARDS).

- **Friction rubs** are crackling, grating sounds heard more often with inspiration than expiration. A friction rub can be heard with pleural effusion, pneumothorax, or pleurisy. It is important to distinguish a pleural friction rub from a pericardial friction rub. (A pericardial friction rub is a high-pitched, rasping, scratchy sound that varies with the cardiac cycle.)

The Older Patient. In elderly people, anatomical and physiological changes associated with aging may manifest in different assessment findings, including increased hyperresonance (caused by increased distensibility of the lungs), decreased chest wall expansion, decreased use of respiratory muscles, increased use of accessory muscles (secondary to calcification of rib articulations), less subcutaneous tissue, possible pronounced dorsal curvature, and basilar crackles in the absence of disease (these should clear after a few coughs). Also be aware that older people may have a decreased ability to hold their breath during the examination.

Respiratory Monitoring

Arterial Blood Gases

Arterial blood gas (ABG) assessment involves analyzing a sample of arterial blood to determine the quality

BOX 15-4 Normal Arterial Blood Gas (ABG) Values

PaO_2: 80 to 100 mm Hg
SaO_2: 93% to 99%
pH: 7.35 to 7.45
$PaCO_2$: 35 to 45 mm Hg
HCO_3: 22 to 26 mEq/L

and extent of pulmonary gas exchange and acid–base status. Normal ABG values are given in Box 15-4.

Measuring Oxygen in the Blood

Oxygen is carried in the blood in two ways. Approximately 3% of oxygen is dissolved in the plasma (PaO_2). The normal PaO_2 is 80 to 100 mm Hg at sea level. For people living at higher altitudes, the normal PaO_2 is lower because of the lower barometric pressure. The remaining 97% of oxygen is attached to hemoglobin in red blood cells (SaO_2). The normal SaO_2 ranges from 93% to 99%. SaO_2 is an important oxygenation value to assess because most oxygen supplied to tissues is carried by hemoglobin.

 The Older Patient. *PaO_2 tends to decrease with age. For patients who are 60 to 80 years of age, a PaO_2 of 60 to 80 mm Hg is normal.[1]*

The relationship between PaO_2 and SaO_2 is depicted by the oxyhemoglobin dissociation curve (Fig. 15-1). At a PaO_2 greater than 60 mm Hg, large changes in the PaO_2 result in only small changes in the SaO_2. However, at a PaO_2 of less than 60 mm Hg, the curve drops sharply, signifying that a small decrease in PaO_2 is associated with a large decrease in SaO_2. Factors such as pH, carbon dioxide concentration, temperature, and levels of 2,3-diphosphoglycerate (2,3-DPG) influence hemoglobin's affinity for oxygen and can cause the curve to shift to the left or to the right (see Fig. 15-1). When the curve shifts to the right, there is a reduced capacity for hemoglobin to hold onto oxygen, resulting in more oxygen released to the tissues. When the curve shifts to the left, there is an increased capacity for hemoglobin to hold oxygen, resulting in less oxygen released to the tissues.

Measuring pH in the Blood

The normal blood pH is 7.35 to 7.45. Box 15-5 reviews terms used in acid–base balance. An acid–base disorder may be either respiratory or metabolic in origin (Table 15-4). If the respiratory system is responsible, serum carbon dioxide levels are affected, and if the metabolic system is responsible, serum bicarbonate levels are affected (see Table 15-4). Occasionally, patients present with both respiratory and metabolic disorders that together cause an acidemia or alkalemia. When this occurs, the ABG reflects a mixed respiratory and metabolic acidosis. Examples of ABG values in mixed disorders are given in Box 15-6.

Interpreting Arterial Blood Gas Results

When interpreting ABG results, three factors must be considered: oxygenation status, acid–base balance, and degree of compensation (Box 15-7). If the patient presents with alkalemia or acidemia, it is important to determine whether the body has tried to compensate for the abnormality. The respiratory system responds to metabolic-based pH imbalances by increasing the respiratory rate and depth (metabolic acidosis) or decreasing the respiratory rate and depth (metabolic alkalosis). The renal system responds to respiratory-based pH imbalances by increasing hydrogen secretion and bicarbonate reabsorption (respiratory acidosis) or decreasing hydrogen secretion and bicarbonate reabsorption (respiratory alkalosis).

ABGs are defined by their degree of compensation: uncompensated, partially compensated, or completely compensated. To determine the level of compensation, the nurse examines the pH, carbon dioxide, and bicarbonate values to evaluate whether the opposite system (renal or respiratory) has worked to try to shift back toward a normal pH. The primary abnormality (metabolic or respiratory) is correlated with the abnormal pH (acidotic or alkalotic). The secondary abnormality is an attempt to correct the primary disorder. By using the rules for defining compensation in Box 15-8, it is possible to determine the compensatory status of the patient's ABGs.

Shift to the left

Alkalosis (↑ pH)
↓ $PaCO_2$
↓ Temperature
↓ 2, 3 DPG

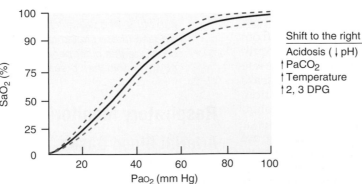

Shift to the right

Acidosis (↓ pH)
↑ $PaCO_2$
↑ Temperature
↑ 2, 3 DPG

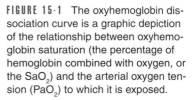

FIGURE 15-1 The oxyhemoglobin dissociation curve is a graphic depiction of the relationship between oxyhemoglobin saturation (the percentage of hemoglobin combined with oxygen, or the SaO_2) and the arterial oxygen tension (PaO_2) to which it is exposed.

BOX 15-5 Acid–Base Terminology

Acid: A substance that can donate hydrogen ions (H⁺).
Example: H_2CO_3 (an acid) $\rightarrow$ H⁺ + HCO_3
Base: A substance that can accept hydrogen ions (H⁺).
Example: HCO_3 (a base) + H⁺ $\rightarrow$ H_2CO_3
Acidemia: Acid condition of the blood in which the pH is less than 7.35
Alkalemia: Alkaline condition of the blood in which the pH is greater than 7.45
Acidosis: The process causing acidemia
Alkalosis: The process causing alkalemia

BOX 15-6 Arterial Blood Gases (ABGs) in Mixed Respiratory and Metabolic Disorders

Mixed Acidosis	Mixed Alkalosis
pH: 7.25	pH: 7.55
$PaCO_2$: 56 mm Hg	$PaCO_2$: 26 mm Hg
HCO_3: 15 mEq/L	HCO_3: 28 mEq/L

TABLE 15-4 Possible Causes and Signs and Symptoms of Acid–Base Disorders

Condition	Possible Causes	Signs and Symptoms
Respiratory Acidosis $PaCO_2$ greater than 45 mm Hg pH less than 7.35	**Inadequate elimination of CO_2 by lungs** Central nervous system (CNS) depression Head trauma Oversedation Anesthesia High cord injury Pneumothorax Hypoventilation Bronchial obstruction and atelectasis Severe pulmonary infections Heart failure and pulmonary edema Massive pulmonary embolus Myasthenia gravis Multiple sclerosis	Dyspnea Restlessness Headache Tachycardia Confusion Lethargy Dysrhythmias Respiratory distress Drowsiness Decreased responsiveness
Respiratory Alkalosis $PaCO_2$ less than 35 mm Hg pH greater than 7.45	**Excessive elimination of CO_2 by the lungs** Anxiety and nervousness Fear Pain Hyperventilation Fever Thyrotoxicosis CNS lesions Salicylates Gram-negative septicemia Pregnancy	Light-headedness Confusion Decreased concentration Paresthesias Tetanic spasms in the arms and legs Cardiac dysrhythmias Palpitations Sweating Dry mouth Blurred vision
Metabolic Acidosis HCO_3 less than 22 mEq/L pH less than 7.35	**Increased acids** Renal failure Ketoacidosis Anaerobic metabolism Starvation Salicylate intoxication **Loss of base** Diarrhea Intestinal fistulas	Headache Confusion Restlessness Lethargy Weakness Stupor/coma Kussmaul's respirations Nausea and vomiting Dysrhythmias Warm, flushed skin
Metabolic Alkalosis HCO_3 greater than 26 mEq/L pH greater than 7.45	**Gain of base** Muscle twitching and cramps Excess use of bicarbonate Lactate administration in dialysis Excess ingestion of antacids **Loss of acids** Vomiting Nasogastric suctioning Hypokalemia Hypochloremia Administration of diuretics Increased levels of aldosterone	Tetany Dizziness Lethargy Weakness Disorientation Convulsions Coma Nausea and vomiting Depressed respiration

BOX 15-7 Interpretation of Arterial Blood Gas (ABG) Results

Approach

1. Evaluate oxygenation by examining the PaO_2 and the SaO_2.
2. Evaluate the pH. Is it acidotic, alkalotic, or normal?
3. Evaluate the $PaCO_2$. Is it high, low, or normal?
4. Evaluate the HCO_3. Is it high, low, or normal?
5. Determine whether compensation is occurring. Is it complete, partial, or uncompensated?

Examples

Sample blood gas

PaO_2	80 mm Hg	Normal
SaO_2	95%	Normal
Ph	7.30	Acidemia
$PaCO_2$	55 mm Hg	Increased (respiratory cause)
HCO_3	25 mEq/L	Normal

Conclusion: Respiratory acidosis (uncompensated)

Sample blood gas

PaO_2	85 mm Hg	Normal
SaO_2	90%	Low
pH	7.49	Alkalemia
$PaCO_2$	40	Normal
HCO_3	29 mEq/L	Increased (metabolic cause)

Conclusion: Metabolic alkalosis with a low saturation (uncompensated)

Pulse Oximetry

The SpO_2 is the arterial oxygen saturation of hemoglobin as measured by pulse oximetry. In pulse oximetry, light-emitting and light-receiving sensors quantify the amount of light absorbed by oxygenated/deoxygenated hemoglobin in the arterial blood. Usually, the sensors are in a clip placed on a finger, ear lobe, or forehead. The value displayed by the oximeter is an average of numerous readings taken over a 3- to 10-second period. Oximetry is not used in place of ABG monitoring. Rather, pulse oximetry is used to assess trends in oxygen saturation when the correlation between arterial blood and pulse oximetry readings has been established.

BOX 15-8 Compensatory Status of Arterial Blood Gases (ABGs)

Uncompensated: pH is *abnormal,* and *either* the CO_2 or HCO_3 is also abnormal. There is no indication that the opposite system has tried to correct for the other.

In the example below, the patient's pH is alkalotic as a result of the low (below the normal range of 35 to 45 mm Hg) CO_2 concentration. The renal system value (HCO_3) has not moved out its normal range (22 to 26 mEq/L) to compensate for the primary respiratory disorder.

PaO_2	94 mm Hg	Normal
pH	7.52	Alkalotic
$PaCO_2$	25 mm Hg	Decreased
HCO_3	24 mEq/L	Normal

Partially compensated: pH is *abnormal,* and *both* the CO_2 and HCO_3 are also abnormal; this indicates that one system has attempted to correct for the other but has not been completely successful.

In the example below, the patient's pH remains alkalotic as a result of the low CO_2 concentration. The renal system value (HCO_3) has moved out its normal range (22 to 26 mEq/L) to compensate for the primary respiratory disorder but has not been able to bring the pH back within the normal range.

PaO_2	94 mm Hg	Normal
pH	7.48	Alkalotic
$PaCO_2$	25 mm Hg	Decreased
HCO_3	20 mEq/L	Decreased

Completely compensated: pH is *normal* and *both* the CO_2 and HCO_3 are abnormal; the normal pH indicates that one system has been able to compensate for the other.

In the example below, the patient's pH is normal but is tending toward alkalosis (greater than 7.40). The primary abnormality is respiratory because the $PaCO_2$ is low (decreased acid concentration). The bicarbonate value of 18 mEq/L reflects decreased concentration of base and is associated with acidosis, not alkalosis. In this case, the decreased bicarbonate has completely compensated for the respiratory alkalosis.

PaO_2	94 mm Hg	Normal
pH	7.44	Normal, tending toward alkalosis
$PaCO_2$	25 mm Hg	Decreased, primary problem
HcO_3	18 mEq/L	Decreased, compensatory response

RED FLAG! *Values obtained by pulse oximetry are unreliable in the presence of vasoconstricting medications, IV dyes, shock, cardiac arrest, severe anemia, and dyshemoglobins (eg, carboxyhemoglobin, methemoglobin).[2]*

End-Tidal Carbon Dioxide Monitoring

End-tidal carbon dioxide ($ETCO_2$) monitoring and capnography measures the level of carbon dioxide at the end of exhalation, when the percentage of carbon dioxide dissolved in the arterial blood ($PaCO_2$) approximates the percentage of alveolar carbon dioxide ($PACO_2$). Therefore, $ETCO_2$ can be used to estimate $PaCO_2$. Although $PaCO_2$ and $ETCO_2$ values are similar, $ETCO_2$ is usually lower than $PaCO_2$ by 2 to 5 mm Hg.[3] The difference between $PaCO_2$ and $ETCO_2$ ($PaCO_2$–$ETCO_2$ gradient) may be attributed to several factors; pulmonary blood flow is the primary determinant.

$ETCO_2$ values are obtained by analyzing samples of expired gas from an endotracheal tube, an oral airway, a nasopharyngeal airway, or a nasal cannula. Because $ETCO_2$ provides continuous estimates of alveolar ventilation, it is useful for monitoring the patient during weaning from a ventilator, in cardiopulmonary resuscitation (CPR), and in endotracheal intubation.

On a capnogram, the waveform is composed of four phases, each one representing a specific part of the respiratory cycle (Fig. 15-2):

1. The first phase is the baseline phase, which represents both the inspiratory phase and the very beginning of the expiratory phase, when carbon dioxide–free air in the anatomical dead space is exhaled. This value should be zero in a healthy adult.
2. The second phase is the expiratory upstroke, which represents the exhalation of carbon dioxide from the lungs. Any process that delays the delivery of carbon dioxide from the patient's lungs to the detector (eg, COPD, bronchospasm, kinked ventilator tubing) prolongs the expiratory upstroke.
3. The third phase, the plateau phase, begins as carbon dioxide elimination rapidly continues and indicates the exhalation of alveolar gases. The

$ETCO_2$ is the value generated at the very end of exhalation, indicating the amount of carbon dioxide exhaled from the least ventilated alveoli.
4. The fourth phase is the inspiratory downstroke. The downward deflection of the waveform is caused by the washout of carbon dioxide that occurs in the presence of the oxygen influx during inspiration.

Mixed Venous Oxygen Saturation

Mixed venous oxygen saturation (SvO_2) is a parameter that is measured to evaluate the balance between oxygen supply and oxygen demand. SvO_2 indicates the adequacy of the supply of oxygen relative to the demand for oxygen at the tissue levels. Normal SvO_2 is 60% to 80%; this means that supply of oxygen to the tissues is adequate to meet the tissue's demand. However, a normal value does not indicate whether compensatory mechanisms were needed to maintain the balance. For example, in some patients, an increase in cardiac output is needed to compensate for a low supply of oxygen.

A pulmonary artery catheter (PAC) with an oximeter built into its tip that allows continuous monitoring of SvO_2 provides ongoing assessment of oxygen supply and demand imbalances. If a catheter with a built-in oximeter is not available, a blood sample drawn from the pulmonary artery port of a PAC can be sent to the laboratory for blood gas and SvO_2 analysis.

A low SvO_2 value may be caused by a decrease in oxygen supply to the tissues or an increase in oxygen use due to a high demand (Table 15-5). A decrease in SvO_2 often occurs before other hemodynamic changes and therefore is an excellent clinical tool in the assessment and management of critically ill patients. Elevated SvO_2 values are associated with increased delivery of oxygen or with decreased demand (see Table 15-5).

Respiratory Diagnostic Studies

Pulmonary function tests measure the ability of the chest and lungs to move air into and out of the alveoli. Pulmonary function tests include volume measurements, capacity measurements, and dynamic measurements (Table 15-6):

- Volume measurements show the amount of air contained in the lungs during various parts of the respiratory cycle.
- Capacity measurements quantify part of the pulmonary cycle.
- Dynamic measurements provide data about airway resistance and the energy expended in breathing (work of breathing).

These measurements are influenced by exercise, disease, age, gender, body size, and posture.

Other diagnostic studies that are often used to evaluate the respiratory system are summarized in Table 15-7.

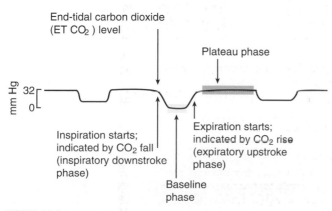

FIGURE 15-2 Capnogram tracing.

TABLE 15-5 Possible Causes of Abnormalities in Mixed Venous Oxygen Saturation (SvO_2)

Abnormality	Possible Cause
Low SvO_2 (less than 60%)	**Decreased oxygen supply** Low hematocrit from anemia or hemorrhage Low arterial saturation and hypoxemia from lung disease, ventilation–perfusion mismatches Low cardiac output from hypovolemia, heart failure, cardiogenic shock, myocardial infarction **Increased oxygen demand** Increased metabolic demand, such as hyperthermia, seizures, shivering, pain, anxiety, stress, strenuous exercise
High SvO_2 (greater than 80%)	**Increased oxygen supply** Supplemental oxygen **Decreased oxygen demand** Anesthesia, hypothermia **Technical problems** False high reading because of wedged PAC Fibrin clot at end of catheter **Decreased oxygen consumption** Sepsis

TABLE 15-6 Volume Measurements, Capacity Measurements, and Dynamic Measurements

Term Used	Symbol	Description	Remarks	Normal Values
Volume Measurements				
Tidal volume	V_T	Volume of air inhaled and exhaled with each breath	Tidal volume may vary with severe disease.	500 mL
Inspiratory reserve volume	IRV	Maximum volume of air that can be inhaled after a normal inhalation		3000 mL
Expiratory reserve volume	ERV	Maximum volume of air that can be exhaled forcibly after a normal exhalation	Expiratory reserve volume is decreased with restrictive disorders, such as obesity, ascites, and pregnancy.	1100 mL
Residual volume	RV	Volume of air remaining in the lungs after a maximum exhalation	Residual volume may be increased with obstructive diseases.	1200 mL
Capacity Measurements				
Vital capacity	VC	Maximum volume of air exhaled from the point of maximum inspiration	Decrease in vital capacity may be found in neuromuscular disease, generalized fatigue, atelectasis, pulmonary edema, and chronic obstructive pulmonary disease (COPD), asthma.	4600 mL
Inspiratory capacity	IC	Maximum volume of air inhaled after normal expiration	Decrease in inspiratory capacity may indicate restrictive disease.	3500 mL
Functional residual capacity	FRC	Volume of air remaining in lungs after a normal expiration	Functional residual capacity may be increased with COPD and decreased in acute respiratory distress syndrome (ARDS).	2300 mL
Total lung capacity	TLC	Volume of air in lungs after a maximum inspiration and equal to the sum of all four volumes (V_T, IRV, ERV, RV)	Total lung capacity may be decreased with restrictive disease (atelectasis, pneumonia) and increased in COPD.	5800 mL

TABLE 15-6 Volume Measurements, Capacity Measurements, and Dynamic Measurements (continued)

Term Used	Symbol	Description	Remarks	Normal Values
Dynamic Measurements				
Respiratory rate (frequency)	f	Number of breaths per minute		15 breaths/min
Minute volume (minute ventilation)		Volume of air inhaled and exhaled per minute; equal to $V_T \times f$		7500 mL/min
Dead space	V_D	The part of the tidal volume that does not participate in alveolar gas exchange; equal to the air contained in the airways (anatomical dead space) plus the alveolar air that is not involved in gas exchange (alveolar dead space); calculated as $P_ACO_2 - PaCO_2$	Alveolar dead space occurs only in disease states (eg, pulmonary embolism, pulmonary hypertension) Anatomic plus alveolar dead space is physiologic dead space	Less than 40% of the V_T
Alveolar ventilation	$\dot{V}_A$	The part of the tidal volume that does participate in alveolar gas exchange; calculated as $(V_T - V_D) \times f$	A measure of ventilatory effectiveness	4500 mL/min

TABLE 15-7 Respiratory Diagnostic Studies

Test and Purpose	Method of Testing	Nursing Implications
Chest Radiography		
Used to assess anatomical and physiological features of the chest and to detect pathological processes.	X-rays pass through chest wall, making it possible to visualize structures. Bones appear as opaque or white; heart and blood vessels appear as gray; lungs filled with air appear black; lungs with fluid appear white.	• Test can be done at the bedside or in the diagnostic center. • Nurse may be asked to help position the patient and ensure that the patient takes a deep breath during the test.
Ventilation–Perfusion Scanning		
A nuclear imaging test used to evaluate a suspected alteration in the ventilation–perfusion relationship in the lung.	To test ventilation, the patient inhales radioactive gas. Diminished areas of ventilation are visible on the scan. To test perfusion, a radioisotope is injected intravenously, enabling visualization of the blood supply to the lungs. When a pulmonary embolus is present, the blood supply beyond the embolus is restricted.	• Test is done in a diagnostic center. • The nurse may need to calm the patient's feeling of claustrophobia due to face mask. • Check for post–procedure allergic reaction.
Bronchoscopy		
Used to examine lung tissue, collect secretions, determine the extent and location of a pathologic process, and obtain a biopsy.	The larynx, trachea, and bronchi are visualized through a fiberoptic bronchoscope.	• The patient often receives sedation or analgesia before the procedure. • Postprocedure complications may include laryngospasm, fever, hemodynamic changes, cardiac dysrhythmias, pneumothorax, hemorrhage, or cardiopulmonary arrest.
Thoracentesis		
Used to remove air, fluid, or both from the chest; to obtain specimens for diagnostic evaluation; or instill medications.	With the patient placed in an upright or sitting position, a needle is placed into the pleural space. A local anesthetic is used at the site to reduce pain.	• Before the test, chest radiograph, coagulation studies, and patient education are done; antianxiety medication may be given. • During the procedure, the nurse helps the patient remain in a position with the arms and shoulders raised (to facilitate needle insertion between the ribs) and monitors the patient's comfort, anxiety, and respiratory status. • Postprocedure complications may include pneumothorax, pain, hypotension, and pulmonary edema.

(continued on page 218)

TABLE 15-7 Respiratory Diagnostic Studies (continued)

Test and Purpose	Method of Testing	Nursing Implications
Sputum Culture Used to identify specific microorganisms and their corresponding drug sensitivity.	The patient is asked to cough up sputum from the lungs.	• The nurse instructs the patient not to place saliva in the container but instead cough up sputum from the lungs.
Pulmonary Angiography Used to visualize the pulmonary vasculature.	A radiopaque contrast material is injected into one or both arms, the femoral vein, or a catheter placed in the pulmonary artery. Positive test is indicated by impaired flow of substance through narrowed vessel or by abrupt cessation of flow.	• The nurse monitors the patient's pulse, blood pressure, and breathing during test. • Possible complications include allergic reaction to dye, pulmonary embolus, and abnormal cardiac rhythm.
Spiral Computed Tomography (CT) Used to screen for tumors, pulmonary embolism, and abdominal aortic aneurysm.	Continuously rotating x-rays send images to a computer to create a 3D composite image.	• Test is done in a diagnostic center. • The nurse monitors for claustrophobia and administers a mild sedative if necessary.

CASE STUDY

Mr. J. is a 75-year-old man who has been admitted to the cardiac care unit with a diagnosis of exacerbated heart failure. He has a history of two myocardial infarctions and underwent a triple coronary artery bypass graft 4 years ago.

On admission to the unit, Mr. J. is profoundly short of breath, restless, and tachycardic. His daughter, who accompanied him to the hospital, reports that Mr. J. is uncharacteristically confused. On physical examination, his vital signs are as follows: RR, 32 breaths/min; HR, 126 beats/min; and BP, 100/64 mm Hg. The nurse notes that Mr. J. is using accessory muscles for breathing, and his jugular veins are visibly distended at 45 degrees. Mr. J.'s mucous membranes are pale, and he has a Glasgow Coma Scale score of 14. On auscultation, the nurse hears coarse crackles in both bases with some audible expiratory wheezing. During assessment of breath sounds, the nurse is able to clearly hear whispered sounds through the stethoscope. Arterial blood gases (ABGs) are PaO_2, 68 mm Hg; $PaCO_2$, 49 mm Hg; HCO_3, 29 mEq/L; and pH, 7.31.

1. What three findings from Mr. J.'s assessment are consistent with a diagnosis of heart failure?

2. Describe some of the differences in respiratory assessment of the older patient.

3. What signs of respiratory distress are apparent, even before auscultating the lungs or obtaining arterial blood gas (ABG) results?

4. Why is Mr. J. tachypneic?

5. Why is the nurse able to hear whispered sounds clearly with the stethoscope? What is this condition called?

6. Interpret the ABG results. Is Mr. J. compensating?

References

1. Miller RD, et al: Chapter 71: Geriatrics: Pulmonary changes. In Miller's Anesthesia, 7th edition. Churchill Livingstone, 2009
2. Wilson B, et al: The accuracy of pulse oximetry in emergency department: patients with severe sepsis and septic shock. BMC Emerg Med 10:9, 2010
3. Respiratory Care. In Best Practices: Evidence-Based Nursing Procedures, 2nd ed. Lippincott Williams & Wilkins, 2007, p. 298–302

Want to know more? A wide variety of resources to enhance your learning and understanding of this chapter are available on the**Point** . Visit **http://thepoint.lww.com/MortonEss1e** to access chapter review questions and more!

Patient Management: Respiratory System

OBJECTIVES

Based on the content in this chapter, the reader should be able to:

1 Describe various bronchial hygiene therapy (BHT) techniques and explain their role in preventing and treating pulmonary complications.

2 Describe the nursing assessment of patients on oxygen therapy.

3 Discuss nursing interventions necessary to prevent complications in a patient with a chest tube drainage system.

4 Describe nursing considerations specific to the major classes of drugs used to treat respiratory disorders.

5 List and define types of surgeries that may be used to treat respiratory system disorders.

Bronchial Hygiene Therapy

Hospitalized patients are often not able to deep breathe, cough, or clear mucus effectively because of weakness, sedation, pain, or an artificial airway. Bronchial hygiene therapy (BHT) aims to improve ventilation and diffusion through secretion mobilization and removal and through improved gas exchange.

BHT methods include coughing and deep breathing, airway clearance adjunct therapies, chest physiotherapy (CPT), and bronchodilator therapy. BHT methods are used individually or in combination, depending on the patient's needs. Physical assessment, chest radiography, and arterial blood gases (ABGs) are used to determine the need for BHT, the appropriate methods to use, and the effectiveness of these interventions. Incentive spirometry may be given before any of the BHT methods to promote mucus removal.

Coughing and Deep Breathing

The objectives of coughing and deep breathing are to promote lung expansion, mobilize secretions, and prevent the complications of retained secretions (atelectasis and pneumonia). Even if crackles or rhonchi are not auscultated, the nurse encourages the high risk patient to cough and deep breathe as a prophylactic measure every hour. These techniques are effective only if the patient is able to cooperate and has the strength to cough productively.

The nurse instructs the patient to sit upright, inhale maximally and cough, and then take a slow, deep breath and hold it for 2 to 3 seconds. Use of incentive spirometry along with coughing and deep-breathing exercises improves inhaled volumes and prevents atelectasis. Effective incentive spirometry provides the patient with immediate visual feedback on the breath depth and encourages the patient to increase breath volume. Ideally, the patient uses the incentive spirometer hourly while awake, completing 10 breaths each session followed by coughing and striving to progressively increase breath volumes.

Airway Clearance Adjunct Therapies

Airway clearance adjunct therapies may be useful for patients who require mucus removal when coughing efforts are limited by a disease process, injury, or surgery.

- **Autogenic drainage ("huff cough").** It is a breathing technique frequently used by patients with cystic fibrosis and other chronic pulmonary diseases associated with the production of large amounts of thick mucus. To practice the technique, the patient takes a series of controlled breaths, exhaling with gentle huffs to unstick the mucus while at the same time suppressing the urge to cough.
- **Oscillating positive expiratory pressure (PEP).** An oscillating PEP device (eg, Acapella valve, Flutter valve) loosens mucus by producing PEP and oscillatory vibrations in the airways so that the mucus can then be cleared with a cough. The nurse manually assists the patient's cough by exerting positive pressure on the abdominal costal margin during exhalation, thus increasing the cough's force.
- **High-frequency chest wall oscillation.** The patient wears a vest-like device that uses air pulses to compress the chest wall, loosening secretions. High-frequency chest wall oscillation has been shown to improve mucus removal and pulmonary function, is well tolerated by surgical patients, and can be self-administered at home.
- **Positive airway pressure (PAP).** PAP devices enable airway recruitment and reduce atelectasis by delivering pressures between 5 and 20 cm H_2O with variable flow of oxygen during therapy. They are used in patients when other airway clearance therapies are not sufficient to reduce or prevent atelectasis.

Chest Physiotherapy

CPT techniques include postural drainage, chest percussion and vibration, and patient positioning. CPT is preceded by bronchodilator therapy and followed by deep breathing and coughing or other BHT techniques. Patients with an artificial airway or an ineffective cough may require suctioning after CPT. No single method of CPT has been shown to be superior, and there are many contraindications to using these techniques.

Studies have questioned the efficacy of CPT, except in segmental atelectasis caused by mucus obstruction and diseases that result in increased sputum production.[1] Bronchoscopy with bronchoalveolar lavage (BAL) is an alternative to CPT for removing mucus plugs that result in atelectasis. The inclusion of CPT in the plan of care must be individualized and evaluated in terms of derived benefit versus potential risks.

Postural Drainage

In postural drainage, gravity facilitates drainage of pulmonary secretions. The positions used depend on the lobes affected by atelectasis or accumulations of fluid or mucus (Fig. 16-1). Postural drainage in all positions is not indicated for all critically ill patients. The nurse must closely monitor the patient who is in a head-down position for aspiration, respiratory distress, and dysrhythmias. Alternate techniques may include gentle chest percussion and vibration.

 RED FLAG! Contraindications to postural drainage include increased intracranial pressure (ICP), tube feeding, inability to cough, hypoxia or respiratory instability, hemodynamic instability, decreased mental status, recent eye surgery, hiatal hernia, and obesity.

Chest Percussion and Vibration

Chest percussion and vibration are used to dislodge secretions. Percussion involves striking the chest wall with the hands formed into a cupped shape. The patient's position depends on the segment of lung to be percussed. Vibration involves manually compressing the chest wall while the patient exhales through pursed lips to increase the velocity and turbulence of exhaled air to loosen secretions. Vibration is used instead of percussion if the chest wall is extremely painful. Critical care unit beds have options to percuss or vibrate, with variable settings for high to low frequency of percussion or vibration. The nurse assesses the patient for tolerance to the level of therapy.

RED FLAG! Contraindications to percussion and vibration include fractured ribs, osteoporosis, chest or abdominal trauma or surgery, pulmonary hemorrhage or embolus, chest malignancy, mastectomy, pneumothorax, subcutaneous emphysema, cervical cord trauma, tuberculosis, pleural effusions or empyema, and asthma.

Patient Positioning

Turning the patient laterally every 2 hours (at minimum) aids in mobilizing secretions for removal with cough or suctioning. Changing the patient's position affects gas exchange, and positioning the patient with the "good" lung down improves oxygenation by improving ventilation to perfusion match.[2]

 RED FLAG! Positioning is altered if the patient has a lung abscess. In this case, the preferred position is with the diseased lung down, because otherwise gravity can cause the abscessed lung's purulent contents to drain into the opposite lung.

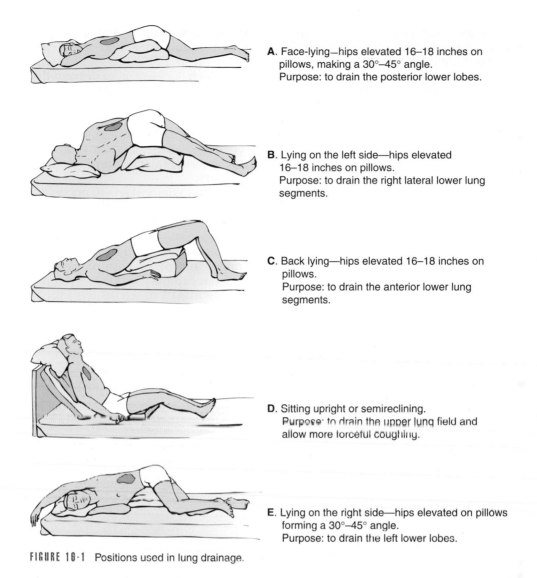

A. Face-lying—hips elevated 16–18 inches on pillows, making a 30°–45° angle.
Purpose: to drain the posterior lower lobes.

B. Lying on the left side—hips elevated 16–18 inches on pillows.
Purpose: to drain the right lateral lower lung segments.

C. Back lying—hips elevated 16–18 inches on pillows.
Purpose: to drain the anterior lower lung segments.

D. Sitting upright or semireclining.
Purpose: to drain the upper lung field and allow more forceful coughing.

E. Lying on the right side—hips elevated on pillows forming a 30°–45° angle.
Purpose: to drain the left lower lobes.

FIGURE 16-1 Positions used in lung drainage.

Continuous lateral rotation therapy (CLRT), defined as continuous lateral positioning of less than 40 degrees for 18 of 24 hours daily, improves oxygenation and blood flow to the lung tissue in affected regions and promotes secretion removal and airway patency.[2] Using lateral rotation therapy beds is more effective than the inconsistent nursing care of turning every 2 hours at minimum.[3] CLRT beds rotate to less than 40 degrees, while kinetic therapy beds rotate to 40 degrees or more. The best evidence-based research involves kinetic therapy beds. The nurse assesses the patient for tolerance to position changes when a CLRT or kinetic therapy bed is in use.

Patients who are ventilated benefit from having the head of the bed elevated 30 degrees at all times.[4] The rationale is to promote lung expansion, prevent the aspiration that can occur in the recumbent position in intubated patients, and prevent ventilator-associated pneumonia (VAP). Rotation therapy may also help reduce pneumonia, although it may not reduce days on the ventilator or the length of hospital stay. For best outcomes, rotation must be continuous and at the maximum for each side.

Prone positioning is an advanced technique used with critically ill ventilated patients who have acute lung injury (ALI) or acute respiratory distress syndrome (ARDS) with a low PaO_2/FiO_2 ratio. Studies have demonstrated improved oxygenation in these patients when placed in the prone position, although this maneuver may not ultimately improve survival.[5] Prone positioning involves multiple personnel and specialized equipment, and must be performed only by specially trained staff to prevent complications.

Progressive mobility, from sitting up in a chair to ambulation, is also used as part of pulmonary hygiene.

Oxygen Therapy

Oxygen therapy is used to correct hypoxemia, decrease the work of breathing, and decrease myocardial work. The goals for all patients on oxygen therapy are a stable arterial oxygen saturation (SaO_2)

level, eupneic respirations, and a decrease in anxiety and shortness of breath. These goals should be accomplished through delivery of the least amount of supplemental oxygen needed, so the nurse continuously monitors the patient on oxygen for desired results, as well as for complications.

 RED FLAG! *Complications of oxygen therapy include respiratory arrest; skin breakdown from straps and masks; dry nasal mucous membranes; epistaxis, infection in the nares; oxygen toxicity; absorptive atelectasis; and carbon dioxide narcosis (manifested by altered mental status, confusion, headache, and somnolence).*

Several methods of oxygen delivery are available (Box 16-1). The choice of delivery method depends on the patient's condition. Low-flow oxygen devices are suitable for patients with normal respiratory patterns, rates, and ventilation volumes. High-flow

oxygen devices are suitable for patients with high oxygen requirements because high-flow devices deliver up to 100% FiO_2 and maintain humidification, which is essential to prevent drying of the nasal mucosa. The nurse monitors the SaO_2 closely for at least 30 to 60 minutes when switching from a low-flow to a high-flow oxygen delivery device, evaluates ABGs as needed, and assesses patient tolerance. If increased distress, desaturation, or both are noted, more extreme interventions (eg, intubation) may be necessary.

Oxygen toxicity starts to occur in patients breathing an FiO_2 of more than 50% for longer than 24 hours. The FiO_2 should be decreased as tolerated to the lowest possible setting as long as the SaO_2 remains greater than 90%. The pathophysiological changes that occur with oxygen toxicity may progress from capillary leaking to pulmonary edema and possibly to ALI or ARDS with prolonged high FiO_2 continues for several days. Patients on a high FiO_2

BOX 16-1   Oxygen Delivery Methods With Delivered Fraction of Inspired Oxygen (FiO_2)

High-Flow Devices

High-Flow Nasal Cannula

Flow (L/min)	FiO_2 (%)
1–35	21–100

Low-Flow Devices

Nasal Cannula

Flow (L/min)	FiO_2 (%)
1	21–25
2	25–28
3	28–32
4	32–36
5	36–40
6	40–44

Facemask

Flow (L/min)	FiO_2 (%)
5–6	40
6–7	50
7–10	60

Face Tent

Air is mixed with the oxygen flow in the mask, resulting in variable delivery with humidification (21% delivered with compressed air and up to 50% delivered with 10 L/min oxygen flow attached). A face tent is often used for patients who cannot tolerate the claustrophobic feeling associated with more traditional masks.

Venturi Mask

Oxygen Flow (Minimal Rate) (L/min)	FiO_2 Setting[a] (%)
4	25
4	28
6	31
8	35
8	40
10	50

[a]*FiO_2 setting is based on venturi setting/adapter used and oxygen flow.*

Nonrebreather Mask

The nonrebreather mask is used in severe hypoxemia to deliver the highest oxygen concentration. The one-way valve on one side allows for the exhalation of carbon dioxide. The mask delivers 80% to 95% FiO_2 at a flow rate of 10 L/min depending on the patient's rate and depth of breathing, with some room air entrained through the open port on the mask. The mask should fit snugly to prevent additional entrainment of room air.

Tracheostomy Collar and T-Piece

The T-piece is a T-shaped adapter used to provide oxygen to either an endotracheal or a tracheostomy tube. The tracheostomy collar may also be used and is generally preferred because it is more comfortable than the T-piece. The strap on the tracheostomy collar is adjusted to keep the collar on top of the tracheostomy. With both the T-piece and tracheostomy collar, the goal is to provide a high enough flow rate (at least 10 L/min with humidification) to ensure that there is a minimal amount of entrained room air. Flow can also be provided by a ventilator.

TABLE 16-1	Indications for Chest Tube Placement	
Indication	**Potential Causes**
Hemothorax	Chest trauma, neoplasms, pleural tears, excessive anticoagulation, postthoracic surgery, post–open lung biopsy
Pneumothorax	
Spontaneous (greater than 20%)	Bleb rupture, lung disease
Tension	Mechanical ventilation, penetrating puncture wound, prolonged clamping of chest tubes, lack of seal in chest tube drainage system
Bronchopleural fistula	Tissue damage, esophageal cancer, aspiration of toxic chemicals, Boerhaave's syndrome (spontaneous esophageal rupture)
Pleural effusion	Neoplasms, cardiopulmonary disease, inflammatory conditions, recurrent infections, pneumonia
Chylothorax	Trauma or thoracic surgery, malignancy, congenital abnormalities

may also develop absorptive atelectasis as a result of less nitrogen in the delivered gas mixture. Because nitrogen is not absorbed, it exerts pressure within the alveoli, keeping the alveoli open. When nitrogen is "washed out," the oxygen replacing it is absorbed, resulting in alveolar collapse (atelectasis).

Chest Tubes

Chest tubes are used to remove air or fluid from the pleural space, restore intrapleural negative pressure, reexpand a collapsed or partially collapsed lung, and prevent reflux of drainage back into the chest. Indications for chest tube placement are listed in Table 16-1.

Equipment

Most chest tubes are multifenestrated transparent tubes with distance and radiopaque markers that facilitate visualization of the tube on chest radiographs (necessary for verifying correct positioning in the pleural space). Larger tubes (20 to 36 French) are used to drain blood or thick pleural drainage. They are placed at about the fifth to sixth intercostal space (ICS) midaxillary. Smaller tubes (16 to 20 French) are used to remove air and are placed at the second to third ICS midclavicular.

Chest tubes are attached to a drainage system. Modern systems are disposable and have three chambers (Fig. 16-2). The first chamber is the collection receptacle, the second chamber is the water seal, and the third chamber is suction. The water

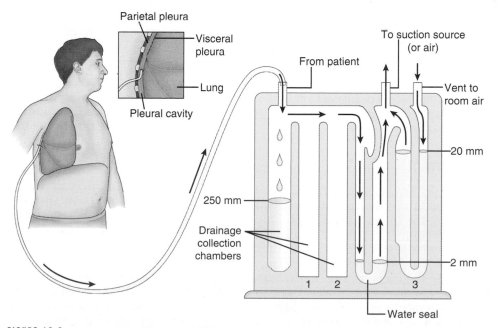

FIGURE 16-2   A disposable chest tube drainage system.

seal chamber acts as a one-way valve, allowing air to escape while preventing air from reentering the pleural space. The fluid level in the water seal chamber fluctuates during respiration. During inspiration, pleural pressures become more negative, causing the fluid level in the water seal chamber to rise. During expiration, pleural pressures become more positive, causing the fluid level to descend. If the patient is being mechanically ventilated, this process is reversed. Intermittent bubbling is seen in the water seal chamber as air and fluid drain from the pleural cavity. Constant bubbling indicates either an air leak in the system or a bronchopleural fistula.

In a disposable system that requires water suction, it is achieved by adding water up to the prescribed level in the suction chamber, usually –20 cm H₂O. It is the height of the water column in the suction chamber, not the amount of wall suction, that determines the amount of suction applied to the chest tube, most commonly –20 cm H₂O. Once the wall suction exceeds the force necessary to "lift" this column of fluid, any additional suction simply pulls air from a vented cap atop the chamber up through the water. The amount of wall suction applied should be sufficient to create a "gently rolling" bubble in the suction control chamber. Vigorous bubbling results in water loss through evaporation, changing suction pressure and increasing the noise level in the patient's room. It is important to assess the system for water loss and to add sterile water as necessary to maintain the prescribed level of suction.

Dry suction (waterless) systems use a spring mechanism to control the suction level and can provide levels of suction ranging from –10 to –40 cm H₂O. The amount of negative pressure is dialed in, again, it is the amount dialed in not the wall suction which determines the amount of suction. Dry suction systems that can deliver higher levels of suction may be necessary in patients with large bronchopleural fistulas, hemorrhage, or obesity. They also afford the patient a quieter environment.

 RED FLAG! *The chest tube drainage system should never be raised above the chest, or the drainage will back up into the chest.*

Chest Tube Placement

The patient is placed in Fowler's or semi-Fowler's position for the procedure. Because the parietal pleura is innervated by the intercostal and phrenic nerves, chest tube insertion is a painful procedure and administration of analgesics is indicated. After insertion, bacteriostatic ointment or petroleum gauze can be applied to the incision site. Petroleum gauze is thought to prevent air leaks; however, it also has the potential to macerate the skin and predispose the site to infection. A 4 × 4 gauze pad with a split is positioned over the tube and taped occlusively to the chest. All connections from the insertion site to

---

BOX 16-2   Chest Tube Drainage System Assessment and Management

1. Assess cardiopulmonary status and vital signs every 2 hours and as needed.
2. Check and maintain tube patency every 2 hours and as needed.
3. Monitor and document the type, color, consistency, and amount of drainage.
4. Mark the amount of drainage on the collection chamber in hourly or shift increments, depending on drainage, and document in output record.
5. Prevent dependent loops from forming in tubing; ensure that the patient does not inadvertently lie on the tubing.
6. Assess for fluctuation of the water level ("tidaling") in the water seal chamber with respiration or mechanical ventilation breaths.
7. Assess for the air leaks, manifested as constant bubbling in the water seal chamber. If constant bubbling is noted, identify the location of the leak by first turning off the suction. Then, beginning at the insertion site, briefly occlude the chest tube or drainage tube below each connection point until the drainage unit is reached.
8. Check that all tubing connections are securely sealed and taped.
9. Ensure water seal chambers are filled to the 2-cm water line. Relieve negative pressure if the water level is above the 2-cm water line.
10. Assess the patient for pain, intervene as needed, and reassess appropriately. Pain management may include the use of analgesics, a lidocaine patch, or nonsteroidal anti-inflammatory drugs (NSAIDs).
11. Assess the actual chest tube insertion site for signs of infection and subcutaneous emphysema.
12. Change the dressing per unit guidelines, when soiled, and when ordered.

---

the drainage collection system are securely taped to prevent air leaks as well as inadvertent disconnection. The proximal portion of the tube is taped to the chest to prevent traction on the tube and sutures if the patient moves. A postinsertion chest radiograph is always ordered to confirm proper positioning. The lungs are auscultated, and the condition of the tissue around the insertion site is evaluated for the presence of subcutaneous air. Ongoing assessment and management of a patient with a chest tube is summarized in Box 16-2.

 RED FLAG! *Occasionally, the chest tube may fall out or be accidentally pulled out. If this occurs, the insertion site should be quickly sealed off using petroleum gauze covered with dry gauze and an occlusive tape dressing to prevent air from entering the pleural cavity.*

RED FLAG! *The most serious complication associated with chest tube placement is tension pneumothorax, which can develop if there is an obstruction in the chest tube that prevents air from leaving (thus allowing it to accumulate in the pleural space.) Clamping chest tubes predisposes patients to this complication and is only recommended as a momentary measure, such as when it is necessary to locate the source of an air leak or replace the chest tube drainage unit.*

Chest Tube Removal

Chest tubes are removed after drainage is minimal. Prior to chest tube removal (12 to 24 hours before), the wall suction is disconnected (ie, the chest tube is placed on water seal). Premature removal of the chest tube may cause reaccumulation of the pneumothorax. Before the chest tube is removed, the patient is premedicated to alleviate pain. The tube is removed in one quick movement during expiration to prevent entraining air back into the pleural cavity. Immediately after tube removal, the lung fields are auscultated for any change in breath sounds, and an occlusive sterile dressing with petroleum gauze is applied over the site. A chest radiograph is obtained to look for the presence of residual air or fluid.

Pharmacotherapy

Bronchodilators

Bronchodilators dilate the airways by relaxing bronchial smooth muscle. Bronchodilator therapy can be delivered through metered-dose inhalers (MDIs) or nebulization. Patient inhalation ensures delivery into the lungs. Assessment before, during, and after the therapy is essential and includes breath sounds, pulse, respiratory rate, and pulmonary function tests to measure improvement in severity of airway obstruction. ABGs also may be indicated.

- **β_2-Adrenergic blockers.** Because of their rapid onset of action, β-adrenergic blockers are the bronchodilators of choice for the treatment of acute exacerbation of asthma or severe bronchial constriction. The bronchodilator effects of β-adrenergic blockers result from stimulation of β_2-adrenergic receptors in the lung bronchial smooth muscle. These agents may also stimulate β_1-adrenergic receptors in the heart, leading to undesired cardiac effects. β_2-selective drugs are more specific for the β_2-receptor, although they retain some β_1 activity. β_2-Adrenergic blockers may be administered orally or inhaled. Inhaled therapy has been shown to produce bronchodilation comparable to that of oral administration, with fewer adverse systemic effects.
- **Anticholinergic agents.** These drugs produce bronchodilation by reducing intrinsic vagal tone to the airways. They also block reflex bronchoconstriction caused by inhaled irritants.
- **Methylxanthines.** The use of methylxanthines in the treatment of bronchospastic airway disease is controversial. Theophylline, the prototype methylxanthine, may be used chronically in the treatment of bronchospastic disease but is usually considered third- or fourth-line therapy. Some patients with severe disease that is not controlled with β-adrenergic blockers, anticholinergics, or anti-inflammatory agents may benefit from theophylline. Aminophylline, the IV form of theophylline, is rarely used in acute exacerbations because of the lack of evidence that it is beneficial in this situation and it produces significant tachycardia.

Anti-Inflammatory Agents

Anti-inflammatory agents may be used prophylactically to interrupt the development of bronchial inflammation. They may also be used to reduce or terminate ongoing inflammation in the airway.

- **Corticosteroids** are the most effective anti-inflammatory agents for the treatment of reversible airflow obstruction. Corticosteroid therapy should be initiated simultaneously with bronchodilator therapy because the onset of action may be 6 to 12 hours. Corticosteroids may be administered parenterally, orally, or as aerosols. In acute exacerbations, high-dose parenteral steroids (eg, IV methylprednisolone) are used and then tapered as the patient tolerates. Short courses of oral therapy may be used to prevent the progression of acute attacks. Long-term oral therapy is associated with systemic adverse effects and should be avoided if possible.
- **Mast cell stabilizers** are thought to stabilize the cell membrane and prevent the release of mediators from mast cells. These agents are not indicated for acute exacerbations of asthma. Rather, they are used prophylactically to prevent acute airway narrowing after exposure to allergens (eg, exercise, cold air). A 4- to 6-week trial may be required to determine efficacy in individual patients. The goal is to reduce the frequency and severity of asthma attacks and enhance the effects of concomitantly administered bronchodilator and steroid therapy. It may be possible to decrease the dose of bronchodilators or corticosteroids in patients who respond to mast cell stabilizers.
- **Leukotriene receptor antagonists** may be used in the management of exercise-induced bronchospasm, asthma, allergic rhinitis, and urticaria. These agents block the activity of endogenous inflammatory mediators, particularly leukotrienes, which cause increased vascular permeability, mucus secretion, airway edema, bronchoconstriction, and other inflammatory cell process activities. Leukotriene receptor antagonists are administered once daily and are usually well tolerated. They are

not administered for acute conditions; rather, they are used as a part of an ongoing program of therapy.[6]

Neuromuscular Blocking Agents

Critically ill patients frequently require pharmacological intervention for analgesia, sedation, anxiety control, and facilitation of mechanical ventilation. If metabolic demands and work of breathing continue to compromise ventilatory or hemodynamic stability after maximization of sedation, neuromuscular blocking (NMB) agents may be required. NMB agents induce muscular paralysis by blocking acetylcholine at the motor endplate. The paralysis prevents the patient from "fighting" the ventilator and increasing the work of breathing. The goal of therapy with NMB agents is to maximize oxygenation and prevent complications such as barotrauma. NMB drugs do not possess analgesic or sedative properties. The patient is awake and aware, but unable to move. When NMB agents are used, sedation and analgesia are required, along with patient and family education. Numerous reports of prolonged paralysis following the use of NMB agents have prompted many facilities to initiate protocols for monitoring with the use of peripheral nerve stimulators.

Thoracic Surgery

Thoracic surgery is indicated as part of the management plan for many disorders involving the lungs and associated structures.

- Wedge resection is performed for the removal of benign or malignant lesions.
- Segmentectomy is the preferred method when patients are a poor risk with limited pulmonary reserve. Bleeding may be extensive following the surgery, and two chest drains are usually in place to drain air or blood.
- Lobectomy may be performed as a treatment for malignant or benign tumors and for infections such as bronchiectasis, tuberculosis, or fungal infection.
- Pneumonectomy is performed to remove one lung, usually because of primary carcinoma or significant infection.
- Lung volume reduction surgery (LVRS) involves resecting parts of the lung to reduce hyperinflation (eg, as part of the treatment for emphysema).
- Lung transplantation may involve one lung or both lungs, and it may be done along with heart transplantation. To be considered a viable candidate for lung transplantation, a patient must have minimal comorbidities and advanced lung disease that is unresponsive to other therapies.

CASE STUDY

Mr. B. is admitted to the critical care unit for the diagnosis of pancreatitis. The physician places a right subclavian central line. Immediately after the line placement, the nurse notes that Mr. B. has increasing dyspnea and tachycardia. Further assessment reveals diminished breath sounds on the right and unequal chest wall expansion. A chest radiograph is obtained and the physician is notified. Mr. B. is diagnosed with a right pneumothorax, and a chest tube connected to a drainage system and –20 cm H_2O suction is placed.

Two days later, the nurse is assessing Mr. B. and notes intermittent bubbling in the water seal chamber, fluctuation of the fluid in the tubing, a small amount of subcutaneous air, and a dry and occlusive dressing. Chest radiographs, obtained daily, demonstrate the presence of a small pneumothorax. The chest tube is still connected to –20 cm H_2O suction.

Five days later, the chest radiograph demonstrates complete resolution of the pneumothorax. The chest tube is taken off of suction and left to water seal for 8 hours. Mr. B. tolerates this without any signs of dyspnea and the chest tube is removed by the physician. The incision site is covered with petroleum gauze and occlusive tape is applied to secure the dressing.

1. What was the cause of the pneumothorax?

2. What is the clinical difference between finding intermittent bubbling and constant bubbling in the water seal chamber?

3. What would be the reasoning for applying a petroleum gauze dressing after removal of the chest tube?

References

1. Nettina SM: Respiratory disorders. In Mills EJ (ed): Lippincott Manual of Nursing Practice, 9th ed. Philadelphia, PA: Lippincott Williams & Wilkins, 2009
2. Staudinger T, et al.: Continuous lateral rotation therapy to prevent ventilator-associated pneumonia. Crit Care Med 38(2):706–707, 2010
3. Swadener-Culpepper, L. Continuous lateral rotation therapy. Critical Care Nurse 30(2):S5–S7, 2010
4. Tolentino-DelosReyes AF, et al.: Am J Crit Care 16(1):20–27, 2007
5. Kopterides P, Siempos I, Armagaidis A, et al.: Prone positioning in hypoxemix respiratory failure: Meta analysis of randomized controlled trials. J Crit Care 24:89–100, 2009
6. Karch AM (ed): Lippincott's Nursing Drug Guide, 2007 ed. Philadelphia, PA: Lippincott Williams & Wilkins, 2007

Want to know more? A wide variety of resources to enhance your learning and understanding of this chapter are available on the**Point** ✳. Visit **http://thepoint.lww.com/MortonEss1e** to access chapter review questions and more!

Common Respiratory Disorders

OBJECTIVES

Based on the content in this chapter, the reader should be able to:

1 Describe the pathophysiology, assessment, and management of pneumonia in the critically ill patient.
2 Describe the pathophysiology, assessment, and management of acute respiratory failure.
3 Differentiate between hypoxemic (type I) acute respiratory failure and hypercapnic (type II) acute respiratory failure.
4 Describe the pathophysiology, assessment, and management of acute respiratory distress syndrome (ARDS).
5 Discuss the pathophysiology, assessment, and management of pleural effusion.
6 Describe the pathophysiology, assessment, and management of pneumothorax.
7 Discuss the pathophysiology, assessment, management, and prevention of pulmonary embolism.
8 Explain the pathophysiology, assessment, and management of an acute exacerbation of chronic obstructive pulmonary disease (COPD).
9 Describe the pathophysiology, assessment, and management of an acute exacerbation of asthma and status asthmaticus.

Pneumonia

Pneumonia is a common infection in both the community and hospital. In the United States, pneumonia is the leading cause of death from infectious disease, the second most common hospital-acquired infection, and the seventh leading cause of death.[1] Critical care nurses encounter pneumonia when it complicates the course of a serious illness or leads to acute respiratory distress. According to guidelines developed by the American Thoracic Society (ATS), patients with severe community-acquired pneumonia (CAP) require admission to the critical

care unit. Severe CAP is defined as the presence of one of two major criteria or the presence of two of three minor criteria (Box 17-1).[2] *Streptococcus pneumoniae* (pneumococcus) is the predominant pathogen in patients with CAP who require hospitalization.

The Older Patient. *The incidence of CAP requiring hospitalization is four times higher in patients older than 65 years than it is in those 45 to 64 years of age.[3] In addition, the cause of CAP in patients older than 65 years is frequently a drug-resistant strain of S. pneumoniae.[2]*

Major Criteria
- Need for mechanical ventilation
- Need for vasopressors for greater than 4 hours (septic shock)
- Acute renal failure (urine output less than 80 mL in 4 hours or serum creatinine greater than 2 mg/dL in the absence of chronic renal failure)
- Increase in size of infiltrates by more than 50% in presence of clinical nonresponse to treatment or deterioration

Minor Criteria
- Respiratory rate greater than 30 breaths/min
- Systolic blood pressure less than or equal to 90 mm Hg
- Diastolic blood pressure less than 60 mm Hg, multilobar disease
- PaO_2/FiO_2 ratio less than 250

Adapted from American Thoracic Society: Guidelines for the management of adults with community-acquired pneumonia. Am J Respir Crit Care Med 163:1730–1754, 2001.

Hospital-acquired pneumonia (HAP) is pneumonia occurring more than 48 hours after admission to a hospital, which excludes infection that is incubating at the time of admission.[4] Ventilator-associated pneumonia (VAP) is the occurrence of pneumonia more than 48 to 72 hours after intubation. HAP and VAP continue to cause morbidity and mortality despite advances in antimicrobial therapy and advanced supportive measures.[4]

Bacteria, viruses, mycoplasmas, fungi, and aspiration of foreign material can cause pneumonia. Etiology varies greatly depending on whether the pneumonia is community acquired or hospital acquired.[5] HAP and VAP may be polymicrobial and multidrug resistant.

Pathophysiology

Pneumonia is an inflammatory response to inhaled or aspirated foreign material or the uncontrolled multiplication of microorganisms invading the lower respiratory tract. This response results in the accumulation of neutrophils and other proinflammatory cytokines in the peripheral bronchi and alveolar spaces.[6] The severity of pneumonia depends on the amount of material aspirated, the virulence of the organism, the amount of bacteria in the aspirate, and the host defenses.[6]

The means by which pathogens enter the lower respiratory tract include aspiration, inhalation, hematogenous spread from a distant site, and translocation. Risk factors that predispose a patient to one of these mechanisms include conditions that enhance colonization of the oropharynx, conditions favoring aspiration, conditions requiring prolonged intubation, and host factors.[6] The risk for clinically significant aspiration is increased in patients who are unable to protect their airways.

Colonization of the oropharynx has been identified as an independent factor in the development of HAP and VAP. Gram-positive bacteria and anaerobic bacteria normally live in the oropharynx. When normal oropharyngeal flora are destroyed, the oropharynx is susceptible to colonization by pathogenic bacteria. Pathogenic organisms that have colonized the oropharynx are readily available for aspiration into the tracheobronchial tree. Gastric colonization may also lead to retrograde colonization of the oropharynx, although the role the stomach plays in the development of pneumonia is controversial. The stomach is normally sterile because of the bactericidal activity of hydrochloric acid. However, when gastric pH increases above normal (eg, with the use of histamine type 2 antagonists or antacids), microorganisms are able to multiply, increasing the risk for retrograde colonization of the oropharynx and pneumonia.[4]

Inhalation of bacteria-laden aerosols from contaminated respiratory equipment is another potential source of pneumonia-causing bacteria. Condensate collection in the ventilator tubing can become contaminated with secretions and serve as a reservoir for bacterial growth.

Assessment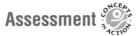

Knowledge of risk factors and symptoms assists in making the diagnosis and identifying the causative organism. A comprehensive cardiovascular and pulmonary assessment is completed, with a focus on the ATS major and minor criteria (see Box 17-1). The nurse assesses for signs of hypoxemia and dyspnea. Patients presenting with new-onset respiratory symptoms (eg, cough, sputum production, dyspnea, pleuritic chest pain) usually have an accompanying fever and chills. Decreased breath sounds and crackles or bronchial breath sounds are heard over the area of consolidation.

 The Older Patient. *Confusion and tachypnea are common presenting symptoms in older patients with pneumonia. The usual symptoms (fever, chills, increased white blood cell (WBC) count) may be absent. Other symptoms include weakness, lethargy, failure to thrive, anorexia, abdominal pain, episodes of falling, incontinence, headache, delirium, and nonspecific deterioration.*

 RED FLAG! *Disorders that may mimic pneumonia clinically include heart failure, atelectasis, pulmonary thromboembolism, drug reactions, pulmonary hemorrhage, and ARDS.*

Diagnostic tests are ordered to determine whether pneumonia is the cause of the patient's symptoms and to identify the pathogen when pneumonia is present. Table 17-1 summarizes the current ATS

TABLE 17-1	Diagnostic Studies in Patients With Severe Community-Acquired Pneumonia (CAP) or Severe Hospital-Acquired Pneumonia (HAP)

Study	Rationale
Chest radiograph (anterior–posterior and lateral)	Identifies the presence, location, and severity of infiltrates (multilobar, rapidly spreading, or cavitary infiltrates indicate severe pneumonia) Facilitates assessment for pleural effusions Differentiates pneumonia from other conditions
Two sets of blood cultures from separate sites	Isolates the etiologic pathogen in 8%–20% of cases
Complete blood count	Documents the presence of multiple-organ dysfunction
Serum electrolyte panel, renal and liver function tests	Helps define severity of illness
Arterial blood gases (ABGs)	Defines severity of illness Determines need for supplemental oxygen and mechanical ventilation
Thoracentesis (if pleural effusion greater than 10 mm identified on lateral decubitus film)	Rules out empyema

Pleural fluid studies, including
  WBC count with differential
  Protein
  Glucose
  Lactate dehydrogenase (LDH)
  pH
  Gram stain and acid-fast stain
  Culture for bacteria, fungi, and mycobacteria	

From data in American Thoracic Society: Guidelines for the management of adults with community-acquired pneumonia. Am J Respir Crit Care Med 163:1730–1754, 2001.

recommendations. Lower respiratory secretions can be easily obtained in intubated patients using endotracheal aspiration and may assist in excluding certain pathogens and modifying initial empirical treatment. Invasive diagnostic techniques, such as bronchoalveolar lavage (BAL) or bronchoscopy with protected specimen brush (PSB), may be used in selected circumstances (eg, nonresponse to antimicrobial therapy, immunosuppression, suspected tuberculosis in the absence of a productive cough, pneumonia with suspected neoplasm or foreign body, or conditions that require lung biopsy).[4] Pneumococcal urinary antigen assay, which returns results within 15 minutes, is recommended as an addition to blood culture testing.[7] The IDSA recommends HIV testing for people between the ages of 15 and 54 years as well.[7]

Management

Antibiotic Therapy

Patients are initially treated empirically, based on the severity of disease and the likely pathogens.[4] Because data show that hospitalized patients with CAP who receive their first dose of antibiotic therapy within 8 hours of arrival at the hospital have reduced mortality at 30 days, initial therapy should be instituted rapidly.[2] Double antibiotic coverage is necessary for patients with severe CAP.[7] Initial therapy should not be changed within the first 48 to 72 hours unless progressive deterioration is evident or initial blood or respiratory cultures indicate a

need to modify therapy.[4] The duration of therapy depends on many factors, including the presence of concurrent illness or bacteremia, the severity of pneumonia at the onset of antibiotic therapy, the causative organism, the risk for multidrug resistance, and the rapidity of clinical response.[4]

Supportive Therapy

Oxygen therapy may be required to maintain adequate gas exchange. Humidified oxygen should be administered by mask or endotracheal tube to promote adequate ventilation. Mechanical ventilation to correct hypoxemia is frequently required in both severe CAP and HAP. Aggressive bronchial hygiene therapy (BHT) and adequate nutritional support are critical.

Acute Respiratory Failure

Acute respiratory failure is a sudden and life-threatening deterioration in pulmonary gas exchange, resulting in carbon dioxide retention and inadequate oxygenation. Acute respiratory failure is defined as an arterial oxygen tension (PaO_2) of 50 mm Hg or less, an arterial carbon dioxide tension ($PaCO_2$) greater than 50 mm Hg, and an arterial pH less than 7.35. Patients with advanced COPD and chronic hypercapnia may exhibit an acute increase in $PaCO_2$ to a high level, a decrease in blood pH, and a significant increase in serum bicarbonate during the onset of acute respiratory failure. Acute respiratory failure

BOX 17-2 Causes of Acute Respiratory Failure

Intrinsic Lung and Airway Diseases

Large Airway Obstruction
- Congenital deformities
- Acute laryngitis, epiglottitis
- Foreign bodies
- Intrinsic tumors
- Extrinsic pressure
- Traumatic injury
- Enlarged tonsils and adenoids
- Obstructive sleep apnea

Bronchial Diseases
- Chronic bronchitis
- Asthma
- Acute bronchiolitis

Parenchymal Diseases
- Pulmonary emphysema
- Pulmonary fibrosis and other chronic diffuse infiltrative diseases
- Severe pneumonia
- Acute lung injury (ALI), acute respiratory distress syndrome (ARDS)

Vascular Disease
- Cardiac pulmonary edema
- Massive or recurrent pulmonary embolism
- Pulmonary vasculitis

Extrapulmonary Disorders

Diseases of the Pleura and the Chest Wall
- Pneumothorax
- Pleural effusion
- Fibrothorax
- Thoracic wall deformity
- Traumatic injury to the chest wall (flail chest)
- Obesity

Disorders of the Respiratory Muscles and the Neuromuscular Junction
- Myasthenia gravis and myasthenia-like disorders
- Muscular dystrophies
- Polymyositis
- Botulism
- Muscle-paralyzing drugs
- Severe hypokalemia and hypophosphatemia

Disorders of the Peripheral Nerves and Spinal Cord
- Poliomyelitis
- Guillain–Barré syndrome
- Spinal cord trauma (quadriplegia)
- Amyotrophic lateral sclerosis
- Tetanus
- Multiple sclerosis

Disorders of the Central Nervous System
- Sedative and narcotic drug overdose
- Head trauma
- Cerebral hypoxia
- Stroke
- CNS infection
- Epileptic seizure: status epilepticus
- Metabolic and endocrine disorders
- Bulbar poliomyelitis
- Primary alveolar hypoventilation
- Sleep apnea syndrome

---

may be caused by a variety of pulmonary and non-pulmonary diseases (Box 17-2). Many factors may precipitate or exacerbate acute respiratory failure (Box 17-3).

BOX 17-3 Precipitating and Exacerbating Factors in Acute Respiratory Failure

- Changes in tracheobronchial secretions
- Disturbances in tracheobronchial clearance
- Viral or bacterial pneumonia
- Drugs: sedatives, narcotics, anesthesia, oxygen
- Inhalation or aspiration of irritants, vomitus, or foreign body
- Cardiovascular disorders: heart failure, pulmonary embolism, shock
- Mechanical factors: pneumothorax, pleural effusion, abdominal distention
- Trauma, including surgery
- Neuromuscular abnormalities
- Allergic disorders: bronchospasm
- Increased oxygen demand: fever, infection
- Inspiratory muscle fatigue

There are three main types of acute respiratory failure:

- **Acute hypoxemic respiratory failure (type I).** Type I acute respiratory failure is the result of abnormal oxygen transport secondary to pulmonary parenchymal disease, with increased alveolar ventilation resulting in a low $PaCO_2$.[8] The principal problem in type I acute respiratory failure is the inability to achieve adequate oxygenation, as evidenced by a PaO_2 of 50 mm Hg or less and a $PaCO_2$ of 40 mm Hg or less. Right-to-left shunt and alveolar hypoventilation are the most clinically significant causes of type I failure.[8]
- **Acute hypercapnic respiratory failure (type II).** Type II acute respiratory failure (ventilatory failure) is the result of inadequate alveolar ventilation secondary to decreased ventilatory drive, respiratory muscle fatigue or failure, and increased work of breathing.[8] Type II acute respiratory failure is characterized by marked elevation of carbon dioxide levels with relative preservation of oxygenation. Hypoxemia results from reduced alveolar pressure of oxygen (PAO_2) and is proportionate to hypercapnia.[8]

- **Combined hypoxemic and hypercapnic respiratory failure (type I and type II).** The combined type of acute respiratory failure develops as a consequence of inadequate alveolar ventilation and abnormal gas transport. Any cause of type I failure may lead to combined failure, especially if increased work of breathing and hypercapnia are involved.

Pathophysiology

A vicious positive feedback mechanism characterizes the deleterious effects of continued hypoxemia and hypercapnia. Mechanisms of hypoxemia in acute respiratory failure are summarized in Table 17-2. Effects of prolonged hypoxemia and hypercapnia include

- Increased pulmonary vascular resistance
- Right ventricular failure (cor pulmonale)
- Right ventricular hypertrophy
- Impaired left ventricular function
- Reduced cardiac output
- Cardiogenic pulmonary edema
- Diaphragmatic fatigue from increased workload of respiratory muscles

Assessment

Presentation of acute respiratory failure varies, depending on the underlying disease, precipitating factors, and degree of hypoxemia, hypercapnia, or acidosis. The classic symptom of hypoxemia is dyspnea,[9] although dyspnea may be completely absent in ventilatory failure resulting from depression of the respiratory center. Other presenting symptoms of hypoxemia include cyanosis, restlessness, confusion, anxiety, delirium, tachypnea, tachycardia, hypertension, cardiac dysrhythmias, and tremor.[9]

The cardinal symptoms of hypercapnia are dyspnea and headache. Other clinical manifestations of hypercapnia include peripheral and conjunctival hyperemia, hypertension, tachycardia, tachypnea, impaired consciousness, papilledema, and asterixis (wrist tremor).[9] Uncorrected carbon dioxide narcosis leads to diminished alertness, disorientation, increased intracranial pressure (ICP), and loss of consciousness. Associated findings in acute respiratory failure may include use of accessory muscles for respiration, intercostal or supraclavicular retraction, and paradoxical abdominal movement if diaphragmatic weakness or fatigue is present.

Arterial blood gas (ABG) analysis is needed to determine PaO_2, $PaCO_2$, and blood pH levels and confirm the diagnosis of acute respiratory failure. Other diagnostic tests that may be ordered to aid in determining the underlying cause may include chest radiography, sputum examination, pulmonary function testing, angiography, ventilation–perfusion scanning, computed tomography (CT), toxicology screening, complete blood count, serum electrolytes, cytology, urinalysis, bronchogram, bronchoscopy, electrocardiography, echocardiography, and thoracentesis.[8] Table 17-3 summarizes key clinical findings and diagnostic tests according to the underlying cause of the respiratory failure.

Management

Treatment of acute respiratory failure warrants immediate intervention to correct or compensate for the gas exchange abnormality and identify the cause. Therapy is directed toward correcting the cause and alleviating the hypoxia and hypercapnia (see Table 17-3).

If alveolar ventilation is inadequate to maintain PaO_2 or $PaCO_2$ levels (due to respiratory or neurological

TABLE 17-2 Mechanisms of Hypoxemia in Acute Respiratory Failure

Mechanism	Comments
Ventilation–perfusion mismatching ("dead space")	Resultant hypoxemia is reversible with supplemental oxygen
Inhalation of a hypoxic gas mixture or severe reduction of barometric pressure (eg, toxic inhalation, oxygen consumption in fire, high altitudes)	Oxygen content of inhaled gas is decreased
Alveolar hypoventilation	Alveolar partial pressure of oxygen (PaO_2) is decreased while alveolar partial pressure of carbon dioxide ($PaCO_2$) is increased
Impaired diffusion (eg, emphysema, diffuse lung injury)	Prevents complete equilibration of alveolar gas with pulmonary capillary blood; small effect is usually easily compensated by a small increase in the fraction of inspired oxygen (FiO_2)
Right-to-left shunt	Indicates closure of air passages, especially the distal airways and alveoli
	Changes in FiO_2 have little effect on the arterial carbon dioxide tension (PaO_2) when the shunt exceeds 30%
Abnormal pulmonary gas exchange, cardiac output that is too high or too low, high metabolic rate	Increased oxygen extraction from arterial blood results in decreased PaO_2
	Oxygen content of mixed venous blood is reduced

TABLE 17-3 Evaluation and Management of Common Causes of Acute Respiratory Failure

Etiology	Key Clinical Findings	Key Diagnostic Tests	Specific Therapy
Acute Hypoxemic (Type I) Respiratory Failure: Increased Alveolar–Arterial Gradient			
Alveoli/interstitium			
Cardiogenic pulmonary edema	Crackles, diaphoresis	CXR: pulmonary edema PA catheter: elevated CVP and PAOP ECG	Diuresis Reduce LVEDP
Acute respiratory distress syndrome (ARDS)	Crackles, PaO_2 less than 55 mm Hg with FiO_2 greater than 60%	CXR: bilateral fluffy white infiltrates PA catheter: normal or low PAOP	Treat underlying cause Ventilation
Pneumonia	Fever, crackles, or diminished breath sounds, egophony	CXR: diffuse or lobar infiltrate CBC: leukocytosis Sputum gram stain, blood culture	Antibiotics: empirical therapy tailored to likely pathogens
Pleural effusion	Egophony	CXR: pleural effusion; contralateral mediastinal shift Thoracentesis	Drainage Treat underlying cause Consider pleurodesis
Atelectasis	Postoperative status Diminished breath sounds	CXR: volume loss, ipsilateral mediastinal shift	Reduce sedation Bronchial hygiene therapy (BHT) Consider bronchoscopy
Pneumothorax	Diminished breath sounds, chest wall asymmetry, tracheal deviation	CXR: pneumothorax; contralateral mediastinal shift	Decompression (chest tube)
Alveolar hemorrhage	Hemoptysis	CXR: localized or diffuse infiltrate; air bronchograms Sputum: hemosiderin-laden macrophages ANCA, anti-GBM, sputum AFB, cytology, Gram stain, urinalysis	Protect uninvolved lung Identify bleeding site and etiology If localized, consider resection, embolization
Pulmonary infarct	Hypercoagulable state, risk for DVT, tachypnea, tachycardia, pleuritic chest pain, hemoptysis	CXR: wedge-shaped peripheral infiltrate Abnormal VQ scan or pulmonary arteriogram	Heparin anticoagulation Consider thrombolysis and IVC filter
Airways			
Asthma	Wheezing (may be absent if severe airflow obstruction)	Reduced PEF, FEV_1, VC	β-Adrenergic blockers, corticosteroid, theophylline Consider HELIOX
Chronic obstructive pulmonary disease (COPD)	Wheezing (infrequent), crackles, sputum production	ABG: hypoxemia, hypercarbia, normal pH	Titrate oxygen carefully to SaO_2 greater than 90% β-Adrenergic blockers, ipratropium bromide, corticosteroid, theophylline, antibiotics (if clinical evidence of infection)
Foreign body	Witnessed aspiration	CXR: frequent right upper lobe pneumonia	Bronchoscopy to localize and remove foreign body
Epiglottitis	Odynophagia, drooling	Lateral neck films	Racemic epinephrine, antibiotics, HELIOX
Vascular disease			
Pulmonary embolus	Hypercoagulable state, risk for DVT, tachypnea, tachycardia, pleuritic chest pain, hemoptysis	CXR: nonspecific Abnormal VQ scan or pulmonary arteriogram	Heparin anticoagulation Consider thrombolysis and IVC filter

TABLE 17-3 Evaluation and Management of Common Causes of Acute Respiratory Failure (continued)

Etiology	Key Clinical Findings	Key Diagnostic Tests	Specific Therapy
Lymphatic disease			
Lymphangitic carcinomatosis	History of neoplasm	CXR: reticular infiltrates Cytology from PA catheter	Treat underlying disease
Acute Hypercapnic (Type II) Respiratory Failure: Normal Alveolar–Arterial Gradient			
Reduced FiO_2	Geographic location (altitude)	Ambient FiO_2	Change location
CNS depression	History of drug overdose, head trauma, or anoxic encephalopathy Comatose	Response to naloxone Toxicology screen Electrolytes (glucose, calcium, sodium) Head CT, EEG	Naloxone, charcoal Correct electrolytes Neurological evaluation
Neuromuscular dysfunction	History of neuromuscular blockade, neck trauma, or neuromuscular disease	Cervical spine films CXR: elevated hemidiaphragms PFTs: reduced VC, NIF, PEF in supine position	Stabilize cervical spine Discontinue paralytics Noninvasive ventilation

AFB, acid-fast bacilli; ANCA, antineutrophilic cytoplasmic antibody; anti-GBM, antiglomerular basement membrane antibody; CBC, complete blood cell count; CNS, central nervous system; CT, computed tomography; CXR, chest x-ray; DVT, deep venous thrombosis; ECG, electrocardiogram; EEG, electroencephalogram; HELIOX, helium and oxygen mixture; IVC, inferior vena cava; LVEDP, left ventricular end-diastolic pressure; NIF, negative inspiratory force; PA, pulmonary artery; PAOP, pulmonary artery occlusion pressure; PEF, peak expiratory flow; PEFR, peak expiratory flow rate; PFTs, pulmonary function tests; VC, vital capacity.

failure), endotracheal intubation and mechanical ventilation may be lifesaving. Box 17-4 lists indications for intubation and ventilation. The initial assessment and the decision to initiate mechanical ventilation should be performed rapidly. Controlled oxygen therapy and mechanical ventilation are used to increase PaO_2 (by increasing the FiO_2) and to normalize pH (by increasing minute ventilation).

In patients with acute hypoxemic respiratory failure, the FiO_2 should be rapidly increased to maintain an arterial oxygen saturation (SaO_2) of 90% or higher. These patients require continuous pulse oximetry monitoring. Once hypoxemia is reversed, oxygen is titrated to the minimum level necessary for correction of hypoxemia and prevention of significant carbon dioxide retention.

Patients with acute hypercapnic respiratory failure are immediately assessed for either an impaired central respiratory drive associated with sedative or narcotic use or for underlying bronchospasm secondary to an asthma exacerbation or COPD. Reversal agents (eg, naloxone) are used in the case

of impaired central respiratory drive, and inhaled bronchodilators and systemic corticosteroids are used in the case of underlying bronchospasm.

Acute Respiratory Distress Syndrome

ARDS is a complex clinical syndrome that carries a high risk for mortality. ARDS may be precipitated by either direct or indirect pulmonary injury (Box 17-5). ARDS is characterized by pathological changes in lung vascular tissue, increased lung edema, and impaired gas exchange that ultimately lead to refractory hypoxemia (Fig. 17-1). ARDS is at the extreme end of a continuum of hypoxic acute lung injury (ALI) that results in respiratory failure (Table 17-4).

Systemic inflammatory response syndrome (SIRS) describes an inflammatory response occurring throughout the body as a result of some systemic insult. (The criteria that define SIRS are given in Box 17-6, and SIRS is discussed in more detail in Chapter 33.)

Often, patients with SIRS develop multisystem organ dysfunction syndrome (MODS) and the respiratory system is usually the earliest organ system involved. The respiratory system dysfunction presents as ARDS.

 RED FLAG! *Critical care nurses must be vigilant for early warning signs of ARDS. Monitoring patients who meet the criteria for SIRS (see Box 17-6) may aid in identifying those who are at risk for ARDS. An unexplained increase in respiratory rate may be a sign of impending ALI or ARDS and should not be taken lightly. Other changes in vital signs include hypotension, tachycardia, and hyper-or hypothermia.*

BOX 17-4 Indications for Intubation and Ventilation in Acute Respiratory Failure

- Depressed mental status or coma
- Severe respiratory distress
- Extremely low or agonal respiratory rate
- Obvious respiratory muscle fatigue
- Peripheral cyanosis
- Impending cardiopulmonary arrest

Direct Injury
- Aspiration (gastric fluids, drowning)
- Infectious pneumonia
- Lung contusions with trauma
- Toxic inhalation
- Upper airway obstruction (relieved)
- Severe acute respiratory syndrome (SARS) coronavirus
- Neurogenic pulmonary edema
- Acute eosinophilic pneumonia
- Bronchiolitis obliterans with organizing pneumonia (BOOP)
- Military tuberculosis

Indirect Pulmonary Injury
- Sepsis
- Burns
- Trauma
- Blood transfusion (transfusion-related acute lung injury [TRALI])
- Lung or bone marrow transplantation
- Drug or alcohol overdose
- Drug reaction
- Cardiopulmonary bypass
- Acute pancreatitis
- Multiple fractures
- Venous air embolism
- Amniotic fluid embolism
- Pancreatitis

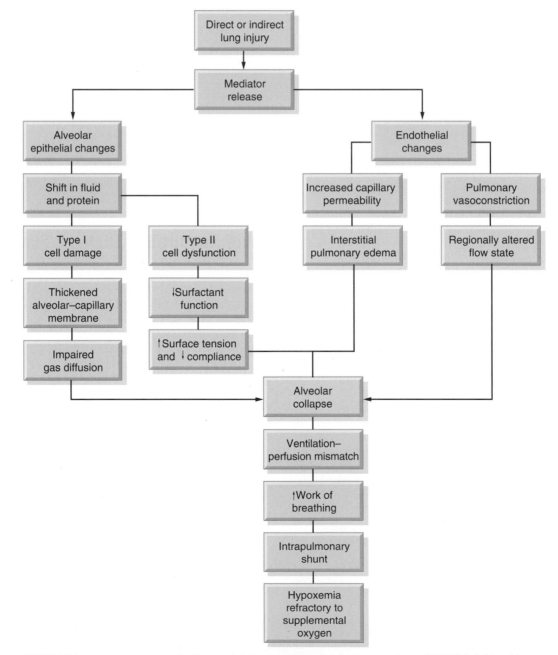

FIGURE 17·1 The pathophysiological cascade in acute respiratory distress syndrome (ARDS) is initiated by injury resulting in mediator release. The multiple effects result in changes to the alveoli, vascular tissue, and bronchi. The ultimate effect is ventilation–perfusion mismatching and refractory hypoxemia.

TABLE 17-4 Comparison of Acute Lung Injury (ALI) and Acute Respiratory Distress Syndrome (ARDS)

Criterion	ALI	ARDS
PaO$_2$/FiO$_2$ ratio, regardless of PEEP level	Less than 300	Less than 200
Chest radiograph	Bilateral infiltrates	Bilateral infiltrates
PAOP	Less than 18 mm Hg or no indication of left atrial hypertension	Less than 18 mm Hg or no indication of left atrial hypertension

PaO$_2$/FiO$_2$ ratio, ratio of arterial oxygen to inspired oxygen; PAOP, pulmonary artery occlusion pressure; PEEP, positive end-expiratory pressure; ALI, Acute lung injury; ARDS, Acute Respiratory Distress Syndrome.
Adapted from Bernard GR, Artigas A, Brigham KL, et al: The American-European Consensus conference on ARDS: Definitions, mechanisms, relevant outcomes, and clinical trials co-ordination. Am J Respir Crit Care Med 149:818–824, 1994.

 The Older Patient. *People who are 65 years of age or older are at increased risk for multisystem organ involvement with less chance of recovering from ARDS; therefore, the mortality rate is increased in this population.*

Pathophysiology

In ARDS, diffuse alveolar–capillary membrane damage occurs, increasing membrane permeability and allowing fluids to move from the vascular space into the interstitial and alveolar spaces. Air spaces fill with blood, proteinaceous fluid, and debris from degenerating cells, causing interstitial and intra-alveolar edema and impairing oxygenation (Fig. 17-2). In addition, inflammatory mediators cause the pulmonary vascular bed to constrict, resulting in pulmonary hypertension and reduced blood flow to portions of the lung.

The pathological changes affect the mechanics of breathing. Surfactant is lost, resulting in alveolar collapse. Lung compliance is reduced as a result of the stiffness of the fluid-filled, nonaerated lung. Mediator-induced bronchoconstriction causes airway narrowing and increased airway resistance. As a result of reduced lung compliance and increased airway resistance, ventilation is impaired. As airway pressures rise, the lung is traumatized, resulting in further lung tissue damage.

BOX 17-6 Systemic Inflammatory Response Syndrome (SIRS) Criteria

SIRS is manifested by two or more of the following:

- Temperature greater than 100.4°F (38°C) or less than 96.8°F (36°C)
- Heart rate greater than 90 beats/min
- Respiratory rate greater than 20 breaths/min or an arterial carbon dioxide tension (PaCO$_2$) less than 32 mm Hg
- White blood cell (WBC) count greater than 12,000 cells/mm^3 or less than 4000 cells/mm^3 OR more than 10% immature (band) forms

ARDS progresses in stages:

- **Stage 1.** The patient exhibits increased dyspnea and tachypnea, but there are few radiographic changes. Within 24 hours, the symptoms of respiratory distress increase in severity, with coarse bilateral crackles on auscultation, and radiographic changes consistent with patchy infiltrates (fluid-filled alveoli alongside collapsed alveoli).
- **Stage 2,** the exudative stage, is marked by mediator-induced interstitial and alveolar edema. The endothelial and epithelial beds are increasingly permeable to proteins. The hypoxia is resistant to supplemental oxygen administration, and mechanical ventilation is usually required to maintain oxygenation.
- **Stage 3,** the proliferative stage, is characterized by hemodynamic instability, generalized edema, the possible onset of hospital-acquired infections, increased hypoxemia, and lung involvement. Evidence of SIRS is present.
- **Stage 4,** the fibrotic stage, is typified by progressive lung fibrosis and emphysematous changes resulting in increased dead space. Fibrotic lung changes result in ventilation management difficulties, with increased airway pressure and development of pneumothoraces.

Assessment

ARDS symptoms typically develop within a few hours to several days after the inciting insult. The clinical presentation includes tachypnea, dyspnea, use of accessory muscles, and severe acute hypoxia resistant to improvement with supplemental oxygen. Patients with acute respiratory failure may exhibit neurological changes (eg, restlessness, agitation) associated with impaired oxygenation and decreased perfusion to the brain.

As pathological changes progress, lung auscultation may reveal crackles and rhonchi secondary to an increase in secretions and narrowed airways. Decreases in SaO$_2$ are early signs of impending decompensation. Lethargy is an ominous sign and indicates the immediate need for interventions to support ventilation and oxygenation. Multisystem

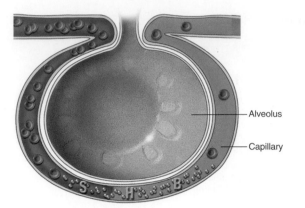

Phase 1. Injury reduces normal blood flow to the lungs. Platelets aggregate and release histamine (H), serotonin (S), and bradykinin (B).

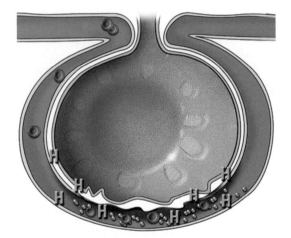

Phase 2. Those substances, especially histamine, inflame and damage the alveolar–capillary membrane, increasing capillary permeability. Fluids then shift into the interstitial space.

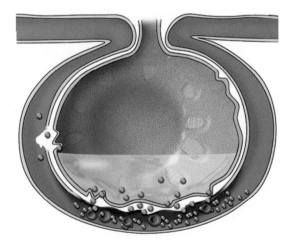

Phase 3. As capillary permeability increases, proteins and fluids leak out, increasing interstitial osmotic pressure and causing pulmonary edema.

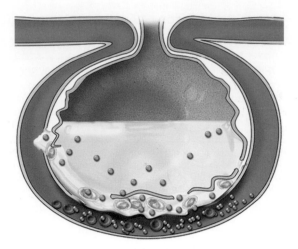

Phase 4. Decreased blood flow and fluids in the alveoli damage surfactant and impair the cell's ability to produce more. As a result, alveoli collapse, impeding gas exchange and decreasing lung compliance.

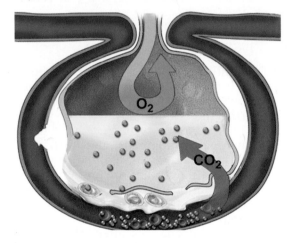

Phase 5. Sufficient oxygen cannot cross the alveolar–capillary membrane, but carbon dioxide (CO_2) can and is lost with every exhalation. Oxygen (O_2) levels decrease in the blood.

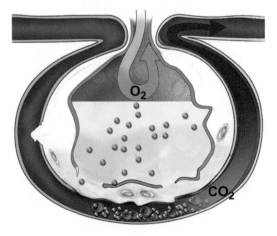

Phase 6. Pulmonary edema worsens, inflammation leads to fibrosis, and gas exchange is further impeded.

FIGURE 17-2 In acute respiratory distress syndrome (ARDS), changes in lung epithelium and vascular endothelium result in fluid and protein movement, changes in lung compliance, and disruption of the alveoli with accompanying hypoxia. (From Anatomical Chart Company: Atlas of Pathophysiology, 3rd ed. Ambler, PA: Lippincott Williams & Wilkins, 2010, pp 81, 83.)

involvement becomes evident as highly perfused organ systems respond to decreased oxygen delivery with diminished function.

Diagnostic criteria for ARDS include a PaO_2/FiO_2 ratio less than or equal to 200, bilateral infiltrates on chest radiograph, and no cardiogenic etiology for the pulmonary edema. Radiographic evidence, brain-type natriuretic peptide (BNP) levels, or a pulmonary artery occlusion pressure (PAOP) less than 18 cm H_2O may be used to rule out a cardiogenic etiology.[10] Cytology of bronchoalveolar fluid may be useful for diagnosing diffuse alveolar damage (DAD), an early feature of ARDS. Because the tissue hypoxia that occurs in ARDS results in anaerobic metabolism, serum lactate levels may be elevated (lactic acid is a by-product of anaerobic metabolism).

Lung compliance and airway resistance can be evaluated by assessing ventilator pressures (ie, mean airway pressure [MAP], peak inspiratory pressure [PIP], plateau pressure) and tidal volume changes during ventilation. Throughout the stages of ARDS, diagnostic tests are also used for ongoing assessment (Table 17-5).

Arterial Blood Gases

Deterioration of ABGs, despite interventions, is a hallmark of ARDS. Initially, hypoxemia may improve with supplemental oxygen; however, refractory hypoxemia and a persistently low SaO_2 eventually develop. Early in acute respiratory failure, dyspnea and tachypnea are associated with a decreased $PaCO_2$ and development of respiratory alkalosis. Hypercarbia develops as gas exchange and ventilation become increasingly impaired.

An intrapulmonary shunt is the common ventilation–perfusion mismatch in ARDS. It involves alveoli that are not being ventilated but are still being perfused. The intrapulmonary shunt fraction may be estimated using the PaO_2/FiO_2 ratio. In general, a PaO_2/FiO_2 ratio greater than 300 is normal, a value of 200 is associated with an intrapulmonary shunt of 15% to 20%, and a value of 100 is associated with an intrapulmonary shunt of more than 20%. Advanced respiratory failure and ARDS are associated with a shunt of 15% or more. As the intrapulmonary shunt increases to 15% and greater, more

TABLE 17-5 Assessment of Acute Respiratory Distress Syndrome (ARDS)

Stage	Physical Examination	Diagnostic Test Results
Stage 1 (first 12 h)	• Restlessness, dyspnea, tachypnea • Moderate to extensive use of accessory respiratory muscles	• ABGs: Respiratory alkalosis (hypocarbia) • CXR: No radiographic changes • Chemistry: Blood results may vary depending on precipitating cause (eg, elevated WBC count, changes in hemoglobin) • Hemodynamics: Elevated pulmonary artery pressure, normal or low pulmonary artery occlusion pressure (PAOP)
Stage 2 (24 h)	• Severe dyspnea, tachypnea, cyanosis, tachycardia • Coarse bilateral crackles • Decreased air entry to dependent lung fields • Increased agitation and restlessness	• ABGs: Decreased arterial oxygen saturation (SaO_2) despite supplemental oxygen administration • CXR: Patchy bilateral infiltrates • Chemistry: Increasing metabolic acidosis depending on severity of onset • Hemodynamics: Increasingly elevated pulmonary artery pressure, normal or low PAOP
Stage 3 (2–10 d)	• Decreased air entry bilaterally • Impaired responsiveness (may be related to sedation necessary to maintain mechanical ventilation) • Decreased gut motility • Generalized edema • Poor skin integrity and breakdown	• ABGs: Worsening hypoxemia • CXR: Air bronchograms, decreased lung volumes • Chemistry: Signs of other organ involvement: decreased platelets and hemoglobin, increased WBC count, abnormal clotting factors • Hemodynamics: Unchanged or becoming increasingly worse
Stage 4 (greater than 10 d)	• Symptoms of MODS, including decreased urine output, poor gastric motility, symptoms of impaired coagulation OR • Single-system involvement of the respiratory system with gradual improvement over time	• ABGs: Worsening hypoxemia and hypercapnia • CXR: Air bronchograms, pneumothoraces • Chemistry: Persistent signs of other organ involvement: decreased platelets and hemoglobin, increased WBC count, abnormal clotting factors • Hemodynamics: Unchanged or becoming increasingly worse

ABGs, arterial blood gases; CXR, chest radiograph; MODS, multisystem organ dysfunction syndrome; WBC, white blood cell.

aggressive interventions, including mechanical ventilation, are required because this level of shunt is associated with profound hypoxemia and may be life threatening.

Radiographic Studies

Another hallmark of ARDS is patchy bilateral alveolar infiltrates on the chest radiograph. These patchy infiltrates progress to diffuse infiltrates, and consolidation ("white out") of the chest. CT of the chest also shows areas of infiltrates and consolidation of lung tissue. Daily chest radiographs are important in the continuing evaluation of the progression and resolution of ARDS and for ongoing assessment of potential complications, especially pneumothoraces.

Management

Treatment is supportive. Contributing factors are corrected, and while the lungs heal, care is taken to prevent further damage. Care "bundles" representing evidence-based protocols that have been shown to reduce major complications in critically ill patients are often employed in the management of ARDS (Box 17-7).[11] A collaborative care guide for the patient with ARDS is given in Box 17-8.

Mechanical Ventilation

Mechanical ventilation is used to deliver appropriate levels of oxygen and allow for removal of carbon dioxide. Lung-protective ventilation strategies limit ventilator-associated lung injury (VALI) and include

---

BOX 17·7   Care "Bundles" in Critical Care

Ventilator-associated pneumonia (VAP) "bundle" basics

- Head of the bed elevated 30 to 45 degrees
- Daily weaning assessment (spontaneous breathing trials)
- Daily sedation withholding
- Weaning protocol
- Deep vein thrombosis (DVT) prophylaxis
- Peptic ulcer prophylaxis

Sepsis "bundle" basics

- Appropriate antibiotic therapy
- Early goal-directed fluid resuscitation
- Steroid administration
- Activated protein C
- DVT prophylaxis
- Peptic ulcer prophylaxis

Other protocols that may be added

- Tight glucose control
- Postpyloric tube feeding
- Subglottic suctioning
- Electrolyte replacement

- Use of the lowest FiO_2 that results in adequate oxygenation (reduces the risk for oxygen toxicity)
- Use of small tidal volumes (6 mL/kg predicted body weight) to minimize airway pressures and prevent or reduce lung damage from barotrauma and volutrauma
- Use of adequate positive end-expiratory pressure (PEEP) to prevent repetitive collapsing and opening of alveolar sacs, facilitating diffusion of gases across the alveolar–capillary membrane and reducing the FiO_2 requirement (recommended values for PEEP are 10 to 15 cm H_2O, but values in excess of 20 cm H_2O are acceptable to reduce FiO_2 requirements or maintain adequate oxygenation)
- Limiting plateau pressures to 30 cm H_2O[12]

The Older Patient. *Decreased maximal oxygen uptake associated with decreased lung volumes puts elderly patients at greater risk for ventilator-associated lung injury (VALI).*

Permissive hypercapnia is a strategy that entails reducing the tidal volume and allowing the $PaCO_2$ to rise without making ventilator changes in respiratory rate or tidal volume. Minimizing the tidal volume, respiratory rate, or both limits the plateau and peak airway pressures and helps to prevent lung injury. A $PaCO_2$ between 55 and 60 mm Hg and a pH of 7.25 to 7.35 are tolerated when achieved gradually. The increase in $PaCO_2$ must be monitored to prevent too rapid a rise, and overall values should be no greater than 80 to 100 mg Hg because of the potential effects on cardiopulmonary function. Permissive hypercapnia is not used for patients with cardiac or neurological involvement.

Several modes of mechanical ventilation are directed toward minimizing airway pressures and iatrogenic lung injury associated with conventional volume-controlled mechanical ventilation:[13]

- **Pressure-controlled ventilation (PCV)** limits the PIP to a set level and uses a decelerating inspiratory airflow pattern to minimize the peak pressure while delivering the necessary tidal volume. Patients on PCV typically require sedation and pharmacological paralysis to prevent attempts at breathing and dyssynchrony with the ventilator.
- **Airway pressure release ventilation (APRV)** is similar to PCV but has the advantage of allowing the patient to initiate breaths; therefore, these patients do not require the same level of sedation or paralysis that is required with PCV.
- **Inverse-ratio ventilation (IRV)** is used to improve alveolar recruitment. Reversal of the normal inspiratory:expiratory (I:E) ratio to 2:1 (and up to 4:1) prolongs inspiration time, preventing complete exhalation. This increases the end-expiratory volume, creating auto-PEEP (intrinsic PEEP) that is added to the applied extrinsic PEEP. Advantages are thought to include reduced alveolar pressures and overall PEEP levels. Sedatives or paralytics

BOX 17-8 COLLABORATIVE CARE GUIDE for the Patient With Acute Respiratory Distress Syndrome (ARDS)

OUTCOMES	INTERVENTIONS
Oxygenation/Ventilation	
A patent airway is maintained. A PaO_2/FiO_2 ratio of 200–300 or more is maintained, if possible.	Auscultate breath sounds q2–4h and PRN. Intubate to maintain oxygenation and ventilation and decrease work of breathing. Suction endotracheal airway when appropriate. Hyperoxygenate and hyperventilate before and after each suction pass.
The patient does not experience ventilator-associated lung injury (VALI).	Maintain a low tidal volume (<6 mL/kg), a plateau pressure ≤30 cm H_2O, and PEEP levels titrated to pressure–volume curve. Monitor airway pressures q1–2h and after suctioning. Administer bronchodilators and mucolytics. Consider a change in ventilator mode to prevent barotrauma and volutrauma.
The patient does not develop atelectasis or VAP and oxygenation is improved.	Turn side to side q2h. Perform chest physiotherapy q4h, if tolerated. Elevate head of bed 30 degrees. Obtain daily chest x-ray.
The patient's oxygenation is maximized, as evidenced by a PaO_2 of 55–80 mm Hg or an SaO_2 of 88%–95%.	Monitor pulse oximetry and end-tidal CO_2. Monitor ABGs as indicated by changes in noninvasive parameters. Monitor intrapulmonary shunt (Qs/Qt and PaO_2/FiO_2 ratio). Increase PEEP and FiO_2 to decrease intrapulmonary shunting, using lowest possible FiO_2. Consider permissive hypercapnia to maximize oxygenation. Monitor for signs of barotrauma, especially pneumothorax. Consider risk for oxygen toxicity and decrease FiO_2 to <60% as soon as able.
Circulation/Perfusion	
Blood pressure, cardiac output, central venous pressure, and pulmonary artery pressures remain stable on mechanical ventilation.	Assess hemodynamic effects of initiating positive-pressure ventilation (eg, potential for decreased venous return and cardiac output). Monitor ECG for dysrhythmias related to hypoxemia. Assess effects of ventilator setting changes (inspiratory pressures, tidal volume, PEEP, and FiO_2) on hemodynamic and oxygenation parameters. Administer intravascular volume as ordered to maintain preload.
Blood pressure, heart rate, and hemodynamic parameters are optimized to therapeutic goals (eg, DaO_2 > 600 mL O_2/m^2).	Monitor vital signs q1–2h. Monitor pulmonary artery pressures and RAP qh and cardiac output, systemic vascular resistance, peripheral vascular resistance, DaO_2, and oxygen consumption (VO_2) q6–12h, if pulmonary artery catheter is in place. Administer intravascular volume as indicated by actual or relative hypovolemia, and evaluate response. Consider monitoring gastric mucosal pH as a guide to systemic perfusion.
Serum lactate is within normal limits.	Monitor lactate as required until it is within normal limits. Administer RBCs, positive inotropic agents, and colloid infusion as ordered to increase oxygen delivery.
Fluids/Electrolytes	
The patient is euvolemic. Urine output is >30 mL/h (or >0.5 mL/kg/h).	Monitor hydration status to reduce viscosity of lung secretions. Monitor I&O. Avoid use of nephrotoxic substances and overuse of diuretics. Administer fluids and diuretics to maintain intravascular volume and renal function.
There is no evidence of electrolyte imbalance or renal dysfunction.	Replace electrolytes as ordered. Monitor BUN, creatinine, serum osmolality, and urine electrolytes as required.

(continued on page 240)

BOX 17-8 COLLABORATIVE CARE GUIDE for the Patient With Acute Respiratory Distress Syndrome (ARDS) (continued)

OUTCOMES	INTERVENTIONS
Mobility/Safety	
The patient does not develop complications related to bed rest and immobility.	Initiate DVT prophylaxis.
	Reposition frequently.
	Mobilize to chair when acute phase is past and hemodynamic stability and hemostasis are achieved.
	Consult physiotherapist.
	Conduct range-of-motion and strengthening exercises when patient is able.
Physiological changes are detected and treated without delay.	Monitor mechanical ventilator alarms and settings and patient parameters (eg, tidal volume) q1–2h.
	Ensure appropriate settings and narrow limits for hemodynamic, heart rate, and pulse oximetry alarms.
There is no evidence of infection; WBC count is within normal limits.	Monitor for SIRS criteria (increased WBC count, increased temperature, tachypnea, tachycardia).
	Use strict aseptic technique during procedures, and monitor others.
	Maintain sterility of invasive catheters and tubes.
	Change chest tube and other dressings and invasive catheters.
	Culture blood and other fluids and line tips when they are changed.
Skin Integrity	
Patient is without evidence of skin breakdown.	Assess skin q4 h and each time patient is repositioned.
	Turn q2 h.
	Consider pressure relief/reduction mattress, kinetic therapy bed, or prone positioning.
	Use Braden Scale to assess risk for skin breakdown.
Nutrition	
Nutritional intake meets calculated metabolic need (eg, basal energy expenditure equation).	Consult dietitian for metabolic needs assessment and recommendations.
	Provide enteral nutrition within 24 h.
	Consider small bowel feeding tube if gastrointestinal motility is an issue for enteral feeding.
	Monitor lipid intake.
	Monitor albumin, prealbumin, transferrin, cholesterol, triglycerides, and glucose.
Comfort/Pain Control	
Patient is as comfortable as possible (as evidenced by stable vital signs or cooperation with treatments or procedures).	Document pain assessment, using numerical pain rating or similar scale when possible.
	Provide analgesia and sedation as indicated by assessment.
	Monitor patient's cardiopulmonary and pain response to medication.
	If patient is receiving NMB for ventilatory control:
	Use peripheral nerve stimulator to assess pharmacological paralysis.
	Provide continuous or routine (q1–2h) IV sedation and analgesia.
Psychosocial	
Patient demonstrates decreased anxiety.	Assess vital signs during treatments, discussions, and the like.
	Cautiously administer sedatives.
	Consult social services, clergy, as appropriate.
	Provide for adequate rest and sleep.
Teaching/Discharge Planning	
Patient and family understand procedures and tests needed for treatment.	Prepare patient and family for procedures (eg, bronchoscopy), pulmonary artery catheter insertion, or laboratory studies.
Patient and family understand the severity of the illness, ask appropriate questions, and anticipate potential complications.	Explain the causes and effects of ARDS and the potential for complications (eg, sepsis, barotrauma, renal failure).
	Encourage patient and family to ask questions related to the ventilator, the pathophysiology of ARDS, monitoring, and treatments.

are required with this therapy to improve patient tolerance.

- **High-frequency ventilation** uses very low tidal volumes delivered at rates that can exceed 100 breaths/min, resulting in lower airway pressures and reduced barotrauma. Deleterious effects of high-frequency ventilation include increased trapping of air in the alveoli (auto-PEEP) and increased MAPs.

Other ventilation therapies, including partial liquid ventilation,[14] and extracorporeal lung-assist technology,[13] while showing effectiveness in some studies, have not demonstrated consistent improvements in patient outcomes in ARDS.

Prone Positioning

Prone positioning improves pulmonary gas exchange by improving ventilation–perfusion matching, facilitates pulmonary drainage in the dorsal lung regions, and aids resolution of consolidated alveoli that are dependent when the patient is in the supine position. The evidence for the effectiveness of proning is variable.[10] There are alternative explanations for the improved oxygenation associated with the positioning, and the question of whether the improvement in oxygenation persists beyond a short time remains controversial. The associated risks include loss of airway control through accidental extubation, loss of vascular access, facial edema and development of pressure areas, and difficulties with cardiopulmonary resuscitation (CPR).

Pharmacotherapy

Pharmacotherapy for patients with ARDS is largely supportive.

- Antibiotic therapy is appropriate in the presence of a known microorganism but should not be used prophylactically because it has not shown to improve outcome.
- Bronchodilators are useful for maintaining airway patency and reducing the inflammatory reaction and accumulation of secretions in the airways. The response to therapy is evaluated by monitoring airway resistance pressures and lung compliance.
- Administration of exogenous surfactant to adults with ARDS has shown some potential but requires further investigation.
- Administration of corticosteroids to decrease the inflammatory response in late stages of ARDS has been used. However, a large randomized controlled clinical trial did not show improvement in 60-day mortality, and therefore the routine use of corticosteroids is not recommended.[10] Corticosteroids continue to be used on a case-by-case basis until further research is completed.
- Diuretics and reduced fluid administration have been studied to reduce lung edema. Although these strategies result in fewer ventilator days and

shorter time spent in the critical care unit, actual mortality is unchanged.[15]

- Neuromuscular blocking (NMB) agents and sedatives (eg, propofol) are used to decrease the work of breathing and facilitate ventilation for patients with ARDS. Frequent assessment of the adequacy of both neuromuscular blockade and sedation is important.

Nutritional Support

Early initiation of nutritional support (via enteral feeding) is essential for patients with ARDS because nutrition plays an active therapeutic role in recovery from critical illness.[16] The mechanism through which enteral feeding improves outcomes remains unproved, but the reduction in mortality in critically ill patients who are enterally fed indicates that this practice is of general benefit. Patients with ARDS usually require 35 to 45 kcal/kg/day. High-carbohydrate solutions are avoided to prevent excess carbon dioxide production. When parenteral nutrition must be used, lipid emulsions are judiciously administered to avoid up-regulation of the inflammatory response (many key mediators of inflammation are derived from lipids). Amino acid supplementation is being reviewed because of the role amino acids play in the immune response.[16]

Prevention of Complications

Complications of ARDS are primarily related to SIRS, VALI, VAP, and immobility imposed by critical illness. Prevention or reduction in the incidence of VAP can be accomplished through the use of in-line suction catheters. The use of an endotracheal tube that allows continuous or intermittent subglottic suctioning (allowing for removal of pooled secretions above the cuff) has been shown to reduce aspiration of secretions associated with VAP.[17] Elevating the head of the bed 30 degrees and post-pyloric feeding tube placement also reduce VAP by reducing microaspiration.

The Older Patient. Because of increased immunosuppression with aging, older patients with ARDS are at greater risk for VAP.

Pleural Effusion

Pleural effusion is the accumulation of pleural fluid in the pleural space due to an increased rate of fluid formation, a decreased rate of fluid removal, or both.[18] Possible underlying mechanisms include

- Increased pressure in the subpleural capillaries or lymphatics
- Increased capillary permeability
- Decreased colloid osmotic pressure of the blood
- Increased intrapleural negative pressure
- Impaired lymphatic drainage of the pleural space

Pleural effusions may be transudative or exudative. Transudative pleural effusions are an ultrafiltrate of plasma, indicating that the pleural membranes are not diseased. The fluid accumulation may be unilateral or bilateral. Causes of transudative pleural effusions include heart failure (the most common cause in the critical care unit), atelectasis, cirrhosis, nephrotic syndrome, malignancy, and peritoneal dialysis.

Seventy percent of pleural effusions are exudative.[19] Exudative pleural effusions result from leakage of fluid with a high protein content across an injured capillary bed into the pleura or adjacent lung. Pneumonia and malignancies are the first and second most common causes of exudative pleural effusions, respectively. Other causes include pulmonary embolism, hemothorax, empyema (gross pus in the pleural space), and chylothorax (chyle or a fatty substance in the pleural space).[19]

Assessment

Subjective findings include shortness of breath and pleuritic chest pain, depending on the amount of fluid accumulation. Objective findings include tachypnea and hypoxemia if ventilation is impaired, dullness to percussion, and decreased breath sounds over the involved area.

Diagnosis can be made by a chest radiograph, an ultrasound, or a CT scan; however, a lateral decubitus chest radiograph permits the best demonstration of free pleural fluid. When a pleural effusion is confirmed radiologically, diagnostic thoracentesis is performed to obtain a sample of pleural fluid for analysis (Table 17-6). Analysis of the pleural fluid is necessary to distinguish transudative from exudative effusions.

Management

Treatment entails addressing the underlying cause. Removal of the pleural effusion by thoracentesis or chest tube placement may be indicated depending on the etiology and size of effusion. The primary indication for therapeutic thoracentesis is relief of dyspnea.

Pneumothorax

A pneumothorax occurs if air enters the pleural space, producing partial or complete lung collapse.

Pathophysiology

During spontaneous breathing, the pleural pressure remains negative in both inspiration and expiration but increased negativity with inspiration. Pressure in the airways is positive during expiration and negative during inspiration. Therefore, airway pressure remains higher than pleural pressure throughout the respiratory cycle. Sudden communication of the pleural space with either alveolar or external air allows gas to enter, changing the pressure from

TABLE 17-6 Assessment of Pleural Fluid

Test	Comment
Red blood cell (RBC) count greater than 100,000/mm³	Trauma, malignancy, pulmonary embolism
Hematocrit greater than 50% of peripheral blood White blood cell (WBC) count	Hemothorax
Greater than 50,000–100,000/mm³	Grossly visible purulent drainage, otherwise total WBC less useful than WBC differential
Greater than 50% Neutrophils	Acute inflammation or infection
Greater than 50% Lymphocytes	Tuberculosis, malignancy
Greater than 10% Eosinophils	Most common: hemothorax, pneumothorax; also benign
Greater than 5% Mesothelial cells	Asbestos effusions, drug reaction, paragonimiasis; tuberculosis *less likely*
Glucose less than 60 mg/dL	Infection, malignancy, tuberculosis, rheumatoid
Amylase greater than 200 units/dL	Pleuritis, esophageal perforation, pancreatic disease, malignancy, ruptured ectopic pregnancy
	Isoenzyme profile: salivary–esophageal disease, malignancy (especially lung)
pH less than 7.2	Isoenzyme profile: pancreatic–pancreatic disease
	Infection (complicated parapneumonic effusion and empyema), malignancy, esophageal rupture, rheumatoid or lupus pleuritis, tuberculosis, systemic acidosis, urinothorax
Triglyceride greater than 110 mg/dL	Chylothorax
Microbiological studies	Etiology of infection
Cytology	Diagnostic of malignancy

Adapted from Sahn SA: State of the art: The pleura. Am Rev Respir Dis 138:184–234, 1988. From Zimmerman LH: Pleural effusions. In Goldstein RH, et al (eds): A Practical Approach to Pulmonary Medicine. Philadelphia, PA: Lippincott-Raven, 1997, p 199.

Open pneumothorax

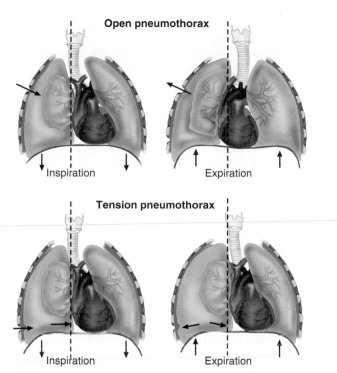

Inspiration   Expiration

Tension pneumothorax

Inspiration   Expiration

FIGURE 17-3 Open (communicating) pneumothorax (*top*) and tension pneumothorax (*bottom*). In an open pneumothorax, air enters the chest during inspiration and exits during expiration. There may be slight inflation of the affected lung due to a decrease in pressure as air moves out of the chest. In tension pneumothorax, air can enter but not leave the chest. As the pressure in the chest increases, the heart and great vessels are compressed, and the mediastinal structures are shifted toward the opposite side of the chest. The trachea is pushed from its normal midline position toward the opposite side of the chest, and the unaffected lung is compressed.

negative to positive (Fig. 17-3). When the pleural pressure increases, the elasticity of the lung causes it to collapse. The lung continues to collapse until either the pressure gradient no longer exists or the pleural defect closes. Lung collapse produces a decrease in vital capacity, an increase in the alveolar–arterial partial pressure of oxygen (P_AO_2–PaO_2) gradient, a ventilation–perfusion mismatch, and an intrapulmonary shunt resulting in hypoxemia.

There are two types of pneumothorax:

- **Spontaneous pneumothorax** is any pneumothorax that results from the introduction of air into the pleural space without obvious cause. Primary spontaneous pneumothorax occurs in the absence of underlying lung disease, and is most common in young, tall men. Family history and cigarette smoking are risk factors.[9] Secondary spontaneous pneumothorax occurs as a complication of underlying lung disease (eg, COPD, asthma, cystic fibrosis, *Pneumocystis carinii* pneumonia, necrotizing pneumonia, sarcoidosis, histiocytosis X).
- **Traumatic pneumothorax** occurs when the pressure of air in the pleural space exceeds the atmospheric pressure. As pressures in the thorax increase, the mediastinum shifts to the contralateral side, placing torsion on the inferior vena cava

and decreasing venous return to the right side of the heart (see Fig. 17-3). The most common causes of a traumatic pneumothorax in critically ill patients are invasive procedures and barotrauma associated with mechanical ventilation.

 RED FLAG! *Tension pneumothorax is a life-threatening condition manifested by hypoxemia (early sign); apprehension; severe tachypnea; deviated trachea on palpation; cardiovascular collapse (manifested by a heart rate greater than 140 beats/min accompanied by peripheral cyanosis, hypotension, or pulseless electrical activity); and increasing peak and MAPs, decreasing compliance, and auto-PEEP in patients receiving mechanical ventilation.*

Assessment

The patient reports the sudden onset of acute pleuritic chest pain localized to the affected lung. The pleuritic chest pain is usually accompanied by shortness of breath, increased work of breathing, and dyspnea. Chest wall movement may be uneven because the affected side does not expand as much as the normal (unaffected) side. Breath sounds are diminished or absent on (unaffected) side. Tachycardia and tachypnea occurs frequently with pneumothoraces.

A chest radiograph is obtained with the patient in the upright or decubitus position. In a patient with a tension pneumothorax, the chest film shows contralateral mediastinal shift, ipsilateral diaphragmatic depression, and ipsilateral chest wall expansion. Chest CT may be used to confirm the size of the pneumothorax. ABGs are used to assess for hypoxemia and hypercapnia.

Management

Supplemental oxygen is administered to all patients with pneumothorax because oxygen accelerates the rate of air resorption from the pleural space.[20] If the pneumothorax is 15% to 20%, no intervention is required, and the patient is placed on bed rest or limited activity.[20] If the pneumothorax is greater than 20%, then a chest tube is placed in the pleural space, located at the midaxillary and is directed toward the second ICS, midclavicular line to assist air removal. In approximately one third of patients with COPD, persistent air leaks require multiple chest tubes to evacuate the pneumothorax.[19]

A tension pneumothorax requires immediate treatment; if untreated, it leads to cardiovascular collapse. When signs and symptoms of tension pneumothorax are present, treatment is not delayed to obtain radiographic confirmation. If a chest tube is not immediately available, a large-bore (16- or 18-gauge) needle is placed into the second intercostal space, midclavicular. After needle insertion, a chest tube is placed and connected to suction. When the tension pneumothorax is relieved, rapid improvement in oxygenation and hemodynamic parameters is seen.

Pulmonary Embolism

Most incidents of pulmonary embolism occur when a thrombus breaks loose and migrates to the pulmonary arteries, obstructing part of the pulmonary vascular tree. Sites of clot formation include upper and lower extremities (deep venous thrombosis [DVT]), the right side of the heart, and the deep vessels of the pelvic region.[21] Although most thrombi form in the calf, 80% to 90% of pulmonary emboli arise from venous thrombi that extend into the proximal popliteal and iliofemoral veins.[22] Nonthrombotic causes of pulmonary embolism include fat, air, and amniotic fluid but are much less common than thromboembolism.[21]

Thrombus formation is frequently bilateral and often asymptomatic. Risk factors for venous thromboembolism are listed in Box 17-9.

Pathophysiology

Three factors, known as Virchow's triad, contribute to thrombus formation: venous stasis, hypercoagulability, and damage to the vein wall. Conditions such as immobility, heart failure, dehydration, and varicose veins contribute to decreased venous return, increased retrograde pressure in the venous system, and stasis of blood with resultant thrombus formation. Hypercoagulability may occur in the presence of trauma, surgery, malignancy, or use of oral contraceptives.

Occlusion of a pulmonary artery by an embolus produces both pulmonary and hemodynamic changes:

- **Pulmonary changes.** Alveoli are ventilated but not perfused producing areas of ventilation–perfusion mismatch and gas exchange is compromised (alveolar deadspace). Accompanying physiological changes include increased minute ventilation, decreased vital capacity, increased airway resistance, and decreased diffusing capacity.[21]
- **Hemodynamic changes.** The severity of hemodynamic change in pulmonary embolism depends on the size of the embolus, the degree of pulmonary vascular obstruction, and the preexisting status of the cardiopulmonary system. Increased right ventricular afterload results from obstruction of the pulmonary vascular bed by embolism. Patients with preexisting cardiopulmonary disease may develop severe pulmonary hypertension from a relatively small reduction of pulmonary blood flow.

Assessment

Both DVT and pulmonary embolism (venous thromboembolisms [VTE]) have nonspecific signs and symptoms and often, no significant signs or symptoms are present, resulting in delayed treatment and

---

BOX 17-9　Risk Factors for Thromboembolism

Strong Risk Factors
- Fracture of the hip, pelvis, or leg
- Hip or knee replacement
- Major general surgery
- Spinal cord injury/paralysis
- Major trauma

Moderate Risk Factors
- Arthroscopic knee surgery
- Central venous lines
- Malignancy
- Heart or respiratory failure
- Hormone replacement therapy, oral contraceptives
- Paralytic stroke
- Postpartum period
- Previous venous thromboembolism
- Thrombophilia

Weak Risk Factors
- Bed rest for more than 3 days
- Immobility due to sitting
- Increasing age
- Laparoscopic surgery
- Obesity
- Antepartum period
- Varicose veins

Risk Stratification for Patients Undergoing Surgery

Low Risk
- Uncomplicated surgery in patients younger than 40 years with minimal immobility postoperatively and no risk factors

Moderate Risk
- Any surgery in patients between the ages of 40 and 60 years
- Major surgery in patients younger than 40 years with no other risk factors
- Minor surgery in patients with one or more risk factors

High Risk
- Major surgery in patients age 60 years and older
- Major surgery in patients between the ages of 40 and 60 years with one or more risk factors

Very High Risk
- Major surgery in patients 40 years and older with previous venous thromboembolism, cancer, or known hypercoagulable state
- Major orthopedic surgery
- Elective neurosurgery
- Multiple trauma or acute spinal cord injury

From Blann AD, Lip GYH: Venous thromboembolism. BMJ 332(7535):215–219, 2006.

EVIDENCE-BASED PRACTICE GUIDELINES
Venous Thromboembolism Prevention

PROBLEM: Almost all critically ill patients have at least one risk factor for venous thromboembolism. Taking measures to prevent venous thromboembolism reduces the morbidity and mortality associated with deep venous thrombosis (DVT) and pulmonary embolism.

EVIDENCE-BASED PRACTICE GUIDELINES

1. Assess all patients on admission to the critical care unit for risk factors for venous thromboembolism and anticipate orders for venous thromboembolism prophylaxis based on risk assessment. (level D)
2. Review daily—with the physician and during multidisciplinary rounds— each patient's current risk factors for venous thromboembolism, including clinical status, the presence of a central venous catheter, the current status of venous thromboembolism prophylaxis, the risk for bleeding, and the response to treatment. (level E)
3. Maximize patient mobility whenever possible and take measures to reduce the amount of time the patient is immobile because of the effects of treatment (eg, pain, sedation, neuromuscular blockade, mechanical ventilation). (level E)
4. Ensure that mechanical prophylaxis devices are fitted properly and in use at all time except when they must be removed for cleaning or inspection of the skin. (level E)
5. Implement regimens for venous thromboembolism prophylaxis as ordered:
   a. Moderate-risk patients (medically ill and postoperative patients): low-dose unfractionated heparin, low-molecular-weight heparin (LMWH), or fondaparinux (level B)
   b. High-risk patients (major trauma, spinal cord injury, orthopedic surgery): LMWH, fondaparinux, or oral vitamin K antagonist (level B)
   c. Patients at high risk for bleeding: mechanical prophylaxis, including graduated compression stockings, intermittent pneumatic compression devices, or both (level B)

KEY

Level A: Meta-analysis of quantitative studies or metasynthesis of qualitative studies with results that consistently support a specific action, intervention, or treatment

Level B: Well-designed, controlled studies with results that consistently support a specific action, intervention, or treatment

Level C: Qualitative studies, descriptive or correlational studies, integrative review, systematic reviews, or randomized controlled trials with inconsistent results

Level D: Peer-reviewed professional organizational standards with clinical studies to support recommendations

Level E: Multiple case reports, theory-based evidence from expert opinions, or peer-reviewed professional organizational standards without clinical studies to support recommendations

Level M: Manufacturer's recommendations only

■ Adapted from American Association of Critical-Care Nurses (AACN) Practice Alert, revised 04/2010.

substantial morbidity and mortality. Patients with lower extremity DVT may present with pain, erythema, tenderness, swelling, and a palpable cord in the affected limb.[22] Signs and symptoms of pulmonary embolism are given in Box 17-10.

 RED FLAG! *In patients with pulmonary embolism, the most common signs and symptoms (in order of frequency) are dyspnea, pleuritic chest pain, hypoxia, cough, apprehension, leg swelling, and pain.*

Management

Anticoagulation with heparin is the mainstay of treatment (Table 17-7). Patients with VTEs are treated with unfractionated IV heparin or adjusted-dose subcutaneous heparin. The heparin dosage should prolong the activated partial thromboplastin time (aPTT) to 2 to 2.5 times normal.

Low-molecular-weight heparin (LMWH) can be substituted for unfractionated heparin in patients with DVT and in stable patients with pulmonary embolism. Treatment with heparin or LMWH continues for at least 5 days, overlapped with oral anticoagulation with warfarin for at least 4 to 5 days.[5] The recommended length of anticoagulation therapy varies, depending on the patient's age, comorbidities, and the likelihood of recurrence of pulmonary embolism or DVT. In most patients, anticoagulation therapy with warfarin or LMWH is continued for 3 to 6 months.[22] Patients with massive pulmonary embolism or severe iliofemoral thrombosis may require a longer period of anticoagulation therapy.[22] In patients with contraindications to anticoagulation therapy (eg, risk for major bleed, drug sensitivity), an inferior vena cava filter is recommended to prevent pulmonary embolism in patients with known lower extremity DVT of a long term, high risk patient.

Thrombolytic therapy is only recommended for patients with acute massive pulmonary embolism who are hemodynamically unstable and not prone to bleeding. Intracranial disease, recent surgery, trauma, and hemorrhagic disease are contraindications to thrombolytic therapy. Heparin is not administered concurrently with thrombolytics; however, thrombolytic therapy is followed by administration of heparin then warfarin.

Chronic Obstructive Pulmonary Disease

COPD is a disease state characterized by airflow limitation that is not fully reversible. The airflow limitation is usually both progressive and associated with an abnormal inflammatory response of the lungs to noxious particles or gases (primarily cigarette smoke) or an inherited deficiency of α_1-antitrypsin.[23] COPD includes two diseases: chronic bronchitis and emphysema (Table 17-8). Most patients with COPD have a combination of the two.

BOX 17-10 Signs and Symptoms of Pulmonary Embolism

Small to Moderate Embolus
- Dyspnea
- Tachypnea
- Tachycardia
- Chest pain
- Mild fever
- Hypoxemia
- Apprehension
- Cough
- Diaphoresis
- Decreased breath sounds over affected area
- Crackles
- Wheezing

Massive Embolus
A more pronounced manifestation of the signs and symptoms of a small to moderate embolus plus:
- Cyanosis
- Restlessness
- Anxiety
- Confusion

- Hypotension
- Cool, clammy skin
- Decreased urinary output
- Pleuritic chest pain associated with pulmonary infarction
- Hemoptysis associated with pulmonary infarction
- Signs of RV strain/failure

Signs of Pulmonary Embolism in Critical Care Patients
- Worsening hypoxemia or hypocapnia in a patient on spontaneous ventilation
- Worsening hypoxemia and hypercapnia in a sedate patient on controlled mechanical ventilation
- Worsening dyspnea, hypoxemia, and a reduction in $PaCO_2$ in a patient with chronic lung disease and known carbon dioxide retention
- Unexplained fever
- Sudden elevation in pulmonary artery pressure or central venous pressure in a hemodynamically monitored patient

TABLE 17-7 American College of Chest Physicians Recommendations for Treatment of Venous Thromboembolism

Agent and Condition	Anticoagulation Guidelines
Unfractionated Heparin	
Suspected VTE	• Obtain baseline aPTT, PT, CBC.
	• Check for contraindications to heparin therapy.
	• Give heparin 5,000 U IV.
	• Order imaging study.
Confirmed VTE	• Rebolus with heparin 80 U/kg IV, and start maintenance infusion at 18 U/kg/h.
	• Check aPTT at 6 h; maintain a range corresponding to a therapeutic heparin level.
	• Start warfarin therapy on day 1 at 5 mg; adjust subsequent daily dose according to INR.
	• Stop heparin after 4–5 d of combined therapy, when INR is greater than 2.0 (2.0–3.0).
	• Anticoagulate with warfarin for at least 3 mo (target INR 2.5; 2.0–3.0).
	• Consider checking platelet count between days 3 and 5.
Low-Molecular-Weight Heparin (LMWH)	
Suspected VTE	• Obtain baseline aPTT, PT, CBC.
	• Check for contraindication to heparin therapy.
	• Give unfractionated heparin: 5,000 U IV.
	• Order imaging study.
Confirmed VTE	• Give LMWH (enoxaparin), 1 mg/kg subcutaneously q12 h.
	• Start warfarin therapy on day 1 at 5 mg; adjust subsequent daily dose according to the INR.
	• Stop LMWH after at least 4–5 d of combined therapy, when INR is greater than 2.0 on 2 consecutive days.
	• Anticoagulate with warfarin for at least 3 mo (goal INR 2.5; 2.0–3.0).

VTE, venous thromboembolism; aPTT, activated partial thromboplastin time; PT, prothrombin time; INR, international normalized ratio; CBC, complete blood count.
From American College of Chest Physicians: Seventh ACCP consensus conference on Antithrombotic and Thrombolytic Therapy. Chest 126(3 suppl):401S, 428S, 2004.

TABLE 17-8   Patterns of Disease in Advanced Chronic Obstructive Pulmonary Disease (COPD)

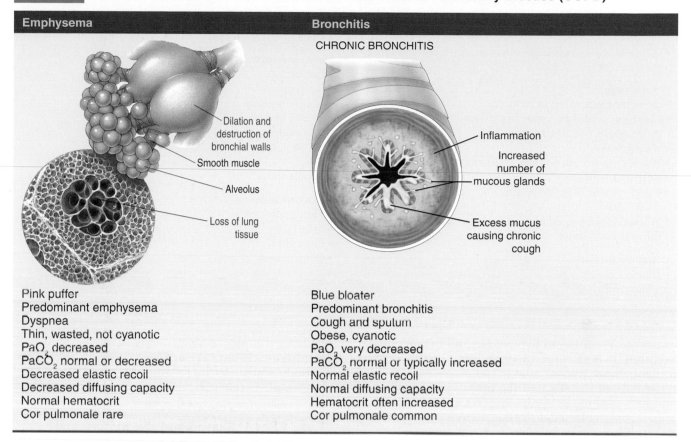

Emphysema	Bronchitis

Labels on Emphysema figure:
- Dilation and destruction of bronchial walls
- Smooth muscle
- Alveolus
- Loss of lung tissue

CHRONIC BRONCHITIS

Labels on Bronchitis figure:
- Inflammation
- Increased number of mucous glands
- Excess mucus causing chronic cough

Emphysema	Bronchitis
Pink puffer	Blue bloater
Predominant emphysema	Predominant bronchitis
Dyspnea	Cough and sputum
Thin, wasted, not cyanotic	Obese, cyanotic
PaO_2 decreased	PaO_2 very decreased
$PaCO_2$ normal or decreased	$PaCO_2$ normal or typically increased
Decreased elastic recoil	Normal elastic recoil
Decreased diffusing capacity	Normal diffusing capacity
Normal hematocrit	Hematocrit often increased
Cor pulmonale rare	Cor pulmonale common

- **Chronic bronchitis** is defined as the presence of a productive cough for at least 3 months per year over 2 consecutive years, in the absence of other medical causes.[23] Chronic airway irritation leads to inflammation of the airways and airway obstruction. Subsequently, edema and hyperplasia occur with excess mucus excretion into the bronchial tree, resulting in a chronic productive cough. Once the airway lumen is occluded by secretions and narrowed by a thickened wall, patients develop airflow obstruction and COPD. Acute bacterial or viral infection in patients with chronic bronchitis can exacerbate symptoms and airway obstruction. Signs and symptoms of an acute exacerbation of chronic bronchitis are summarized in Box 17-11. Often patients wait to seek medical treatment until they are in severe distress.
- **Emphysema** is defined as a loss of lung elasticity and abnormal, permanent enlargement of the airspaces distal to the terminal bronchioles with destruction of the alveolar walls and capillary beds without obvious fibrosis.[23] Emphysema is believed to result from the breakdown of elastin by proteases (enzymes that digest proteins). These proteases, especially elastase, are released from neutrophils, alveolar macrophages, and other inflammatory cells.[23] The enlargement of the airspaces in emphysema results in hyperinflation

of the lungs and increased total lung capacity. In severe emphysema, air is trapped in the lungs during forced expiration, leading to pulmonary hyperinflation. Spontaneous pneumothorax may occur related to rupture of thinned parenchyma. An acute exacerbation of COPD may necessitate admission to the critical care unit (Box 17-12).[24]

Pathophysiology

In COPD, pathophysiological changes usually occur in the following order: mucus hypersecretion, ciliary dysfunction, airflow limitation, pulmonary hyperinflation, gas exchange abnormalities, pulmonary hypertension, and hypertrophy of the right ventricle (cor pulmonale).[25] The central airways, peripheral airways, lung parenchyma, and pulmonary vasculature are affected.[23]

The peripheral airways become the major site of obstruction in patients with COPD. Structural changes in the airway wall are the most important cause of increased peripheral airway resistance. Inflammatory changes such as airway edema and mucus hypersecretion also contribute to narrowing of the peripheral airways.

In advanced COPD, peripheral airway obstruction, parenchymal destruction, and pulmonary vascular irregularities reduce the lung's capacity for gas

BOX 17·11 Manifestations of Severe Exacerbations of Chronic Bronchitis

Constitutional
- Temperature frequently subnormal
- White blood cell (WBC) count varies—may be slightly elevated, normal, or decreased

Respiratory
- Copious sputum expectoration
- Changes in sputum color from whitish to yellow or green (signs of infection)
- Hemoptysis
- Worsening breath sounds, wheezes, or rhonchi
- Resting respiratory rate greater than 16 breaths/min
- Development of acute respiratory acidosis (pH less than 7.30)
- Worsening of forced expiratory time (greater than the normal 4 seconds)

Cardiovascular
- Diaphoresis
- Tachycardia

- Blood pressure varies: normal, increased, or decreased
- Vasoconstriction initially followed by vasodilation

Neurological
- Headache
- Confusion
- Hallucinations
- Depression
- Drowsiness
- Somnolence
- Coma
- Papilledema

Neuromuscular
- Fine tremors
- Asterixis
- Flaccidity
- Convulsions

exchange, resulting in hypoxemia and hypercapnia.[23] Ventilation–perfusion mismatching is the driving force behind hypoxemia in patients with COPD, regardless of the stage of the disease. As hypoxemia and hypercapnia progress late in COPD, pulmonary hypertension often develops, causing cor pulmonale. Right-sided heart failure leads to further venous stasis and thrombosis that may result in pulmonary embolism.

Assessment

Elements of the history and physical examination for a patient with COPD are summarized in Box 17-13. On ABG analysis, patients with COPD typically have chronic hypoxemia and hypercapnia,

resulting initially in respiratory acidosis. However, because the respiratory acidosis develops over time, the body adjusts by increasing the bicarbonate level to normalize the pH. Uncompensated respiratory

BOX 17·13 Features of the History and Physical Examination for Chronic Obstructive Pulmonary Disease (COPD)

History
- Exposure to risk factors
- Medical history (eg, asthma, allergy, sinusitis, nasal polyps, respiratory infections in childhood, other respiratory diseases)
- Family history of COPD or other chronic respiratory disease
- Pattern of symptom development
- History of exacerbations or previous hospitalizations for respiratory disorder
- Comorbidities
- Current medical treatments
- Impact of disease on patient's life

Physical Examination

Inspection
- Central cyanosis
- Barrel-shaped chest
- Flattening of the hemidiaphragms
- Resting respiratory rate greater than 20 breaths/min
- Pursed-lip breathing
- Ankle or lower leg edema

Auscultation
- Reduced breath sounds
- Wheezing
- Inspiratory crackles

BOX 17·12 Indications for Critical Care Unit Admission for Patients With Acute Exacerbation of Chronic Obstructive Pulmonary Disease (COPD)

- Severe dyspnea that responds inadequately to initial emergency therapy
- Confusion, lethargy, coma
- Persistent worsening hypoxemia (PaO_2 less than 50 mm Hg), or severe/worsening hypercapnia ($PaCO_2$ greater than 70 mm Hg), or severe/worsening respiratory acidosis (pH less than 7.30) despite supplemental oxygen and noninvasive positive-pressure ventilation

From Pauwels RA, et al: Global strategy for the diagnosis, management, and prevention of chronic obstructive pulmonary disease: National Heart, Lung, and Blood Institute and World Health Organization global initiative for chronic obstructive lung disease (GOLD). Am J Respir Crit Care Med 163:1256–1276, 2001.

acidosis in a patient with a history of COPD indicates acute respiratory compromise or failure.

Management

Table 17-9 summarizes therapeutic guidelines for the various stages of COPD.

Nutritional support

Malnutrition is a common problem in patients with COPD and is present in more than 50% of patients with COPD admitted to the hospital. Because improving the nutritional state of patients with COPD can lead to increased respiratory muscle strength, a complete nutritional assessment is conducted and appropriate nutritional care provided.[25]

Pharmacotherapy

Bronchodilators (β-adrenergic agonist) are the cornerstone of symptom management in patients with COPD. These agents increase the forced expiratory volume in 1 second (FEV_1) by widening the smooth muscle tone of the airways rather than by altering the elastic recoil properties of the lung.[26] The choice of bronchodilator therapy depends on the patient's response in terms of symptom relief and side effects. Combination therapy (anticholinergics, corticosteroids, β_2 selective bronchodilators), rather than an increased dose of a single agent, may lead to improved efficacy and a decreased risk for side effects.

Regular treatment with inhaled or intravenous glucocorticosteroids for COPD is appropriate only for patients with symptomatic disease and a documented spirometric response to glucocorticosteroids, or in patients with an FEV_1 less than 50% predicted and repeated exacerbations requiring treatment with antibiotics or oral glucocorticosteroids. Extended treatment with glucocorticosteroids may alleviate symptoms but does not alter the long-term decline in FEV_1 typically seen in patients with COPD. The dose–response relationships and long-term safety of inhaled glucocorticosteroids in COPD are not fully known, and long-term treatment with oral glucocorticosteroids is not recommended.[23]

Oxygen Therapy

Oxygen therapy is initiated for patients with severe (stage III) COPD if

TABLE 17-9   Therapeutic Guidelines for the Stages of Chronic Obstructive Pulmonary Disease (COPD)

Stage	Characteristics	Recommended Treatment
0: At Risk	• Chronic symptoms (cough, sputum) • Exposure to risk factor(s) • Normal spirometry	• Avoidance of risk factor(s) • Influenza vaccination • Smoking cessation • Short-acting bronchodilator when needed
I: Mild COPD	• FEV_1/FVC less than 70% • FEV_1 greater than or equal to 80% predicted • With or without symptoms	
II: Moderate COPD	IIA: • FEV_1/FVC less than 70% • 50% less than or equal to FEV_1 less than 80% predicted • With or without symptoms	• Regular treatment with one or more bronchodilators • Rehabilitation • Inhaled glucocorticosteroids if significant symptoms and lung function response
	IIB: • FEV_1/FVC less than 70% • 30% less than or equal to FEV_1 less than 50% predicted • With or without symptoms	• Regular treatment with one or more bronchodilators • Rehabilitation • Inhaled glucocorticosteroids if significant symptoms and lung function response or if repeated exacerbations
III: Severe COPD	• FEV_1/FVC less than 70% • FEV_1 less than 30% predicted or presence of respiratory failure or right-sided heart failure	• Regular treatment with one or more bronchodilators • Inhaled glucocorticosteroids if significant symptoms and lung function response or if repeated exacerbations • Treatment of complications • Rehabilitation • Long-term oxygen therapy if respiratory failure • Consider surgical treatments

FEV_1, forced expiratory volume in 1 second; FVC, forced vital capacity.
From Pauwels RA, et al: Global strategy for the diagnosis, management, and prevention of chronic obstructive pulmonary disease: National Heart, Lung, and Blood Institute and World Health Organization global initiative for chronic obstructive lung disease (GOLD). Am J Respir Crit Care Med 163:1256–1276, 2001.

- The PaO_2 is at or below 55 mm Hg or the SaO_2 is at or below 88%, with or without hypercapnia
- The PaO_2 is between 55 and 60 mm Hg or the SaO_2 is below 90% and there is evidence of pulmonary hypertension, heart failure, or polycythemia.[26]

Patients with COPD normally tolerate higher levels of carbon dioxide because their chemoreceptors no longer respond to the normally accepted partial pressure of carbon dioxide (PCO_2) levels and serum pH. Instead, their primary drive to breathe comes from their oxygen levels. Because of the risk for carbon dioxide retention from loss of respiratory drive, there has historically been a hesitation to administer oxygen to patients with COPD. However, in the face of acute exacerbation, prevention of tissue hypoxia overrules any concern regarding carbon dioxide retention. If successful oxygenation (SaO_2 greater than or equal to 90%) is not obtained without a progression of respiratory acidosis, intubation and mechanical ventilation are usually indicated.[26]

Surgical Therapy

Surgical interventions may include lung volume reduction surgery (LVRS) and lung transplantation. LVRS is a surgical procedure for emphysema in which parts of the lung are resected to reduce hyperinflation, thereby improving the mechanical efficiency of the respiratory muscles, increasing the elastic recoil of the lungs, and ultimately improving expiratory flow rate.[27] The target for LVRS, as determined by CT and ventilation–perfusion scanning, is the hyperinflated portion of the diseased lung with well-demarcated areas of trapped air or dead space.[27] For patients awaiting lung transplantation, LVRS provides a means to obtain immediate symptomatic improvement by significantly increasing oxygenation and decreasing arterial carbon dioxide.[23] Contraindications to LVRS include active smoking, marked obesity or cachexia, and an inability to undertake pulmonary rehabilitation successfully.[23] Morbidity in LVRS is related to persistent postoperative air leaks, difficulty with postoperative weaning from the ventilator, and postoperative nosocomial pulmonary infections.[27]

For end-stage COPD, the only definitive surgical treatment is single-lung transplantation. Because of the short supply of donor lungs, lung transplantation is usually reserved for patients younger than 60 years with α_1-protease inhibitor deficiency.[23]

Acute Asthma

Asthma is defined as airway hyperresponsiveness to a variety of stimuli, reversible airflow limitation, and inflammation of the airway submucosa.[28] It is manifested as variable airway obstruction that resolves either spontaneously or after bronchodilator administration.

Asthma severity can be classified based on frequency of symptoms and pulmonary function tests (Table 17-10). Common triggers of asthma exacerbations are given in Box 17-14. These irritants stimulate the receptors in the walls of the larynx and large bronchi, which induces bronchoconstriction.

TABLE 17-10 **Classification of Asthma Severity**

	Symptoms	Nighttime Symptoms	Lung Function
Mild intermittent	Symptoms less than or equal to two times a week Asymptomatic and normal PEF between exacerbations Exacerbations brief (few hours to few days); intensity may vary	Less than or equal to two times a month	FEV_1 or PEF greater than or equal to 80% predicted PEF variability less than or equal to 20%
Mild persistent	Symptoms greater than two times a week but less than one time a day Exacerbations may affect activity	Greater than two times a month	FEV_1 or PEF greater than 80% predicted PEF variability 20%–30%
Moderate persistent	Daily symptoms Daily use of inhaled short-acting β_2-adrenergic blockers Exacerbations affect activity Exacerbations greater than or equal to two times a week; may last days	Greater than one time a week	FEV_1 or PEF greater than 60% to less than 80% predicted PEF variability greater than 30%
Severe persistent	Continual symptoms Limited physical activity Frequent exacerbations	Frequent	FEV_1 or PEF less than or equal to 60% predicted PEF variability greater than 30%

FEV_1, forced expiratory volume in 1 second; PEF, peak expiratory flow.
Adapted from National Asthma Education and Prevention Program, Expert Panel Report 2: Guidelines for the Diagnosis and Management of Asthma. National Institutes of Health publication no. 97-4051. Bethesda, MD: National Institutes of Health, 1997.

BOX 17-14 Common Asthma Triggers

- Viral respiratory infections
- Environmental allergens (domestic dust mite, tobacco smoke, animals with fur, cockroach, outdoor and indoor pollens and mold, perfume, wood-burning stoves)
- Temperature, humidity
- Occupational and recreational allergens or irritants
- Medications (aspirin, nonsteroidal anti-inflammatory drugs, β-adrenergic blockers)
- Food (sulfites)
- Emotions
- Exercise
- Stress

From National Heart, Lung, and Blood Institute, National Institutes of Health: Global Initiative for Asthma. Bethesda, MD: National Heart, Lung, and Blood Institute, 2003, p 249.

Pathophysiology

Inflammation may be present throughout the bronchial tree, from the large airways to the alveoli. This inflammation is characterized by mast cell activation, inflammatory cell infiltration, edema, denudation and disruption of the bronchial epithelium, collagen deposition beneath the basement membrane, goblet cell hyperplasia (which contributes to mucus hypersecretion), and smooth muscle thickening (Fig. 17-4). This inflammatory process contributes to airway hyperresponsiveness, airflow limitation, pathological damage, and associated respiratory symptoms (ie, wheezing, shortness of breath, and chest tightness).

Assessment

The severity of an acute asthma exacerbation is evaluated on the basis of the clinical signs and symptoms and functional assessment (Table 17-11). Signs and symptoms of an asthma exacerbation include mouth breathing, dark discoloration beneath the lower eyelids ("allergic shiners"), edematous or pale nasal mucosa, clear nasal discharge, tearing and periorbital edema, wheezing on lung auscultation, hyperexpansion of the thorax, use of accessory muscles, and tachypnea. Additional findings, including tachycardia, retractions, restlessness, anxiety, inspiratory or expiratory wheezing, hypoxemia, hypercapnia, cough, sputum production, expiratory prolongation, cyanosis, and an elevated pulsus paradoxus (systolic blood pressure in expiration exceeding that in inspiration by more than 10 mm Hg), may be observed in patients having a severe attack.[28]

RED FLAG! *Status asthmaticus, an acute refractory asthma attack that does not respond to rigorous therapy with β_2-adrenergic blockers, is a medical emergency. Patients present with acute anxiety, markedly labored breathing, tachycardia, and diaphoresis. Deterioration of pulmonary function results in alveolar hypoventilation with subsequent hypoxemia, hypercapnia, and acidemia. A rising $PaCO_2$ in a patient with an acute asthmatic attack is often the first objective indication of status asthmaticus.*

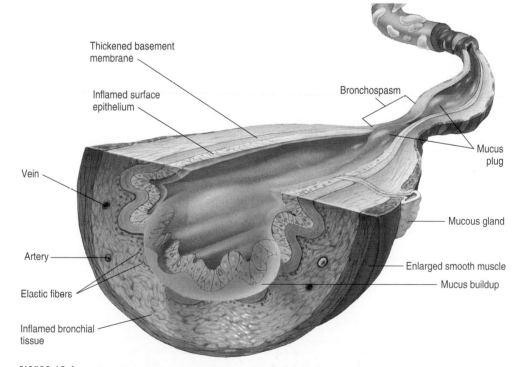

FIGURE 17-4 Asthmatic bronchus. (From Anatomical Chart Company: Atlas of Pathophysiology. Springhouse, PA: Springhouse, 2010, p 85.)

TABLE 17-11 Classification of Severity of Asthma Exacerbations

	Mild	Moderate	Severe	Impending Respiratory Failure
Symptoms				
Breathlessness	With activity	With talking	At rest	At rest
Speech	Sentences	Phrases	Words	Mute
Signs				
Body position	Able to recline	Prefers sitting	Unable to recline	Unable to recline
Respiratory rate	Increased	Increased	Often greater than 30/min	Greater than 30 breaths/min
Use of accessory respiratory muscles	Usually not	Commonly	Usually	Paradoxical thoracoabdominal movement
Breath sounds	Moderate wheezing at mid- to end-expiration	Loud wheezes throughout expiration	Loud inspiratory and expiratory wheezes	Little air movement without wheezes
Heart rate (beats/min)	Less than 100	100–120	Greater than 120	Relative bradycardia
Pulsus paradoxus (mm Hg)	Less than 10	10–25	Often greater than 25	Often absent
Mental status	May be agitated	Usually agitated	Usually agitated	Confused or drowsy
Functional Assessment				
PEF (% predicted or personal best)	Greater than 80	50–80	Less than 50 or response to therapy lasts less than 2 h	Less than 50
SaO_2 (%, room air)	Greater than 95	91–95	Less than 91	Less than 91
PaO_2 (mm Hg, room air)	Normal	Greater than 60	Less than 60	Less than 60
$PaCO_2$ (mm Hg)	Less than 42	Less than 42	Greater than or equal to 42	Greater than or equal to 42

PEF, peak expiratory flow.
Adapted from National Asthma Education and Prevention Program, Expert Panel Report 2: Guidelines for the Diagnosis and Management of Asthma. National Institutes of Health publication no. 97-4051. Bethesda, MD: National Institutes of Health, 1997.

Management

The main goal of treatment is to gain control quickly. Medications used in the treatment of asthma include bronchodilators, anti-inflammatory drugs (eg, corticosteroids, cromolyn, nedocromil), 5-lipoxygenase inhibitors, leukotriene antagonists, and anti-IgE antibody. A stepwise pharmacological approach is recommended in treating patients with asthma (Fig. 17-5).

The treatment of status asthmaticus involves the institution of multiple therapeutic modalities. All patients with status asthmaticus require oxygen therapy (to counteract hypoxemia) and fluid resuscitation (to counteract dehydration). Pharmacological agents include methylxanthines, sympathomimetic amines, and corticosteroids.[28] If pulmonary function cannot be improved and respiratory failure ensues, patients may require intubation and assisted ventilation.

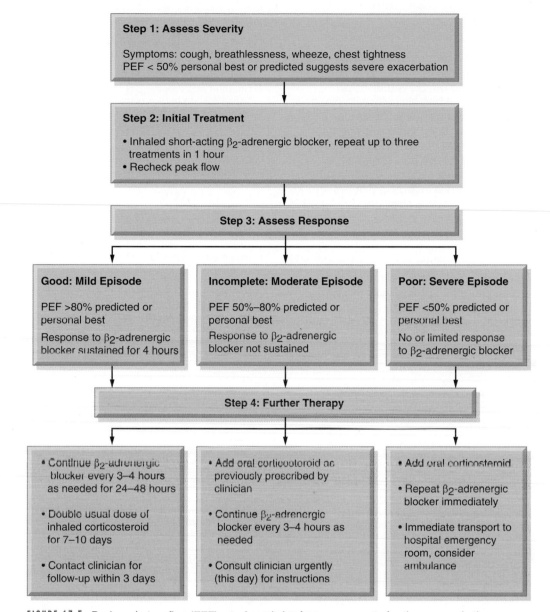

Step 1: Assess Severity

Symptoms: cough, breathlessness, wheeze, chest tightness
PEF < 50% personal best or predicted suggests severe exacerbation

Step 2: Initial Treatment

• Inhaled short-acting β_2-adrenergic blocker, repeat up to three treatments in 1 hour
• Recheck peak flow

Step 3: Assess Response

Good: Mild Episode

PEF >80% predicted or personal best

Response to β_2-adrenergic blocker sustained for 4 hours

Incomplete: Moderate Episode

PEF 50%–80% predicted or personal best

Response to β_2-adrenergic blocker not sustained

Poor: Severe Episode

PEF <50% predicted or personal best

No or limited response to β_2-adrenergic blocker

Step 4: Further Therapy

• Continue β_2-adrenergic blocker every 3–4 hours as needed for 24–48 hours

• Double usual dose of inhaled corticosteroid for 7–10 days

• Contact clinician for follow-up within 3 days

• Add oral corticosteroid as previously prescribed by clinician

• Continue β_2-adrenergic blocker every 3–4 hours as needed

• Consult clinician urgently (this day) for instructions

• Add oral corticosteroid

• Repeat β_2-adrenergic blocker immediately

• Immediate transport to hospital emergency room, consider ambulance

FIGURE 17-5 Peak expiratory flow (PEF) rate–based plan for management of asthma exacerbations. (Modified from National Asthma Education Program: Expert Panel Report II. Guidelines for the diagnosis and management of asthma. Washington, DC: U.S. Department of Health and Human Services, 1997. NIH Publ. No. 97-4051. From Givelber RJ, O'Connor GT: Asthma. In Goldstein RH, Connell JJ, Karlinsky JB, et al.: [eds]: A Practical Approach to Pulmonary Medicine. Philadelphia, PA: Lippincott-Raven, 1997, pp 68–84.)

CASE STUDY

Ms. S. presents to the urgent care clinic with her 75-year-old father, stating that her father just "doesn't seem right." On speaking to Mr. S., you discover that he is oriented to self but has difficulty with place and time. He states that he has "felt a little under the weather for a couple of days." His daughter confirms that he has complained of shortness of breath, chills, and lack of appetite for the past 2 or 3 days. Exploration of Mr. S.'s medical history reveals that he had an inferior wall myocardial infarction 5 years ago, and he smoked two packs of cigarettes per day for 45 years but quit smoking 5 years ago. Ms. S. is unsure of the medications her father is currently taking.

Mr. S. is a tall, thin, frail elderly man who appears chronically ill and mildly distressed. He has a productive cough, with thick yellow sputum with green streaks. He rests leaning over the bedside table, and breathes using pursed lips and accessory respiratory muscles. Physical examination reveals diminished bilateral breath sounds in the lung bases and 1+ pitting edema in the lower extremities. Mr. S.'s vital signs are as follows: temp, 101.2°F; HR, 130 beats/min; BP, 142/86 mm Hg; and RR, 28 breaths/min. A chest radiograph reveals blunted costophrenic angles and diffuse infiltrates in the left lower lobes.

1. What respiratory disorders would be included in Mr. S.'s differential diagnosis?

2. What additional diagnostic studies would be useful?

3. What potential infectious organisms should be considered?

4. What treatment modalities would be involved in the plan of care for Mr. S.?

References

1. Hoyert DL, Kung H, Smith BL: Death: Preliminary data for 2003. Natl Vital Stat Rep 53(15):1–48, 2005
2. American Thoracic Society. Infectious diseases Society of America/American Thoracic Society of Consensus Guidelines on management of community acquired pneumonia in adults, 2007
3. Miskovich-Riddle L, Keresztes P: CAP management guidelines. Nurse Pract 31(1):43–53, 2006
4. American Thoracic Society: Guidelines for the management of adults with hospital-acquired, ventilator-associated, and healthcare-associated pneumonia. Am J Respir Crit Care Med 171(4):388–416, 2005
5. Lutfiyya MN, Henley E, Chang LF, et al.: Diagnosis and treatment of community-acquired pneumonia. Am Fam Physician 73(3):442–450, 2006
6. Guidelines for the management of adults with hospital acquired pneumonia, ventilator acquired pneumonia and healthcare associated pneumonia. Am J Crit Care Med 171:388–416, 2005
7. Mandell LA, Bartlett JG, Dowell SF, et al.: Update of practice guideline for the management of community acquired pneumonia in immunocompetent adults. Clin Infect Dis 37(11):1405–1433, 2003
8. Christie HA, Goldstein LS: Respiratory failure and the need for ventilatory support. In Wilkins RL, Stoller JK, Scanlan CL, et al.: (eds): Egan's Fundamentals of Respiratory Care, 9th ed. St. Louis, MO: Mosby, 2008, pp 913–927
9. Chesnutt MS, Prendergast TJ: Lung. In Tierney L, McPhee SJ, Papadakis MA (eds): Current Medical Diagnosis and Medical Treatment, 46th ed. New York: McGraw-Hill, 2007, pp 222–315
10. Ware LB, Matthay MA: Clinical practice. Acute pulmonary edema. N Engl J Med 353:2788–2796, 2005
11. Winters B, Dorman T: Patient-safety and quality initiatives in the intensive-care unit. Curr Opin Anaesthesiol 19:140–145, 2006
12. Kallet RH, Jasmer RM, Pittet JF, et al.: Clinical implementation of the ARDS network protocol is associated with reduced hospital mortality compared with historical controls. Crit Care Med 33:925–929, 2005
13. Bein T, Weber F, Philipp A, et al.: A new pumpless extracorporeal interventional lung assist in critical hypoxemia/hypercapnia. Crit Care Med 34:1372–1377, 2006
14. Kacmarek RM, Wiedemann HP, Lavin PT, et al.: Partial liquid ventilation in adult patients with acute respiratory distress syndrome. Am J Respir Crit Care Med 173:882–889, 2005
15. National Heart, Lung, and Blood Institute Acute Respiratory Distress Syndrome (ARDS) Clinical Trials Network; Wiedemann HP, Wheeler AP, Bernard GR, et al: Comparison of two fluid-management strategies in acute lung injury. N Engl J Med 354:2564–2575, 2006
16. Pontes-Arruda A, DeMichele S: Enteral nutrition with anti-inflammatory lipids in acute lung injury/acute distress syndrome. Yearbook of Intensive Care and Emergency Medicine. 695–704
17. Speroni K, et al.: Comparative effectiveness of standard endotracheal tube vs endotracheal tube with continuous subglottic suction on ventilator associated pneumonia rates. Nurs Econ 29(1):15–21, 2011
18. Porth C: Disorders of ventilations and gas exchange. In Pathophysiology: Concepts of Altered Health States, 7th ed. Philadelphia, PA: Lippincott Williams & Wilkins, 2005, pp 689–724
19. Des Jardin T, Burton GG: Pleural diseases. In Clinical Manifestations and Assessments of Respiratory Diseases, 5th ed. Philadelphia, PA: Elsevier Mosby, 2006, pp 318–327
20. Des Jardin T, Burton GG: Pneumothorax. In Clinical Manifestations and Assessments of Respiratory Diseases, 5th ed. Philadelphia, Elsevier Mosby, 2006, pp 306–316
21. West JB: Pulmonary Pathophysiology: The Essentials, 7th ed. Philadelphia, PA: Lippincott Williams & Wilkins, 2007
22. Blann AD, Lip GYH: Venous thromboembolism. BMJ 332(7535):215–219, 2006
23. American Thoracic Society: Standards for the Diagnosis and Management of Patients with COPD. New York: Author, 2004
24. American Lung Association: Chronic obstructive pulmonary disease (COPD) fact sheet (chronic bronchitis and emphysema), 2006. Retrieved from http://www.lungusa.org/
25. Geerts WH, Pineo GF, Heit JA, et al.: Prevention of venous thromboembolism: The seventh ACCP conference on antithrombotic and thrombolytic therapy. Chest 126(3):338S–400S, 2004
26. Petty TL: Chronic obstructive pulmonary disease. In Hanley ME, Walsh CH (eds): Current Diagnosis and Treatment in Pulmonary Medicine. New York: McGraw-Hill, 2003, pp 82–91
27. Weder W, Michaele T, Konrad B: Lung volume reduction surgery in nonheterogenous emphysema. Thorac Surg Clin 19(2): 193–199, 2009
28. John J, Idell S: Managing severe exacerbations of asthma. Emerg Med 38(4):20–32, 2006

Renal System

FIVE

CHAPTER
18

Patient Assessment: Renal System

OBJECTIVES

Based on the content in this chapter, the reader should be able to:

1 Describe the components of the history for renal assessment.
2 Describe the components of the physical examination for renal assessment.
3 Describe laboratory tests used to evaluate renal function.
4 Describe diagnostic studies used to evaluate renal function.

Assessment of the renal system facilitates early identification of renal dysfunction, which can result in fluid, electrolyte, and acid–base imbalances.

History

Information about the patient's present illness, past health history, family history, and personal and social history helps to determine the cause, severity, treatment, and management of renal dysfunction (Box 18-1)

Physical Examination

Because renal dysfunction can affect many organ systems, a head-to-toe assessment is indicated. Patients with renal dysfunction usually have significant problems with fluid and electrolyte balance; therefore, the nurse makes careful note of signs of fluid imbalance (Box 18-2) throughout the examination.

- **Vital signs.** The nurse assesses the blood pressure and pulse pressure (noting the presence of pulsus paradoxus); the respiratory rate, rhythm, depth, and effort; and the temperature. An elevated temperature may indicate infection or hypovolemia. Patients with chronic kidney disease tend to have low temperatures because they are often immunocompromised.
- **Skin and mucous membranes.** The nurse inspects the skin on the extremities and trunk for color and evidence of excoriation, bruising, or bleeding; palpates for moistness, dryness, temperature, and edema; checks skin turgor; and inspects the tongue and oral mucosa.

BOX 18-1 Renal Health History

History of the Present Illness

Complete analysis of the following signs and symptoms (using the NOPQRST format, see Chapter 12, Box 12-2):

- Frequency
- Urgency
- Hesitancy
- Burning
- Dysuria
- Hematuria
- Incontinence
- Lower back pain
- Change in color, odor, or amount of urine
- Thirst
- Change in weight
- Edema

Past Health History

- **Past acute and chronic medical problems, including treatments and hospitalizations:** renal failure, renal calculi, renal cancer, glomerulonephritis, Wegener's granulomatosis, polycystic kidney disease, dialysis (type, frequency, and duration), urinary tract infections, systemic lupus erythematosus, sickle cell anemia, cancer, AIDS, hepatitis C, heart failure, diabetes, hypertension
- **Risk factors:** age, trauma, heavy use of nonsteroidal anti-inflammatory drugs (NSAIDs), use of heroin or cocaine
- **Past surgeries:** kidney transplantation, placement of dialysis fistula
- **Past diagnostic tests and interventions:** urinalysis, cystoscopy, intravenous pyelography (IVP), renal ultrasound, renal biopsy, magnetic resonance imaging (MRI), diagnostic tests that have used contrast material

- **Medications, including prescription drugs, over-the-counter drugs, vitamins, herbs, and supplements:** diuretics, aminoglycosides, antibiotics, angiotensin-converting enzyme (ACE) inhibitors, angiotensin-receptor blockers (ARBs), NSAIDs
- **Allergies and reactions to medications, foods, contrast, latex, or other materials:** radiopaque contrast material
- **Transfusions, including type and date**

Family History

- **Health status or cause of death of parents and siblings:** hereditary nephritis, polycystic kidney disease, diabetes, hypertension

Personal and Social History

- Tobacco, alcohol, and substance use: heroin, cocaine
- Environment: exposure to nephrotoxic substances (eg, organic acids, pesticides, lead, mercury)
- Diet: restrictions, supplements, caffeine intake
- Sleep patterns: disruptions owing to need to get up to urinate

Review of Other Systems

- **HEENT:** periorbital edema
- **Cardiovascular:** hypertension, heart failure, vascular disease
- **Respiratory:** Goodpasture's syndrome
- **Gastrointestinal:** hepatitis, cirrhosis
- **Musculoskeletal:** rhabdomyolysis, muscle weakness
- **Neurological:** numbness, tingling, burning, tremors, memory loss
- **Endocrine:** diabetes mellitus
- **Hematological:** sickle-cell anemia
- **Immune:** systemic lupus erythematosus
- **Integument:** dryness, itching

- **Chest.** The nurse observes and palpates the precordial area for heaves, pulsations, and thrills; auscultates the heart for third or fourth heart sounds, murmurs, clicks, or a pericardial friction rub (often caused by fluid overload); and auscultates the anterior and posterior lung fields for breath sound quality and the presence of adventitious breath sounds (also indicative of fluid overload).
- **Kidneys.** The nurse places the stethoscope above and to the left and right of the umbilicus to auscultate the renal arteries for bruits, which may indicate renal artery stenosis (see Chapter 24,

BOX 18-2 Signs of Hypervolemia and Hypovolemia

Hypervolemia

Increased Vascular Volume
- Elevated blood pressure
- Crackles, rhonchi, moist rales, cough
- Jugular venous distention
- Liver congestion and enlargement

Increased Extravascular Volume
- Pitting edema of the feet, ankles, hands, or fingers
- Periorbital edema

- Sacral edema
- Ascites

Hypovolemia
- Low blood pressure
- Orthostatic hypotension
- Decreased pulse pressure
- Rapid, weak, thready pulse
- Dry skin and mucous membranes
- Sunken eyes

TABLE 18-1 Assessing Pitting Edema

Scale	Description	Depth of Indentation	Return to Baseline
4 +	Severe	8 mm	2–5 min
3 +	Moderate	6 mm	1–2 min
2 +	Mild	4 mm	10–15 s
1 +	Trace	2 mm	Disappears rapidly

From Rhoads J: Advanced Health Assessment and Diagnostic Reasoning. Philadelphia, PA: Lippincott Williams & Wilkins, 2006, p 253.

Fig. 24-4). To identify ascites, the nurse measures the abdominal girth and may check for a fluid wave or shifting dullness.

- **Extremities.** The nurse checks the quality of the peripheral pulses, inspects the color and shape of the nails, assesses the capillary refill time, and assesses for pitting edema (Table 18-1). If the patient has an arteriovenous graft or fistula for dialysis, the nurse palpates for a thrill and auscultates for the presence of a bruit to assess graft patency, and assesses circulation to the extremity distal to the access. If the patient has temporary dialysis access, the catheter insertion site is inspected for signs of inflammation or infection.

- **Electrolytes.** Patients with renal impairment may be at risk for electrolyte abnormalities (eg, hypocalcemia, hyperkalemia). The nurse observes for tremors; tests for paresthesia, numbness, and weakness; and checks for Chvostek's sign (twitching of the facial muscles in response to tapping the facial nerve in front of the auditory meatus) and Trousseau's sign (spasm of the hands in response to arm compression). Positive Chvostek's or Trousseau's signs are suggestive of hypocalcemia and hypomagnesemia.

Laboratory Studies

Urine Studies

Changes in characteristics of urine can indicate kidney damage, infection, excretion of drugs, or the kidney's compensation for systemic homeostatic imbalance.[1] Urine labs are summarized in Table 18-2.

TABLE 18-2 Urine Laboratory Studies

Test	Normal Values or Findings	Abnormal Findings	Possible Causes of Abnormal Findings
Specific gravity	• Between 1.005 and 1.030, with slight variations from one specimen to the next	Below-normal (dilute) specific gravity	Diabetes insipidus, glomerulonephritis, pyelonephritis, acute renal failure (pre-renal), alkalosis, water excess
		Above-normal (concentrated) specific gravity	Dehydration, nephrosis, hemorrhage; presence of high-molecular-weight substances (eg, protein, glucose, mannitol, radiopaque contrast material) in urine (falsely high), SIADH
		Fixed specific gravity	Severe renal damage (acute tubular necrosis, acute nephritis, chronic renal failure)
pH	• Between 4.5 and 7.5	Alkaline pH (above 7.5)	Fanconi's syndrome (chronic renal disease) urinary tract infection, metabolic or respiratory alkalosis
		Acidic pH (below 4.5)	Renal tuberculosis, phenylketonuria, acidosis (compensating)
Protein	• No protein	Proteinuria	Damage to capillary structure, glomerulosclerosis, acute or chronic glomerulonephritis, nephrolithiasis, polycystic kidney disease, acute or chronic renal failure, diabetic nephropathy
Ketones	• No ketones	Ketonuria	Diabetes mellitus, starvation, conditions causing acutely increased metabolic demands and decreased food intake (eg, vomiting, diarrhea)
Glucose	• No glucose	Glycosuria	Diabetes mellitus (serum glucose greater than 200 mg/dL)
Red blood cells (RBCs)	• 0–3 RBCs/high-power field	Numerous RBCs	Urinary tract infection, obstruction, inflammation, trauma, or tumor; glomerulonephritis; renal hypertension; lupus nephritis; renal tuberculosis; renal vein thrombosis; hydronephrosis; pyelonephritis; parasitic bladder infection; polyarteritis nodosa; hemorrhagic disorder

(continued on page 258)

TABLE 18-2 **Urine Laboratory Studies** (continued)

Test	Normal Values or Findings	Abnormal Findings	Possible Causes of Abnormal Findings
Epithelial cells	• Few epithelial cells	Excessive epithelial cells	Renal tubular degeneration
White blood cells (WBCs)	• 0–4 WBCs/high-power field	Numerous WBCs	Urinary tract inflammation, especially cystitis or pyelonephritis
		Numerous WBCs and WBC casts	Renal infection (eg, acute pyelonephritis and glomerulonephritis, nephrotic syndrome, pyogenic infection, lupus nephritis)
Casts	• No casts (except occasional hyaline casts)	Excessive casts	Renal disease
		Excessive hyaline casts	Renal parenchymal disease, inflammation, glomerular capillary membrane trauma
		Epithelial casts	Renal tubular damage, nephrosis, eclampsia, chronic lead intoxication
		Fatty, waxy casts	Nephrotic syndrome, chronic renal disease, diabetes mellitus
		RBC casts	Renal parenchymal disease (especially glomerulonephritis), renal infarction, subacute bacterial endocarditis, sickle cell anemia, blood dyscrasias, malignant hypertension, collagen disease
Crystals	• Some crystals	Numerous calcium oxalate crystals	Hypercalcemia
		Cystine crystals (cystinuria)	Inborn metabolic error
Yeast cells	• No yeast crystals	Yeast cells in sediment	External genitalia contamination, vaginitis, urethritis, prostatovesiculitis
Parasites	• No parasites	Parasites in sediment	External genitalia contamination
Creatinine clearance	• Males (age 20): 90 mg/min/173 m² of body surface	Above-normal creatinine clearance	Little diagnostic significance
	• Females (age 20): 84 mL/min/1.73 m² of body surface	Below-normal creatinine clearance	Reduced renal blood flow (associated with shock or renal artery obstruction), acute tubular necrosis, acute or chronic glomerulonephritis, advanced bilateral renal lesions (as in polycystic kidney disease, renal tuberculosis, and cancer), nephrosclerosis, heart failure, severe dehydration
	• Older patients: normally decreased concentrations by 6 mL/min/decade after age 40 y		
Osmolality	• 300–900 mOsm/kg/24 h	High urine osmolality	Presence of high-molecular-weight substances in urine (falsely high), syndrome of inappropriate antidiuretic hormone (SIADH)
		Below-normal osmolality	Renal failure (acute tubular necrosis, glomerulonephritis), diabetes insipidus
Urine sodium concentration	• 10–20 mEq/L	Greater than 30–40 mEq/L	Acute renal failure (acute tubular necrosis, glomerulonephritis), ischemia, toxicity (eg, antibiotics, contrast material), cerebral salt wasting syndrome
		Less than 10 mEq/L	Poor renal perfusion (eg, heart failure, hypovolemia)
Fractional excretion of sodium (FE$_{Na}$)	• 1%	Less than 1%	Prerenal azotemia (underperfusion)
		Greater than 1%	Acute renal failure
Myoglobin	• No myoglobin	Presence of myoglobin	Skeletal muscle breakdown (crush injuries), burns, trauma, compartment syndrome

Modified from Critical Care Nursing Made Incredibly Easy, 2nd ed. Philadelphia, PA: Lippincott Williams & Wilkins, 2008, pp. 505–506.

- **Urinalysis.** Urinalysis involves examining the physical characteristics of urine (color, clarity, and odor), performing a chemical analysis of the urine, and examining the urine under a microscope for abnormal substances (eg, cells, casts, crystals, microorganisms).
- **Urine volume.** Trends in urine production can provide important clues to the body's recruitment of compensatory responses (eg, the renin–angiotensin–aldosterone system to compensate for hypovolemia).
- **Specific gravity and osmolality.** The specific gravity of the urine is an indication of the kidneys' ability to concentrate and dilute the urine. Urine osmolality, which measures the number of solute particles present in the urine, is a more accurate measurement of urine concentration than specific gravity.
- **Urine sodium concentration.** States of poor kidney perfusion are usually associated with a decrease in urine sodium concentration. This is a compensatory reaction that occurs when the renin–angiotensin–aldosterone system is activated, resulting in increased reabsorption of sodium and water. In intrarenal failure and other conditions that are characterized by damage to the tubular transport mechanisms, the urine sodium concentration is usually greater than normal.

RED FLAG! When the urine pH is alkaline, the urine sodium concentration does not reflect sodium balance accurately. In this case, the chloride concentration becomes a better indicator of volume status.

- **Fractional excretion of sodium (FE$_{Na}$).** This test gives a more precise estimation of the amount of filtered sodium remaining in urine and is more accurate in predicting tubular injury than the urine sodium concentration because it removes the confounding effect of water.[2] FE$_{Na}$ is calculated using the following formula:

$$FE_{Na} = \frac{U_{Na} \times P_{Cr}}{P_{Na} \times U_{Cr}}$$

where U and P are urinary and plasma concentrations of sodium and creatinine, respectively.

- **Creatinine clearance.** Creatinine is a by-product of normal muscle metabolism and is excreted in urine primarily as the result of glomerular filtration. Creatinine clearance is defined as the amount of blood cleared of creatinine in 1 minute and is an excellent clinical indicator of renal function. The amount of creatinine excreted in the urine is directly related to muscle mass. Because men tend to have a higher proportion of muscle than women, the creatinine and creatinine clearance can be higher in men than women. To obtain an accurate creatinine clearance, the nurse collects all urine made in a 24-hour period and obtains

a blood specimen (usually at the midpoint of the urine collection). The creatinine clearance, usually expressed in milliliters per minute, is calculated by the following formula:

$$CrCl = \frac{U_{Cr} \times V}{P_{Cr}}$$

where U$_{Cr}$ is urine creatinine concentration; V, urine volume; and P$_{Cr}$, plasma creatinine concentration.

The creatinine clearance may be estimated using the Cockcroft–Gault formula when there is difficulty collecting a 24-hour urine sample or when spot-checking creatinine clearance will assist prompt treatment (eg, in drug nephrotoxicity):

$$CrCl = \frac{(140 - age \times weight\ (kg)}{72 \times P_{Cr}\ (mg/dL)}$$

where P$_{Cr}$ is plasma creatinine.

Many labs are now routinely reporting the glomerular filtration rate (GFR) using estimate formulas for creatinine clearance based on a single serum creatinine level. An estimate may be made when there is difficulty collecting a 24-hour urine or spot checking to identify an issue early for treatment.

The Older Patient. *With aging, renal blood flow and the total number of functioning glomeruli decreases, resulting in a GFR decrease of about 7 to 10 mL/min per decade after 40 years of age.*

The Older Patient. *In an older patient, a 24-hour urine study or an isotopic renal scan is the most accurate way to assess creatinine clearance and GFR. Formulas that estimate GFR based on onetime creatinine levels are not as accurate in elderly patients. When an older patient's true GFR is known, therapy (eg, drug dosages) can be guided more safely.*

Blood Studies

Expected values for blood studies commonly used to evaluate renal function are summarized in Table 18-3.

TABLE 18-3 **Bloodwork to Evaluate Renal Function**

Diagnostic Test	Normal Values
Creatinine	0.6–1.2 mg/dL
BUN	8–20 mg/dL
BUN:Creatinine ratio	10:1 to 15:1
Osmolality	275–295 mOsm/kg
Hemoglobin	Men: 13.5–17.5 g/dL
	Women: 12–16 g/dL
Hematocrit	Men: 40%–52%
	Women: 37%–48%
Uric acid	2–8.5 mg/dL

BOX 18-3 Factors Affecting Blood Urea Nitrogen (BUN) Levels

Elevated BUN
- Increase urea production, which can result from
  - Increased protein intake (tube feedings and some forms of hyperalimentation)
  - Increased tissue breakdown (as with crush injuries)
  - Febrile illnesses
  - Steroid or tetracycline administration
  - Reabsorption of blood from the intestine in patients with intestinal hemorrhage
- Dehydration
- Decreased renal perfusion (eg, secondary to shock or heart failure)

Decreased BUN
- Decreased protein intake
- Liver disease
- Large volume of urine secondary to excessive fluid intake

BOX 18-4 Factors Affecting the Blood Urea Nitrogen (BUN): Creatinine Ratio

Decreased BUN:Creatinine Ratio (Less than 10:1)
- Liver disease
- Protein restriction
- Excessive fluid intake

Increased BUN:Creatinine Ratio (Less than 10:1)
- Volume depletion
- Decreased "effective" blood volume
- Catabolic states
- Excessive protein intake

- **Serum creatinine.** When kidneys are damaged by a disease process, creatinine clearance decreases, and serum creatinine concentration rises. When a patient has rapidly changing renal function and oliguria (eg, acute renal failure), serum creatinine levels are more reliable indicators of renal function than the creatinine clearance. In patients with rhabdomyolysis, conversion of muscle creatine to creatinine causes the serum creatinine level to be elevated out of proportion to the reduced GFR. In this situation, serum creatinine is less reliable as an indicator of renal function.
- **Blood urea nitrogen (BUN).** The BUN level, another indicator of kidney function, is influenced by many factors (Box 18-3). At low urine flow rates, more sodium and water, and consequently more urea, are reabsorbed. Therefore, when the patient is volume depleted, BUN tends to increase out of proportion to any change in renal function (creatinine levels). However, BUN can be of significant clinical value when compared with the serum creatinine concentration, BUN:creatinine ratio (Box 18-4).
- **Osmolality.** All substances in solution contribute to osmolality. Serum osmolality is primarily determined by the concentration of sodium and its accompanying anions, urea, and glucose. Therefore, when these concentrations are known, serum osmolality can be calculated by the following formula:

$$\text{Osmolality} = 2(\text{Na}) + \frac{\text{Glucose}}{18} + \frac{\text{BUN}}{2.8}$$

The calculated osmolality normally is within 10 mOsm of the measured osmolality. Normally, the serum osmolality remains quite constant because water can move freely between blood, interstitial fluid, and tissues. A decrease in serum osmolality can occur only when serum sodium is decreased. An increase in serum osmolality can occur whenever serum sodium, urea, or glucose is elevated or when abnormal compounds are present in the blood, such as drugs, poisons, or metabolic waste products (eg, lactic acid).

- **Serum electrolytes.** The kidney's role is central in maintaining fluid volume and ionic composition of body fluids. When the kidneys properly regulate the excretion of water and ions, homeostasis is achieved. When they fail to adapt adequately, imbalances occur. Because minor shifts in electrolytes can be lethal, the nurse must monitor all electrolyte values closely.
- **Hematocrit and hemoglobin.** False elevations of hematocrit can be seen with dehydration or after dialysis. Low hematocrits may result from hypervolemia. Many patients with chronic kidney disease produce insufficient amounts of erythropoietin, which can result in chronic anemia and decreased hemoglobin levels.
- **Uric acid.** Uric acid is a nitrogenous end product of protein and purine metabolism. Humans produce only small quantities of uric acid under normal conditions. Serum uric acid values may be elevated because of excessive production from cell breakdown or inadequate excretion by the kidney.

Diagnostic Studies

- **Radiological studies** used to evaluate structure and function of the renal system are summarized in Table 18-4.
- **Renal biopsy** is the most invasive but most definitive diagnostic tool used in comprehensive renal evaluation.[3] It is used to define histology, provide etiological clues for diagnosis, assess prognosis, and guide therapy. Possible indications for renal biopsy are given in Box 18-5. Contraindications include serious bleeding disorders, excessive obesity, and severe hypertension. Complications include retroperitoneal bleeding or bleeding into the urinary tract, inadvertent biopsy of other abdominal viscera, and tears in the diaphragm or pleura.

TABLE 18-4 Radiological Studies Used to Evaluate the Renal System

Diagnostic Test	Description	Purpose
Kidney–ureter–bladder (KUB) radiograph, abdominal radiograph	Standard x-rays capture image	Detects abnormal calcifications and renal size
Tomography	Standard x-rays capture a series of cross-sectional scans made along a single axis; a computer then uses the scans to create a three-dimensional image.	Determines renal outlines and abnormalities
Intravenous pyelography (IVP)	Contrast material is injected intravenously and then collected in the renal system, turning areas bright white.	Detects anatomical abnormalities of the kidneys and ureters
Retrograde pyelography	Contrast material is injected through a urinary catheter; typically performed at the same time as cystoscopy.	Assesses renal size, evaluates ureteral obstruction, and localizes and diagnoses tumors and obstructions
Antegrade pyelography	Contrast material is injected into ureter to visualize structures of upper urinary tract.	Distinguishes cysts from hydronephrosis
Renal arteriography and venography	A vessel (artery or vein) is accessed and contrast material is injected to visualize structures "downstream."	Evaluates possible renal arterial stenosis, renal mass lesions, renal vein thrombosis, and venous extension of renal cell carcinoma
Digital subtraction angiography	Radiographs of the renal vessels are obtained before and after contrast material is injected; tissues and blood vessels on the first image are digitally subtracted from second image, leaving a clear picture of the major arteries.	Reveals significant narrowing or obstruction of the major vessels
Ultrasonography	Sound waves are used to create images.	Delineates renal outlines Measures longitudinal and transverse dimensions of the kidneys Evaluates mass lesions Examines perinephric area Detects and grades hydronephrosis
Radionuclide scintillation imaging (renal scan)	A small amount of a radioactive tracer is injected into the bloodstream to produce images of blood flow through the kidneys.	Measures kidney function
Static imaging	A radioactive tracer is used to provide static images of the renal parenchyma.	Gives information about the size, shape, and position of the kidneys; identifies scar tissue
Dynamic imaging	A radioactive tracer is followed through vascular, renal parenchymal, and urinary tract compartments.	Gives information about blood flow to the kidneys and how well each kidney is producing urine; indicates obstructions to urine output
Magnetic resonance imaging (MRI)	Uses nonionizing radiofrequency signals to acquire images; best suited for noncalcified tissue.	Determines anatomical abnormalities

BOX 18-5 Possible Indications for Renal Biopsy

- Hematuria, proteinuria, or both accompanied by a decreased glomerular filtration rate (GFR)
- Nephrotic syndrome
- Systemic disease with renal abnormalities
- Acute renal failure accompanied by azotemia lasting more than 3 weeks, moderate proteinuria, anuria, or eosinophilia or eosinophiluria
- Posttransplant decrease in GFR

- **Renal angiography** may be used to evaluate renal blood flow when precise measurements are required. An introducer (sheath) is inserted percutaneously into the femoral artery, a small catheter is passed to the bifurcation of the renal arteries, and contrast material is injected to permit radiological visualization of blood flow. Following removal of the sheath, nursing care entails maintaining pressure on the site, regularly assessing the site for bleeding, and assessing perfusion (pulses, color, refill) distal to the site.

CASE STUDY

Mrs. R. is a 28-year-old woman who was admitted to the emergency department after being involved in a motor vehicle crash. The time required to extricate Mrs. R. from the vehicle was prolonged. During the trauma evaluation, Mrs. R is noted to have bilateral lower extremity fractures and crush injuries. During physical examination, Mrs. R.'s vital signs are as follows: temp, 35.6°C; HR, 135 beats/min; RR, 24 breaths/min; and BP, 102/68 mm Hg. Oxygen saturation is 95% on oxygen at 100% by nonrebreather mask. Additional injuries include a grade two splenic laceration, traumatic brain injury, and bilateral rib fractures. Mrs. R.'s lower extremity fractures are repaired, and she is brought to the critical care unit for further assessment and management. Initial bloodwork obtained on arrival to the unit reveals the following: sodium, 135 mEq/L; chloride, 99 mEq/L; potassium, 3.4 mEq/L; carbon dioxide, 20 mEq/L; glucose, 156 mg/dL; BUN, 10 mg/dL; creatinine, 0.7 mg/dL; and hematocrit, 30%.

On posttrauma day 2, Mrs. R is endotracheally intubated and sedated. She has palpable distal pulses. Her vital signs are stable. Her urine is pink tinged and output over the past several hours has been averaging 20 to 25 mL/hour. Bloodwork reveals a BUN of 22 mg/dL and a creatinine of 1.2 mg/dL. Other studies remain relatively unchanged. Mrs. R. is given a diagnosis of acute renal failure.

1. Explain why Mrs. R. is experiencing renal insufficiency. Describe the influence of Mrs. R.'s trauma on her renal function.

2. What interventions may be required to improve Mrs. R.'s renal function?

3. What other assessments or diagnostic tests may be indicated?

References

1. Dains J, Baumann L, Scheibel P: Advanced Health Assessment and Clinical Diagnosis in Primary Care. Elsevier Health Sciences, 2007
2. Darmon M, et al.: Diagnostic performance of fractional excretion of urea in the evaluation of critically ill patient with acute kidney injury: multicenter cohort study. Crit Care 15:178, 2011
3. Scheckner B, et al.: Diagnostic yield of renal biopsies: A retrospective single center review. BMC Nephrology 10:11, 2009

Want to know more? A wide variety of resources to enhance your learning and understanding of this chapter are available on the**Point** ✴. Visit **http://thepoint.lww.com/MortonEss1e** to access chapter review questions and more!

Patient Management: Renal System

OBJECTIVES

Based on the content in this chapter, the reader should be able to:

1 Describe drug classes used in the pharmacologic management of renal dysfunction.

2 Explain the basic physiological principles involved in dialysis.

3 Describe the nursing care of a patient undergoing hemodialysis, continuous renal replacement therapy (CRRT), and peritoneal dialysis.

Pharmacotherapy

Diuretics

Diuretics (Table 19-1) promote fluid removal through increased urine production. The ultimate goal of diuretic therapy is to improve cardiopulmonary status. It may be necessary to use combination therapy (using drugs from different classes) to achieve the desired therapeutic end point. Overdiuresis is the most common side effect of diuretics in responsive kidneys. The nurse must monitor fluid balance, especially when diuretic regimens are altered or initiated. A reduction in the effective circulatory volume can worsen acute renal failure, increase the heart's workload, and cause metabolic alterations. The most effective management strategy is to replace only the volume required to achieve adequate perfusion.

Inotropes

A failing heart can cause reduced blood flow to the kidney and potentiate acute renal failure. Inotropes (eg, dopamine, dobutamine) may be administered to improve forward flow when the cause of decreased

effective circulatory volume is reduced cardiac contractility. In addition, when infused at lower doses (1 to 3 mcg/kg/min), dopamine stimulates the dopaminergic receptors in the kidney, increasing renal blood flow and promoting natriuresis.

Dialysis

Dialysis is a life-maintaining therapy that replaces renal function in acute and chronic renal failure. Critical care nurses may care for patients with acute renal failure who require dialysis and for patients already on some form of chronic dialysis who subsequently become critically ill. The three most common forms of dialysis are hemodialysis, continuous renal replacement therapy (CRRT), and peritoneal dialysis (Table 19-2).

All forms of dialysis make use of the principles of diffusion and osmosis to remove waste products and excess fluid from the blood. A semipermeable membrane is placed between the blood and a specially formulated solution called dialysate. The dialysate solution is composed of water and the major electrolytes of normal serum. Dissolved substances

TABLE 19-1   **Medications Used to Produce Diuresis**

Medication	Mechanism of Action	Nursing Implications
Loop diuretics furosemide (Lasix) ethacrynic acid (Edecrin) bumetanide (Bumex)	Act primarily in the thick segment of the medullary and cortical ascending limbs of loop of Henle.	• Monitor daily weights, intake and output, signs and symptoms of volume depletion. • May cause hypokalemia, hyponatremia, hypocalcemia, and hypomagnesemia.
Thiazides chlorothiazide (Diuril) hydrochlorothiazide (HCTZ)	Inhibit sodium reabsorption in distal tubule and, to a lesser extent, inner medullary collecting duct.	• Monitor calcium levels; loop diuretic may be indicated if calcium levels are persistently elevated. • Potassium supplements or extradietary potassium may be necessary when these agents are used routinely.
Potassium-sparing diuretics spironolactone (Aldactone) triamterene (Dyrenium) amiloride (Midamor)	Spironolactone inhibits action of aldosterone, thereby reducing sodium reabsorption while increasing potassium reabsorption. Triamterene acts on distal renal tubule to depress exchange of sodium. Amiloride is thought to inhibit sodium entry into cell from luminal fluid.	• Potassium supplements are contraindicated, as are salt substitutes containing potassium. • Often combined with thiazides for effective diuresis; hypokalemic tendency of thiazides may offset hyperkalemic tendency of triamterene and spironolactone.
Carbonic anhydrase inhibitors acetazolamide (Diamox)	Decrease proximal tubular sodium reabsorption and facilitate excretion of bicarbonate.	• Not very effective when administered alone • May cause metabolic acidosis; monitor pH and bicarbonate.
Osmotic diuretics mannitol	Nonreabsorbable polysaccharide that pulls water into vascular space, thereby increasing glomerular flow	• Monitor serum osmolality; withhold therapy if serum osmolality is greater than 300–305 mmol/L.

Adapted from Metheny NM: Fluid and Electrolyte Balance: Nursing Considerations. Philadelphia, PA: Lippincott Williams & Wilkins, 2000, p 53, with permission.

TABLE 19-2   **Comparison of Hemodialysis, Continuous Renal Replacement Therapy (CRRT), and Peritoneal Dialysis**

	Hemodialysis	CRRT	Peritoneal Dialysis
Access	Arteriovenous fistula or graft; dual-lumen venous catheter	Arteriovenous fistula or graft; dual-lumen venous catheter	Temporary or permanent peritoneal catheter
Anticoagulation requirements	Systemic heparinization or frequent saline flushes	Systemic anticoagulation with heparin or citrate may be indicated depending on the patient's coagulation studies before starting therapy.	May only need heparin intraperitoneally Not absorbed systemically
Length of treatment	3–4 h, three to five times per wk, depending on patient acuity	Continuous throughout the day; may last as many days as needed	Continuous (cycled) or intermittent exchanges; time between exchanges =1–6 h
Indications	End stage renal disease (ESRD) Complications of acute renal failure (eg, uremia, fluid overload, acidosis, hyperkalemia, drug overdose)	Patients with a high risk for hemodynamic instability who do not tolerate the rapid fluid shifts that occur with hemodialysis Patients who require large amounts of hourly IV fluids or parenteral nutrition Patients who need more than the usual 3–4h hemodialysis treatment to correct the metabolic imbalances of acute renal failure	Acute renal failure when hemodialysis is not available or access to bloodstream is not possible Initial treatment for renal failure while the patient is being evaluated for a hemodialysis program

TABLE 19-2	Comparison of Hemodialysis, Continuous Renal Replacement Therapy (CRRT), and Peritoneal Dialysis (continued)		
	Hemodialysis	**CRRT**	**Peritoneal Dialysis**
Contraindications	Coagulopathies, hypotension, extremely low cardiac output, inability to tolerate abrupt changes in volume status	Hemodynamic stability	Postabdominal surgery status, abdominal adhesions and scars, peritonitis
Advantages	Quick, efficient removal of metabolic wastes and excess fluid	Best choice for a patient who is hemodynamically unstable because less blood is outside body than with hemodialysis and blood flow rates are slower; amount of fluid removed can still be achieved but over a much longer period of time Good for hypercatabolic patients who receive large amounts of IV fluids	Continuous removal of wastes and fluid Better hemodynamic stability Fewer dietary restrictions Less complicated and less need for highly skilled personnel
Disadvantages	May require frequent vascular access procedures Places strain on a compromised cardiovascular system Potential blood loss from bleeding or clotted lines Requires specially trained staff to perform therapy	Requires vascular access Potential blood loss from clotting or equipment leaks Requires specially trained staff to perform therapy	Waste products may be removed too slowly in a catabolic patient. Risk for peritonitis Long periods of immobility

(eg, urea, creatinine) diffuse across the membrane from the area of greater concentration (blood) to the area of lesser concentration (dialysate). Water molecules move across the membrane by osmosis to the dialysate, which contains varying concentrations of dextrose or sodium to produce an osmotic gradient. This process of fluid moving across a semipermeable membrane in relation to forces created by osmotic and hydrostatic pressures is called ultrafiltration.

 RED FLAG! *Because medications can be removed from the blood during dialysis, the nurse must consider the patient's dialysis schedule when timing the administration of medications. Medications that are commonly removed during dialysis are listed in Box 19-1.*

Hemodialysis

Equipment and Setup

In hemodialysis, water and excess waste products are removed from the blood as it is pumped by the dialysis machine through an extracorporeal circuit (Fig. 19-1A) into a device called a dialyzer, which acts as an artificial kidney (see Fig. 19-1B). Within the dialyzer, blood and dialysate flow past a semipermeable membrane in opposite directions from each other (countercurrent flow); as blood travels through the dialyzer, it is constantly exposed to a fresh flow of dialysate. This countercurrent flow maintains the concentration gradient (ie, the difference in the concentration of the blood and the dialysate) and

provides the most efficient dialysis. Waste substances (eg, urea, creatinine) diffuse from the blood to the dialysate. Excess water is removed by a pressure differential created between the blood and the dialysate.

Because hemodialysis uses an extracorporeal circuit, access to the patient's circulation is required. This can be achieved in a variety of ways:

- **Dual-lumen venous catheter.** A dual-lumen venous catheter (one lumen for blood outflow

BOX 19-1 Examples of Commonly Hemodialyzed Medications

Acetaminophen	Fluconazole	Morphine
Acyclovir	Ganciclovir	Nitroprusside
Allopurinol	Gentamicin	Penicillin
Amoxicillin	Imipenem	Phenobarbital
Ampicillin	Lisinopril	Piperacillin
Captopril	Lithium	Procainamide
Cefazolin	Mannitol	Salsalate
Cefepime	Meropenem	Sotalol
Cefoxitin	Metformin	Streptomycin
Ceftazidime	Methotrexate	Sulfamethoxazole
Cimetidine	Methylprednisolone	Theophylline
Enalapril	Metoprolol	Tobramycin
Esmolol	Metronidazole	Valacyclovir

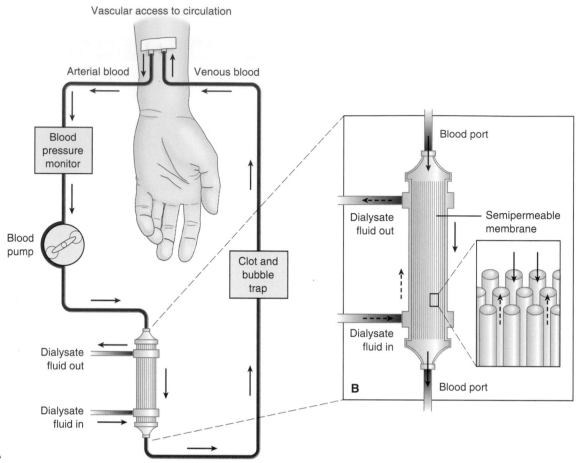

Vascular access to circulation

FIGURE 19-1 Hemodialysis system. **A:** Blood from an artery is pumped into a dialyzer (**B**), where it flows through the cellophane tubes, which act as the semipermeable membrane (*inset*). The dialysate, which has the same chemical composition as the blood except for urea and waste products, flows in around the tubules. The waste products in the blood diffuse through the semipermeable membrane into the dialysate. (From Smeltzer SC, Bare BG, Hinkle JL, et al: Brunner & Suddarth's Textbook of Medical-Surgical Nursing, 12th ed. Philadelphia, PA: Lippincott Williams & Wilkins, 2010, p 1334.)

and one for blood return) is inserted into a large central vein (eg, the femoral, internal jugular, or subclavian). Dual-lumen catheters are used for critically ill patients who require acute dialysis and for patients on chronic dialysis who are waiting for more permanent vascular access. Whenever venous catheters are used, care must be taken to avoid accidental dislodgment during hemodialysis. Catheters left in place between dialysis treatments usually are filled with a concentrated heparin–saline solution after dialysis and capped to prevent clotting. Procedures for cleaning and dressing of the insertion site are the same as for other central lines and require strict aseptic technique.

 RED FLAG! *Dual-lumen catheters should never be used for any purpose other than hemodialysis without first checking with dialysis unit personnel.*

- **Arteriovenous fistula.** To create an arteriovenous fistula, a surgeon anastomoses an artery and a vein, creating a fistula (artificial opening) between them (Fig. 19-2A). Arterial blood flowing into the venous system results in marked dilation of the vein, which can then be punctured easily with a 15- or 16-gauge dialysis fistula needle. Two venipunctures are made at the time of dialysis: one for blood outflow and one for blood return. Most arteriovenous fistulas are developed and ready to use 1 to 3 months after surgery. Although arteriovenous fistulas usually have a long life, complications may occur. These include thrombosis, aneurysm or pseudoaneurysm, and "steal syndrome" (ie, shunting of blood from the artery to the vein leading to ischemia, pain, and coldness of the hand). Teaching points for the patient with an arteriovenous fistula are summarized in Box 19-2.
- **Synthetic graft.** Synthetic grafts, made from a highly porous form of Teflon called polytetrafluoroethylene (PTFE), are used when a patient's own vessels are not adequate for fistula formation and to patch areas of arteriovenous fistulas that have stenosed or developed areas of aneurysm. The graft

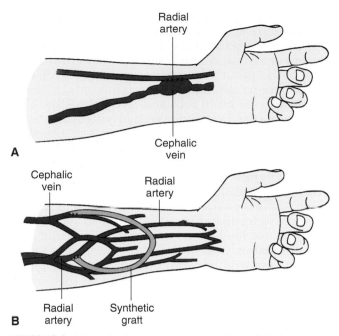

FIGURE 19-2 Methods of vascular access for hemodialysis. **A:** Arteriovenous fistula. **B:** Synthetic graft.

is anastomosed between an artery and a vein and is used in the same manner as an arteriovenous fistula (see Fig. 19-2B). Venipuncture of a new synthetic graft is avoided for 2 to 4 weeks while the patient's tissue grows into the graft. Complications include thrombosis, infection, aneurysm formation, and stenosis at the site of anastomosis.

BOX 19-2 **Patient Teaching: Arteriovenous Fistula**

- Wash the fistula site with antibacterial soap each day and always before dialysis.
- Refrain from picking the scab that forms after completion of dialysis therapy.
- Check for redness, feeling of excess warmth, or the beginning of a pimple on any area of access.
- Ask the dialysis care team to rotate needles at the time of dialysis treatment.
- Check blood flow several times each day by feeling for a pulse or thrill. If you cannot feel a pulse or thrill, or if there is a change, call your healthcare provider or dialysis center.
- Avoid wearing tight clothes or jewelry on the access arm. Also avoid carrying anything heavy or doing anything that will put pressure on the access site.
- Avoid sleeping with your head on the arm where the access site is located.
- Remind caregivers not to use a blood pressure cuff on, or draw blood from, the arm where the access site is located.
- Apply only gentle pressure to the access site after the needle is removed. Too much pressure stops flow of blood to the access site.

Nursing interventions for a patient with dialysis vascular access are summarized in Box 19-3.

The use of an extracorporeal circuit also necessitates anticoagulation, because blood in the dialyzer and blood lines clots rapidly. Heparin is most commonly used because it is simple to administer, increases clotting time rapidly, is monitored easily, and may be reversed with protamine. Citrate, which chelates calcium to inactivate the coagulation cascade, may also be used.

Typically, the circuit is initially primed with a dose of heparin, followed by smaller intermittent doses administered at a constant rate by an infusion pump. This results in systemic anticoagulation, in which the clotting times of the patient and the dialyzer essentially are the same. Systemic anticoagulation does not usually present a risk unless the patient has overt bleeding (eg, gastrointestinal bleeding, epistaxis, hemoptysis), has had surgery within the last 3 to 7 days, or has uremic pericarditis. In these situations, regional anticoagulation may be used. In regional anticoagulation, the patient's clotting time is kept normal while the clotting time of the dialyzer is increased. This can be accomplished by infusing the anticoagulant at a constant rate into the dialyzer and simultaneously neutralizing its effects with protamine sulfate (for heparin) or calcium chloride (for citrate) before the blood returns to the patient.

BOX 19-3 **Nursing Interventions for the Patient With Dialysis Vascular Access**

Dual-Lumen Venous Catheter
- Verify central line catheter placement radiographically before use.
- Do not inject IV fluids or medication into the catheter. Both lumens of the catheter usually are filled with concentrated heparin.
- Do not unclamp the catheter unless preparing for dialysis therapy. Unclamping the catheter can cause blood to fill the lumen and clot.
- Maintain sterile technique in handling vascular access.
- Observe the catheter exit site for signs of inflammation or catheter kinking.

Arteriovenous Fistula or Graft
- Do not take blood pressure or draw blood from the access limb.
- Listen for bruit and palpate for thrill every 8 hours.
- Avoid placing tight clothing or restraints on the access limb.
- Check access patency more frequently in hypotensive patients (hypotension can predispose to clotting).
- In the event of postdialysis bleeding from the needle site, apply just enough pressure to stop the flow of blood and hold until bleeding stops. Do not occlude the vessel.

RED FLAG! *When citrate is used for anticoagulation, calcium is replaced via infusion through the venous return line or peripherally to maintain normal ionized calcium levels.[1] Therefore, the patient needs to be closely monitored for calcium abnormalities—hypercalcemia and hypocalcemia.*

Nursing Care of a Patient Receiving Hemodialysis

Before dialysis, the nurse consults with other caregivers and reviews the patient's history, clinical findings, and laboratory test results. Assessment of the patient's blood pressure, pulse, weight, intake and output, tissue turgor, and hemodynamic parameters (eg, pulmonary artery occlusion pressure [PAOP], central venous pressure [CVP]) is important for determining the patient's fluid balance. The nurse also assesses the patient's response to previous dialysis treatments and the patient's level of understanding of the procedure. Providing a basic explanation of the procedure can allay some of the anxiety experienced by the patient and family. It is important to stress that dialysis is being used to support normal body function, rather than to "cure" the kidney disease process.

A dialysis nurse is in constant attendance during acute hemodialysis. During the dialysis procedure, the critical care nurse collaborates with the dialysis nurse to coordinate patient care. Throughout the dialysis treatment, the patient's blood pressure and pulse are monitored and recorded at least every half hour when the patient's condition is stable. If hypotension develops, saline, blood, or plasma expanders are administered to correct blood pressure. Medications that can be given during dialysis may be infused through the medication port in the dialyzer. After the prescribed treatment time, dialysis is terminated by clamping off blood from the patient and rinsing the circuit with saline to return the patient's blood.

Following the treatment, the patient's weight is obtained and compared to the predialysis weight to determine the amount of fluid removed. Blood samples for laboratory tests are drawn 2 to 3 hours after the dialysis treatment to assess the degree to which electrolyte and acid–base imbalances have been corrected. Blood drawn immediately after dialysis may show falsely low levels of electrolytes, urea nitrogen, and creatinine because it takes time for these substances to move from inside the cell to the plasma.

Complications of Hemodialysis

Complications that can develop during or after hemodialysis include the following.

- **Disequilibrium syndrome.** Uremia must be corrected slowly to prevent disequilibrium syndrome, characterized by signs and symptoms of cerebral edema (eg, headache, nausea, restlessness, mild mental impairment, vomiting, confusion, agitation, seizures). This syndrome is thought to occur as the plasma concentration of solutes that play a role in serum osmolality (eg, urea, nitrogen) is lowered. Because of the blood–brain barrier, solutes are removed much more slowly from brain cells. The plasma becomes hypotonic in relation to the brain cells, resulting in a shift of water from plasma to the brain cells and cerebral edema. This syndrome can be avoided by dialyzing patients for shorter periods (eg, 1 to 2 hours on 3 or 4 consecutive days) or by using alternative therapies (eg, CRRT).

- **Hypovolemia.** The rapid removal of fluid during dialysis can lead to volume depletion and hypotension. Little is gained if IV fluids are given to correct the problem; therefore, it is better to reduce the volume overload slowly over two or three dialyses.

- **Hypotension.** The use of antihypertensive drugs in patients who undergo dialysis may precipitate hypotension during dialysis. To avoid this, many dialysis units hold antihypertensive drugs 4 to 6 hours before dialysis. Sedatives may also cause hypotension and should be avoided, if possible.

- **Hypertension.** Fluid overload, kidney injury, and anxiety are common causes of hypertension during dialysis. Hypertension caused by fluid overload can usually be corrected by ultrafiltration (ie, adjusting the concentration of solutes in the dialysate to promote movement of water from the blood to the dialysate). Some patients who are normotensive before dialysis become hypertensive during dialysis. The increase in blood pressure may occur gradually or abruptly. The cause is not well understood, but it may be the result of renin production in response to ultrafiltration and an increase in renal ischemia. Patients must be carefully monitored because the vasoconstriction caused by the renin response is limited. Once the decrease in blood volume surpasses the body's ability to maintain blood pressure through vasoconstriction, hypotension can occur precipitously. Restrict fluids and sodium before and during the dialysis treatment to control hypertension.

- **Muscle cramps.** Excess fluid removal can result in diminished intravascular volume and reduced muscle perfusion, leading to muscle cramps. During dialysis, cramps may be treated by lowering the rate of ultrafiltration and administering hypertonic solutions, normal saline boluses, mannitol, or glucose to increase muscle perfusion.[1]

- **Dysrhythmias and angina.** Fluid and electrolyte removal can precipitate dysrhythmias and angina in patients with underlying cardiac disease. Decreasing the rate of fluid removal may help. Medication may be needed to control cardiac rhythm.

Continuous Renal Replacement Therapy
Equipment and Setup

CRRT is similar to hemodialysis in that blood circulates outside the body through a highly porous filter and water, electrolytes, and small- to medium-sized molecules are removed by ultrafiltration and dialysis. The extracorporeal circuit is similar to the hemodialysis circuit (Fig. 19-3), and access to the patient's circulation is the same as that used for short-term hemodialysis. However, unlike hemodialysis, CRRT is accompanied by a simultaneous reinfusion of a physiological solution, and it occurs continuously for an extended period. The CRRT device often includes a weighing system so that fluids can be intricately balanced hour to hour. The ultrafiltration rate is titrated to reach an hourly goal (set by the physician) and is based on the patient's cardiac and pulmonary status. Indications for CRRT are given in Box 19-4. Treatment is usually terminated when the patient becomes hemodynamically stable or shows signs of recovering renal function.

Specific types of CRRTs include continuous venovenous hemofiltration (CVVH) and continuous venovenous hemofiltration with dialysis (CVVHD).

- CVVH is used when a patient primarily needs excess fluid removed. With CVVH, blood is driven through the filter. Dialysate is not used; solutes are "dragged" across the filter along with excess fluid

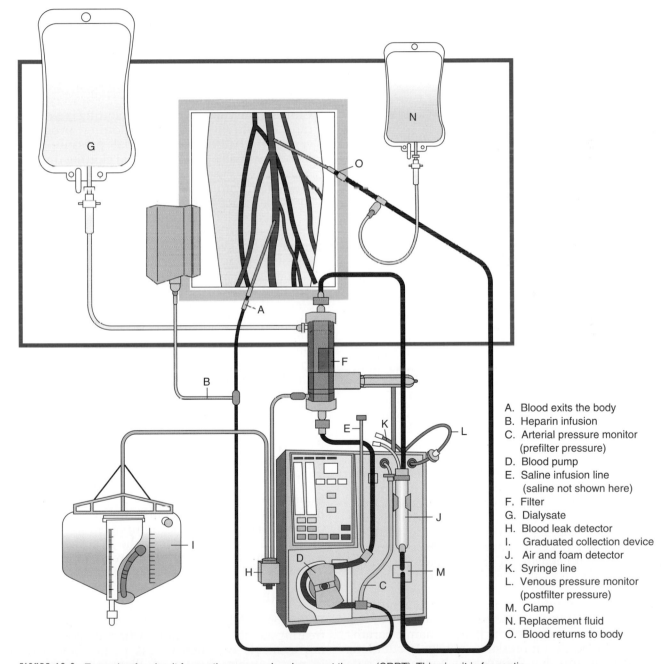

A. Blood exits the body
B. Heparin infusion
C. Arterial pressure monitor
   (prefilter pressure)
D. Blood pump
E. Saline infusion line
   (saline not shown here)
F. Filter
G. Dialysate
H. Blood leak detector
I. Graduated collection device
J. Air and foam detector
K. Syringe line
L. Venous pressure monitor
   (postfilter pressure)
M. Clamp
N. Replacement fluid
O. Blood returns to body

FIGURE 19-3 Example of a circuit for continuous renal replacement therapy (CRRT). This circuit is for continuous venovenous hemofiltration with dialysis (CVVHD). (Courtesy of Baxter Health Care Corporation, Renal Division, McGaw Park, IL.)

as a result of hydrostatic pressure. Replacement fluid may be connected either before or after the filter, depending on the patient and facility protocol.
- CVVHD entails the addition of dialysis to the CVVH process. Adding the dialysate increases removal of wastes such as urea.

Nursing Care of a Patient Receiving Continuous Renal Replacement Therapy

Critical care nurses who receive training in the procedure and complete a competency assessment and validation can perform and manage CVVH and CVVHD. Prior to initiating therapy, the nurse obtains the patient's baseline vital signs, central venous pressure readings (if available), breath sounds, heart sounds, weight, intake, and output. Vital signs are assessed every half hour during treatment. Electrolytes, urea nitrogen, creatinine, and glucose levels are drawn before the procedure is started and then at least twice daily.

Anticoagulation, if indicated, is administered as therapy begins. For patients with low platelet counts, saline flushes without low-dose heparin may be used to prevent circuit clotting, the most common mechanism for interruption of CRRT. Alternatively, citrate may be used. Evidence suggests that the use of citrate in patients who are receiving CRRT is associated with fewer life-threatening bleeding complications than heparin.[2,3] For some patients, saline flushes may be used along with anticoagulation.

The nurse measures blood and dialysate flows, calculates net ultrafiltration and replacement fluid, titrates anticoagulants, assesses the integrity of the vascular access, and monitors hemodynamic parameters and blood circuit pressures hourly. In addition, the nurse ensures that the goal for hourly fluid balance is met by comparing total intake and output. The amount of replacement fluid is determined by

the difference between desired and net fluid balance. Fluid balance and replacement are carefully documented in the patient's medical record.

The nurse monitors the patient for hypotension and electrolyte imbalances. If hypotension occurs, the nurse administers saline boluses (100 to 200 mL), reduces ultrafiltration by raising the collection device, and, if necessary, obtains an order for 5% albumin. Electrolyte imbalances can be corrected by altering the composition of the replacement fluid or by custom mixing the dialysate.

The nurse also monitors for mechanical problems with vascular access or the circuit, which can interrupt treatment:

- **Access problems.** A clot or kink in the arterial or venous lumen of the catheter manifests as lowered arterial and venous pressures. If obstruction is suspected, treatment is temporarily halted and each lumen is flushed to determine patency. If blood flow still cannot be established, the physician must replace the catheter.
- **Clotting.** An early sign of filter clotting is a reduced rate of ultrafiltration. As clotting progresses, venous pressure rises, arterial pressure drops, blood lines will appear dark, and clotting times will be low. To prevent filter clotting, the nurse flushes the system with saline as often as needed to assess the appearance of the filter and circuit. The nurse also checks clotting times at initiation of therapy and at prescribed intervals throughout the treatment. If the system is clotting, as much blood as possible should be returned to the patient before changing the system, unless clotting is extensive.
- **Air in the circuit.** Air can enter the circuit if the connections are loose or a prefilter infusion line runs dry. The air collects in the drip chamber, setting off the air detector alarm and triggering the clamp on the venous line to close. Before resetting the line clamp, the nurse detects the source of the air and then ensures that all bubbles have been tapped out of the drip chamber, all connections are tight, and there is no danger of air entering the patient's bloodstream.

Complications of Continuous Renal Replacement Therapy

Complications of CRRT include hypotension and hypothermia. Advancements in the technologies used to perform CRRT have improved the precision of fluid balance and reduced the hypothermia that can develop with any extracorporeal therapy.

Peritoneal Dialysis

Peritoneal dialysis is an alternative method of treating acute renal failure when hemodialysis is not available or when access to the bloodstream is not possible. Peritoneal dialysis and hemodialysis operate on the same principle of diffusion. However, in peritoneal dialysis, the peritoneum is

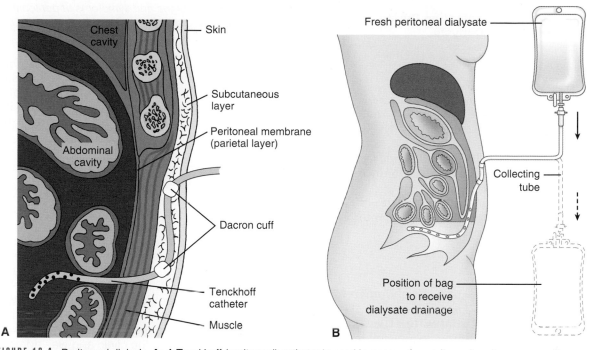

FIGURE 19-4 Peritoneal dialysis. **A:** A Tenckhoff (peritoneal) catheter is used to access the peritoneal cavity. A Dacron cuff wrapped around the catheter helps to reduce complications related to infection. **B:** Dialysate flows by gravity into the peritoneal catheter and then into the peritoneal cavity. After a prescribed period of time, the fluid is drained by gravity and discarded. (From Smeltzer SC, Bare BG, Hinkle JL, et al.: Brunner & Suddarth's Textbook of Medical–Surgical Nursing, 12th ed. Philadelphia, PA: Lippincott Williams & Wilkins, 2010, p 1341.)

the semipermeable membrane, and osmosis is used to remove fluid, rather than the pressure differentials used in hemodialysis.

Equipment and Setup

Peritoneal dialysate must be sterile. Like dialysates used in hemodialysis, peritoneal dialysates contain electrolytes and dextrose to promote osmosis. The dextrose concentration varies. Use of 2.5% or 4.25% solutions usually is reserved for more fluid removal and occasionally for better solute clearance.

 RED FLAG! *A dialysate warming device should always be used to warm dialysate. Dialysate should not be warmed in a microwave oven because microwaves heat fluids unevenly.*

The peritoneal cavity is accessed with a Tenckhoff (peritoneal) catheter (Fig. 19-4A). Over the course of 5 to 10 minutes, the warmed dialysate flows into the patient's abdominal cavity by gravity (see Fig. 19-4B). After the dialysate is infused, the tubing is clamped, and the solution remains in the abdominal cavity for 30 to 45 minutes. A receptacle for the used dialysate is positioned below the level of the abdominal cavity, and the dialysate is then allowed to drain out of the peritoneal cavity by gravity in a steady, forceful stream. Drainage should take no more than 20 minutes. This cycle is repeated continuously for the prescribed time (12 to 36 hours, depending on the purpose of the treatment and the patient's condition).

Automated peritoneal dialysis systems ("cyclers") may be used in the critical care setting. These systems have built-in monitors and automatic timing devices that cycle the infusion and removal of peritoneal fluid. Most also have a log that retains cycle-by-cycle information on ultrafiltration. The cycler is programmed to deliver a set amount of dialysate per exchange for a certain length of time. When the time is up, the peritoneal cavity is automatically drained and then refilled.

 RED FLAG! *If cardiac arrest occurs in a patient receiving peritoneal dialysis, the patient's abdomen must be drained immediately to maximize the efficiency of chest compressions.*

Nursing Care of a Patient Receiving Peritoneal Dialysis

Nursing responsibilities during peritoneal dialysis include maintaining accurate records of intake and output and weights, preventing infection and maintaining the sterility of the system (Box 19-5), and detecting and correcting mechanical problems before they result in physiological problems. Common mechanical problems include:

- **Slow influx or drainage of dialysate.** If the dialysate enters the peritoneal cavity too slowly, the catheter may need to be repositioned. If it drains too slowly, the catheter tip may be buried in the omentum or clogged with fibrin. Turning the patient from side to side, elevating the head of

BOX 19-5 Preventing Infection During Peritoneal Dialysis

- Maintain aseptic technique throughout dialysis procedure.
- Use sealed plastic dialysate bags.
- Change dialysis tubing regularly per protocol.
- Swab or soak tubing connections and injection ports with bactericidal solution before adding medications or breaking closed system.
- Change exit site dressing daily using aseptic technique until healing occurs. Assess daily for increased inflammation or drainage.
- If infection is suspected, obtain appropriate culture, and begin antibiotic therapy according to protocol or physician's order.

the bed, and gently massaging the abdomen may facilitate drainage.

- **Incomplete recovery of dialysate.** The amount of dialysate removed should equal or exceed the amount of dialysate instilled (about 1000 to 2000 mL). If, after several exchanges, the volume drained is less (by 500 mL or more) than the amount instilled, the cause must be investigated. Incomplete removal of dialysate can lead to hypertension and fluid overload.

 RED FLAG! Signs of fluid retention include abdominal distention, complaints of fullness, and increased weight.

- **Leakage around the catheter.** A leaking catheter must be corrected because it acts as a pathway for bacteria to enter the peritoneum. Superficial leakage after surgery may be controlled with extra sutures and a decrease in the amount of dialysate instilled into the peritoneum. Increased intra-abdominal pressure (eg, from vomiting, coughing, or jarring movements) can also cause leaking.

 RED FLAG! Because dialysis effluent is considered a contaminated fluid, gloves must be worn while handling it.

 RED FLAG! Blood-tinged effluent is expected in the initial outflow but should clear after a few exchanges. Gross bleeding at any time is an indication of a more serious problem and must be investigated immediately.

Complications of Peritoneal Dialysis

Complications of peritoneal dialysis include hypotension (if excessive fluid is removed), hypertension and fluid overload (if not enough fluid is removed), hypokalemia, hyperglycemia, and mild abdominal discomfort (most likely caused by distention and chemical irritation of the peritoneum). More severe abdominal pain may be a sign of peritonitis, one of the more serious complications of peritoneal dialysis.

 RED FLAG! Signs and symptoms of peritonitis include low-grade fever, abdominal pain, and cloudy effluent.

If peritonitis is suspected, treatment with a broad-spectrum antibiotic (either added to the dialysate or administered IV) begins as soon as a sample of peritoneal fluid is obtained for culture and sensitivity. Marked improvement should be seen after 8 hours of antibiotic therapy.

CASE STUDY

Mr. D. is a 65-year-old man with a history of diabetes and hypertension. A year ago, he began experiencing some shortness of breath and was diagnosed with heart failure. He has been treated with the following medications: furosemide, 20 mg PO once daily; KCl, 20 mEq PO once daily; metformin, 500 mg PO twice daily; enalapril, 10 mg PO once daily; and metoprolol, 25 mg PO twice daily. His shortness of breath has worsened over the past 2 days. He was seen in the clinic and was admitted for evaluation. Admission data are as follows: temp, 97.3°F; HR, 120 beats/min; BP, 87/50 mm Hg; RR, 18 breaths/min; and oxygen saturation by pulse oximetry (SpO_2), 94% (on 50% FiO_2). Laboratory test results are Na^+, 130 mEq/L; K^+, 5.4 mEq/L; creatinine 4.5 mg/dL; blood urea nitrogen (BUN), 50 mg/dL; and glucose, 162 mg/dL. Urine sodium levels are high and urine osmolality and urine specific gravity are low. The nurse observes that Mr. D.'s urine output is decreased, and the urine is dark amber in color with sediment. Mr. D. is diagnosed with acute renal failure and based on the laboratory data, the physician decides to initiate continuous venovenous hemodialysis with dialysis (CVVHD).

1. Which type of dialysis access will most likely be used in Mr. D.?
2. Discuss the probable reasoning for treating Mr. D. with continuous venovenous hemofiltration with dialysis (CVVHD).
3. Describe nursing concerns when a patient is receiving CVVHD.

References

1. Nissenson AR, Fine RN: Clinical Dialysis, 4th ed. New York, NY: McGraw-Hill Medical, 2005
2. Filippo M, et al.: Citrate anticoagulation for continuous renal replacement therapy in critically ill patients: Success and limits. Int J Nephrol 2011
3. Oudemans-van Straaten, et al.: Citrate anticoagulation for continuous venovenous hemofiltration. Crit Care Med 37(2):545–552, 2009

Want to know more? A wide variety of resources to enhance your learning and understanding of this chapter are available on thePoint. Visit **http://thepoint.lww.com/MortonEss1e** to access chapter review questions and more!

CHAPTER 20

Common Renal Disorders

OBJECTIVES

Based on the content in this chapter, the reader should be able to:

1 Differentiate among the three types of acute kidney injury in terms of causes, pathophysiology, and assessment findings.
2 Discuss the nursing care of a patient with acute kidney injury or end-stage renal disease (ESRD).

Acute Kidney Injury

Acute kidney injury is a clinical syndrome in which a rapid loss of renal function (ie, over hours to a few days) results in derangements of fluid, electrolyte, and acid–base balance. The hallmark of acute kidney injury is a decreased glomerular filtration rate (GFR), resulting in azotemia (ie, the accumulation of urea, creatinine, and other nitrogenous end products in the blood). Acute kidney injury exists when one of the following criteria is met:

• An increase in serum creatinine of 26 μmol/L within 48 hours or a 1.5-fold increase from the reference creatinine level (ie, the lowest creatinine value recorded within the past 3 months)
• A urine output of less than 0.5 mL/kg/h for more than 6 consecutive hours[1]

The staging system for acute kidney injury (Table 20-1) was developed to reflect the clinical significance of relatively small increases in serum creatinine.

The Older Patient. *In an elderly patient, a minimal increase in serum creatinine that would be within normal limits for a young adult may actually signify major renal impairment. In elderly people, muscle mass is decreased, which can lower the baseline serum creatinine level.*

Acute kidney injury occurs in 15% to 18% of hospitalized patients, and in as many as 66% of those treated in critical care units.[1-3] In general, patients with acute kidney injury are older and have a great number of comorbid conditions.[1] Regardless of the underlying etiology, acute kidney injury is associated with increased in-hospital morbidity, mortality, and costs along with increased long-term mortality and morbidity.[1,2,4] Patients with acute kidney injury who are treated with renal replacement therapy have a mortality rate between 50% and 60%.[1,3,5] However, among patients who require renal replacement therapy but recover, 80% are independent of dialysis by the time of discharge.[1]

Etiology and Pathophysiology

Precipitating causes of acute kidney injury can be organized into three general categories—prerenal, intrinsic, and postrenal (Box 20-1).

Prerenal Acute Kidney Injury

Prerenal acute kidney injury can be precipitated by any physiological event that results in renal hypoperfusion (see Box 20-1). Decreased renal perfusion activates the renin–angiotensin–aldosterone system (Fig. 20-1), resulting in increased vascular volume and increased arterial blood pressure. These effects

TABLE 20-1 Acute Dialysis Quality Initiative (ADQI) and Acute Kidney Injury Network (AKIN) Staging System for Acute Kidney Injury

Stage	Serum Creatinine Level	Urine Output
1	Increase greater than or equal to 26 μmol/L within 48 h or increase greater than or equal to 1.5–1.9 times the reference serum creatinine level	Urine output less than 0.5 mL/kg/h for greater than 6 consecutive hours
2	Increase greater than 2–2.9 times the reference serum creatinine level	Urine output less than 0.5 mL/kg/h for greater than 12 h
3	Increase greater than or equal to 3 times the reference serum creatinine level or an increase greater than or equal to 354 μmol/L or the patient requires continuous renal replacement therapy (CRRT), irrespective of stage	Urine output less than 0.3 mL/kg/h for greater than 24 h or anuria for 12 h

help the body preserve circulatory volume and maintain adequate blood flow to essential organs such as the heart and the brain. In the kidneys, angiotensin II also helps maintain GFR, both by increasing efferent arteriolar resistance and by inducing intrarenal vasodilator prostaglandins that dilate the afferent arteriole, thus increasing hydrostatic pressure in the glomeruli.[6] In this way, the kidneys can preserve the GFR over a wide range of mean arterial pressures. However, when renal perfusion is severely compromised, this capacity for autoregulation is overwhelmed, and the GFR decreases.

BOX 20-1 Precipitating Causes of Acute Kidney Injury

Prerenal

Decreased Intravascular Volume
- Dehydration
- Hemorrhage
- Hypovolemia (gastrointestinal losses, diuretics, diabetes insipidus)
- Hypovolemic shock
- Third spacing (burns, peritonitis)

Decreased "Effective Renal Perfusion"
- Sepsis
- Cirrhosis
- Neurogenic shock

Heart Disease
- Heart failure
- Myocardial infarction
- Cardiogenic shock
- Valvular heart disease

Renal Artery Stenosis or Thromboembolism

Drugs
- Angiotensin-converting enzyme (ACE) inhibitors
- Nonsteroidal anti-inflammatory drugs (NSAIDs)
- Calcineurin inhibitors (tacrolimus, cyclosporine)

Intrinsic

Glomerular Disease (Acute Glomerulonephritis)

Vascular Disease
- Malignant hypertension
- Microangiopathic hemolytic–uremic syndrome (HUS)
- Thrombotic thrombocytopenic purpura (TTP)
- Scleroderma

- Eclampsia
- Atheroembolic disease
- Acute cortical necrosis

Interstitial Disease
- Allergic interstitial nephritis
- Acute pyelonephritis

Tubular Disease
- Obstruction (multiple myeloma, acute urate nephropathy, ethylene glycol or methanol toxicity)
- Acute tubular necrosis (ATN)
- Kidney transplant rejection

Postrenal

Ureteral Obstruction
- Intrinsic (stones, transitional cell carcinoma of the ureter, blood clots, stricture)
- Extrinsic (ovarian cancer; lymphoma; metastatic cancer of the prostate, cervix, or colon; retroperitoneal fibrosis)

Bladder Problems
- Tumors
- Blood clots
- Neurogenic bladder (spinal cord injury, diabetes mellitus, ischemia, drugs)
- Stones

Urethral Obstruction
- Prostate cancer or benign prostatic hypertrophy
- Stones
- Stricture
- Blood clots
- Obstructed indwelling catheter

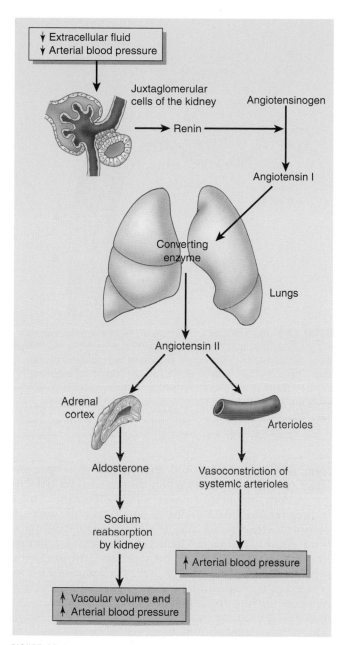

FIGURE 20-1 The renin–angiotensin–aldosterone system.

 RED FLAG! *In the presence of conditions such as hypovolemia, preexisting renal insufficiency, liver disease, heart failure, and renal artery disease, the use of nonsteroidal anti-inflammatory drugs (NSAIDs) and angiotensin-converting enzyme (ACE) inhibitors can induce prerenal acute kidney injury by disrupting the kidney's autoregulatory mechanisms. NSAIDs can inhibit prostaglandin-mediated afferent arteriolar vasodilation, and ACE inhibitors can prevent increased efferent arteriolar resistance.*

Characteristic changes in urine volume and composition occur in prerenal acute kidney injury: the volume is reduced to less than 400 mL/d (less than 17 mL/h), the sodium concentration is low (less than 20 mEq/L), and the specific gravity is increased (greater than 1.020). Improved renal perfusion leads to normalization of these laboratory values. This ability to reverse prerenal acute kidney injury confirms the diagnosis.

Intrinsic Acute Kidney Injury

Intrinsic acute kidney injury is characterized by damage to the renal parenchyma (see Box 20-1). Consistent with the diversity of causes, there are various pathophysiological pathways that can lead to intrinsic acute kidney injury (Fig. 20-2).

A common cause of hospital-acquired intrinsic acute kidney injury is acute tubular necrosis (ATN). The course of ATN can be divided into four clinical phases:

- **Onset phase.** The onset phase of ATN begins with a toxic or ischemic insult and lasts until cell injury occurs. This can take hours to days, depending on the cause, and is heralded by an increase in serum creatinine. The major goal during this phase is to determine the cause of the ATN and begin treatment to minimize irreversible tubular damage.
- **Oliguric/nonoliguric phase.** The second phase of ATN is characterized as either oliguric (less than 400 mL of urine/d) or nonoliguric (more than 400 mL of urine/d). This phase usually lasts for 7 to 14 days, although it may last longer depending on the extent of renal injury.[6] The main goal during this period is to support renal function until the injury heals. The nonoliguric presentation of ATN is most often associated with toxic injury and is characterized by a renal concentrating defect (inability to concentrate the urine). Nonoliguric ATN is typically of short duration, lasting an average of 5 to 8 days. The

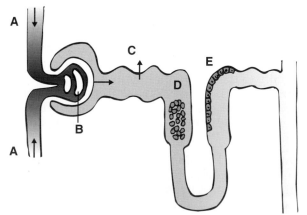

FIGURE 20-2 Potential mechanisms of intrinsic acute kidney injury include (**A**) decreased filtration pressure due to renal arteriolar constriction, (**B**) decreased glomerular capillary permeability, (**C**) increased proximal tubule permeability with back leak of filtrate, (**D**) obstruction of urine flow by necrotic tubular cells, and (**E**) increased sodium delivery to the macula densa, which causes an increase in renin–angiotensin production and vasoconstriction at the glomerular level.

BOX 20-2 Clinical Manifestations of Oliguric Acute Tubular Necrosis (ATN)

Fluid overload
Azotemia
Electrolyte abnormalities
　Hyperkalemia
　Hyperphosphatemia
　Hypocalcemia
Metabolic acidosis
Uremic signs and symptoms
　Gastrointestinal (anorexia, nausea, vomiting, metallic taste in mouth)
　Neuromuscular (mental status changes, muscle cramps)
　Integumentary (pruritus, uremic frost)
　Uremic fetor (the smell of urine or ammonia on the breath)

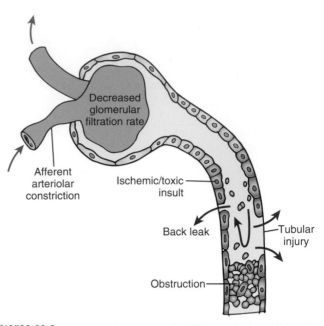

FIGURE 20-3 In acute tubular necrosis (ATN), necrosis and sloughing of tubular epithelial cells as a result of an ischemic or toxic insult leads to obstruction of the lumen and increased intraluminal pressure. These changes, combined with afferent arteriolar vasoconstriction, result in decreased glomerular filtration. In addition, tubular injury and increased intraluminal pressure cause fluid to "back-leak" from the tubular lumen into the interstitium.

oliguric presentation of ATN (Box 20-2) is most often caused by ischemia. Patients with oliguric ATN are less likely to recover renal function than those with nonoliguric ATN, and have a higher associated mortality rate.

- **Diuretic phase.** The diuretic phase of ATN lasts 1 to 2 weeks and is characterized by a gradual increase in urine output as renal function starts to return. The degree of diuresis, which can exceed 10 L/d, is primarily determined by the state of hydration at the time the patient enters this stage. Although the urine output may be normal or elevated, renal concentrating ability is still impaired, putting the patient at risk for fluid volume deficits and electrolyte abnormalities (eg, hyponatremia, hypokalemia). Primary goals during this stage are maintenance of hydration, prevention of electrolyte depletion, and continued support of renal function.
- **Recovery phase.** The recovery phase of ATN lasts from several months to a year, the time it takes for renal function to return to normal or near-normal levels. If significant tubular damage has occurred, especially to the basement membrane (which cannot regenerate), residual renal impairment may persist. A major goal during this phase is preventing recurrence through follow-up care and patient education.

Ischemic Acute Tubular Necrosis

Ischemic ATN results from a prolonged prerenal condition that causes hypoperfusion. Thus, prerenal acute kidney injury and ischemic ATN are a continuum, underscoring the importance of prompt recognition and treatment of the prerenal state. When renal hypoperfusion is severe enough to overwhelm autoregulation and persists for a sufficient time (the exact duration of which is unpredictable and varies with clinical circumstances), the hypoxic renal tubular epithelial cells sustain irreversible damage, so that tubular function does not improve even when

renal perfusion is restored. Profound renal vasoconstriction, which results when damaged renal vascular endothelial cells release vasoconstrictors, may reduce renal blood flow by as much as 50%, further compromising renal oxygen delivery and adding to the ischemic damage.[6] Ischemia decreases adenosine triphosphate (ATP) production, robbing the cells of their major energy supply. Because energy is needed to maintain proper intracellular electrolyte concentrations, this results in electrolyte disturbances—including increased intracellular calcium, which has been shown to predispose the cells to injury and dysfunction.[6,7] Further cellular damage occurs during reperfusion, due to release of oxygen free radicals. Eventually, these cellular insults cause the tubular cells to swell and become necrotic. The necrotic cells then slough off and may obstruct the tubular lumen (Fig. 20-3).

Toxic Acute Tubular Necrosis

Toxic ATN results from concentration of a nephrotoxin in the renal tubular cells, leading to necrosis. The necrotic cells then slough off into the tubular lumen, where they may cause obstruction and impair glomerular filtration. In toxic ATN, unlike in ischemic ATN, the basement membrane of the tubular cells usually remains intact, and the necrotic areas are more localized. This may partially explain why nonoliguria occurs more often with toxic ATN, and why the healing process is often more rapid. Although there are many potential nephrotoxins (Box 20-3), aminoglycoside antibiotics

BOX 20-3 Common Nephrotoxins

- Drugs, including antimicrobials (aminoglycosides, amphotericin), cyclosporine, anesthetics, chemotherapeutic agents
- Heavy metals (mercury, lead, cisplatinum (cisplatin), uranium, cadmium, bismuth, arsenic)
- Radiopaque contrast material
- Heme pigments (myoglobin, hemoglobin)
- Organic solvents (carbon tetrachloride)
- Fungicides and pesticides
- Plant and animal substances (mushrooms, snake venom)

and radiopaque contrast material are among the most common causes of toxic ATN in hospitalized patients.

- **Aminoglycosides.** The onset of aminoglycoside-induced acute kidney injury is usually delayed, often beginning 7 to 10 days after drug therapy is initiated. Aminoglycoside toxicity is dose dependent. Several studies have suggested that a single daily dose may result in less nephrotoxicity than the same total amount of aminoglycoside in three divided doses.[8,9]

 RED FLAG! *Risk factors for aminoglycoside toxicity include renal impairment, volume depletion, advanced age, concurrent use of other nephrotoxic agents, and liver dysfunction.[8,10]*

- **Contrast material.** Contrast-induced acute kidney injury is a sudden decline of renal function following intravascular injection of contrast material. Contrast-induced acute kidney injury usually begins within 48 hours of IV contrast administration, peaks in 3 to 5 days, and returns to baseline in another 3 to 5 days. The risk for contrast-induced acute kidney injury can be reduced by ensuring aggressive hydration with IV saline or sodium bicarbonate before and after contrast administration, administering *N*-acetylcysteine (NAC) preprocedure, stopping any nephrotoxic drugs 24 hours before contrast injection, using the lowest effective contrast dose, using hypo or iso-osmolar nonionic contrast material instead of ionic hyperosmolar agents, and avoiding short intervals between contrast procedures.[11,12] Although contrast-induced acute kidney injury typically is nonoliguric, transient, and reversible, in high-risk patients it may cause severe kidney injury requiring permanent dialysis or kidney transplantation.

 RED FLAG! *Patients at greatest risk for contrast-induced acute kidney injury are those with diabetes mellitus, intravascular volume depletion, heart failure, or multiple myeloma; elderly patients; and those who receive a large contrast load.[11]*

Postrenal Acute Kidney Injury

Postrenal acute kidney injury results from obstruction of urine flow (see Box 20-1). Obstruction can occur anywhere in the urinary tract, from the renal collecting ducts to the external urethral orifice. Because a single well-functioning kidney is adequate to maintain homeostasis, the development of postrenal acute kidney injury requires blockage of both kidneys (ie, urethral or bladder neck obstruction or bilateral ureteral obstruction), or unilateral ureteral obstruction in patients with a single kidney. Urinary tract obstruction causes congestion and retrograde pressure through the renal collecting system, slowing the tubular fluid flow rate and decreasing the GFR. As a result, reabsorption of sodium, water, and urea is reduced, leading to a lower urine sodium concentration, higher urine osmolality, and elevated serum creatinine and blood urea nitrogen (BUN) levels. With prolonged pressure from urinary obstruction, the entire collecting system dilates, compressing and damaging nephrons. These changes can be avoided by prompt removal of the obstruction. After obstruction is relieved, there is often a profound diuresis that may be as great as 5 to 8 L/d.[7] If electrolytes and water are not replenished as needed, this diuresis can lead to hemodynamic compromise, renal ischemia, and ATN.

 The Older Patient. *In elderly men, the high prevalence of prostatic enlargement (benign or malignant) increases susceptibility to postrenal acute kidney injury.*

Assessment

Clues to the type and exact cause of the acute kidney injury are obtained by correlating history and physical examination findings (Box 20-4) with the results of laboratory and diagnostic studies.

Laboratory assessment of acute kidney injury includes both blood and urine tests. A comparison of laboratory values in prerenal acute kidney injury, postrenal acute kidney injury, and ATN is given in Table 20-2.

- **Urinalysis.** Urine sodium concentration, osmolality, and specific gravity reflect the concentrating ability of the kidney, and are especially helpful in distinguishing between prerenal acute renal failure and ATN. In prerenal failure, the hypoperfused kidney actively reabsorbs sodium and water in an attempt to increase circulatory volume. Consequently, the urine sodium level and fractional sodium excretion (FE_{Na}) are low, while the urine osmolality and specific gravity are high. In contrast, in ATN, where there is parenchymal damage to the kidney, the tubular cells can no longer effectively reabsorb sodium or concentrate the urine. As a result, the urine sodium concentration and FE_{Na} are high, and the urine specific gravity is low (approximately 1.010).

Prerenal

History	Physical Examination
Any event or condition that could contribute to decreased renal perfusion (see Box 20-1, p. 274)	Poor skin turgor, dry mucous membranes, weight loss, reduced jugular venous distention (suggestive of decreased renal perfusion related to dehydration or hypovolemia)
A history of atherosclerotic disease	Edema, ascites, weight gain (suggestive of decreased renal perfusion related to vasodilation, third spacing, cardiovascular disease, or liver disease)

Intrinsic

History	Physical Examination
Any prolonged prerenal event or condition	Signs of streptococcal throat infection
Exposure to nephrotoxins	Signs of lupus (eg, butterfly rash)
Systemic diseases (eg, lupus, vasculitis, recent streptococcal infections)	Signs of embolism (eg, discolored toes, bluish mottling of the skin of the extremities)
History of trauma or prolonged loss of consciousness History of extremity trauma (could suggest a cause of heme pigment toxicity, such as rhabdomyolysis) History of cardiac catheterization, anticoagulation, or thrombolytic therapy	

Postrenal

History	Physical Examination
History of abdominal tumors or calculi	Bladder distention
History of benign or malignant prostatic enlargement	Abdominal mass Enlarged or nodular prostate gland Kinked or obstructed indwelling urinary catheter

RED FLAG! Diuretics may alter the urine's chemical composition; therefore, it is best to obtain the urine sample before diuretics are administered. In patients who have already received diuretics, the fractional excretion of urea nitrogen (FE_{UN}) may be helpful in distinguishing prerenal acute kidney injury from ATN. Urea, like sodium, is reabsorbed in a prerenal hypoperfused kidney; but unlike sodium, its reabsorption is primarily passive and is not inhibited by loop or thiazide diuretic administration.[13] In prerenal acute kidney injury, the FE_{UN} is less than 35%, whereas normally and in ATN, it is greater than 50%.

• **BUN and creatinine levels.** In prerenal acute kidney injury, the BUN:creatinine ratio increases from the normal ratio of 10:1 to more than 20:1, and may be as high as 40:1. This is caused by dehydration (which increases primarily the BUN) and by passive reabsorption of urea as the tubules become more permeable to sodium and water. In contrast, in ATN and in postrenal acute kidney injury, the BUN and creatinine tend to increase proportionally, maintaining a more normal ratio.

TABLE 20-2 Comparison of Laboratory Findings in Acute Prerenal Failure, Acute Postrenal Failure, and Acute Tubular Necrosis (ATN)

Value	Prerenal	Postrenal	ATN
Urine volume	Oliguria	May alternate between anuria and polyuria	Anuria, oliguria, or nonoliguria
Urine osmolality	Increased (greater than 500 mOsm/kg H_2O)	Varies; increased or equal to serum osmolality	Decreased (250–300 mOsm/kg H_2O)
Urine specific gravity	Increased (greater than 1.020)	Varies	Approximately 1.010
Urine sodium	Less than 20 mEq/L	Varies	Greater than 40 mEq/L
Urine sediment	Normal, few hyaline casts	Normal, may contain crystals	Granular casts, tubular epithelial cells
Fractional excretion of sodium (FE_{Na})	Less than 1%	Greater than 1%	Greater than 1% (often greater than 3%)
BUN:creatinine ratio	Greater than 20:1	10:1 to 15:1	10:1 to 15:1

BOX 20·5 Causes of Chronic Kidney Disease

- Diabetes mellitus
- Hypertension
- Glomerulonephritis
  - Primary (immunoglobulin A nephropathy, postinfectious glomerulonephritis)
  - Secondary (HIV nephropathy, lupus, cryoglobulinemia, Wegener's granulomatosis, Goodpasture's syndrome, polyarteritis nodosa, amyloidosis)
- Interstitial nephritis (allergic interstitial nephritis, pyelonephritis)
- Microangiopathic vascular disease (atheroembolic disease, scleroderma)
- Congenital disease
- Genetic disease (polycystic kidney disease, medullary cystic kidney disease)
- Obstructive uropathy
- Neoplasms
- Transplant rejection
- Hepatorenal syndrome

Diagnostic studies used in the evaluation of acute kidney injury include renal ultrasonography (to identify or rule out obstruction), computed tomography (CT) and magnetic resonance imaging (MRI) (to evaluate for masses, vascular disorders, and filling defects in the collecting system), renal angiography (to evaluate for renal artery stenosis or thromboembolism), and renal biopsy (to evaluate for non-ATN intrinsic acute kidney injury, especially if urinalysis reveals significant proteinuria or unexplained hematuria).

Chronic Kidney Disease

Chronic kidney disease is a slowly progressive, irreversible deterioration in renal function that results in the kidney's inability to eliminate waste products and maintain fluid and electrolyte balance. Ultimately, it leads to end-stage renal disease (ESRD) and the need for renal replacement therapy, renal transplantation, or both to sustain life. There is an association between renal and cardiovascular disease, and in patients with ESRD, cardiovascular disease is the leading cause of morbidity and mortality.[7]

Although chronic kidney disease has many causes (Box 20-5), diabetes and hypertension are the two most common (accounting for more than 36% and 24% of ESRD cases, respectively).[14] Because predictable complications and management strategies are correlated with the level of kidney dysfunction, regardless of underlying etiology, staging of chronic kidney disease is based on the GFR (Table 20-3).

Regardless of the underlying cause, common morphologic features seen in chronic kidney disease include fibrosis, loss of native renal cells, and infiltration by monocytes and macrophages.[15,16] Abnormal glomerular hemodynamics, hypoxia, and proteinuria contribute to these pathologic changes.

- **Abnormal glomerular hemodynamics.** Because each of the more than one million nephrons in each kidney is an independent functioning unit, as renal disease progresses, nephrons can lose function at different times. When an individual nephron becomes dysfunctional, nephrons in close proximity compensate, increasing their individual filtration rates by increasing blood flow and hydrostatic pressure in their glomerular capillaries. This hyperfiltration response in the nondiseased nephrons enables the kidneys to maintain excretory and homeostatic functions, even when up to 70% of the nephrons are damaged. However, eventually, the intact nephrons reach a point of maximal filtration, so that any additional loss of glomerular mass is accompanied by an incremental reduction of GFR and subsequent accumulation of filterable toxins. Although hyperfiltration is an adaptive response to nephron loss, over time it can actually accelerate nephron loss because the hyperfiltration causes endothelial injury, stimulates profibrotic cytokines, leads to infiltration by monocytes and macrophages, and causes detachment of glomerular epithelial cells. In addition, hyperfiltration promotes hypertrophy of the nondiseased nephrons, increasing wall stress and causing injury.[7]
- **Hypoxia.** In chronic kidney disease, loss of peritubular capillaries results in reduced capillary

TABLE 20·3 Stages of Chronic Kidney Disease

Stage	Description	GFR (mL/min/1.73 m²)
1	Kidney damage[a] with normal or increased GFR	Greater than or equal to 90
2	Kidney damage with mildly decreased GFR	60–89
3	Moderately decreased GFR	30–59
4	Severely decreased GFR	15–29
5	Kidney failure	Less than 15 or dialysis

GFR, glomerular filtration rate.

[a]Kidney damage is defined as pathologic abnormalities or markers of damage, including abnormal blood or urine tests or imaging studies.

Adapted from Jacobs C, Opolinsky D. The Little Handbook of Dialysis. Boston, MA: Jones and Bartlett Publishers, 2010.

perfusion of the tubules. The resultant hypoxia favors the release of proinflammatory and profibrotic cytokines, leading to fibrosis and cell injury.

- **Proteinuria.** This is the result of glomerular hypertension and abnormal glomerular permeability. The filtered protein is partially reabsorbed and accumulates in the proximal tubule cells, leading to inflammation and fibrosis.[14]

Increasing evidence shows that early detection and treatment of chronic kidney disease may delay or prevent progression to ESRD. Measures to slow the progression of chronic kidney disease include managing the underlying cause (eg, strict control of blood glucose levels in patients with diabetes, strict control of blood pressure in patients with hypertension) and avoiding secondary insults to the kidney that can rapidly accelerate nephron loss (Box 20-6).

Complications of Impaired Renal Function

Impaired renal function has wide-reaching effects on the body. Acute kidney injury and chronic kidney disease share many of the same clinical manifestations and complications.

Cardiovascular Complications

Common cardiovascular complications seen in patients with impaired renal function include hypertension, hyperkalemia-induced heart dysrhythmias, and pericarditis.

Hypertension

Hypertension, a complication of both acute kidney injury and chronic kidney disease, results from excess water and sodium retention, overactivation of the sympathetic nervous system, and stimulation of the renin–angiotensin–aldosterone system. Blood pressure control is essential to prevent end-organ damage and reduce the risk for life-threatening cardiovascular events. Management strategies may include fluid and sodium restriction, administration of diuretics and antihypertensive agents, and dialysis to remove excess fluid.

BOX 20·6   Secondary Insults That Can Accelerate Chronic Kidney Disease Progression

- Altered renal perfusion
- Hypovolemia
- Nonsteroidal anti-inflammatory drugs (NSAIDs)
- Nephrotoxic agents
- Urinary obstruction
- Urinary infection
- Hypercalcemia
- Hyperlipidemia

Cardiac Dysrhythmias

In both acute kidney injury and chronic kidney disease, hyperkalemia occurs when the decreased GFR impairs the kidneys' ability to excrete excess potassium. Hyperkalemia causes characteristic electrocardiographic (ECG) abnormalities (Fig. 20-4) and, if not recognized and treated, can lead to life-threatening cardiac dysrhythmias.

Mild hyperkalemia (less than 6 mEq/L without ECG changes) can be treated with dietary potassium restriction, diuretics, and oral or rectal potassium-binding resins (eg, sodium polystyrene sulfate). For patients with substantial ECG changes, IV calcium gluconate or chloride is administered to antagonize the effects of potassium on the heart. IV insulin and dextrose administration and IV bicarbonate administration promote movement of potassium into cells. Finally, potassium-binding resins and diuretics are used to facilitate the removal of potassium from the body. If these measures do not control hyperkalemia, dialysis must be initiated.

Pericarditis

Uremic pericarditis (inflammation of the pericardial membrane that occurs primarily in ESRD) is usually (but not always) aseptic. Although its exact etiology is unknown, it is associated with the accumulation of uremic toxins, treatment with the antihypertensive agent minoxidil, heparin administration, and bacterial or viral infection. Treatment entails aggressive dialysis therapy, usually daily, until symptoms resolve. Because anticoagulation during dialysis may precipitate or enhance bleeding into the pericardial space, either low-dose, regional, or no heparin may be prescribed. Systemic steroids and NSAIDs may be used to reduce inflammation, but have variable results.

 RED FLAG! *Pericardial effusion associated with pericarditis can lead to tamponade if fluid accumulates in the pericardial sac. Tamponade, a life-threatening complication, requires urgent pericardiocentesis to relieve the pressure on the heart.*

Pulmonary Complications

Pulmonary edema secondary to fluid overload, heart failure, or both is a frequent complication in patients with oliguric acute kidney injury or ESRD. Other pulmonary complications in patients with impaired renal function include pleural effusions, pulmonary infections, pleuritic inflammation and pain, and uremic pneumonitis. Pleuritic inflammation and uremic pneumonitis are seen most frequently in ESRD and are due to the effect of uremic toxins on the lungs and inadequate dialysis.

Hematological Complications

Hematological complications in acute kidney injury and chronic kidney disease include an increased bleeding tendency and anemia. The increased

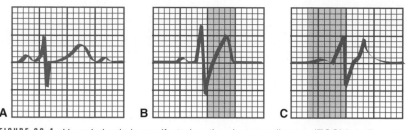

FIGURE 20-4 Hyperkalemia is manifested on the electrocardiogram (ECG) by tall, narrow, peaked T waves; flat, wide P waves; and widening of the QRS complex. **A:** Waveform produced when potassium levels fall within the normal range (3.5 to 5 mEq/L). **B:** When the serum potassium level rises above 5.5 mEq/L, the T wave begins to peak (*highlighted area*). The P wave and QRS complex are normal. **C:** When the potassium level exceeds 6.5 mEq/L, the P wave grows wider and flatter, and the QRS complex widens (*highlighted area*).

bleeding tendency in patients with impaired renal function is attributable to impaired platelet aggregation and adhesion and an altered platelet response to clotting factor VII. These alterations are thought to be due to uremia, but their exact pathophysiological mechanisms are unknown.

Anemia in patients with renal injury is attributable to three main mechanisms: erythropoietin deficiency, decreased red blood cell (RBC) survival time, and blood loss due to increased bleeding tendency. Erythropoietin, a glycoprotein that stimulates RBC production in response to hypoxia, is produced in the kidney; as nephrons are damaged, synthesis of erythropoietin is impaired. Decreased RBC survival time in renal injury is the result of a mild hemolysis, possibly related to dialysis therapy or the effect of uremia on erythrocytes. To counteract anemia, recombinant human erythropoietin (rHuEPO), darbepoetin (an analogue of rHuEPO), or blood products may be administered. The full effect of rHuEPO or darbepoetin takes weeks to achieve; hence, in patients with profound anemia, RBC transfusion is indicated. In addition, rHuEPO or darbepoetin administration may result in blood pressure elevation, in some cases requiring modification of antihypertensive therapy.

Gastrointestinal Complications

In both acute kidney injury and chronic kidney disease, gastrointestinal bleeding is a potentially life-threatening complication. In patients with acute kidney injury, gastrointestinal bleeding may have many causes, including platelet and blood-clotting abnormalities, the use of anticoagulation during dialysis, physiological stress, and increased ammonia production in the gastrointestinal tract from urea breakdown. Other gastrointestinal complications associated primarily with chronic kidney disease include anorexia, nausea, vomiting, diarrhea, constipation, gastroesophageal reflux disease (GERD), stomatitis, a metallic taste in the mouth, and uremic fetor (the smell of urine or ammonia on the breath).

Neuromuscular Complications

Neuromuscular complications, seen primarily in advanced chronic kidney disease, include sleep disturbances, cognitive disturbances, lethargy, muscle irritability, restless legs syndrome, and peripheral neuropathies, including burning feet syndrome (ie, paresthesias and numbness in the soles of the feet and lower parts of the legs).

Infection

Infection is a major cause of mortality in patients with acute kidney injury and chronic kidney disease, because patients with impaired renal function are immunocompromised. The immune impairment is thought to be due to malnutrition and the effects of uremia on leukocytes (ie, depressed T-cell and antibody–mediated immunity, impaired phagocytosis, and decreased leukocyte chemotaxis and adherence).[7] Preventive measures include frequent handwashing and removing invasive catheters as soon as possible (or avoiding their use altogether). In addition, the nurse closely monitors for signs and symptoms of infection.

 RED FLAG! Baseline body temperature is decreased in uremic patients, and any increase above baseline is significant.

Musculoskeletal Complications

In patients with impaired renal function, disturbances in calcium and phosphate balance set the stage for bone disease (Fig. 20-5). As the GFR declines, serum phosphate levels begin to rise. The excess phosphate binds calcium, lowering serum levels of ionized calcium. In response to decreased ionized calcium levels, the parathyroid glands secrete parathyroid hormone (PTH). PTH causes reabsorption of calcium and phosphate salts from the bones, thus increasing the serum calcium level at the expense of bone mineral density and mass and resulting in the condition known as high-turnover renal osteodystrophy. Eventually, as calcium and phosphate continue to be reabsorbed from bones, their serum levels rise concomitantly. Calcium phosphate crystals can form and precipitate in various parts of the body (eg, the brain, eyes, gums, heart valves, myocardium, lungs, joints, blood vessels, and skin), leading to metastatic calcifications. Other musculoskeletal complications include bone pain, fractures, pseudogout (from deposits of calcium in synovial fluid), periarthritis (from calcifications in the soft tissues around the joints), proximal muscle weakness, and spontaneous tendon ruptures.

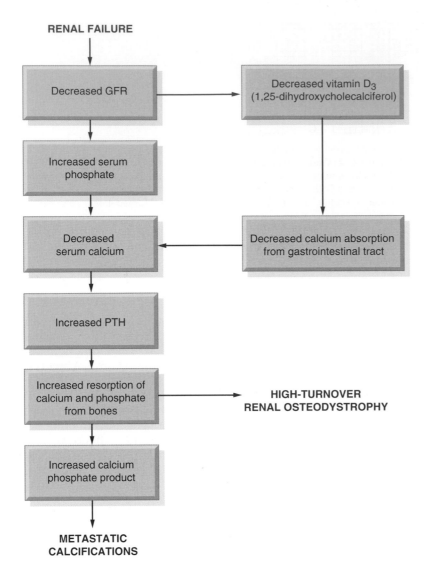

RENAL FAILURE

Decreased GFR

Decreased vitamin D₃
(1,25-dihydroxycholecalciferol)

Increased serum
phosphate

Decreased calcium absorption
from gastrointestinal tract

Decreased
serum calcium

Increased PTH

Increased resorption of
calcium and phosphate
from bones

**HIGH-TURNOVER
RENAL OSTEODYSTROPHY**

Increased calcium
phosphate product

**METASTATIC
CALCIFICATIONS**

FIGURE 20-5 Effects of renal injury on the skeletal system. GFR, glomerular filtration rate; PTH, parathyroid hormone.

Integumentary Complications

Xerosis (dryness), pruritus, and lesions (eg, pale bronze skin discolorations, ecchymosis, purpura, bullous dermatosis) may be seen in patients with impaired renal function. Uremic frost (a white, powdery substance on the skin that is caused by crystallization of urea) is usually only seen in severely uremic patients. In patients with an arteriovenous fistula or graft, a benign proliferation of blood vessels called pseudo-Kaposi's sarcoma may develop in the area of the fistula, graft, or hands as a reaction to increased venous pressure.

 RED FLAG! *Because many medications and their metabolites are excreted by the kidneys, extreme caution must be used when administering medication to patients with impaired renal function. Depending on the patient's GFR, adjustments may need to be made in the drug dosage, the interval between drug dosages, or both. In addition, due to instability of the GFR, frequent monitoring of the GFR is necessary to determine accurate dosages.*

Management of Impaired Renal Function

In both acute kidney injury and chronic kidney disease, management includes treating the primary insult as well as the complications that result from loss of kidney function. In addition, many patients with acute or chronic kidney injury require renal replacement therapy (see Chapter 19). A collaborative care guide for the patient with renal injury is presented in Box 20-7.

Managing Fluid Balance

Management of fluid balance is of primary importance in patients with impaired renal function.

• **Acute kidney injury.** In prerenal acute kidney injury and the onset phase of ischemic ATN, if the cause of the inadequate renal perfusion is an intravascular volume deficit, prompt administration of replacement fluids is indicated. Fluid

BOX 20-7 COLLABORATIVE CARE GUIDE for the Patient With Impaired Renal Function

OUTCOMES	INTERVENTIONS
Oxygenation/Ventilation The patient has adequate gas exchange as evidenced by: • ABGs within normal limits • SpO2 >92% • Clear breath sounds • Normal respiratory rate and depth • Normal chest x-ray	• Monitor ABGs and continuous pulse oximetry. • Monitor acid–base status. • Monitor for signs and symptoms of pulmonary distress from fluid overload. • Provide routine bronchial hygiene therapy (BHT), including suctioning, chest percussion, incentive spirometry, and turning. • Mobilize out of bed to chair. • Support the patient with oxygen therapy, mechanical ventilation, or both as indicated. Involve respiratory therapist.
Circulation/Perfusion The patient's BP, HR, and hemodynamic parameters are within normal limits. The patient has adequate tissue perfusion as evidenced by: • Adequate hemoglobin levels • Euvolemic status • Optimal urine output depending on phase of acute renal failure • Appropriate level of consciousness	• Monitor vital signs q1–2h. • Monitor PAOP and CVP qh and cardiac output, systemic vascular resistance, and peripheral vascular resistance per protocol and acuity level, if pulmonary artery catheter is in place. • Assess vital signs continuously or every 15 min during dialysis. • Monitor hemoglobin and hematocrit levels daily. • Assess for evidence of tissue perfusion (pain, pulses, color, temperature) and for signs of decreased organ perfusion (eg, altered level of consciousness, ileus, decreasing urine output). • Administer intravascular crystalloids or blood products as indicated.
Fluids/Electrolytes The patient is euvolemic. The patient achieves normal electrolyte balance. The patient achieves optimal renal function.	• Monitor fluid status, including I&O (fluid restriction), daily weights, urine output trends, vital signs, CVP, and PAOP. • Monitor for signs and symptoms of hypervolemia (hypertension, pulmonary edema, peripheral edema, jugular venous distention, and increased CVP). • Monitor serum electrolytes daily. • Monitor renal parameters, including urine output, BUN, serum creatinine, acid–base status, urine electrolytes, urine osmolality, and urine specific gravity. • Administer fluids and diuretics to maintain intravascular volume and renal function per order. • Replace electrolytes as ordered, if low. • Treat the elevated electrolytes as ordered. • Treat the patient with, and monitor response to, dialysis therapies if indicated. • Monitor and maintain dialysis access for chosen intermittent or continuous dialysis method. *Continuous Veno–Veno Dialysis* • Monitor and regulate ultrafiltration rate hourly based on the patient's response and fluid status. • Provide fluid replacements as ordered. • Assess and troubleshoot hemofilter and blood tubing hourly • Protect vascular access from dislodgment. • Change filter and tubing per protocol. • Monitor vascular access for infection. *Peritoneal Dialysis* • Slowly infuse warmed dialysate. • Drain after appropriate dwell time. • Assess drainage for volume and appearance. • Send cultures daily. • Assess access site for infection. *Intermittent Hemodialysis* • Assess shunt for thrill and bruit q12h. • Avoid constrictions (ie, blood pressures), phlebotomy, and IV fluid administration in arm with shunt. • Assess for infection. • Monitor perfusion of related extremity.

(continued on page 284)

BOX 20-7   COLLABORATIVE CARE GUIDE for the Patient With Impaired Renal Function
(continued)

OUTCOMES	INTERVENTIONS
Mobility The patient remains free of complications related to bedrest and immobility.	• Initiate DVT prophylaxis. • Reposition frequently. • Mobilize to chair when possible. • Consult physical therapist. • Conduct range-of-motion and strengthening exercises.
Protection/Safety The patient is protected from possible harm.	• Assess need for wrist restraints if the patient is intubated, has a decreased level of consciousness, is unable to follow commands, or is acutely agitated, or for affected extremity during hemodialysis. Explain need for restraints to the patient and family members. If restrained, assess response to restraints and check skin integrity and perfusion q1–2h. Follow facility protocol for use of restraints. • Use siderails on bed and safety belts on chairs as appropriate. • Follow seizure precautions.
Skin Integrity The patient is without evidence of skin breakdown.	• Assess skin integrity and all bony prominences q4h. • Turn q2h. • Consider a pressure relief/reduction mattress. Use Braden scale to assess risk for skin breakdown. • Use superfatted or lanolin-based soap for bathing and apply emollients for pruritus. • Treat pressure ulcers according to facility protocol. Involve enterostomal nurse in care.
Nutrition The patient is adequately nourished as evidenced by • Stable weight not <10% below or >20% above ideal body weight • An albumin level of 3.5–4.0 g/dL • A total protein level of 6–8 g/dL • A total lymphocyte count of 1000–3000×10^6/L	• Consult dietitian to direct and coordinate nutritional support. • Observe sodium, potassium, protein, and fluid restriction as indicated. • Provide small, frequent feedings. • Provide parenteral or enteral feeding as ordered. • Monitor albumin, prealbumin, total protein, hematocrit, hemoglobin, and WBC counts, and monitor daily weights to assess effectiveness of nutritional therapy.
Comfort/Pain Control The patient is as comfortable as possible (as evidenced by stable vital signs or cooperation with treatments or procedures).	• Monitor for signs and symptoms of respiratory distress related to fluid overload and support oxygenation as needed. Keep head of bed elevated and teach breathing techniques to minimize respiratory distress, such as pursed-lip breathing. • Plan fluid restrictions over 24 h allowing for periodic sips of water and ice chips to minimize thirst. • Provide frequent mouth and skin care. • Document pain assessment, using numerical pain rating or similar scale when possible. • Provide a quiet environment and frequent reassurance. • Observe for complications that may cause discomfort, such as infection of vascular access device, peritonitis or inadequate draining during peritoneal dialysis, and gastrointestinal disturbances (nausea, vomiting, diarrhea, constipation). • Administer analgesics, antiemetics, antidiarrheals, laxatives (nonmagnesium and nonphosphate containing), stool softeners, antihistamines, sedatives, or anxiolytics as needed and monitor response.

BOX 20-7 COLLABORATIVE CARE GUIDE for the Patient With Impaired Renal Function
(continued)

OUTCOMES	INTERVENTIONS
Psychosocial	
The patient demonstrates a decrease in anxiety, as evidenced by patient self-report and objective observations (eg, vital signs within normal limits)	• Assess vital signs. • Explore patient and family concerns. • If the patient is intubated, develop interventions for effective communication. • Arrange for flexible visitation to meet needs of the patient and family. • Provide for adequate rest and sleep. • Provide frequent information and updates on condition and treatment, and explain equipment. Answer all questions. • Consult social services and clergy as appropriate. • Administer sedatives and antidepressants as appropriate and monitor response.
Teaching/Discharge Planning	
The patient and family members understand procedures and tests needed for treatment during acute renal failure and maintenance of a patient with chronic disease. The patient and family members understand the severity of the illness, ask appropriate questions, and anticipate potential complications. In preparation for discharge to home, the patient and family members demonstrate an understanding of renal replacement therapy, fluid and dietary restrictions, and the medication regimen	• Prepare the patient and family members for procedures, such as insertion of dialysis access, dialysis therapy, or laboratory studies. • Explain the causes and effects of renal failure and the potential for complications, such as hypertension and fluid overload. • Encourage family members to ask questions related to the pathophysiology of renal failure, dialysis, and dietary or fluid restrictions. • Make appropriate referrals and consults early during hospitalization. • Initiate family education regarding home care of the patient on dialysis, what to expect, maintenance of renal function, and when to seek medical attention.

ABGs, arterial blood gases; BHT, bronchial hygiene therapy; BP, blood pressure; HR, heart rate; RAP, right atrial pressure; PAOP, pulmonary artery occlusion pressure; CVP, central venous pressure; DVT, deep venous thrombosis; WBC, white blood cell; BUN, blood urea nitrogen.

administration is also indicated to replace fluid losses in the diuretic phase of ATN and after relief of obstruction in postrenal acute kidney injury, due to the profound diuresis that occurs. Diuretics are also used to increase urinary flow and help alleviate fluid overload or prevent tubular obstruction.

> **RED FLAG!** In any oliguric state, caution must be taken to prevent fluid overload. In a sustained oliguric state (eg, the oliguric phase of ATN), fluid administration is restricted to the previous day's urine output volume plus 500 to 800 mL to account for insensible losses.

• **Chronic kidney disease.** In chronic kidney disease, fluid and salt restriction is a mainstay of therapy to prevent fluid overload. Sodium is restricted to less than 2400 mg/d, and fluid intake is limited to 500 mL plus the previous day's 24-hour urine output. Diuretics may also be used to manage volume overload in the early stages of chronic kidney disease; however, by the time the patient develops ESRD, extensive renal damage prevents an adequate response. Patients with ESRD require dialysis to manage fluid overload and ongoing assessment of fluid status is imperative.

Managing Acid–Base Alterations

Acute kidney injury and chronic kidney disease typically result in metabolic acidosis because of the nephrons' progressive inability to secrete and excrete hydrogen ions and reabsorb bicarbonate ions. In chronic kidney disease, metabolic acidosis begins to manifest in stage 3. Although the metabolic acidosis seen in chronic kidney disease is usually mild, it is associated with many adverse consequences, including fatigue, protein catabolism, and bone demineralization (which occurs as bone phosphate and carbonate are pulled into the blood for use as buffers against excess hydrogen ion). In critically ill patients with acute kidney injury, metabolic acidosis may be intensified by concurrent conditions such as lactic acidosis or diabetic ketoacidosis (DKA).

BOX 20-8 Goals of Nutritional Therapy in Patients With Renal Disease

- Minimize uremic symptoms.
- Reduce the incidence of fluid, electrolyte, and acid–base imbalances.
- Minimize symptoms of anemia.
- Decrease susceptibility to infections.
- Limit catabolism.
- Reduce cardiovascular risk.
- Manage other comorbid conditions.

Treatment with alkalinizing medications (eg, Bicitra, sodium bicarbonate tablets), dialysis, or both, is warranted when the plasma bicarbonate level is less than 22 mEq/L. Because of potential complications (eg, extracellular volume excess, metabolic alkalosis, hypokalemia), the use of IV sodium bicarbonate is reserved for severe acidosis (evidenced by a blood pH less than 7.2 or a plasma bicarbonate level less than 12 to 14 mEq/L). Intractable acidosis is an indication for dialysis.

 RED FLAG! *Too rapid correction of metabolic acidosis may lead to overcorrection (ie, metabolic alkalosis), resulting in a suppressed respiratory drive and hypoventilation. Overcorrection can also lead to acute hypocalcemia and tetany (because alkalosis increases calcium binding, reducing the levels of ionized calcium in the blood).*

Providing Nutritional Support

The goals of nutritional therapy in patients with renal disease are listed in Box 20-8. Renal diets typically restrict fluid, sodium, potassium, and phosphate intake, and may include supplementation of iron, vitamins, and calcium. Critically ill patients with renal disease need a high-calorie diet (35 to 45 kcal/kg/d). Most of the calories should come from a combination of carbohydrates and lipids, with adequate protein intake to prevent catabolism. Protein restriction to decrease uremic symptoms is controversial; if prescribed, it should never compromise anabolic goals, which would put the patient at risk for malnutrition.

Providing Psychosocial Support

Patients with acute kidney injury or chronic kidney disease often experience fear, anxiety, depression, feelings of powerlessness, and body image disturbances. Patients and their families may have difficulty coping owing to stress, limited resources or support, interruptions in usual family roles, or a combination of these factors. Nursing interventions include providing information, involving the patient and family in care, and involving other members of the interdisciplinary team (eg, social services) as needed.

CASE STUDY

Mr. H., a 72-year-old African American, is brought to the emergency department by paramedics. According to the paramedics, Mr. H.'s daughter found her father unconscious in his home. Two days ago, when she last saw him, he "seemed slightly more confused than normal but otherwise okay." His past medical history is notable for hypertension, type 2 diabetes mellitus, chronic kidney disease (stage 3), "mild" dementia, and benign prostatic enlargement. He takes the following medications daily: aspirin, 81 mg; lisinopril, 5 mg; amlodipine, 10 mg; atorvastatin, 20 mg; glipizide XL, 5 mg; and tamsulosin, 0.4 mg. His baseline serum creatinine and estimated GFR, determined in a routine clinic visit less than 2 weeks ago, are 2.0 mg/dL and 56 mL/min/1.73 m², respectively.

On presentation, Mr. H. is responsive to painful stimuli. His vital signs are BP, 80/40 mm Hg; HR, 130 beats/min and regular; RR, 28 breaths/min; and rectal temp, 101.3°F. Physical examination shows dry mucous membranes; clear breath sounds bilaterally; tachycardia without any rubs, gallops, or murmurs; a soft abdomen, but grimacing on deep palpation, with normal active bowel sounds in all quadrants, and no organomegaly or masses; and no edema in the extremities or diminished distal pulses.

Initial laboratory studies are notable for the following: Na⁺, 158 mEq/L; K⁺, 5.8 mEq/L; chloride, 98 mEq/L; bicarbonate, 14 mEq/L; blood urea nitrogen (BUN), 127 mg/dL; creatinine, 8.5 mg/dL; WBC count, 20,000/mm³ with 85% neutrophils; hemoglobin, 14 g/dL; hematocrit, 47%; urinalysis—specific gravity, 1.030, +1 protein, +1 blood; and urine microscopy—too numerous to count WBCs, 3 to 5 RBCs, dark muddy granular casts, and renal tubular epithelial cells. Arterial blood gases (ABGs) on room air are pH, 7.2; PaCO₂, 25 mm Hg; and PaO₂, 75 mm Hg. A chest radiograph shows no infiltrates. An ECG shows sinus tachycardia, left ventricular hypertrophy, and no ischemic changes. Additional diagnostic testing reveals a normal total creatine phosphokinase and serum troponin.

Mr. H. is admitted to the critical care unit. His blood pressure remains tenuous despite 2.5 L of normal saline, and he is placed on a dopamine infusion to keep the mean arterial pressure (MAP) greater than 65 mm Hg. His first hospital day is notable for persistent fever (T_max = 102.2°F) and hemodynamic instability. Blood and urine cultures return positive for *Escherichia coli* and antibiotic therapy is initiated. Repeat laboratory studies on critical care unit day 1 reveal the following: Na⁺, 148 mEq/L; K⁺, 6 mEq/L; chloride, 105 mEq/L; bicarbonate, 12 mEq/L; BUN, 134 mg/dL; and creatinine 8.7 mg/dL. Urine output for the first 24 hours is 50 mL.

Renal ultrasound reveals abnormalities. Repeat ABGs on 50% oxygen are now pH, 7.2;

$PaCO_2$, 33 mm Hg; and PaO_2, 83 mm Hg. Mr. H. is intubated. A chest radiograph obtained after intubation shows prominent pulmonary arteries with diffuse alveolar infiltrates, consistent with pulmonary edema. The nephrologist is consulted and recommends continuous renal replacement therapy (CRRT).

1. What is the cause of Mr. H.'s acute kidney injury?

2. Is Mr. H.'s acute kidney injury prerenal or intrinsic?

3. What acid–base disorder does Mr. H. have? Explain your answer.

4. Why does the nephrologist recommend dialysis for Mr. H?

References

1. Hoste E, Schurgers M: Epidemiology of acute kidney injury: How big is the problem? Crit Care Med 36(4):S146–S151, 2008
2. Lafrance J-P, Miller D: Acute kidney injury associates with increased long-term mortality. J Am Soc Nephrol 21(2):345–352, 2010
3. Lewington A, Sayed A: Acute kidney injury: how do we define it? Ann Clin Biochem 47(1):4–7, 2010
4. Coca S, Yusuf B, Shlipak M, et al.: Long-term risk of mortality and other adverse outcomes after acute kidney injury: A systemic review and meta-analysis. Am J Kidney Dis 53(6):961–973, 2009
5. Goldberg R, Dennen P: Long-term outcomes of acute kidney injury. Adv Chronic Kidney Dis 15(3):297–307, 2008
6. Lameire N: The pathophysiology of acute renal failure. Crit Care Clin 21(2):197–210, 2005
7. Counts C (ed): Core Curriculum for Nephrology Nursing, 5th ed. Pitman, NJ: AJ Jannetti, 2008
8. Pannu N, Nadim M: An overview of drug-induced acute kidney injury. Crit Care Med 36(4):S216–S223, 2008
9. Prescott W, Nagel J: Extended-interval once-daily dosing of aminoglycosides in adult and pediatric patients with cystic fibrosis. Pharmacotherapy 30(1):95–108, 2010
10. Taber S, Pasko D: The epidemiology of drug-induced disorders: The kidney. Expert Opin Drug Saf 7(6):679–690, 2008
11. McCullough P: Contrast-induced acute kidney injury. J Am Coll Cardiol 51(15):1419–1428, 2008
12. Caixeta A, Mehran R: Evidence-based management of patients undergoing PCI: Contrast-induced acute kidney injury. Catheter Cardiovasc Interv 75:(suppl 1):S15–S20, 2010
13. Diskin C, Stokes T, Dansby L, et al.: The comparative benefits of the fractional excretion of urea and sodium in various azotemic oliguric states. Nephron Clin Pract 114(2):C145–C150, 2010
14. U.S. Renal Data System: USRDS 2009 Annual Data Report: Atlas of End-Stage Renal Disease in the United States. Bethesda, MD: National Institutes of Health, National Institute of Diabetes and Digestive and Kidney Diseases, 2009
15. Coresh J, Byrd-Holt D, Astor B, et al.: Chronic kidney disease awareness, prevalence, and trends among U.S. adults, 1999–2000. J Am Soc Nephrol 16(1):180–188, 2005
16. Macconi D. Targeting the renin-angiotensin system for remission/regression of chronic kidney disease. Histol Histopathol 25:655–668, 2010

Want to know more? A wide variety of resources to enhance your learning and understanding of this chapter are available on **thePoint**. Visit **http://thepoint.lww.com/MortonEss1e** to access chapter review questions and more!

Nervous System

SIX

Patient Assessment: Nervous System

OBJECTIVES

Based on the content in this chapter, the reader should be able to:

1 Perform a comprehensive neurological assessment.
2 Identify abnormal assessment findings consistent with neurological compromise.
3 Analyze assessment findings and evaluate the effect of neurological dysfunction on the patient.
4 Identify preprocedure and postprocedure nursing interventions appropriate to selected neurodiagnostic tests.

Changes in neurological status may be the first indication that a patient's condition is worsening. The nurse is responsible for recognizing these changes, correlating findings to the pathophysiological process, and intervening appropriately.

History

Elements of the neurologic history are summarized in Box 21-1.

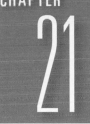 *The Older Patient. When assessing an older adult, it is necessary to ascertain the person's previous level of functioning to assess the person's status adequately.*

Physical Examination

Mental Status

The mental status examination evaluates level of consciousness and arousal, orientation to the environment, and thought content (Table 21-1). The degree of a patient's awareness of, and response to, the environment is the most sensitive indicator of nervous system function. Responsiveness is evaluated in terms of the patient's arousal to external stimuli and is described in terms of gradations of responses (Box 21-2).

Assessment of the patient's ability to communicate is an important aspect of the mental status examination. Use of language requires comprehension

BOX 21-1 Neurological Health History

History of the Present Illness

Complete analysis of the following signs and symptoms (using the NOPQRST format):

- Dizziness, syncope, or seizures
- Headaches
- Vision or auditory changes, including sensitivity to light and tinnitus
- Difficulty swallowing or hoarseness
- Slurred speech or word finding difficulty
- Confusion, memory loss, or difficulty concentrating
- Gait disturbances
- Motor symptoms, including weakness, paresthesia, paralysis, decreased range of motion, and tremors

Past Health History

- **Relevant childhood illnesses and immunizations:** febrile seizures, birth injuries, physical abuse or trauma, meningitis
- **Past acute and chronic medical problems, including treatments and hospitalizations:** tumors, traumatic head injuries, hypertension, thrombophlebitis or deep venous thrombosis (DVT), coagulopathies, sinusitis, meningitis, encephalitis, diabetes, cancer, psychiatric disorders
- **Risk factors:** diabetes, smoking, hypercholesterolemia, hypertension, drug use, alcohol use, cardiovascular disease
- **Past surgeries:** peripheral vascular surgeries; carotid endarterectomy; aneurysm clipping; evacuation of hematoma; head, eyes, ears, nose, or throat (HEENT) procedures
- **Past diagnostic tests and interventions:** electroencephalography, brain scan, carotid Doppler, head and neck computed tomography (CT), magnetic resonance imaging (MRI), thrombolytic therapy, cardiac catheterization

- **Medications, including prescription drugs, over-the-counter drugs, vitamins, herbs, and supplements:** anticonvulsants, anticoagulants, psychotropic agents, oral contraceptives, β-adrenergic blockers, calcium channel blockers, antihyperlipidemics, hormone replacement therapy
- **Allergies and reactions to medications, foods, contrast, latex, or other materials**
- **Transfusions, including type and date**

Family History

- **Health status or cause of death of parents and siblings:** coronary artery disease (CAD), peripheral vascular disease, cancer, hypertension, diabetes, stroke, hyperlipidemia, coagulopathies, seizures, psychiatric disturbances

Personal and Social History

- Tobacco, alcohol, and substance use
- Environment: exposure to chemicals and toxins; physical, verbal, or emotional abuse

Review of Other Systems

- **HEENT:** visual changes, tinnitus, headache
- **Cardiovascular:** hypertension, syncope, palpitations, intermittent claudication
- **Respiratory:** shortness of breath, infections, cough, dyspnea
- **Gastrointestinal:** weight loss, change in bowel habits, nausea or vomiting, diarrhea
- **Genitourinary:** change in bladder habits, painful urination, sexual dysfunction
- **Musculoskeletal:** sensitivity to temperature changes, varicosities, loss of hair on extremities, change in sensation

TABLE 21-1 Mental Status Examination

Functions	Test	Implications
Orientation	*Time:* Patient states year, month, date, season, day of week. *Place:* Patient indicates state, county, city of residency, or hospital name, floor, or room number.	May be altered by a multitude of neurologic conditions
Attention	Digit span, serial 7's; recitation of months of the year in reverse order	May be impaired in delirium, frontal lobe damage, and dementia
Memory	*Short-term:* Patient recalls three items after 5 min. *Long-term:* Patient recalls facts such as mother's maiden name, events of previous day.	May be impaired in conditions such as dementia, stroke, and delirium
Language	*Naming:* Patient identifies objects as the nurse points to them. *Comprehension:* Patient responds to simple and complex commands. *Repetition:* Patient repeats phrases such as "no ifs, ands, or buts." *Reading:* Patient reads and explains a short passage. *Writing:* Patient writes a brief sentence.	Requires integration of visual, semantic, and verbal aspects of language Dysfunction may be associated with lesions of left frontal cerebral cortex (Broca's area); patient's responses may also depend on educational level.
Spatial/perceptual	Patient copies drawings of a cross or square; draws a clock face. Patient is asked to point out right and left side of self. Patient demonstrates actions such as putting on a coat or blowing out a match.	Dysfunction may be associated with parietal lobe lesions.

BOX 21-2 Clinical Terminology for Grading Responsiveness

Awake and alert (full consciousness): normal; may be somewhat confused on first awakening but is fully oriented when aroused

Lethargic: drowsy but follows simple commands when stimulated

Obtunded: arousable with stimulation; responds verbally with a word or two; follows simple commands; otherwise drowsy

Stuporous: very hard to arouse; inconsistently may follow simple commands or speak single words or short phrases; limited spontaneous movement

Semicomatose: movements are purposeful when stimulated; does not follow commands or speak coherently

Comatose: may respond with reflexive posturing when stimulated or may have no response to any stimulus

BOX 21-3 The Glasgow Coma Scale

Response		Score[a]
Best eye-opening response	Spontaneously	4
	In response to speech	3
	In response to pain	2
	No response	1
Best verbal response	Oriented	5
	Confused conversation	4
	Inappropriate words	3
	Garbled sounds	2
	No response	1
Best motor response	Obeys commands	6
	Localizes stimuli	5
	Withdrawal from stimulus	4
	Abnormal flexion (decorticate)	3
	Abnormal extension (decerebrate)	2
	No response	1

[a]A total score of 3 to 8 suggests severe impairment, 9 to 12 suggests moderate impairment, and 13 to 15 suggests mild impairment. A low GCS score may be a predictor of poor functional recovery.

of verbal and nonverbal symbols and the ability to use those symbols to communicate with others. Evaluation of the patient's understanding normally is accomplished through the spoken word. Table 21-2 summarizes patterns of speech deficits.

The Glasgow Coma Scale (GCS) is a reliable tool for assessing arousal and level of consciousness (Box 21-3). This scoring system was designed as a guide for rapid evaluation of the acutely ill or severely injured patient whose status may change quickly. The GCS allows the examiner to record objectively the patient's response to the environment in three major areas (eye opening, verbalization, and movement), with the best response scored in each category. The best eye-opening response and

best verbal response are used to assess arousal and level of consciousness. The intubated patient is usually noted to have a verbal score of 1T, in recognition of the patient's inability to speak secondary to the presence of the endotracheal tube.

TABLE 21-2 Patterns of Speech Deficits

Type	Deficit Locations	Speech Patterns
Receptive (fluent) dysphasia	Left parietal–temporal lobes (Wernicke's area)	• Impaired understanding of spoken word despite normal hearing • Fluent speech that lacks coherent content • May have normal-sounding speech rhythm but no intelligible words • May use invented, meaningless words (neologism), word substitution (paraphasia), or repetition of words (perseveration, echolalia)
Expressive (nonfluent) dysphasia	Left frontal area (Broca's area)	• Inability to initiate sounds • Usually associated with impaired writing skills • Comprehension usually intact • Slow speech with poor articulation
Global dysphasia	Diffuse involvement of frontal, parietal, and occipital areas	• Inability to understand spoken or written words • Nonfluent speech
Dysarthria	Corticobulbar tracts; cerebellum	• Loss of articulation, phonation • Loss of control of muscles of lips, tongue, palate • Slurred, jerky, or irregular speech but with appropriate content

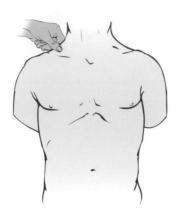

A. Trapezius squeeze

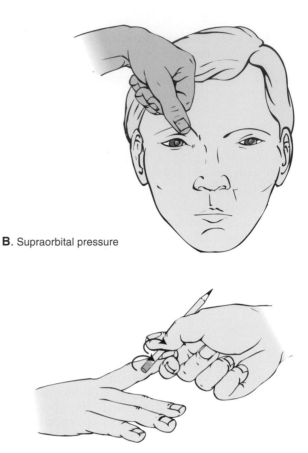

B. Supraorbital pressure

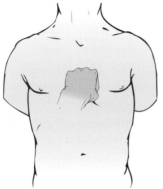

C. Sternal rub

D. Nailbed pressure

FIGURE 21-1 Methods of applying a painful stimulus. The trapezius squeeze **(A)**, application of supraorbital pressure **(B)**, and sternal rub **(C)** are used first; if these actions do not elicit a motor response, application of pressure to the nail bed **(D)** may be used.

Motor Function

Evaluation of motor function entails evaluating the motor response to stimuli, as well as motor strength and coordination.

Motor Response to Stimuli

To elicit the patient's best, or maximal response, stimuli must be applied in a systematic and escalating fashion:

1. Calling the patient's name (in the same manner used to wake a person who is sleeping).
2. Shouting the patient's name (as when waking a "sound sleeper").
3. Shaking the patient.
4. Applying a painful stimulus (Fig. 21-1). The painful stimulus should be applied for 15 to 30 seconds before the patient is considered not to have a motor response. Figure 21-2 depicts possible motor responses to pain.

This staged approach affords the patient the opportunity to demonstrate increasing wakefulness or the best response.

Motor Strength and Coordination

Muscle weakness is a cardinal sign of dysfunction in many neurological disorders. A drift test is used to detect weakness. The upper extremities are tested by having the patient hold the arms straight out with palms upward and eyes closed, while observing for any downward drift or pronation of the forearms (pronator drift). The lower extremities are tested by having the patient lie in bed and raise the legs, one at a time, while observing for a drift of the legs back to the bed.

Extremity strength is tested by evaluating the patient's ability to overcome resistance that is applied to various muscle groups (Box 21-4). Motor function for each extremity is reported as a fraction, with 5 as the denominator and maximal strength (Box 21-5). In patients who do not follow commands or are comatose, it is important to note what, if any, stimuli initiate a response and to describe or grade the type of response obtained to determine motor strength.

 The Older Patient. *Factors that can affect motor function in older patients include decreased strength, alterations in gait, changes in posture, and increased tremors.*

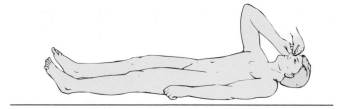

NORMAL

Localizing pain. An appropriate response is to reach up above shoulder level toward the stimulus. A focal motor deficit (eg, hemiplegia) may prevent a bilateral response.

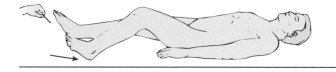

Withdrawal. An appropriate response is to pull the extremity or body away from the stimulus.

ABNORMAL

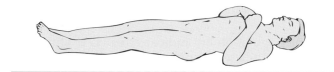

Decorticate posturing. One or both arms in full flexion on the chest. Legs may be stiffly extended.

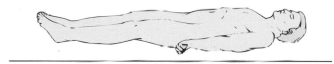

Decerebrate posturing. One or both arms stiffly extended. Possible extension of the legs.

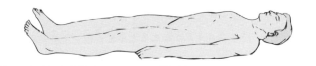

Flaccid. No motor response in any extremity.

FIGURE 21-2 Motor responses to pain.

Each extremity may also be assessed for size, muscle tone, and smoothness of passive movement. Assessment findings may include the "clasp-knife" phenomenon, in which initially strong resistance to passive movement suddenly decreases. "Lead-pipe" rigidity (ie, steady, continuous resistance to passive movement) is characteristic of diffuse hemispheric damage. "Cogwheel" rigidity (ie, a series of small, regular, jerky movements felt on passive movement) is characteristic of Parkinson's disease.

Hemiparesis (weakness) and hemiplegia (paralysis) are unilateral symptoms resulting from a

---

BOX 21-4 **Assessment of Upper and Lower Extremity Muscle Strength**

To evaluate muscle strength, the muscle groups of the upper and lower extremity are assessed individually, initially without resistance, and then against resistance.

Upper Extremity
Upper extremity muscle strength is evaluated by asking the patient to perform the following sequence of movements:
• Shrug the shoulders (trapezius and levator scapulae muscles)
• Raise the arms (deltoid muscle)
• Flex the elbow (biceps muscle)
• Extend the elbow (triceps muscle)

• Extend the wrist (extensor carpi radialis longus muscle)

Lower Extremity
Lower extremity muscle strength is evaluated by asking the patient to perform the following sequence of movements:
• Raise the leg (iliopsoas muscle)
• Extend the knee (quadriceps muscle)
• Dorsiflex and plantar flex the foot (anterior tibialis and gastrocnemius muscles, respectively)
• Flex the knee (hamstring muscle)

BOX 21-5 Motor Function Scale

Score	Interpretation
0/5	No muscle contraction
1/5	Flicker or trace of contraction
2/5	Moves but cannot overcome gravity
3/5	Moves against gravity but cannot overcome resistance applied by examiner
4/5	Moves with some weakness against resistance applied by examiner
5/5	Normal power and strength

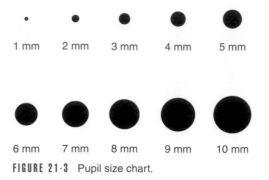

FIGURE 21-3 Pupil size chart.

contralateral brain lesion. Paraplegia (bilateral paralysis) results from a spinal cord lesion or from peripheral nerve dysfunction. Quadriplegia is associated with cervical spinal cord lesions, brainstem dysfunction ("locked in syndrome"), and large bilateral lesions in the cerebrum.

The cerebellum is responsible for smooth synchronization, balance, and ordering of movements. Some of the more common tests for cerebellar synchronization of movement with balance include the following:

- **Romberg test.** The patient stands with feet together and hands at their side, first with the eyes opened, then with the eyes closed. Swaying when the eyes are closed indicates impaired balance. (To prevent the patient from falling, the nurse stands close by.)
- **Finger-to-nose test.** The patient touches one finger to the nurse's finger and then touches his or her own nose. Overshooting or past-pointing the mark is called dysmetria. The nurse tests both sides individually.
- **Rapidly alternating movement (RAM) test.** The patient opposes each finger and thumb in rapid succession or performs rapid pronation and supination of the hand on the leg. Inability to perform RAMs is termed adiadochokinesia; performing RAMs poorly or clumsily is termed dysdiadochokinesia.
- **Heel-to-shin test.** The patient extends the heel of one foot down the anterior aspect of the shin, moving from the knee to the ankle.

Pupillary Changes

Pupils are examined for size (Fig. 21-3), shape, and equality bilaterally. The equality of pupils is assessed before shining a bright light in the eye. The nurse then directs the light into one eye, and notes the briskness of pupillary constriction (direct response). The other pupil also should constrict at the same time (consensual response). The nurse then repeats the procedure with the other eye. Anisocoria (unequal pupils) is normal in a small percentage of the population but indicates neural dysfunction if it is a change from normal.

Pupil reactivity is also assessed with respect to accommodation. To test accommodation, the nurse holds a finger 8 to 12 in in front of the patient's face. The patient focuses on the finger as the nurse moves it toward the patient's nose. The pupils should constrict as the object gets closer.

The normal response to testing is documented as PERRLA, or **p**upils **e**qual, **r**ound, **r**eactive to **l**ight and **a**ccommodation. Abnormal responses are shown in Fig. 21-4. Common causes of abnormal pupillary changes are listed in Box 21-6.

 The Older Patient. *In older patients, vision may be decreased, pupils may be less reactive, and gaze may be impaired.*

Vital Signs

Changes in temperature, heart rate, and blood pressure are considered late findings in neurological deterioration. Changes in respiratory rate, on the other hand, can indicate progression of neurological impairment and are frequently seen early in neurological deterioration.

- **Respirations.** Abnormal respiratory patterns (Fig. 21-5, p. 296) may be correlated with areas of injury in the brain and frequently are a direct indication of increasing intracranial pressure (ICP). Airway management and mechanical ventilation are often required.
- **Temperature.** Diffuse cerebral damage can result in alterations in temperature, which is normally regulated in the hypothalamus. Central nervous system (neurogenic) fevers may be very high and differentiate themselves from other causes of fever by the sudden elevation their resistance to antipyretic therapy.
- **Heart rate and rhythm.** Brain injury may lead to episodes of tachycardia and can predispose the patient to ventricular or atrial dysrhythmias. Bradycardia, a late sign indicative of impending herniation, may be seen with increasing ICP.

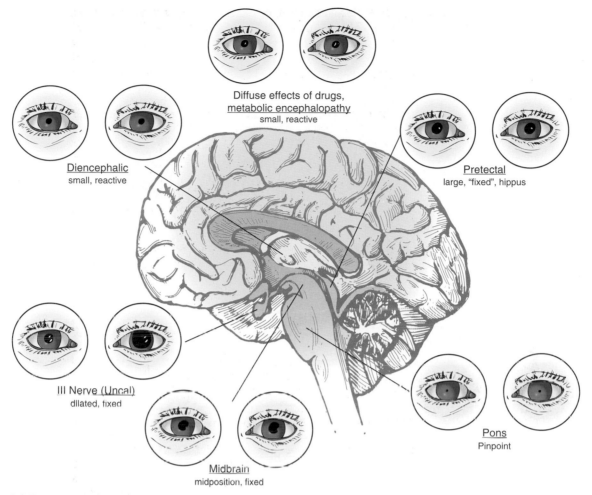

FIGURE 21-4 Abnormal pupils. (Adapted from Saper C: Brain stem modulation of sensation, movement, and consciousness. In Kandel ER, Schwartz JH, Jessel TM (eds): Principles of Neural Science, 4th ed. New York: McGraw-Hill, 2000, pp 871–909, with permission.)

- **Blood pressure.** Damage to the medulla or encroaching edema secondary to injury in other areas results in alterations in blood pressure. Sustained elevation of systolic blood pressure with a widened pulse pressure is a late sign of increasing ICP and impending herniation.

BOX 21-6 Common Causes of Pupil Abnormalities

Sluggish or absent response to light
- Increased intracranial pressure (ICP)
- Glaucoma

Pinpoint pupils
- Opiates
- Medications for glaucoma
- Damage in the pons area (brainstem)

Dilated pupils
- Herniation syndromes
- Seizures
- Cocaine, crack, phencyclidine (PCP)
- Fear, panic attack, extreme anxiety

Cranial Nerve Function

Cranial nerve assessment varies depending on whether the patient is conscious or unconscious. Assessment of the cranial nerves in the unconscious patient is important because it provides data regarding brainstem function. All cranial nerves are ipsilateral, except the trochlear nerve (CN IV), which is contralateral.

- **CN I (olfactory nerve).** To test CN I, the nurse occludes one of the patient's nostrils and places an aromatic substance (eg, soap, coffee, cinnamon) near the other nostril. The patient is asked to identify the substance with the eyes closed. The test is then repeated with the other nostril. Ammonia is not used because the patient will respond to irritation of the nasal mucosa rather than to the odor. This test is usually deferred unless the patient reports an inability to smell.
- **CN II (optic nerve).** Assessment of CN II involves evaluation of visual acuity and visual fields. Gross visual acuity is checked by having the patient read ordinary newsprint (the nurse takes note of the patient's preinjury need for glasses). Visual fields are tested by having the patient look straight

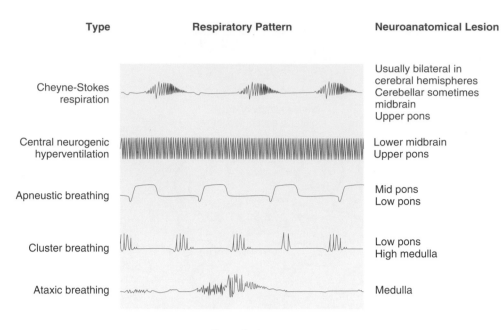

Type	Respiratory Pattern	Neuroanatomical Lesion
Cheyne-Stokes respiration		Usually bilateral in cerebral hemispheres Cerebellar sometimes midbrain Upper pons
Central neurogenic hyperventilation		Lower midbrain Upper pons
Apneustic breathing		Mid pons Low pons
Cluster breathing		Low pons High medulla
Ataxic breathing		Medulla

├─One minute─┤

FIGURE 21-5 Injury to the brainstem can result in various abnormal respiratory patterns.

ahead with one eye covered. The nurse moves a finger from the periphery of each quadrant of vision toward the patient's center of vision as well as from the center to the peripheral. The patient should indicate when he or she sees the examiner's finger. The test is performed for both eyes, and the results are compared with the examiner's visual fields, which are assumed to be normal. An optic nerve lesion or optic tract lesion can produce partial or complete blindness (Table 21-3).

- **CN III (oculomotor nerve), IV (trochlear nerve), and VI (abducens nerve).** These cranial nerves are checked together because they innervate extraocular muscles involved in eye movement. CN III innervates the muscles that move the eyes up, down, and medially, as well as the muscles that elevate the eyelid. CN IV innervates the muscles that move the eyes down and in, and CN VI innervates the muscles that move the eyes laterally. In a conscious patient, these nerves are tested by having the patient follow the nurse's finger as the nurse moves it in all directions of gaze (Fig. 21-6). Diplopia, nystagmus, and disconjugate deviation may indicate dysfunction of CN III, IV, or VI. In a patient who is unable to follow commands, observation of ocular position can provide information about the site of brain dysfunction. If both eyes are conjugately deviated to one side, dysfunction may exist either in the frontal lobe on that side or in the contralateral pontine area of the brainstem. Downward deviation suggests a dysfunction in the midbrain.

- **CN V (trigeminal nerve).** CN V has three divisions: ophthalmic, maxillary, and mandibular. The sensory portion of CN V controls sensation to the cornea and face. The motor portion controls the muscles of mastication. CN V may be partially tested by checking the

TABLE 21-3 Patterns of Visual Field Defects

Visual Field Defect	Left	Right	Description
Anopsia			Blindness in one eye (resulting from complete lesion of the optic nerve before the optic chiasm)
Bitemporal hemianopsia (central vision)			Blindness in both lateral visual fields (resulting from lesions around the optic chiasm, such as pituitary tumors or aneurysms of the anterior communicating artery)
Homonymous hemianopsia			Half-blindness involving both eyes with loss of visual field on the same side of each eye (resulting from lesion of temporal or occipital lobe with damage to the optic tract or optic radiations). Blindness occurs on the side opposite the lesion. Here, the lesion occurred in the right side of the brain, resulting in loss of vision in the left visual field of both eyes.
Quadrant deficit			Blindness in the upper or lower quadrant of vision in both eyes (resulting from a lesion in the parietal or temporal lobe)

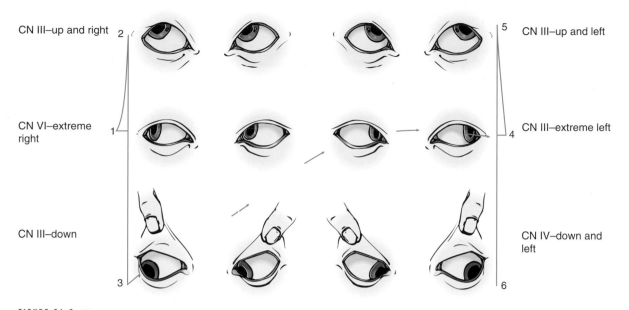

CN III–up and right 2

CN VI–extreme right 1

CN III–down 3

CN III–up and left 5

CN III–extreme left 4

CN IV–down and left 6

FIGURE 21-6 The six cardinal directions of gaze. The nurse leads the patient's gaze in the sequence numbered 1 through 6. CN III, oculomotor nerve; CN IV, trochlear nerve; CN VI, abducens nerve

corneal reflex; if it is intact, the patient blinks when the cornea is stroked with a wisp of cotton or when a drop of normal saline is placed in the eye. Care must be taken not to stroke the eyelashes, because this can cause the eye to blink regardless of the presence of a corneal reflex. Facial sensation is tested by comparing light touch and pinprick on symmetrical sides of the face. The nurse also observes the patient's ability to chew or clench the jaw.

- **CN VII (facial nerve).** The motor portion of CN VII controls muscles of facial expression. Testing is performed by asking the patient to raise the eyebrows, smile, or grimace. With a central lesion, there is muscle paralysis of the lower half of the face on the same side of the lesion, but the muscles around the eyes and forehead are unaffected (Fig. 21-7A). With a peripheral lesion (eg, Bell's palsy), there is complete paralysis of the facial muscles (including the forehead) on the same side as the lesion (see Fig. 21-7B). In a comatose patient, motor function of the facial muscles and jaw can be ascertained by observing spontaneous muscle activity such as yawning, grimacing, or chewing. Symmetry of movement may be assessed by noting facial drooping or flattening of the nasolabial folds (see Fig. 21-7C).

- **CN VIII (acoustic nerve).** CN VIII is divided into the vestibular and cochlear branches, which control equilibrium and hearing, respectively. The vestibular branch of the nerve may not be evaluated routinely. However, the nurse remains alert to reports of dizziness or vertigo from the patient. The cochlear branch of the nerve is tested by air and bone conduction. A vibrating tuning fork is placed on the mastoid process; after the patient can no longer hear the fork, he or she should be able to hear it for a few seconds longer when it is placed in front of the ear (Rinne test). The patient may report ringing in the ears (tinnitus) or decreased hearing if this nerve is damaged.

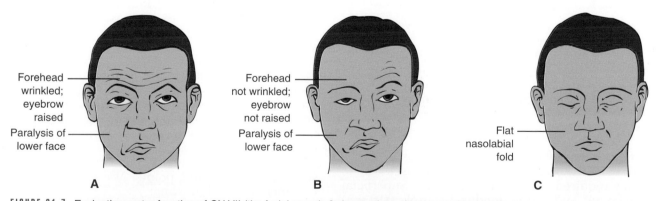

Forehead wrinkled; eyebrow raised

Paralysis of lower face

A

Forehead not wrinkled; eyebrow not raised

Paralysis of lower face

B

Flat nasolabial fold

C

FIGURE 21-7 Evaluating motor function of CN VII (the facial nerve). **A:** In a patient with a central lesion, there is paralysis of the lower face on the side opposite the lesion. The muscles of the upper face are not affected. **B:** In a patient with a peripheral lesion, there is paralysis of the upper and lower face on the same side as the lesion. **C:** Flattening of the nasolabial fold may also be an indication of CN VII dysfunction

TABLE 21-4	Quick Screening Test for Cranial Nerve Function		
	Nerve	**Reflex**	**Procedure**
II III	Optic Oculomotor	Pupil constriction (protection of the retina)	Shine a light into each eye and note whether the pupil on that side constricts (direct response). Next, shine a light into each eye and note whether the opposite pupil constricts (consensual response).
V VII	Trigeminal Facial	Corneal reflex (protection of the cornea)	Approaching the eye from the side and avoiding the eyelashes, touch the cornea with a wisp of cotton. Alternatively, use a drop of sterile water or normal saline. The patient should blink.
IX X	Glossopharyngeal Vagus	Airway protection	Touch the back of the throat with a tongue depressor. The patient should gag or cough. Perform a swallow evaluation.

The Older Patient. *In an older patient with undetected hearing impairment, changes in Rinne test findings may be noted. These findings can lead to the erroneous assumption that the person has more neurological deficits than actually exist.*

- **CN IX (glossopharyngeal nerve) and X (vagus nerve).** CN IX supplies sensory fibers to the posterior third of the tongue as well as the uvula and soft palate. CN X innervates the larynx, pharynx, and soft palate and conveys autonomic responses to the heart, stomach, lungs, and small intestine. These cranial nerves can be tested by eliciting a gag reflex, observing the uvula for symmetrical movement when the patient says "ah," or observing midline elevation of the uvula when both sides are stroked. Inability to cough forcefully, difficulty with swallowing, and hoarseness may be signs of dysfunction.
- **CN XI (spinal accessory nerve).** CN XI controls the trapezius and sternocleidomastoid muscles. CN XI function can be tested by having the patient shrug the shoulders or turn the head from side to side against resistance.
- **CN XII (hypoglossal nerve).** CN XII controls tongue movement. This nerve can be checked by having the patient protrude the tongue. The examiner checks for deviation from midline, tremor, and atrophy. If deviation is noted secondary to nerve damage, it will be to the side of the cerebral lesion.

Performing a complete test of cranial nerve function can be time-consuming and may not be required for every patient. A partial screening assessment (Table 21-4) may be performed, focusing on nerves in which dysfunction may indicate serious problems or interfere with activities of daily living (ADLs).

Reflexes

A reflex occurs when a sensory stimulus evokes a motor response. Cerebral control and consciousness are not required for a reflex to occur. Superficial (cutaneous) and deep tendon (muscle stretch) reflexes are tested on symmetrical sides of the body and compared by noting the strength of contraction elicited on each side.

Superficial reflexes occur when certain areas of skin are lightly stroked or tapped, causing contraction of the muscle groups beneath. An example is the plantar reflex. A sensory stimulus is applied by briskly stroking the outer edge of the sole and across the ball of the foot with a dull object, such as a tongue blade or key. The normal motor response is downward (plantar) flexion of the toes. Upward flexion (dorsiflexion) of the big toe, with or without fanning of the other toes, is called Babinski's sign and is an abnormal response that may indicate a lesion in the corticospinal tract.

Deep tendon reflexes are elicited by briskly tapping a tendon insertion site with a reflex hammer. Hyperreflexia (increased reflex) is associated with upper motor neuron dysfunction (central nervous system injuries), whereas areflexia (absence of reflexes) is associated with lower motor neuron dysfunction (peripheral nerve injuries). Deep tendon reflexes are tested on the biceps, brachioradial, triceps, patellar, and Achilles tendons and are commonly graded on a scale of 0 to 4:

4+: A very brisk response; indicates evidence of disease, electrolyte imbalance, or both; associated with clonic contractions

3+: A brisk response; possibly indicative of disease

2+: A normal response

1+: A response in the low-normal range

0: No response; possibly indicates disease or electrolyte imbalance

Sensation

The final component of the neurological examination involves a sensory assessment. With the patient's eyes closed, multiple and symmetrical areas of the body are tested, including the trunk and extremities. The nurse notes the patient's ability to perceive the sensation (sharp vs dull), comparing distal areas with proximal areas and comparing right and left sides at corresponding points. Assessment of sensation includes the following:

- **Light Touch** is assessed using a cotton wisp or cotton swab.
- **Pain** is assessed using a pin.

- **Temperature** is assessed using glass tubes of hot and cold water or an alcohol swab.
- **Proprioception** (limb position) is tested by moving the patient's finger (eg, up or down) and asking the patient to identify the direction of the movement.
- **Vibration** is assessed by placing a tuning fork over a bony prominence.

Two-point discrimination (ie, the patient's ability to distinguish between two closely located points) and extinction (ie, the patient's ability to recognize simultaneous touch on bilateral extremities) is also tested.

 The Older Patient. *In older patients, changes in sensory function may include decreased reflexes, decreased vibratory and position sense, and decreased two-point discrimination.*

In a comatose patient, it is impossible to perform a complete test for sensation, because the patient's cooperation is required. However, use of painful stimuli to elicit a response gives a gross indication of whether some degree of sensory function remains intact.

Neurodiagnostic Studies

Many diagnostic tests are available to help diagnose neurological and neurosurgical problems (Table 21-5). Nursing responsibilities include preparing the patient and family for the diagnostic procedure, and monitoring the patient for complications during and after the procedure. Many neurodiagnostic tests require the patient be transported to the imaging department or to another facility. When this is the case, the nurse may be required to remain with the patient during the procedure to monitor neurological status and vital signs.

TABLE 21-5 **Neurodiagnostic Tests**

Test and Purpose	Method of Testing	Nursing Implications
Radiography Identify linear skull fractures; vertebral fractures; alignment of spine (assess for subluxation)	X-ray beams are passed through the patient's body to produce images of bony structures.	Plain films of the skull and spine require careful patient positioning; the nurse must be alert for complications related to patient position and the length of the procedure. In patients with spinal cord injury, care must be taken to ensure stabilization of the neck (eg, applying a hard cervical collar, logrolling).
Computed tomography (CT) Used in the initial workup of seizures, headache, and altered level of consciousness; for the diagnosis of suspected hemorrhage, tumors, and other lesions; and to detect shift of structures due to tumors, hematomas, or hydrocephalus; serial CTs allow the healthcare team to follow neurological progression and facilitate rapid intervention	A scanner takes a series of radiographic images all around the same axial plane. A computer then creates a composite picture of various tissue densities visualized. The images may be enhanced with the use of IV contrast media. The denser the material (eg, bones of the skull), the whiter it appears.	The patient must remain as immobile as possible; sedation may be required. The scan may not be of the best quality if the patient moves during the test, or if the x-ray beams were deflected by a metal object (eg, traction tongs, intracranial pressure [(ICP] monitoring devices). If contrast is being used, ascertain preexisting allergies.
Magnetic resonance imaging (MRI) Creates a graphic image of bone, fluid, and soft tissue structures; identifies tumors	A selected area of the patient's body is placed inside a powerful magnetic field. The hydrogen atoms inside the patient are temporarily "excited" and caused to oscillate by a sequence of radiofrequency pulsations. The sensitive scanner measures these minute oscillations, and a computer-enhanced image is created.	This test is contraindicated in patients with previous surgeries where hemostatic or aneurysm clips made of ferrous metal were implanted. The powerful magnetic field can cause metal objects to move out of position, placing the patient at risk for bleeding or hemorrhage. Other contraindications include cardiac pacemakers, prosthetic valves, bullet fragments, and orthopedic pins made of ferrous metal. Inform the patient that the procedure is very noisy. Use caution if the patient is claustrophobic.

(continued on page 300)

TABLE 21-5 Neurodiagnostic Tests (continued)

Test and Purpose	Method of Testing	Nursing Implications
Diffusion-weighted imaging (DWI), perfusion-weighted imaging (PWI) DWI shows diffusion of water through brain and PWI uses contrast media to show blood flow through vessels; both allow early recognition of ischemic areas (within 30 min); used to differentiate reversible tissue injury from irreversible tissue injury	Radiofrequency energy, magnetic fields, and computer software are used to create detailed, cross-sectional images of the brain	Same as for MRI
Positron emission tomography (PET); single-photon emission computed tomography (SPECT) Used to measure cerebral metabolism and cerebral blood flow regionally	The patient either inhales or receives by injection a radioactively tagged substance (eg, oxygen, glucose). A gamma scanner measures the radioactive uptake of these substances, and a computer produces a composite image indicating where the radioactive material is located, corresponding to areas of cellular metabolism.	The patient receives only minimal radiation exposure because the half-life of the radionuclides used is from a few minutes to 2 h. Testing may take a few hours. The patient must remain immobile throughout the test. The procedure is very expensive.
Cerebral angiography Used to visualize the structure of the cerebral circulation, enabling assessment of vessel patency, narrowing, occlusion, structural abnormalities; displacement; and alterations in blood flow	Radiopaque contrast is injected by a catheter into the patient's cerebral arterial circulation. The contrast medium is directed into each common carotid artery and each vertebral artery, and serial radiographs are then taken. Test may be performed with computed tomography angiography (CTA) or magnetic resonance angiography (MRA); this method is less invasive because it does not require arterial cannulation	Preparation includes informing the patient about the location of the catheter insertion (usually the femoral artery), notifying the patient that a local anesthetic will be used, and explaining that the patient can expect to feel a warm, flushed feeling when the contrast medium is injected. Post procedure care includes assessing the puncture site for swelling, redness, and bleeding; checking the skin color, temperature, and peripheral pulses of the extremity distal to the puncture site for signs of arterial insufficiency; and monitoring for major complications (ie, stroke, vasospasm, renal failure secondary to contrast load), bleeding, or hematoma at insertion site.
Digital subtraction angiography Used to examine extracranial circulation (arterial, capillary, and venous) and determine vessel size, patency, narrowing, and degree of stenosis or displacement	A plain radiograph is taken of the patient's cranium, and then radiopaque contrast is injected into a large vein and serial radiographs are taken. A computer converts the images into digital form and "subtracts" the plain radiograph from the ones with the contrast. The result is an enhanced radiographic image of contrast medium in the arterial vessels.	There is less risk to the patient for bleeding or vascular insufficiency because the injection of contrast is intravenous rather than intra-arterial. The patient must remain absolutely motionless during the examination (even swallowing will interfere with the results).
Radioisotope brain scan (cerebral blood flow studies) Used to diagnose intracranial lesions, cerebral infarction or contusion, and brain death	A radioactive isotope is injected intravenously, and a scanning device produces films of areas of concentration of the isotope.	Minimal patient preparation is required. The isotope may not be readily available within the facility. Any movement by the patient will make the test difficult to interpret.

Test and Purpose	Method of Testing	Nursing Implications
Myelography Used to examine the spinal subarachnoid space for partial or complete obstructions resulting from bone displacements, spinal cord compression, or herniated intervertebral disks	A contrast substance (either air or dye) is injected into the lumbar subarachnoid space and then fluoroscopy, conventional radiographs, or CT scans are used to visualize selected areas.	Patient preparation is similar to that for a lumbar puncture; the patient should also be advised that a special table that tilts up and down is used during the procedure. *Postprocedure care* Oil-based contrast dye: • Flat in bed for 24 h • Force fluids • Observe for headache, fever, back spasms, nausea, and vomiting Water-based contrast dye: • Head of bed elevated for 8 h • Keep the patient quiet for first few hours • Do not administer phenothiazines • Observe for headache, fever, back spasms, nausea, vomiting, and seizures
Electroencephalography Used to detect and localize abnormal electrical activity occurring in the cerebral cortex; has diagnostic applications (eg, seizures, sleep disorders); also used as a confirmatory test for brain death and for monitoring induced coma	Electrical impulses generated by the brain cortex are sensed by electrodes on the surface of the scalp and recorded.	Reassure the patient that an electrical shock or pain will not be felt during the test. Oil, dirt, creams, and sprays on the hair or scalp can cause electrical interference and an inaccurate recording. Electrical devices (eg, cardiac monitor, ventilator) may also cause interference.
Cortical evoked potentials, somatosensory evoked potentials (SSEPs), brainstem auditory evoked response (BAER), visual evoked potentials (VEPs) Provide a detailed assessment of neuron transmission along particular pathways	A specialized device senses central or cortical cerebral electrical activity via skin electrodes in response to peripheral stimulation of specific sensory receptors (eg, those for vision, hearing, or tactile sensation). A computer graphically displays the signals and also measures the characteristic peaks and intervals between them.	May be used in both conscious and unconscious patients and can be performed at the bedside. The patient must be as motionless as possible during some phases of these tests to minimize musculoskeletal interference. Depending on the sensory pathway being tested, the patient may be instructed to watch a series of geometric designs or listen to a series of clicking noises.
Transcranial Doppler sonography (TCD) Used to approximate cerebral blood flow and monitor cerebral autoregulation	High-frequency ultrasonic waves are directed from a probe toward specific cerebral vessels. The ultrasonic energy is aimed through cranial "windows," areas in the skull where the bony table is thin (temporal zygoma) or where there are small gaps in the bone (orbit or foramen magnum). The reflected sound waves are analyzed for shifts in frequency, indicating flow velocity.	The test is noninvasive and may be performed at the bedside by the physician or ultrasound technician in 30–60 min. There are no known adverse effects, and the procedure may be repeated as often as necessary. The testing is accomplished with the patient initially supine, and later on lying on the side with head flexed forward.
Lumbar puncture Used to obtain a cerebrospinal fluid (CSF) sample for laboratory analysis and to measure CSF pressure	A hollow needle is positioned in the subarachnoid space at L3–L4 or L4–L5 level to sample CSF and measure pressure.	This test is contraindicated in patients with suspected increased ICP because a sudden reduction in pressure from below may cause brain structures to herniate, leading to death. The patient is positioned on the side with knees and head flexed. Some pressure may be felt as the needle is inserted. The patient should be instructed not to move suddenly or cough. After this procedure, keep the patient flat for 8–10 h to prevent headache. Encourage liberal fluid intake. Assess complications: headache, difficulty voiding. This test should be avoided if the patient is anticoagulated due to the risk of an epidural hematoma.

Determination of Brain Death

Brain death is the irreversible loss of all brain function. Although the neurologic examination to determine brain death is performed by a physician, nurses play a primary role in assisting the physician and communicating with the family. To fulfill these responsibilities, nurses must understand the methods and criteria for determining brain death.

The brain death examination seeks to confirm three cardinal findings: coma or unresponsiveness, absence of brainstem reflexes, and apnea. Electrolyte abnormalities, hypothermia or hyperthermia, severe hypotension, or the presence of medications in amounts that could cause coma must be resolved before brain death testing can be performed. Tests specific for brain death include, but are not limited to, motor testing; evaluation of pupillary responses; evaluation of the corneal, cough, and gag reflexes; apnea testing; evaluation of the oculocephalic reflex ("doll's eyes" phenomenon); and evaluation of the oculovestibular reflex (caloric ice-water test) (Box 21-7). When testing reflexes, if the reflex is not present, the test is negative. If the reflex is intact,

---

BOX 21-7 Apnea, Oculocephalic Reflex, and Oculovestibular Reflex Tests

Apnea Test

To perform an apnea test:

1. Preoxygenate the patient.
2. Disconnect the patient from the ventilator and provide oxygen, 8 to 12 L/min by tracheal cannula.
3. Observe the patient for spontaneous respirations over the next 10 minutes. The patient is considered apneic if there is no respiratory movement and the $PaCO_2$ is greater than 60 mm Hg.

 RED FLAG! *If the patient becomes unstable (hypotension, dysrhythmias, or both), immediately reconnect the patient to the ventilator and obtain an ABG.*

4. After 10 minutes, obtain arterial blood gases (ABGs); the $PaCO_2$ must be greater than 60 mm Hg for an accurate test.
5. Reconnect the patient to the ventilator.

Oculocephalic Reflex Test (Doll's Eyes Phenomenon)

Neutral position

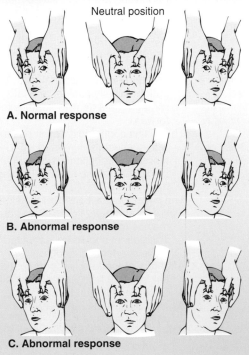

A. Normal response

B. Abnormal response

C. Abnormal response

The patient's head is quickly rotated from one side to the other while observing the patient's eyes for movement. In a normal response (A), the eyes turn together to the side opposite the head movement. In an abnormal response (B), the eyes turn together to the same side as the head movement or (C) remain fixed in the midline position.

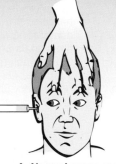 **RED FLAG!** *This test is never performed in a patient with a suspected or known spinal cord injury, or in a patient who is awake.*

Oculovestibular Reflex Test (Caloric Ice-Water Test)

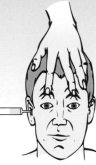

A. Normal response   **B. Abnormal response**

The patient's head is elevated 30 degrees and each ear is irrigated separately with 30 to 50 mL of ice water. In a normal response (A), the eyes exhibit horizontal nystagmus with slow, conjugate movement toward the irrigated ear followed by rapid movement away from the stimulus. In an abnormal response (B), the eyes remain fixed in midline position, indicating midbrain and pons dysfunction.

 RED FLAG! *This test is never performed in a patient who does not have an intact eardrum, a patient who has blood or fluid collected behind the eardrum, or a patient who is awake.*

the test is positive and the patient does not meet the criteria for brain death.

Confirmatory tests for brain death, such as cerebral angiography, transcranial Doppler (TCD) sonography, electroencephalography, brainstem auditory evoked response (BAER), and somatosensory evoked potential (SSEP), can be used if any doubt exists after a full clinical examination has been completed. The American Academy of Neurology (2010) recommends the clinical evaluation for brain death only be required once and not be repeated.[1] Time of death is recorded at the time that brain death is declared.

Reference

1. Eelco F, et al: American Academy of Neurology guidelines brain death. Neurology 74:1911–1918, 2010.

Want to know more? A wide variety of resources to enhance your learning and understanding of this chapter are available on **thePoint**✳. Visit **http://thepoint.lww.com/MortonEss1e** to access chapter review questions and more!

CASE STUDY

Ms. J., a 66-year-old woman, is admitted to the critical care unit after her son brought her to the emergency department because she was experiencing the sudden onset of dizziness, an unsteady gait, weakness in her left arm and leg, and a severe headache. She has a past medical history of hypertension, diabetes, hypercholesterolemia, and smoking. The initial neurological examination reveals a pleasant, anxious woman who answers questions appropriately and follows all commands. However, she exhibits questionable mild weakness of the left arm when performing hand grasps.

An hour later, the nurse observes that Ms. J. is somewhat somnolent and difficult to arouse. Her pupils are equal and reactive to light and accommodation. However, she is able to open her eyes only to repeated verbal stimuli. She does not follow commands and only moves her extremities to painful stimuli by pulling away from the stimuli. She is oriented only to self.

1. After the initial neurological examination, what additional neurological assessment might the nurse perform in order to better characterize the extremity weakness?

2. What is Ms. J.'s Glasgow Coma Scale score and what might this suggest?

3. What diagnostic tests might be ordered?

4. What nursing interventions are appropriate?

Patient Management: Nervous System

OBJECTIVES

Based on the content in this chapter, the reader should be able to:

1 Discuss intracranial dynamics affecting intracranial pressure, including the Monro–Kellie doctrine, compliance, autoregulation, and cerebral perfusion.

2 Discuss the clinical consequences of increased intracranial pressure.

3 Discuss indications for intracranial pressure monitoring.

4 Describe nursing interventions that ensure accuracy of intracranial pressure readings and waveforms.

5 Interpret data obtained through intracranial pressure monitoring.

6 Identify strategies to manage increased intracranial pressure.

7 Describe surgical interventions for treating intracranial disorders and the critical care nurse's role in caring for a patient undergoing intracranial surgery.

Intracranial Pressure Monitoring and Control

Intracranial pressure (ICP) is the pressure within the cranial vault. A normal ICP measurement ranges between 0 and 15 mm Hg. An ICP measurement greater than 20 mm Hg is considered an elevated ICP, or intracranial hypertension.

Intracranial Dynamics

The contents of the cranium can be described as three volumes: the intracranial circulation (blood), the cerebrospinal fluid (CSF), and the brain parenchyma. Because the bony cranium is rigid and non-expendable, any increase in one of the volumes must be compensated by a decrease in another to maintain normal pressure (Monro–Kellie doctrine). As long as the total intracranial volume remains the same, ICP remains constant. Increases in volume that exceed

the compensatory capabilities of the brain lead to an increase in ICP:

- **Cerebral blood flow.** Cerebral autoregulation is a protective mechanism that enables the brain to receive a consistent blood flow over a range of systemic blood pressures. In cerebral autoregulation, vessel diameter changes in response to changes in arterial pressures (ie, vessels dilate to increase cerebral blood flow and constrict to decrease cerebral blood flow). Extremes of blood pressure and brain tissue damage can result in the inability of the cerebral vessels to autoregulate. In patients with impaired autoregulation, any activity that causes an increase in blood pressure (eg, coughing, suctioning, restlessness) can increase cerebral blood flow and ICP. Other factors that induce cerebral vasodilation, thereby increasing cerebral blood volume and ICP, include hypoxia, hypercapnia, and acidosis. Hypercapnia is the most potent cerebral vasodilator.

BOX 22-1 Cerebral Edema

Cerebral edema leading to increased intracranial pressure (ICP) is a process common to multiple neurological illnesses.

- **Vasogenic edema.** The most common type of cerebral edema is vasogenic edema, which is characterized by a disruption in the blood–brain barrier and the inability of the cell walls to control movement of water in and out of the cells. Capillary permeability allows fluid to leak into the extracellular space, resulting in interstitial edema. Common processes leading to vasogenic edema include brain tumors, cerebral abscess, stroke, and cerebral trauma.
- **Cytotoxic edema.** Cytotoxic edema is characterized by swelling of the individual neurons and brain cells. Eventually the cell membrane cannot maintain an effective barrier, and both water and sodium enter the cell, causing swelling, loss of function, and cellular death. Cytotoxic edema occurs in association with anoxic and hypoxic injuries.

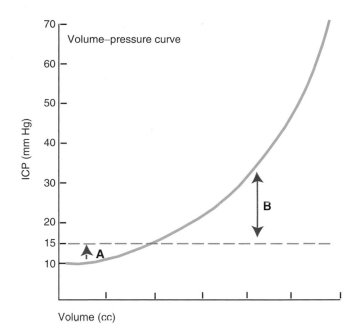

FIGURE 22-1   The intracranial volume–pressure curve demonstrates the relationship between changes in intracranial volume and changes in intracranial pressure (ICP). **A:** The ICP remains within the normal range of 0 to 15 mm Hg as long as compliance is normal and fluid can be displaced by the additional volume. **B:** Once the compensatory system is exhausted, a small additional volume causes a greater increase in pressure.

- **CSF circulation.** CSF is produced in the ventricles and circulates between the ventricles and the subarachnoid space. Increased ICP can result from overproduction of CSF, obstruction of flow, or decreased reabsorption of CSF.
- **Parenchyma.** Changes in the brain parenchyma that may increase volume include an expansile mass (eg, tumor, intracerebral hemorrhage) and cerebral edema (Box 22-1).

The ability of the intracranial contents to compensate for changes in volume depends on the location of the lesion, the rate of expansion, and compliance. A more gradual increase of volume in the cranium is better tolerated then a rapid increase in volume. Compensatory mechanisms to maintain normal ICP include shunting of CSF into the spinal subarachnoid space (by partial collapse of cisterns and ventricles), increased CSF absorption, decreased CSF production, and shunting of and compression of the venous sinuses which shunt the venous blood out of the skull. During the compensatory period, ICP remains fairly constant. However, once these compensatory mechanisms have been exhausted, pressure increases rapidly (Fig. 22-1).

With increased ICP, shifting of brain tissue toward open spaces in the skull occurs and the blood supply to brain tissue is altered, leading to ischemia, anoxic injury, and possible herniation (ie, the displacement of tissue through structures within the skull). Herniation is classified according to the compartment in which it is occurring. In the critical care setting, the most common types of herniation are uncal and central (Fig. 21-2). Uncal herniation is herniation of the medial temporal lobe (uncus) through the tentorium, where it pushes against the brainstem.

Central herniation (supratentorial) describes the downward displacement of the diencephalon and parts of the temporal lobes through the tentorium, causing compression of the brainstem. Or central herniation (infratentorial) describes a downward displacement of the brainstem into the spinal canal.

Clinical Manifestations of Increased Intracranial Pressure

RED FLAG! Early recognition of signs of increased ICP can help prevent progression to herniation. The most sensitive sign of an increased ICP is a change in level of consciousness.

Increased ICP is manifested by deterioration in all aspects of neurological functioning. Initially, the patient may be restless, confused, or combative. The level of consciousness decompensates, ranging from lethargy to obtundation to coma. Pupillary reactions become sluggish or fixed. Motor function also declines, and the patient begins to show abnormal motor activity (posturing) or absent motor activity. Changes in vital signs are considered a late finding. Variations in respiratory patterns occur, eventually resulting in complete apnea. Cushing's triad (increased systolic pressure, bradycardia, and widened pulse pressure) is considered a sign of impending herniation. Clinical manifestations of increased ICP and herniation are compared in Table 22-1.

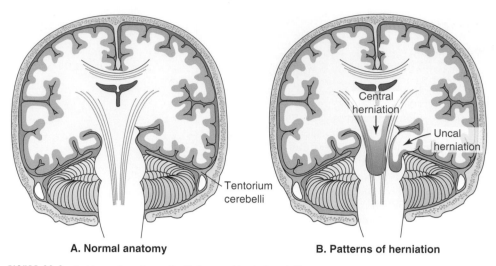

Central
herniation

Uncal
herniation

Tentorium
cerebelli

A. Normal anatomy   **B. Patterns of herniation**

FIGURE 22-2   **A:** Normal anatomy. **B:** Patterns of brain herniation.

Intracranial Pressure Monitoring

ICP monitoring is an invasive technique that provides information about the pressure within the cranial vault and the likelihood of cerebral herniation, facilitates calculation of cerebral perfusion pressure (CPP), assists in guiding treatments to lower the ICP (eg, mannitol, barbiturates), and allows for the drainage of CSF to lower the ICP. For ICP monitoring to be safe and effective, the indications for monitoring, methods of monitoring, and risks versus benefits must be taken into account for each patient. Other factors that affect patient selection include findings on clinical and radiographic evaluation, the patient's diagnosis and prognosis, and the availability of the appropriate level of critical care. Indications and contraindications for ICP monitoring are summarized in Box 22-2.

Various devices are used to monitor ICP. Monitoring systems are named according to where the tip of the catheter is placed (Fig. 22-3). Monitoring can be performed with a fluid-filled system connected to an external transducer or a fiberoptic system, which uses a catheter with a fiberoptic transducer at the end. Fiberoptic systems are versatile; the fiberoptic catheter can be inserted into the ventricle, the subarachnoid space, or the brain parenchyma to monitor pressure. However, the fiberoptic catheter is fragile, and fiberoptic systems are associated with higher costs than fluid-filled systems. Advantages and disadvantages of various types of ICP monitoring systems are summarized in Table 22-2.

 RED FLAG! To prevent infection when a patient is undergoing ICP monitoring, maintain aseptic technique when assembling, manipulating, or accessing fluid-filled systems.

Ensuring Accuracy

Leveling

If a fiberoptic catheter is used, the transducer is located at the tip of the catheter and does not require any external leveling. If an external transducer is used, it must be leveled appropriately to maintain consistency among measurements. The most common external landmark for leveling the transducer is either the external auditory canal (EAC) or the outer canthus of the eye.

TABLE 22-1   **Increased Intracranial Pressure (ICP) Versus Herniation**

	Increased ICP	Herniation
Level of arousal	Increased stimulus required	Unarousable
Motor function	Subtle motor weakness or pronator drift	Dense motor weakness, posturing or absent response
Pupillary response	Sluggish pupillary response	One or both pupils may dilate or become pinpoint and nonreactive, depending on the location of injury
		• One pupil dilating and becoming nonreactive while the other continues to react to light indicates uncal herniation on the ipsilateral side of the nonreactive pupil
		• Bilateral, dilated nonreactive pupils indicate central herniation
Vital signs	May be stable or labile	Cushing's triad (increased systolic blood pressure, bradycardia, widened pulse pressure)

BOX 22-2 Indications and Contraindications for Intracranial Pressure (ICP) Monitoring

Possible Indications
- Stroke
- Brain tumor
- Postcardiac arrest
- Craniotomy
- Coma
- Severe brain injury (GCS score of 3 to 8)
- Subarachnoid hemorrhage
- Intracerebral hemorrhage
- Ischemic infarction
- Hydrocephalus

Relative Contraindications
- Coagulopathy
- Systemic infection
- Central nervous system (CNS) infection
- Infection at the site of device insertion

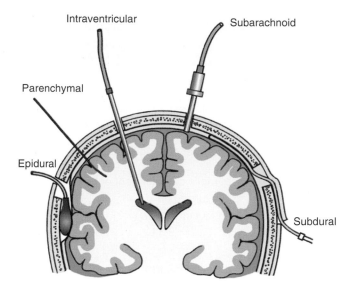

FIGURE 22-3 Intracranial pressure (ICP) monitoring systems.

RED FLAG! *A transducer that is too low will produce falsely high ICP measurements, whereas a transducer that is too high will produce falsely low measurements. Erroneous measurements can result in the patient receiving unnecessary treatments, or not receiving appropriate and necessary treatments.*

Troubleshooting
To ensure accurate measurements and reduce morbidity, the nurse must be alert to problems associated with ICP monitoring systems that could cause incorrect ICP measurements (Table 22-3).

TABLE 22-2 Advantages and Disadvantages of Intracranial Pressure (ICP) Monitoring Systems

Monitoring System	Advantages	Disadvantages
Intraventricular	• Very accurate • True central direct measure of ICP • Allows for CSF drainage to decrease ICP • Can obtain CSF samples • Can be used to administer intrathecal medications	• Transducer must be repositioned with changes in elevation of the head of the bed • High risk for CNS infection • Difficult insertion in patients with small or displaced ventricles • Risk for intracerebral bleeding or edema along the cannula track • Greater risk of CSF leak, catheter displacement or obstruction
Parenchymal	• Ease of insertion • Provides true brain pressures	• CNS infections less common • Unable to obtain CSF samples or drain CSF
Epidural	• Low risk for infections • Not necessary to reposition the transducer with changes in elevation of the head of the bed	• Not as accurate • Unable to recalibrate once device is placed • Unable to obtain CSF samples or drain CSF
Subarachnoid	• More accurate than epidural • Easier to insert than intraventricular	• Unable to obtain CSF samples or drain CSF • Risk for infection • Risk for CSF leak • Requires an intact skull
Lumbar	• Simple-to-do single readings • No penetration of the brain parenchyma • Decreased risk for infection • Can sample CSF • Permits direct pressure management	• Contraindicated with evidence of increased ICP • Transducer must be repositioned with changes in height of bed

TABLE 22-3 Troubleshooting Intracranial Pressure (ICP) Monitoring Systems

Problem	Cause	Intervention
No waveform	Air between the transducer diaphragm and pressure source	Eliminate air bubbles with sterile saline.
	Occlusion of intracranial measurement device with blood or debris	Flush intracranial catheter, using sterile technique, as directed by physician: 0.25 mL sterile saline is often used.
	Transducer connected incorrectly	Check connection, and be sure the appropriate connector for amplifier is in use.
	Fiberoptic catheter bent or broken	Assist with replacing fiberoptic catheter.
	Trace turned off	Turn power on to trace.
False high-pressure reading	Transducer too low	Place the venting port of the transducer at the level of the external auditory canal. For every inch (2.54 cm) the transducer is below the pressure source, there is an error of approximately 2 mm Hg.
	External transducer incorrectly zeroed	With transducer correctly positioned, rezero. Transducer should be zeroed q4h and before the initiation of treatment based on a pressure change.
	Monitoring system incorrectly calibrated with external transducer	Repeat calibration procedures.
	Air in system (air may attenuate or amplify pressure signal)	Remove air from monitoring line.
High-pressure reading	Airway not patent: an increase in intrathoracic pressure may increase $PaCO_2$	Suction patient. Position. Initiate chest physiotherapy. Draw arterial blood gases (ABGs); hypoxia and hypercarbia cause increases in ICP.
	Ventilator setting incorrect, positive end-expiratory pressure (PEEP)	Check ventilator settings.
	Patient position	Elevate head of bed 30 degrees unless contraindicated (eg, due to fracture) to facilitate venous drainage. Limit knee flexion. Avoid acute hip flexion.
	Excessive muscle activity, hyperthermia, or infection	Initiate measures to control muscle movement (eg, relaxants, paralyzing agents), infection, and pyrexia.
	Fluid and electrolyte imbalance secondary to fluid restrictions and diuretics	Draw blood for serum electrolytes, serum osmolality. Note pulmonary artery pressure. Evaluate input and output with specific gravity.
	Blood pressure: vasopressor responses occur in some patients with elevating ICP.	Use measures to maintain adequate continuous positive pressure.
	Low blood pressure associated with hypovolemia, shock, and barbiturate coma may increase cerebral ischemia.	
False low-pressure reading	Air bubbles between transducer and cerebrospinal fluid (CSF)	Eliminate air bubbles with sterile saline.
	Transducer level too high	Place the venting port of the transducer at the level of the external auditory canal. For every inch (2.54 cm) the transducer is above the level of the pressure source, there will be an error of approximately 2 mm Hg.
Low-pressure reading	Transducer incorrectly zeroed or calibrated	Rezero and calibrate monitoring system.
	Collapse of ventricles around catheter	If external ventricular drainage (EVD) is being used, there may be inadequate positive pressure. Check to make sure a positive pressure of 15–20 mm Hg exists. Drain CSF slowly.
	Otorrhea or rhinorrhea	These conditions cause a false low-pressure reading secondary to decompression. Document the correlation between drainage and pressure changes.
	Leakage of fluid from connections	Eliminate all fluid leakage.
	Dislodgment of catheter from ventricle into brain	Contact physician.
	Occlusion of the end of a subarachnoid screw by brain tissue	Contact physician; in most cases, screw must be removed.

RED FLAG! *Flushing the catheter using a syringe and sterile 0.9% normal saline from an IV bag may be necessary if there is a dampened waveform or occlusion in the tubing. Never use heparinized saline or bacteriostatic water. Always flush the catheter away from the patient's head; do not flush the catheter toward the patient's head with the stopcocks open. Flush devices (used in hemodynamic monitoring) are never used in ICP monitoring.*

Data Interpretation

The ICP monitor displays digital values and waveforms. ICP waveforms are monitored as well as the actual ICP reading. A normal ICP waveform may demonstrate three descending peaks that correlate with hemodynamic changes (Fig. 22-4):

- **P1,** the pressure wave, which is fairly consistent in shape and amplitude, originates from choroid plexus pulsations and correlates with systole.
- **P2,** the tidal wave, is more variable in shape and amplitude and ends on the dicrotic notch (which signals the beginning of diastole). P2 most directly reflects the state of intracerebral compliance. As the mean ICP rises (signaling decreasing intracerebral compliance), P2 progressively elevates, causing the pulse wave to appear more rounded. When intracerebral compliance is decreased, P2 is equal to or higher than P1.
- **P3,** the dicrotic wave, follows the dicrotic notch and tapers down to the diastolic position unless retrograde venous pulsations cause a few more peaks.

Some patients experience periods of elevated ICP. The severity is determined by the degree of ICP elevation and the length of time the ICP remains elevated. Sustained periods (greater than 5 minutes) of ICPs greater than 20 mm Hg are considered significant and can be extremely dangerous. Sustained periods of ICPs greater than 60 mm Hg are usually fatal. Plotting ICP measurements over time produces trend patterns that are frequently referred to as A, B, or C waves (Fig. 22-5).

- **A waves (plateau waves)** are produced by spontaneous, rapid increases of pressure ranging from 20 to 50 mm Hg over a period of 20 minutes or more. Periods of elevated ICP that produce A waves are associated with deteriorating neurological status.
- **B waves** are produced by ICPs up to 50 mmHg over an extended period of time (usually longer than 5 minutes but less than 20 minutes). The resulting trend pattern is characterized by small, sharp, rhythmic waves. B waves correspond with decreased intracerebral compliance and are an early indication of deteriorating neurological status.
- **C waves** are produced by ICPs as high as 20 to 25 mm Hg that persist for less than 5 minutes. The resultant pattern is characterized by small, rhythmic waves. C waves are considered normal responses to changes in ICP and are not treated.

Cerebral Oxygenation Monitoring

Monitoring the amount of oxygen the brain tissue is receiving is an important component of monitoring and managing increased ICP. Patients with brain injury or increased ICP are at risk for hypoperfusion and ischemia of the brain tissue. Neuronal demand for oxygen is governed by the cell's metabolic needs, which increase during neuronal activity

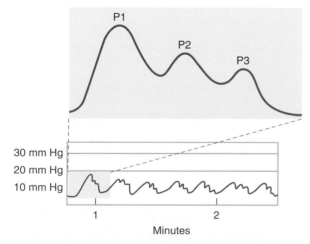

FIGURE 22-4 The intracranial pressure (ICP) waveform. Each pulse wave on the tracing is comprised of three descending peaks, termed P1, P2, and P3.

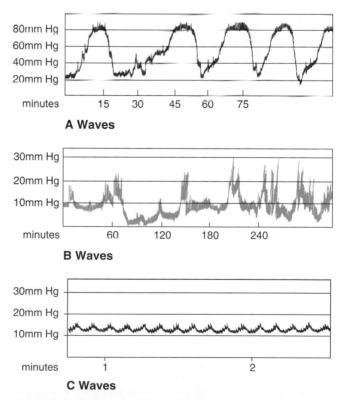

FIGURE 22-5 Plotting of extended periods of increased intracranial pressure (ICP) measurements over time results in patterns called A waves, B waves, and C waves.

TABLE 22-4 Interpretation of Mixed Venous Oxygen Saturation (SjO2) Readings

Reading	Interpretation
Normal (50–75%)	Oxygen consumption and delivery are balanced.
Decreased (less than 50%)	Decreased oxygen delivery Increased oxygen utilization
Increased (greater than 85%)	Hyperemia with increased cerebral blood flow Shunting of blood away from neurons Decrease in cerebral metabolic rate for oxygen ($CMRO_2$), indicative of cell death or brain death

temperature, and the partial pressure of oxygen in brain tissue ($PtiO_2$) are inserted into the brain parenchyma. The normal $PtiO_2$ is 25 to 35 mm Hg. The goal is to maintain a $PtiO_2$ of greater than 20 mm Hg.

• **Jugular venous bulb oximetry** is an invasive technique for studying oxygen delivery and oxygen consumption in the brain that involves placing a sampling catheter in the internal jugular vein, with the tip of the catheter at the jugular venous bulb. Blood samples from this location measure the mixed venous oxygen saturation (SjO_2) of blood leaving the brain. Interpretation of SjO_2 readings is summarized in Table 22-4. It is important to note that SjO_2 is a measure of global cerebral oxygenation and is not sensitive to small areas of focal ischemia.

Managing Increased Intracranial Pressure

Although no single management routine is appropriate for all patients, the goals of treatment for the patient with increased ICP are to reduce ICP, optimize CPP, and avoid brain herniation. Nursing responsibilities related to minimizing ICP are summarized in Table 22-5.

Measures to reduce ICP are usually initiated when the patient's ICP increases to approximately 20 mm Hg or greater. First-tier (conventional) therapies include CSF drainage, mannitol, respiratory support, and sedation and analgesia. Second-tier therapies, employed for refractory increased ICP, include neuromuscular blockade, barbiturate coma, optimized hyperventilation, hypothermia, and decompressive craniectomy. Figure 22-6 provides an algorithm for the treatment of increased ICP.

or injury. Methods of monitoring cerebral oxygenation include CPP monitoring, brain tissue oxygen monitoring, and jugular venous bulb oximetry:

• **CPP monitoring.** The CPP can be calculated at the bedside to estimate cerebral blood flow: CPP = MAP – ICP, where MAP is the mean arterial pressure and ICP is the intracranial pressure A normal CPP is 60 to 100 mm Hg. A CPP of 40 to 60 mm Hg indicates hypoperfusion, and a CPP of less than 40 mm Hg indicates anoxia. The ICP and CPP are recorded hourly.

• **Brain tissue oxygen monitoring.** CPP, while useful, does not measure all aspects of brain perfusion, oxygen delivery, and oxygen demand. CPP calculations provide only an estimate of the amount of oxygen the brain tissue is receiving, whereas brain tissue oxygen monitoring allows for regional precise measurement. In brain tissue oxygen monitoring, sensors that directly measure the ICP, the brain

TABLE 22-5 Nursing Care of Patients at Risk for Increased Intracranial Pressure (ICP)

Nursing Responsibility	Nursing Action	Rationale
Ensure adequate ventilation	• Assess respiratory patterns and rate.	• Indicates neurological changes, pain status, and patency of airway
	• Suctioning: Preoxygenate with 100% O_2, one or two catheter passes, no more than 10 s per catheter insertion.	• Prevents increased CO_2 (vasodilator that increases ICP); decreases coughing stimulation and increased intrathoracic pressure
	• Monitor continuous pulse oximetry and blood gases.	• Alerts nurse to airway and respiratory problems
Manage blood pressure	• Administer vasopressors or antihypertensives as ordered to manipulate MAP and maintain an effective CPP.	• Blood pressure is directly related to cerebral blood volume, perfusion pressure, ischemia, and compliance
Perform neurological assessments	• Evaluate patient's baseline neurological status at beginning of shift (preferably with previous shift registered nurse [RN])—mental status; pupil shape, size, and response; motor function.	• Subtle changes from baseline indicate deterioration and the need for early intervention.
	• Assess vital signs—note trends (review ordered parameters for notification of physician).	• MAP directly correlates with ICP in patient with loss of autoregulation.
	• Review nursing actions and emergency algorithm for neurologic deterioration.	• Ensures optimal patient care and decreases secondary injury from prolonged ICP

TABLE 22-5 **Nursing Care of Patients at Risk for Increased Intracranial Pressure (ICP)** (continued)

Nursing Responsibility	Nursing Action	Rationale
Positioning	• Place head of bed flat or at 30° to 45° elevation per orders.	• Promotes cerebral perfusion or facilitates venous drainage; orders based on physiological process
	• Maintain head in neutral position.	• Promotes jugular outflow
	• Avoid hip flexion.	• Decreases intrathoracic pressure and ICP
	• Assess agitation in restrained patients.	• Increases ICP
	• Turn patient q2h, instructing patient to exhale with turn.	• Prevents skin breakdown and avoids Valsalva maneuver during repositioning
	• Carry out passive range-of-motion exercises.	• Prevents contractures while avoiding Valsalva-inducing isometric contractions
	• Avoid clustering of patient activities (eg, turning, bathing, suctioning).	• Prevents prolonged ICP spikes
	• Minimize unpleasant environmental stimuli—speak with soft voice, use caution with unpleasant conversations, decrease noise, use therapeutic touch.	• Unpleasant stimuli cause elevations in ICP
Transport patient with invasive ICP monitor	• Confirm time of test or possibility of completing as portable study.	• Avoids excessive delays in uncontrolled and potentially overstimulating environment
	• Prepare respiratory therapy and other assistants during transport.	• Adequate oxygenation remains a priority; multiple lines necessitate additional personnel
	• Gather transport supplies (sedation if ordered, transport monitor, antihypertensives).	• Adverse patient responses during travel can increase ICP
	• Assist with transfer of patient to diagnostic table with RN at head of bed monitoring device.	• Ensures patient protection and provides for monitor equipment recalibration for accuracy of monitoring
	• Monitor and record hemodynamics and ICP dynamics during study.	• Monitors patient response to procedure
Temperature control	• Check temperature frequently (oral or rectal route preferred if no contraindications).	• Cerebral metabolic rate increases with elevated body temperature.
	• Confirm orders for early treatment of fever and aggressively treat.	• Increased cerebral blood flow increases ICP
	• Provide gradual cooling with cooling blanket, closely monitored.	• Shivering increases ICP
Glycemic control	• Monitor serum glucose and fingersticks as ordered (q4–6h)—adhere closely to sliding scale protocols in nondiabetic patients.	• Alterations in glucose can produce changes in metabolic rate; elevated glucose worsens neurological outcomes.
	• Maintain euvolemia with normal saline; avoid hypotonic solutions.	• Hypotonic solutions increase cerebral edema.
Bowel and bladder regimens	• Administer daily stool softeners as ordered.	• Reduces risk for straining and increased intra-abdominal pressure, which increases ICP
	• Avoid enemas.	• Prevents Valsalva maneuver
	• Assess patency of Foley catheters.	• Important to monitor amount of diuresis, especially in patients treated with osmotic diuretics
	• Document strict intake and output.	• Important to maintain euvolemia
Seizure prevention and treatment	• Implement seizure precautions per hospital protocol.	• Seizure activity markedly elevates the cerebral metabolic rate and cerebral blood flow.
	• Monitor serum anticonvulsant drug levels.	• Maintains therapeutic levels

Cerebrospinal Fluid Drainage

Intraventricular catheters are widely used in the critical care setting because they allow both monitoring of the ICP and draining of CSF to lower the ICP (Fig. 22-7). When an intraventricular catheter is being used for external ventricular drainage (EVD) of CSF, the physician order will state whether the drainage is to be intermittent or continuous. If intermittent drainage is ordered, the physician will specify the ICP level at which drainage should be initiated (eg, ICP greater than 20 mm Hg). If continuous drainage is ordered, the physician will specify the level of the drainage system (eg, 10 cm above the external auditory canal). The height of the drainage system determines the rapidity and amount of drainage; the lower the drainage system, the more rapid and the greater amount of drainage.

RED FLAG! *Because the rate of CSF drainage is determined by the level of the drainage system relative to the patient, it is very important to maintain the ordered level consistently.*

RED FLAG! *To ensure accuracy of ICP measurements, it is important to turn off the stopcock to drainage before obtaining the ICP measurement in most monitoring systems.*

Mannitol

Mannitol, a hypertonic crystalloid solution that decreases cerebral edema by increasing intravascular osmolality, is typically administered as a bolus IV infusion over 10 to 30 minutes in doses ranging from 0.25 to 2 g/kg body weight. The immediate plasma-expanding effect of mannitol reduces blood viscosity, which in turn increases cerebral blood flow and cerebral oxygen metabolism, permitting

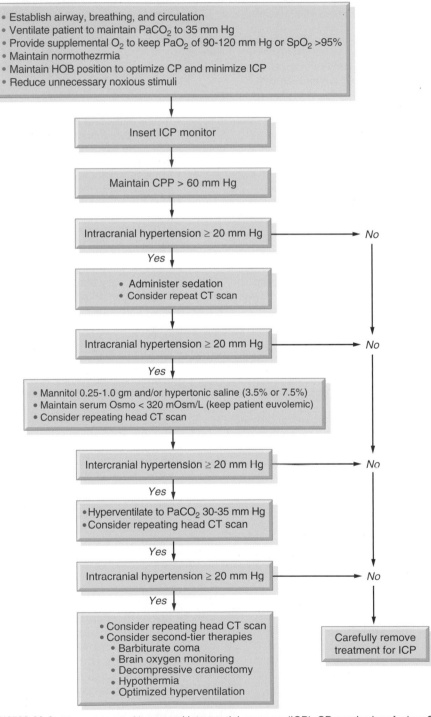

FIGURE 22-6 Management of increased intracranial pressure (ICP). CP, cerebral perfusion; CPP, cerebral perfusion pressure; HOB, head of bed.

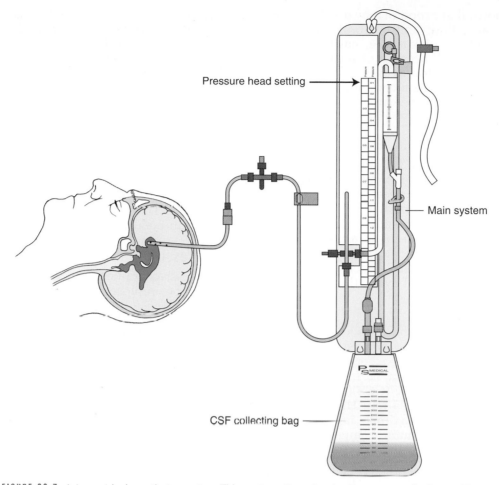

FIGURE 22-7 Intraventricular catheter system. This system allows for simultaneous monitoring and treatment of increased intracranial pressure (ICP) by intermittently draining cerebrospinal fluid (CSF). (Courtesy of Medtronic Neurologic Technologies, Goleta, California.)

cerebral arterioles to decrease in diameter. This lowers cerebral blood volume and ICP, while maintaining constant cerebral blood flow. Hypertonic saline (3.5% or 7.5%) is also effective for this application.[1] Because mannitol induces diuresis, isotonic crystalloid solutions may be infused to correct or prevent hypovolemia.

RED FLAG! *If mannitol is administered in large doses and serum osmolality is greater than 320 mOsm, there is a significant risk for acute tubular necrosis (ATN) and renal failure. redOsmolality measurements must be obtained every 6 to 8 hours and mannitol must be held if the serum osmolality exceeds 320 mOsm.*

Respiratory Support

Increased ICP can cause erratic breathing patterns. Many patients with elevated ICP or altered level of consciousness require mechanical ventilation to maintain adequate oxygenation and manage carbon dioxide levels. However, positive-pressure ventilation and high levels of positive end-expiratory pressure (PEEP) increase intrathoracic pressures. Increased intrathoracic pressures decrease venous

drainage from the brain and lower cardiac output, thereby decreasing cerebral blood flow and increasing the ICP.

Suctioning is performed only as necessary, and care must be taken to avoid hypoxemia and increased intrathoracic pressures. Limiting the duration of passes of the suction catheter to no more than 5 to 10 seconds and limiting the number of passes to one or two avoids overstimulation of the cough reflex and decreases the incidence of increased intrathoracic pressure and ICP.

Sedation and Analgesia

Analgesics and sedatives may be administered to

- Reduce agitation, discomfort, and pain
- Facilitate mechanical ventilation by suppressing coughing
- Limit responses to stimuli, such as suctioning, which may increase ICP

Propofol is a fat-soluble anesthetic that is administered as a continuous infusion to decrease agitation in the critically ill patient. Due to the respiratory depression that can occur with propofol, patients must be intubated and mechanically ventilated.

Studies have shown that propofol may decrease ICP, CPP, cerebral blood flow, and cerebral metabolic function.[2] Propofol is quick-acting, easily titrated to patient response, and, because of its short half-life, easily discontinued for frequent neurological assessments. Hypotension is a common side effect; therefore, frequent blood pressure monitoring is necessary.

Neuromuscular Blockade

Neuromuscular blockade is a "last resort" therapy to decrease the brain's demand for oxygen and lower the ICP. Neuromuscular blockade necessitates mechanical ventilation with full support. For a conscious patient, the inability to move and communicate is frightening; therefore, concurrent administration of analgesia and sedation is mandatory. Complications associated with neuromuscular blockade include tachycardia, hypotension, and dysrhythmias.

Barbiturate Coma

For the patient with severe and refractory elevated ICP, a barbiturate coma may be induced to decrease metabolic activity and preserve brain function. Criteria for the induction of a barbiturate coma include a Glasgow Coma Scale (GCS) score of less than 7; an ICP greater than 25 mm Hg at rest for 10 minutes; and failed maximal interventions, including CSF drainage, mannitol, analgesia, and sedation. Barbiturate coma is typically used for less than 72 hours.

Before the administration of barbiturates, a secure airway with mechanical ventilation; ICP, blood pressure, and cardiac monitoring; and continuous electroencephalogram (EEG) monitoring must be established. EEG monitoring is used to establish barbiturate dosing (the barbiturate is dosed to the ordered level of burst suppression). Barbiturate serum levels alone are poor guides for evaluating therapeutic efficacy and systemic toxicity.

Barbiturates are discontinued with any of the following clinical findings:

- ICP less than 15 mm Hg for 24 to 72 hours
- Systolic blood pressure less than 90 mm Hg despite the use of vasopressors
- Progressive neurological impairment, as evidenced by deterioration of brainstem auditory evoked responses (BAER)
- Cardiac arrest

At the time of discontinuation, the barbiturate is tapered gradually over 24 to 72 hours.

Hyperventilation

Normocapnia (an arterial carbon dioxide tension [$PaCO_2$] of 35 to 40 mm Hg) is essential for the maintenance of stable ICP. Hyperventilation decreases the $PaCO_2$, resulting in cerebral vasoconstriction and a lowering of ICP. Hyperventilation to achieve a $PaCO_2$ of 30 to 35 mm Hg may become necessary for brief periods when there is acute neurological deterioration, or if increased ICP is refractory to other therapies. However, in the absence of a malignant increase in ICP, hyperventilation therapy should be avoided because it can compromise cerebral perfusion during a time of critically reduced cerebral blood flow.[3]

Hypothermia

Hypothermia is controversial but continues to be studied as a means for reducing the brain's metabolic demands during peak times of cerebral edema and brain injury. It is currently recommended therapy for the postresuscitation patient who remains unconscious. There are currently no recommendations for routine use in other neurological patients.

Decompressive Craniectomy

Decompressive craniectomy (surgical decompression) may be employed to manage refractory intracranial hypertension. In decompressive craniectomy, part of the skull (called a "bone flap") is removed to relieve brain swelling. The bone flap is replaced at a later date, after the swelling has decreased. Studies of patients with massive cerebral edema and refractory intracranial hypertension after ischemic stroke have shown varying results when comparing outcomes after surgical decompression and outcomes after best medical management.[4] However, the procedure remains widely used for patients with malignant cerebral edema after traumatic brain injury.

Intracranial Surgery

Intracranial surgery may be performed to

- Obtain tissue for pathological diagnosis
- Remove an abnormal mass or space-occupying lesion (eg, tumor, cyst, hemorrhage) and reduce mass effect
- Repair an abnormality (eg, aneurysm)
- Place a device (eg, shunt, reservoir)

Craniotomy

In craniotomy, a section of the skull is removed to facilitate accessing the brain underneath, and then replaced. Craniotomy is performed to remove space-occupying lesions (eg, tumors, cysts, vascular malformations), to evacuate hematomas, or to reverse herniation. Craniotomy may also be used to clip an aneurysm. Adjunct modalities may be used during surgery to maximize safety and efficiency:

- Ultrasonography can distinguish abnormal lesions from normal brain tissue and edema, enabling identification of residual abnormal tissue before closing.
- Stereotaxy uses a rigid head frame to locate the lesion and establish appropriate coordinates. Next, a contrast-enhanced computed tomography

(CT) scan or magnetic resonance imaging (MRI) scan displays an axial image of the lesion with a number of coordinates to indicate entry points. Frameless stereotaxy can be performed using CT or MRI before the procedure to place markers (fiducials) on the scalp. Stereotaxy enhances surgical safety and effectiveness by reducing craniotomy size, minimizing brain manipulation, and maximizing lesion resection.

- Cortical mapping is used for masses in eloquent areas of the brain (ie, the brainstem and the speech, motor, and visual areas) and can be performed using "awake" craniotomy or functional MRI.
- Somatosensory evoked potentials are recorded during surgery under general anesthesia to assess the relationship between the motor strip and the lesion to be resected. Direct cortical stimulation in "awake" craniotomies provides localization of the sensory–motor cortex and is also used to maximize lesion removal and minimize neurological deficits.

Major risks of intracranial surgery include cerebral edema and intracerebral hemorrhage. Postoperative management of the patient who has undergone a craniotomy includes monitoring for these complications. If there is a significant neurological change from the baseline examination, radiographic evaluation for hemorrhage or cerebral edema is indicated. Other postoperative interventions include early ambulation to avoid pulmonary and cardiovascular complications; physical and occupational therapy evaluations; speech and cognitive assessments (when indicated); deep vein thrombosis (DVT) and pulmonary embolism prophylaxis; and wound evaluation and care.

Transsphenoidal and Transnasal Surgeries

Transsphenoidal and transnasal surgeries are used in many centers to remove pituitary tumors and cysts. If there is evidence of a CSF leak at the time of surgery, the cavity is packed with fat tissue, typically taken from the patient's abdomen. These procedures are usually well tolerated. Postoperative care is aimed at increasing mobility, monitoring respiration, evaluating fluid and electrolyte balance, and observing for evidence of CSF leak and pneumocephalus (air within the cranium). Nasal splints are removed 2 to 4 days after surgery.

Carotid Endarterectomy

In patients with high-grade carotid stenosis (greater than 70%), carotid endarterectomy may be performed to prevent a stroke. Carotid endarterectomy is a surgical procedure in which atherosclerotic plaque that has accumulated inside the carotid artery is surgically removed, restoring blood flow.

Brain injury, local nerve injury, or both may occur. Several cranial nerves traverse the surgical area and can be exposed to trauma. Perioperative stroke occurs in approximately 3% of patients. Neurological assessment includes monitoring level of consciousness, pupil reactivity, eye movement, orientation, appropriateness of response, and motor function (flexion, extension, and hand grips) for the first 24 hours.

Hyperperfusion syndrome occurs in patients with high-grade stenosis. Theoretically, the hemisphere distal to the stenotic area has experienced hypoperfusion that causes the small blood vessels to remain maximally dilated with a loss of autoregulation. Once the stenosis is repaired, autoregulation is still paralyzed, but a marked increase in blood flow occurs that cannot be controlled with vasoconstriction to protect the capillaries. Edema or hemorrhage to the area results. Strict blood pressure control is imperative.

CASE STUDY

Mr. H., a 56-year-old retired man, collapsed while watching television. Before collapsing, he experienced the acute onset of right arm and leg weakness, right facial weakness, and difficulty speaking. Mr. H. was transported by ambulance to the closest hospital and evaluated for suspected acute stroke. In the emergency department (ED), the stroke work-up suggests a large ischemic infarct involving the middle cerebral artery (MCA). Mr. H. is ineligible for thrombolytic therapy because the time of symptom onset was unknown. His wife gives the following history:

- Allergies: none
- Medical history: family history of stroke, obesity, cigarette smoking, hypertension, hypercholesterolemia
- Surgical history: none
- Social history: retired military computer analyst, married with supportive wife, three biological children, aged 28, 26, and 25, and all healthy; social ingestion of alcohol; smoking history 1 pack per day for 35 years
- Medications: lisinopril, 20 mg/d; atorvastatin (Lipitor), 10 mg/d

Mr. H. is admitted to the neuroscience critical care unit for acute stroke management. Because of his large left MCA stroke, he is at risk for cerebral edema, seizure, and worsening of his stroke. During the first 24 hours, he shows no change in neurological status, and his vital signs remain stable. On day 2, his neurological examination shows a decrease in level of consciousness, a decrease in heart rate to 55 beats/min, and an increase in blood pressure to 200/110 mm Hg. He requires immediate intubation for airway protection. The nurse suspects that Mr. H. is experiencing increased ICP due to either cerebral edema or hemorrhagic conversion of the ischemic stroke territory. Laboratory samples are sent for testing, and a stat CT scan is obtained. The neurology specialist and neurosurgeon are notified of the rapid change in Mr. H.'s status.

The CT scan reveals massive cerebral edema with midline shift (no hemorrhage noted). On arrival back at the neuroscience critical care unit, Mr. H. is given his first dose of mannitol, and based on osmolality levels, the dose is repeated every 6 hours. The neurosurgeon places an intraventricular catheter for external ventricular drainage (EVD) under sterile conditions at the bedside. Mr. H.'s initial ICP is 32 mm Hg. The nurse monitors his ICP and CPP on an hourly basis and provides nursing interventions to assist in decreasing ICP and improving CPP, including maintaining a quiet environment, limiting nursing activities, and avoiding flexion and extension of the neck. The patient's blood pressure decreases, and he does not require antihypertensive medications.

On day 3, Mr. H. experiences a generalized tonic–clonic seizure, which is treated with diazepam and a phenytoin load, with daily phenytoin administration. He is taken to CT, and the scan is negative for hemorrhage. On day 4, his ICP has been less than 15 mm Hg for more than 24 hours, and the intraventricular catheter is removed. On day 5, he is extubated. He is alert enough to understand what is being said to him. At this time, Mr. H. is formally evaluated by physical, speech, and occupational therapists. Because he fails a swallowing evaluation, a PEG tube is placed.

During his hospital stay, Mr. H. receives prophylaxis for stress ulcers and DVT, as well as aspirin for stroke prevention. His lipid panel reveals that his atorvastatin needs to be increased. He remains on lisinopril for hypertension. Diagnostic studies to determine the stroke etiology include a transthoracic echocardiogram, which reveals a normal ejection fraction, no right-to-left shunting, and no valvular abnormalities or vegetation. A carotid duplex ultrasound does not reveal significant carotid stenosis.

Until discharge, Mr. H.'s vital signs and clinical status remain stable. His residual neurological deficits include significant hemiparesis on the right side and dysarthria. Mr. H. is transferred to a stroke rehabilitation facility for aggressive stroke rehabilitation.

1. Describe other noninvasive approaches that the nurse might incorporate into Mr. H.'s care in order to reduce intracranial pressure (ICP).

2. Describe the potential complications that Mr. H. might experience while the intraventricular catheter for ICP monitoring is in place.

3. Does the neurological worsening that Mr. H. experiences on day 2 occur at a "typical" time point for patients with neurological injury? Explain.

References

1. Hinson H, Stein D, Sheth K: Hypertonic saline and mannitol therapy in critical care neurology. J Intensive Care Med 26:4, 2011
2. Section VII Neurosurgical Anesthesia: Fleisher L (ed): Evidence-based Practice of Anesthesiology, 2nd ed. Philadelphia, PA: Elsevier, 2009
3. Brain Trauma Foundation, American Association of Neurological Surgeons, Joint Section on Neurotrauma and Critical Care: Guidelines for the management of severe traumatic brain injury, 2007
4. Cooper D, et al.: Decompressive craniectomy in diffuse traumatic brain injury. N Eng J Med 364:1493–1502, 2011

Want to know more? A wide variety of resources to enhance your learning and understanding of this chapter are available on thePoint✻. Visit **http://thepoint.lww.com/MortonEss1e** to access chapter review questions and more!

Common Neurosurgical and Neurological Disorders

OBJECTIVES

Based on the content in this chapter, the reader should be able to:

1 Describe the pathophysiology, assessment, and management of traumatic brain injury (TBI) in the critically ill patient.
2 Describe the pathophysiology, assessment, and management of brain tumors.
3 Describe the pathophysiology, assessment, and management of two common causes of cerebral hemorrhage, aneurysm, and arteriovenous malformation.
4 Describe the pathophysiology, assessment, and management of stroke in the critically ill patient.
5 Describe the pathophysiology, assessment, and management of seizures in the critically ill patient.
6 Describe the assessment and management of spinal cord injury in the critically ill patient.

Traumatic Brain Injury

Traumatic brain injury (TBI) occurs when the head strikes an object or an object strikes the head. It can also be an object penetrates the skull and enters the brain tissue. Leading causes of TBI include falls, motor vehicle crashes (MVCs), and gunshot wounds. Typical mechanisms of injury (Fig. 23-1) include:

- **Acceleration injuries:** a moving object strikes the stationary head
- **Acceleration–deceleration injuries:** the head in motion strikes a stationary object
- **Coup–contrecoup injuries:** the brain "bounces" back and forth within the skull, striking both sides of the brain
- **Rotation injuries:** the brain twists within the skull, resulting in stretching and tearing of blood vessels and shearing of neurons

- **Penetration injuries:** a sharp object disrupts the integrity of the skull and penetrates the brain tissue

The resultant injuries range from mild to severe (Table 23-1). Many patients die from their injuries or are left in a coma or persistent vegetative state. TBI can have a profound and lasting effect on the patient and family. For example, emotional and behavioral changes may affect interpersonal relationships and family roles, or neurologic deficits may affect the patient's ability to resume a chosen career or return to work at all.

Primary Brain Injury

Primary brain injuries are injuries occurring at the time of trauma. Primary injuries include scalp lacerations, fractures, concussions, contusions,

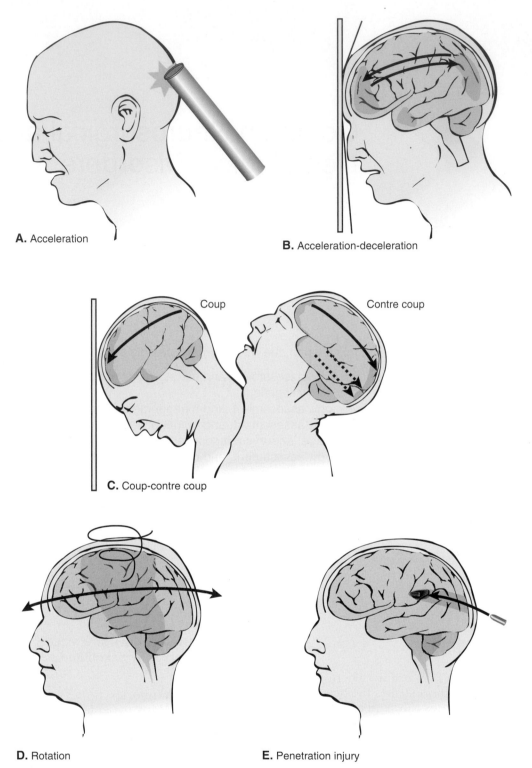

A. Acceleration

B. Acceleration-deceleration

Coup   Contre coup

C. Coup-contre coup

D. Rotation   **E.** Penetration injury

FIGURE 23-1 Typical mechanisms of traumatic brain injury (TBI).

hematomas, subarachnoid hemorrhage, diffuse axonal injury (DAI), and cerebrovascular injury.

Scalp Laceration

A scalp laceration frequently causes significant bleeding (due to the vascularity of the scalp) and may be associated with underlying injuries to the skull and brain. The scalp is gently palpated to assess for deformation of the skull. Scalp lacerations can be sutured at the bedside or may require surgical repair, depending on the size and extent of injury. Avulsed areas of the scalp may require surgical reimplantation.

Skull Fracture

Depressed skull fractures are fractures in which bone fragments are driven into the underlying meninges

TABLE 23-1 Defining the Severity of Head Injury

Severity	Description
Mild	GCS score 13–15 May have lost consciousness or exhibited amnesia or a neurological deficit for 5–60 min No abnormality on CT scan and length of hospital stay less than 48 h
Moderate	GCS score 9–12 Loss of consciousness or amnesia for 1–24 h May have abnormality on CT scan
Severe	GCS score 3–8 Loss of consciousness or amnesia for more than 24 h May have a cerebral contusion, laceration, or intracranial hematoma

GCS, Glasgow Coma Scale.

and brain tissue. Patients with depressed skull fractures may require surgery to debride bone fragments, repair the skull or dura, evacuate a hematoma, or repair adjacent structures such as sinuses or blood vessels.[1] Injury to the dura places the patient at risk for meningitis; therefore, careful monitoring for signs and symptoms of infection is important.

Basilar skull fractures occur at the base, or floor of the skull, typically in the areas of the anterior and middle fossae. Clinical signs of a basilar skull fracture include Battle's sign (bruising behind the ear) or "raccoon eyes" (periorbital edema and bruising). Drainage of cerebrospinal fluid (CSF) from the ear (otorrhea) or nose (rhinorrhea) indicates injury to the dura. Otorrhea typically signifies a fracture in the middle fossa, and rhinorrhea occurs with a fracture in the anterior fossa. Dabbing the drainage from the ear or nose with gauze may reveal the "halo" sign (layering of fluids, with blood on the inside and CSF in a yellowish ring on the outside). CSF leaks typically heal spontaneously; however, a lumbar drain may be used to reduce pressure on the dural tear and promote healing. In some cases, the damaged region of dura must be surgically repaired. A loose gauze dressing can be applied to the ear or nose to quantify the amount and character of drainage while allowing unobstructed drainage of the fluid. The skin around the drainage site is kept clean, and the patient is instructed not to blow his or her nose.

 RED FLAG! In patients with basilar skull fractures, nasogastric and nasotracheal intubation are contraindicated because of the risk for passing the tube through the cribriform fracture into the brain.

Concussion

A concussion is a temporary alteration in mental status resulting from trauma. The patient may or may not lose consciousness. Often patients are unable to recall events leading up to the traumatic event, and occasionally short-term memory is affected. Concussions are not associated with structural abnormalities on radiographic imaging. Recovery after a concussion is usually complete; however, some patients develop postconcussive syndrome (headaches, decreased attention span, short-term memory impairment, dizziness, irritability, emotional lability, fatigue, visual disturbances, noise and light sensitivity, and difficulties with executive functions). Postconcussive syndrome can last for months and as long as 1 year after the injury.[2]

Contusion

Cerebral contusions result from laceration of the microvasculature that causes bruising of, or bleeding into, the brain tissue. Cerebral contusions can range from mild to severe depending on the location, size, and extent of brain tissue injury. The diagnosis of cerebral contusion is made using computed tomography (CT). Complications of a cerebral contusion include intracerebral hematoma development and cerebral edema. Cerebral edema peaks 24 to 72 h after injury, causing increased intracranial pressure (ICP).

Hematoma

Intracranial hematomas may be epidural, subdural, or intraparenchymal (Fig. 23-2).

Epidural Hematoma

An epidural hematoma is a collection of blood between the dura and inside surface of the skull, often caused by laceration of the middle meningeal artery. Patients may have a period of lucidity followed by a loss of consciousness. The rapidly expanding mass can cause uncal herniation. Prompt recognition and surgical evacuation of the hematoma is necessary.

Subdural Hematoma

A subdural hematoma is an accumulation of blood below the dura and above the arachnoid layer covering the brain. Tearing of the bridging veins (veins that pass from the surface of the brain to the inner surface of the dura) or disruption of venous sinuses can cause a subdural hematoma. Subdural hematomas can be categorized based on the time from injury to the onset of symptoms:

- **Acute.** Signs and symptoms of increasing ICP (eg, headache, focal neurological deficit, unilateral pupillary abnormalities, decreasing level of consciousness) manifest 24 to 48 hours after injury. The need for surgical evacuation is determined based on the size and location of the hematoma and the degree of neurological dysfunction.
- **Subacute.** Onset of signs and symptoms is delayed (2 days to 2 weeks after injury). Disruption of smaller blood vessels may lead to a slower accumulation of blood, causing the delay in symptom onset. In some cases, cortical atrophy (often

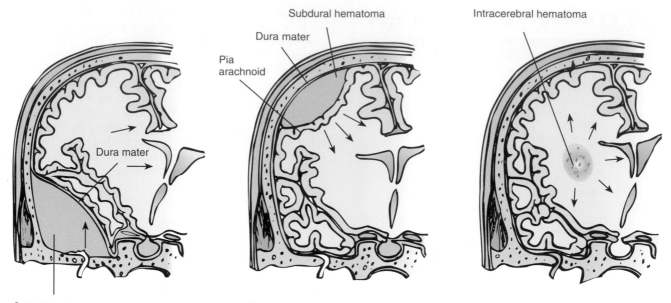

Subdural hematoma
Dura mater
Pia arachnoid
Intracerebral hematoma
Dura mater

A. Epidural hematoma **B.** Subdural hematoma **C.** Intraparenchymal hematoma

FIGURE 23-2 Cerebral hematomas.

associated with advanced age and alcoholism) may allow for a greater amount of fluid to collect before symptoms of increased ICP manifest. Surgical hematoma evacuation may be performed electively according to the degree of neurologic dysfunction.

- **Chronic.** Chronic subdural hematomas result from a small bleed or slow capillary leak. Cortical atrophy causes tension on bridging veins and can increase the risk for chronic subdural hematoma. The slow accumulation of fluids and brain atrophy accounts for the delayed presentation of signs and symptoms, which include headache, lethargy, confusion, and seizures. Surgical intervention may include drilling burr holes into the skull or craniotomy to remove the hematoma. Drains may be placed intraoperatively to prevent reaccumulation of fluid. The head of the patient's bed is kept flat to decrease tension placed on bridging veins. When the head of the bed is raised, it must be raised slowly to prevent rebleeding because as the head is elevated, the brain settles downward.

Intraparenchymal Hematoma

An intraparenchymal hematoma is a collection of blood within the brain parenchyma. Traumatic causes of intraparenchymal hematoma include depressed skull fractures and penetrating injuries. Medical management aims to manage cerebral edema and promote adequate cerebral perfusion. Surgical management is indicated in patients with a deteriorating neurologic examination referable to the injured region of brain tissue, and in patients with increased ICP that is uncontrolled with maximal medical therapies.

Subarachnoid Hemorrhage

Traumatic subarachnoid hemorrhage occurs with tearing or shearing of microvessels in the arachnoid layer, resulting in hemorrhage into the subarachnoid space (which contains the CSF). Blood in the subarachnoid space irritates the brainstem, causing abnormal activity in the autonomic nervous system that may produce cardiac dysrhythmias and hypertension. Hydrocephalus may result when blood in the subarachnoid space impedes reabsorption of CSF. Cerebral vasospasm, a less common complication, may also occur.

Diffuse Axonal Injury

DAI is characterized by a direct tearing or shearing of axons, which worsens during the first 12 to 24 hours as cerebral edema develops. DAI is thought to occur with rotational and acceleration–deceleration forces. DAI can be classified as mild, moderate, or severe:

- **Mild DAI** is associated with a coma lasting no longer than 24 hours.
- **Moderate DAI** is characterized by a coma lasting longer than 24 hours with transient flexor or extensor posturing.
- **Severe DAI** is characterized by prolonged coma, fever, diaphoresis, and severe extensor posturing.

DAI is not easily identified through radiographic imaging; however, small punctate hemorrhages may be visualized deep in the white matter. Magnetic resonance imaging (MRI) may be helpful in identifying neuronal damage after 24 hours.

Cerebrovascular Injury

Carotid or vertebral artery dissection must be considered when a patient presents with neurological deficits unexplained by other brain injuries. Arterial dissection is caused by shearing of the innermost (intima) or middle (media) vessel layers. Damage to the intima can result in clot formation or an intimal flap, either of which can occlude the vessel, resulting in stroke. To detect this type of injury, cerebral angiography may be ordered for patients who have sustained injury to the neck or have unexplained focal neurological deficits.

 RED FLAG! *Early identification of cerebrovascular injury, exclusion of concomitant hemorrhage, and initiation of anticoagulation therapy (if warranted) can prevent stroke in patients with cerebrovascular injury.*

Secondary Brain Injury

Secondary brain injury occurs after the initial traumatic event and causes additional brain injury. Secondary processes (eg, hypoxemia, hypotension, anemia, cerebral edema, cerebral ischemia, uncontrolled increased ICP, hypercarbia, hyperthermia, seizures, hyperglycemia, local or systemic infection) can cause or exacerbate secondary brain injury.

- Cerebral edema commonly occurs in patients with TBIs 24 to 48 hours after the primary insult and typically peaks at 72 hours.[3] If cerebral edema is not aggressively treated, herniation may ensue. Serial neurologic examinations that include evaluation of level of consciousness and motor and cranial nerve function are necessary to identify increased ICP and prevent herniation.
- Cerebral ischemia, a major cause of morbidity and mortality, may be a result of direct vascular injury, loss of autoregulation, or cerebral edema that causes compression or occlusion of blood vessels within the brain. Several studies have suggested that cerebral blood flow may decrease up to 50% during the first 24 to 48 hours after TBI.[4] Continuous surveillance of end-tidal carbon dioxide ($ETCO_2$) or frequent assessment of the arterial carbon dioxide tension ($PaCO_2$) is important to prevent cerebral ischemia.
- Seizures during the early stages of TBI can have severe negative effects on ICP and cerebral metabolic demands. Evidence-based guidelines support the use of antiseizure medication in the first 7 days after TBI.[5] Seizures that occur after this initial period (late posttraumatic seizures) are not prevented by prophylactic administration of antiseizure medications.[5]
- Hyperthermia (temperature greater than 100°F [37.5°C]) in a patient with severe TBI increases metabolic demands and may compound secondary brain injury. Inducing hypothermia may be beneficial in improving functional outcome, although further research is required before this practice is recognized as a standard.[5] Currently, induced hypothermia is used on a case-by-case basis.

 RED FLAG! *Preventing and mitigating secondary brain injury maximizes the patient's chances for positive functional outcomes.*

Management

Initial assessment and treatment of the patient with TBI begins immediately after the insult. Prehospital management of TBI focuses on rapid systems assessment and definitive airway management (Fig. 23-3). Airway management is essential for early correction of hypoxia and hypercarbia, which exacerbate secondary brain injury and affect morbidity and mortality in patients with TBI.

Following transfer of the patient to the critical care unit, management continues to focus on preventing or mitigating secondary brain injury, as well as providing supportive care, preventing or managing multisystemic complications, and providing family support. A collaborative care guide for a patient with TBI is given in Box 23-1.

Caring for the Patient in a Coma or Persistent Vegetative State

Many patients with TBI will be in a coma or persistent vegetative state:

- **Coma** is an alteration in consciousness caused by damage to both hemispheres of the brain or the brainstem. Coma results from disruption of the reticular activating system (RAS), which is a physiological region encompassing nuclei from the medulla to the cerebral cortex. The RAS is responsible for wakefulness, heightened arousal, and alertness. Consciousness can be placed on a continuum from full consciousness to coma, and states of coma can be subdivided into light coma, coma, and deep coma. The duration of coma depends on the type and severity of brain injury. The Ranchos Los Amigos Scale (Table 23-2) can be used to describe the patient's level of awareness and ability to interact with the environment. Coma (sensory) stimulation (Box 23-2) may increase the patient's level of arousal and attention, and lead to better functional outcomes.

 RED FLAG! *Coma stimulation is only appropriate for patients with stable, normal ICPs.*

- **Persistent vegetative state (irreversible coma, coma vigil)** is characterized by a period of sleep-like coma followed by a return to the awake state with an inability to respond to the environment. In a persistent vegetative state, higher cortical functions of the cerebral hemispheres have been damaged permanently, but the lower functions of the brainstem remain intact. The patient's eyes open spontaneously and may appear as if they are opening in response to verbal stimuli. Sleep–wake cycles exist, and the patient maintains normal cardiovascular and respiratory control. Also seen are involuntary lip smacking, chewing, and roving eye movements. A diagnosis of persistent vegetative state cannot be made for at least 4 weeks after onset of TBI and coma.[6]

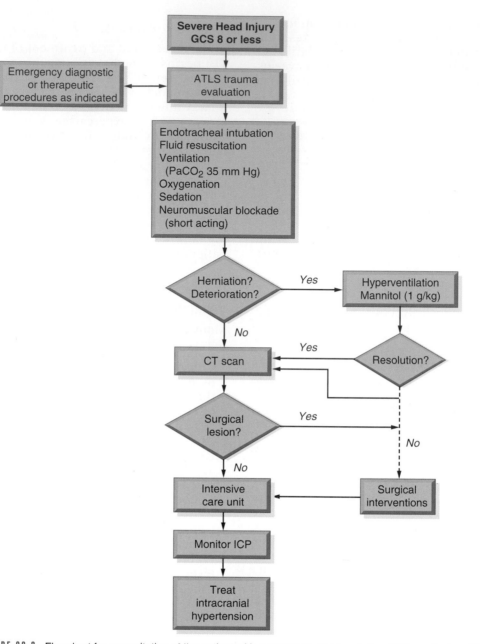

FIGURE 23-3 Flowchart for resuscitation of the patient with a severe head injury before ICP monitoring. GCS, Glasgow Coma Scale; ATLS, advanced trauma life support; CT, computed tomography; ICP, intracranial pressure. © 2000 Brain Trauma Foundation, Inc. Used with permission.

Preventing and Managing Multisystemic Complications

Sympathetic Storming

Patients with severe TBI may experience sympathetic storming as a result of an imbalance of the sympathetic and parasympathetic nervous systems. Sympathetic storming is characterized by diaphoresis; agitation, restlessness, or posturing; hyperventilation; tachycardia; and fever. Stressful events (eg, suctioning, turning, loud noises) can trigger a storming episode.[7] The diagnosis of sympathetic storming is typically based on the appearance of suggestive signs and symptoms, and treatment focuses on finding a medication regimen that suppresses the sympathetic nervous system while avoiding adverse effects such as hypotension and bradycardia. Agents commonly used as part of the medication regimen include α-adrenergic blockers, β-adrenergic blockers, opiates, sedatives, γ-aminobutyric acid agonists, and dopamine agonists.

Disorders of Sodium Imbalance

Disorders of sodium imbalance are common in the patient with TBI (Table 23-3).

BOX 23-1 COLLABORATIVE CARE GUIDE for the Patient With a Traumatic Brain Injury (TBI)

OUTCOMES	INTERVENTIONS
Oxygenation/Ventilation A patent airway is maintained. Lungs are clear to auscultation. Arterial pH, Pao_2, and Sao_2 are maintained within normal limits. $ETCO_2$ or Pco_2 is maintained within prescribed range. There is no evidence of atelectasis or pneumonia on chest x-ray.	• Auscultate breath sounds q2–4h and PRN. • Hyperoxygenate before and after each suction pass. • Avoid suction passes >10 s. • Monitor ICP and CPP during suctioning and chest physiotherapy. • Provide meticulous oral hygiene. • Monitor for signs of aspiration. • Encourage nonintubated patients to use incentive spirometer, cough, and deep breathe q4h and PRN. • Turn side-to-side q2h. • Move patient out of bed to chair one to two times per day when ICP has been controlled.
Circulation/Perfusion Patient exhibits normal sinus rhythm without ectopy or ischemic changes. Patient does not experience thromboembolic complications.	• Monitor for myocardial ischemia and dysrhythmias due to sympathetic activation and catecholamine surges. • Prevent DVT with the use of pneumatic compression devices, compression hose, and subcutaneous heparin. • Implement early mobilization. Facilitate moving to a chair one to two times per day. • Monitor blood pressure continuously by arterial line or frequently by noninvasive cuff. • Monitor oxygen delivery (hemoglobin, Sao_2, cardiac output). • Administer RBCs, inotropes, IV fluids as indicated.
Cerebral Perfusion/Intracranial Pressure CPP > 60 mm Hg. ICP < 20 mm Hg. Patient does not experience seizure activity.	• Monitor ICP and CPP q1h. • Make neurological checks q1–2h. • Elevate the head of bed to 30 degrees unless contraindicated. • Maintain proper body alignment, keeping the head in a neutral position, and avoiding sharp hip flexion. • Maintain normothermia. • Maintain a quiet environment, cluster care, and provide rest periods. • Provide sedation as necessary and as prescribed. • Administer prophylactic antiepileptic agents as prescribed to prevent seizure activity.
Fluids/Electrolytes Serum electrolytes are within normal limits. Serum osmolality remains within prescribed range.	• Maintain strict documentation of I&O; consider insensible losses due to intubation, fever, and the like. • Monitor serum electrolytes, glucose, and osmolality as ordered. • Consider need for electrolyte replacement therapy and administer per physician order or protocol.
Mobility/Safety There are minimal and transient changes in ICP/CPP during treatments or patient care activities, and ICP/CPP returns to baseline within 5 min. Patient does not experience complications related to prolonged immobilization (eg, DVT, pneumonia, ankylosis). Patient does not harm self by dislodging medical equipment or falling.	• Provide range of motion and functional splinting for paralyzed limbs or patients in a coma. • Relieve pressure on pressure points (by repositioning) at least q2h. • Consider use of a specialty mattress based on skin and risk factor assessments. • Keep bed rails in the upright position. • Provide restraints if necessary to prevent dislodgment of medical devices per facility protocol.

TABLE 23-2   Ranchos Los Amigos Scale

Level	Guidelines for Interacting With Patient
1. **No response** to any stimuli occurs. 2. **Generalized response.** Stimulus response is incoherent, limited, and nonpurposeful with random movements or incomprehensible sounds. 3. **Localized response.** Stimulus response is specific but inconsistent; patient may withdraw or push away, may make sounds, may follow some simple commands, or may respond to certain family members.	• Assume that the patient can understand all that is said. Converse with, not about, the patient. • Do not overwhelm the patient with talking. Leave some moments of silence between verbal stimuli. • Manage the environment to provide only one source of stimulation at a time. If talking is taking place, the radio or television should be turned off. • Provide short, random periods of sensory input that are meaningful to the patient. A favorite television program or tape recording or 30 min of music from the patient's favorite radio station will provide more meaningful stimulation than constant radio accompaniment, which becomes as meaningless as the continual bleep of the cardiac monitor.
4. **Confused–agitated.** Stimulus response is primarily to internal confusion with increased state of activity; behavior may be bizarre or aggressive; patient may attempt to remove tubes or restraints or crawl out of bed; verbalization is incoherent or inappropriate; patient shows minimal awareness of environment and absent short-term memory.	• Be calm and soothing when handling the patient. Approach with gentle touch to decrease the occurrence of defensive emotional and motor reflexes. • Watch for early signs that the patient is becoming agitated (eg, increased movement, vocal loudness, resistance to activity). • When the patient becomes upset, do not try to reason with him or her or "talk him or her out of it." Talking will be an additional external stimulus that the patient cannot handle. • If the patient remains upset, either remove him or her from the situation or remove the situation from him or her.
5. **Confused, inappropriate–nonagitated.** Patient is alert and responds consistently to simple commands; however, patient has a short attention span and is easily distracted; memory is impaired and patient exhibits confusion of past and present events; patient can perform previously learned tasks with maximal structure but is unable to learn new information; may wander off with vague intention of "going home."	• Present the patient with only one task at a time. Allow time to complete it before giving further instructions. • Make sure that you have the patient's attention by placing yourself in view and touching the patient before talking. • If the patient becomes confused or resistant, stop talking. Wait until he or she appears relaxed before continuing with instruction or activity.
6. **Confused–appropriate.** Patient shows goal-directed behavior but still needs external direction; can understand simple directions and reasoning; follows simple directions consistently and requires less supervision for previously learned tasks; has improved past memory depth and detail and basic awareness of self and surroundings.	• Use gestures, demonstrations, and only the most necessary words when giving instructions. • Maintain the same sequence in routine activities and tasks. Describe these routines to the patient and relate them to time of day.
7. **Automatic–appropriate.** Patient is able to complete daily routines in structured environment; has increased awareness of self and surroundings but lacks insight, judgment, and problem-solving ability.	• Supervision is still necessary for continued learning and safety. • Reinforce the patient's memory of routines and schedules with clocks, calendars, and a written log of activities.
8. **Purposeful–appropriate.** Patient is alert, oriented, and able to recall and integrate past and recent events; responds appropriately to environment; still has decreased ability in abstract reasoning, stress tolerance, and judgment in emergencies or unusual situations.	• The patient should be able to function without supervision. • Consideration should be given to job retraining or a return to school.

BOX 23-2 Sensory (Coma) Stimulation

Sound
- Explain to the patient what you are going to do.
- Play the patient's favorite television or radio program for 10 to 15 minutes. Alternatively, play a tape recording of a familiar voice of a friend or family member.
- During the program, do not converse with others in the room or perform other activities of patient care. The goal is to minimize distractions so the patient may learn to attend to the stimulus selectively.
- Another approach is to clap your hands or ring a bell. Do this for 5 to 10 seconds at a time, moving the sound to different locations around the bed.

Sight
- Place a brightly colored object in the patient's view. Present only one object at a time.
- Alternatively, use an object that is familiar, such as a family photo or favorite poster.

Touch
- Stroke the patient's arm or leg with fabrics of various textures. Alternatively, the back of a spoon can simulate smooth texture and a towel rough texture.
- Rubbing lotion over the patient's skin will also stimulate this sense. For some, firm pressure may be better tolerated than very light touch.

Smell
- Hold a container of a pleasing fragrance under the patient's nose. Use a familiar scent, such as perfume, aftershave, cinnamon, or coffee.
- Present this stimulation for very short periods (1 to 3 minutes maximum).
- If a cuffed tracheostomy or endotracheal tube is in place, the patient will not be able to appreciate this stimulation fully.

- **Diabetes insipidus** occurs as a result of a decrease in antidiuretic hormone (ADH) secretion, leading to hypovolemia and hypernatremia.
- **Syndrome of inappropriate antidiuretic hormone secretion (SIADH),** in which ADH is released in excessive amounts, results in hemodilution, hypervolemia and hyponatremia.
- **Cerebral salt-wasting syndrome** (centrally mediated excessive renal excretion of sodium and water) may cause hyponatremia in normovolemia to hypovolemia.

Cardiovascular Complications
Myocardial stunning and a transient decrease in cardiac function may occur in severe TBI. Serum cardiac enzymes, electrocardiography, echocardiography, and hemodynamic monitoring may be used to evaluate myocardial function and guide therapy in the critical phases of TBI. The release of large amounts of thromboplastin in response to brain injury can cause disorders of coagulation, such as disseminated intravascular coagulation (DIC). Immobility can place patients with TBI at risk for deep venous thrombosis (DVT) and pulmonary embolism.

Pulmonary Complications
Patients with TBI are at increased risk for pneumonia, acute respiratory distress syndrome (ARDS), pulmonary embolism, and neurogenic ("flash") pulmonary edema. Neurogenic pulmonary edema, which has a sudden onset, may result from injury to the brainstem, increased ICP, or an increase in sympathetic nervous system that causes a catecholamine surge at the time of trauma. Treatment of neurogenic pulmonary edema includes the judicious use of low-dose diuretics. Early mobility is critical for preventing pulmonary complications such as pulmonary embolism and pneumonia.

Caring for the Family
Bond et al.[8] surveyed the needs of family members of patients with severe TBI and identified the following four needs:

- The need for specific, truthful information
- The need for information to be consistent
- The need to be actively involved in the care of the patient
- The need to be able to make sense of the entire experience

TABLE 23-3 Disorders of Sodium Imbalance

	Diabetes Insipidus	Syndrome of Inappropriate Antidiuretic Hormone Secretion (SIADH)	Cerebral Salt-Wasting Syndrome
Urinary output	Increased	Decreased	Increased
Specific gravity	Decreased	Increased	Decreased
Volume status	Decreased	Increased	Decreased
Serum sodium	Increased	Decreased	Decreased
Treatment	Administration of exogenous vasopressin, fluid replacement	Fluid restriction, judicious sodium replacement	Fluid and sodium replacement

Providing emotional support and supporting the family in the process of gathering information and making decisions are essential nursing responsibilities. Measures such as providing accurate and timely information, coordinating available support services (eg, social care, pastoral support) and seeking to involve the family in patient care (eg, encouraging family members to assist in providing sensory stimulation) help to meet the needs of the family, as well as the patient.

A patient's condition may be so severe that brain death is the final outcome. The concept of brain death is often confusing for families because death is so commonly associated with cardiopulmonary death. When communicating with the family about brain death, the language used is very important, and care must be taken to assess the understanding and coping mechanisms of family members. Many patients who are declared brain dead are candidates for organ donation. Discussions about brain death should be separated in time from conversations regarding the opportunities for organ donation.

Brain Tumors

A brain tumor is broadly described as any neoplasm arising within the cranium. Tumors may be primary or metastatic. Tumors are classified according to cell type and location and graded according to degree of malignancy. Table 23-4 summarizes common brain tumors.[9] Prognostic factors include the tumor classification and grade, the tumor's location, the patient's age and general health status, and the time elapsed before detection.

Pathophysiology

Although many brain tumors are low grade or "benign," their location or type may impede complete surgical removal. The physical presence of the tumor can cause vasogenic edema (due to disruption of the blood–brain barrier), shifting of surrounding structures, or both, resulting in ICP that can lead to brain herniation and death.

TABLE 23-4   World Health Organization (WHO) Classification and Grading of Common Intracranial Tumors

Classification/Grade	Description	Symptoms	Treatment/Prognosis
Neuroepithelial Gliomas (Approximately 50% of Primary Tumors)			
Astrocytoma			
WHO grade I—pilocytic astrocytoma	85% cerebellar; slow growing; well circumscribed; cystic; benign	Increased intracranial pressure (ICP); focal neurologic signs	Treated with craniotomy for tumor removal
WHO grade II—astrocytoma	Infiltrative; slow growing	Seizures; acute or subtle onset of symptoms	Radiation therapy (RT) for residual tumor; may withhold RT after gross total resection; young age is good prognostic factor
WHO grade III—anaplastic astrocytoma	Hypercellular; malignant	May have acute onset of symptoms	RT with or without chemotherapy; high recurrence rate; age and overall health affect prognosis
WHO grade IV—glioblastoma multiforme	Poorly differentiated, with high mitotic rate; highly malignant; most common glioma in adults	Rapid onset of symptoms; increased ICP or focal signs	Infiltrative nature: complete removal of all cells not possible; RT with chemotherapy; experimental protocols; recurrence in virtually all cases; median survival: 12–18 mo
Oligodendroglioma	Well differentiated; calcified; infiltrative; slow growing; some tumors are malignant (anaplastic)	Seizures; headaches; subtle onset of symptoms	RT with residual tumor; may withhold after gross total resection; RT with or without chemotherapy for anaplastic oligodendroglioma
Mixed glioma (oligoastrocytoma)	May behave more or less aggressively, depending on features	Dependent on location and degree of malignancy	Variable outcome
Ependymoma	Young adult patients; originates from lining of the ventricles; frequently in posterior fossa; usually benign	May present with hydrocephalus; symptoms related to location	RT for residual or recurrent disease; craniospinal RT for evidence of spinal disease only; good prognosis
Peripheral Nerve Tumors (Approximately 8% of Primary Brain Tumors)			
Vestibular schwannoma (acoustic neuroma)	Cerebellopontine angle; benign; encapsulated; seen in association with neurofibromatosis, type 2	Decreased hearing; tinnitus; balance problems; may have other cranial nerve deficits	Curable with surgery; excellent prognosis; cranial nerve deficits may be permanent or temporary; affect quality of life

Classification/Grade	Description	Symptoms	Treatment/Prognosis
Meningeal Tumors (Approximately 30% of Primary Brain Tumors)			
Meningioma	Composed of arachnoid cells; attached to dura; usually benign; well circumscribed; may be vascular; common locations: falx convexity; olfactory groove; sphenoid ridge; parasellar region; optic nerve	Headaches may occur from dural stretching; seizures and focal neurologic signs	Degree of resection (and recurrence) associated with location; excellent prognosis with gross total resection; atypical and malignant meningiomas have more aggressive features and less favorable outcomes
Lymphomas and Hematopoietic Tumors (Approximately 3% of Primary Brain Tumors)			
Malignant central nervous system lymphoma	Arise in central nervous system without systemic lymphoma; commonly suprasellar; diffuse brain infiltration; may be periventricular and may involve leptomeninges; solitary or multiple	Neurologic or neuropsychiatric symptoms	Diagnosis commonly via stereotactic biopsy or cerebrospinal fluid (CSF) cytology; steroids may decrease or temporarily obliterate lesion on computed tomography (CT) or magnetic resonance imaging (MRI); RT with or without chemotherapy; high-dose methotrexate used as single agent; some studies defer RT; increasing incidence in immunocompetent persons; decreasing in AIDS patients; possible improved survival with newer treatments
Sellar Tumors (Approximately 7% of Primary Brain Tumors)			
Pituitary adenoma	6.3% of sellar tumors; benign; originate from adenohypophysis; classification by hormonal content; microadenoma less than or equal to 1 cm; macroadenoma greater than or equal to 1 cm	Hypersecretion • Prolactin: amenorrhea, galactorrhea • Growth hormone: acromegaly • Adrenocorticotropic hormone: Cushing's syndrome • Thyroid-stimulating hormone: hyperthyroidism (rare) Hyposecretion caused by compression of the pituitary gland Visual field deficits (bitemporal hemianopia); headache; pituitary apoplexy: acute hemorrhage or infarct of gland—emergency treatment indicated	*Surgical:* transsphenoidal for approximately 95% of surgical cases; *medical:* appropriate in some cases of prolactin-secreting and growth hormone–secreting tumors; RT for recurrence or for hypersecretory tumors, when medical management has failed
Craniopharyngioma	Benign, calcified, cystic tumors	Endocrine abnormalities; visual impairment; cognitive and/or personality changes; may have increased ICP	Gross total resection affects prognosis; RT for residual tumor
Metastatic Tumors (Occur in 20–40% of Cancer Patients)			
	Originate from primary systemic tumors; discrete, round, ring-enhancing; 50% are solitary; lung and breast are most common primary sites	Symptoms are location dependent	Prognosis dependent on number of tumors, tumor location, systemic disease, and patient age; improved prognosis with gross total resection and RT

Assessment

A patient with a brain neoplasm may present with one or more general or focal signs or symptoms. The most common general signs and symptoms of brain tumors are related to increasing ICP and include headaches, seizures, nausea with or without vomiting, papilledema, mental status changes, and cognitive changes. History taking and symptom evaluation contribute to the accurate diagnosis of a brain tumor. Of significance are the duration, frequency, and severity of symptoms, as well as whether the symptoms occur at a particular time of day or following certain activities. Because patients may minimize or be unaware of subtle

neurological deficits, family involvement in this discussion is useful. The physical examination aids in further localizing the lesion. Focal neurological deficits may be temporary (resulting from tumor compression) or permanent (resulting from tumor destruction) and are directly related to tumor location (Fig. 23-4).

Imaging studies such as CT and MRI are typically ordered to localize the lesion and assess the amount of edema and mass effect on surrounding structures. MRI is the preferred diagnostic tool because it shows tumors in three dimensions (axial, coronal, and sagittal). An electroencephalogram (EEG) is used to confirm the presence of seizure activity, which may be useful in determining

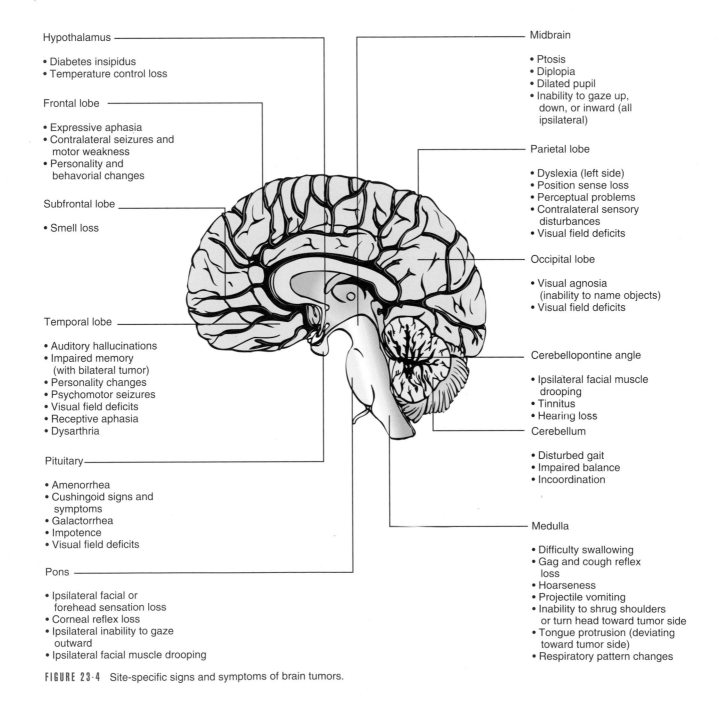

Hypothalamus
- Diabetes insipidus
- Temperature control loss

Frontal lobe
- Expressive aphasia
- Contralateral seizures and motor weakness
- Personality and behavorial changes

Subfrontal lobe
- Smell loss

Temporal lobe
- Auditory hallucinations
- Impaired memory (with bilateral tumor)
- Personality changes
- Psychomotor seizures
- Visual field deficits
- Receptive aphasia
- Dysarthria

Pituitary
- Amenorrhea
- Cushingoid signs and symptoms
- Galactorrhea
- Impotence
- Visual field deficits

Pons
- Ipsilateral facial or forehead sensation loss
- Corneal reflex loss
- Ipsilateral inability to gaze outward
- Ipsilateral facial muscle drooping

Midbrain
- Ptosis
- Diplopia
- Dilated pupil
- Inability to gaze up, down, or inward (all ipsilateral)

Parietal lobe
- Dyslexia (left side)
- Position sense loss
- Perceptual problems
- Contralateral sensory disturbances
- Visual field deficits

Occipital lobe
- Visual agnosia (inability to name objects)
- Visual field deficits

Cerebellopontine angle
- Ipsilateral facial muscle drooping
- Tinnitus
- Hearing loss

Cerebellum
- Disturbed gait
- Impaired balance
- Incoordination

Medulla
- Difficulty swallowing
- Gag and cough reflex loss
- Hoarseness
- Projectile vomiting
- Inability to shrug shoulders or turn head toward tumor side
- Tongue protrusion (deviating toward tumor side)
- Respiratory pattern changes

FIGURE 23-4 Site-specific signs and symptoms of brain tumors.

whether anticonvulsants are needed. Magnetic resonance angiography (MRA) images the vascular anatomy and vessels that feed certain tumors. Functional MRI (fMRI) is used to functionally map areas of the brain, and is often ordered when the tumor is located in the dominant hemisphere or motor strip as part of the preoperative assessment of language, motor, and sensory function in relation to tumor location. Positron emission tomography (PET) is used to differentiate low-grade from high-grade (and more metabolically active) tumors. PET is also used in previously treated patients to differentiate radiation necrosis from high-grade tumors.

Definitive diagnosis can only be achieved by obtaining a tissue sample for histopathological evaluation. Tissue samples may be obtained using stereotactic biopsy (Box 23-3) or craniotomy. Stereotactic biopsy entails localizing the tumor (using CT or MRI to establish entry points), drilling a small hole in the skull, and passing a needle through to the tumor to obtain tissue or fluid for sampling. Craniotomy provides for both definitive diagnosis and surgical resection of the lesion.

Management

When possible, craniotomy may be performed to resect the tumor. In some cases, angiography and embolization are performed within 24 to 48 hours of surgery for highly vascular tumors such as meningiomas. Surgical complications may be severe and require critical care monitoring and management (Table 23-5). Postoperative nursing responsibilities include frequent monitoring of neurological status and vital signs, incision care, ICP monitoring (if present), and airway management.

Some tumors are managed with surgery only, whereas other brain tumors are treated with adjuvant therapies, either because they are not able to be surgically resected or because their aggressive nature precludes complete resection. For most brain tumors, radiation therapy is the first-line treatment after biopsy or craniotomy. Chemotherapy may also be administered. However, chemotherapeutic agents administered orally or intravenously can cause systemic toxicities and often cannot cross the blood–brain barrier in sufficient amounts to provide benefit. Alternatively, a biodegradable polymer wafer that delivers a continuous infusion of a chemotherapeutic agent over a period of 2 to 3 weeks may be placed in the tumor resection cavity at the time of craniotomy. Alternatively, chemotherapy may be given in conjunction with radiation or at the time of tumor recurrence.

Cerebral Hemorrhage

Cerebral hemorrhage may be caused by a ruptured cerebral aneurysm or arteriovenous malformation (AVM).

Cerebral Aneurysm

Cerebral aneurysms may be congenital or degenerative arterial lesions. Most aneurysms arise in the anterior circulation of the circle of Willis (Fig. 23-5). In the posterior circulation, the most common locations are the basilar artery tip and the posterior inferior cerebellar artery.[10] Symptoms occur when the aneurysm ruptures and bleeds into the subarachnoid space or becomes large enough to exert pressure on surrounding brain structures (giant intracranial aneurysm).

Pathophysiology

As the intimal layers of the vessel weaken, high-velocity blood flow begins to create a whirlpool effect, stretching the wall of the vessel. As the wall of the vessel expands, it becomes progressively weaker and may eventually rupture. Hemorrhage from an aneurysm usually occurs into the subarachnoid space. The force of the rupturing vessel can be so great that it can push blood into the brain tissue, causing an intracerebral hematoma.

Approximately 20% to 40% of patients with ruptured cerebral aneurysms die before receiving medical care. Of those who survive the initial bleeding, 35% to 40% bleed again if left untreated, with a mortality rate of about 42%. Rebleeding most often occurs within the first 24 to 48 hours.

Assessment

Approximately half of patients have some warning signs before an aneurysm ruptures, including headache; lethargy; neck pain; a "noise in the head;" and optic, oculomotor, or trigeminal cranial nerve dysfunction. When an aneurysm ruptures and bleeds into the subarachnoid space, patients typically report experiencing a horrific headache, typically described as "the worst headache of their life." Other signs and symptoms of a ruptured aneurysm or aneurysms that present with mass effect include nausea, vomiting, focal neurologic deficits, and coma. Signs of meningeal irritation include a stiff and painful

TABLE 23-5 Critical Care Management of the Patient With Brain Tumor Complications

Diagnosis	Management
Increased intracranial pressure (ICP)	• Corticosteroids • IV fluids (avoid hypotonic solutions) • Elevate head of bed and maintain adequate body alignment • Avoid hypotension and control hypertension; arterial line useful • Keep well oxygenated; may need to intubate • Judicious use of mannitol to expand plasma volume and draw fluid out of the brain • Sedation to reduce activity and decrease hypertension • Intraventricular catheter may be necessary to monitor ICP and drain cerebrospinal fluid (CSF) • Cautious use of mild hyperventilation for short periods only if persistent elevated ICP • Surgical intervention may be required for hematoma
Wound infection, intracranial abscess, or bone flap infection	• Bloodwork, including complete blood count (CBC) and blood cultures • Computed tomography (CT) scan, magnetic resonance imaging (MRI), and in some cases magnetic resonance spectroscopy to identify abscess • Surgical removal of abscess or bone flap, when feasible • Appropriate wound cultures, when possible • Antibiotic therapy • Infectious disease consultation for appropriate drug, dose, and duration
Hyponatremia or hypernatremia	• Evaluate for possible diabetes insipidus, syndrome of inappropriate antidiuretic hormone (SIADH) secretion, or cerebral salt-wasting syndrome • For hyponatremia: fluid restriction and diuresis (SIADH only), administration of hypertonic saline • For hypernatremia: fluids, vasopressin (for diabetes insipidus)
Intracranial hemorrhage	• Immediate CT scan to evaluate for early signs of intracranial bleeding • Monitor blood pressure • Check laboratory values: prothrombin time (PT), partial thromboplastin time (PTT), platelets • Management of increased ICP • May need to intubate and ventilate • Surgery may be necessary to remove blood clot
Thromboembolism: deep venous thrombosis (DVT) and pulmonary embolism	• Heparinization *only after* CT scan has ruled out intracranial bleeding; alternatively, vena cava filter (Greenfield filter) may be used • Mechanical compression devices used instead of anticoagulants in patients at high risk for intracerebral hemorrhage
Seizures	• Monitor for seizures • Protect patient from injury • Administer antiepileptics • Monitor therapeutic levels
Gastric ulceration	• Histamine type 2 receptor (H_2) blockers or proton pump inhibitors (to prevent gastrointestinal symptoms associated with long-term corticosteroid use)

Courtesy of Michael Torbey.

neck, photophobia, blurred vision, irritability, fever, positive Kernig's sign (pain in the neck when the thigh is flexed and the leg is extended at the knee), and positive Brudzinski's sign (involuntary flexion of the knees when the neck is flexed toward the chest). Aneurysms are graded according to their severity on the Hunt and Hess scale (Table 23-6).[11]

The diagnosis of a cerebral aneurysm usually is made on the basis of history, physical examination, and various diagnostic studies. A CT scan reveals subarachnoid hemorrhage in most cases when it is obtained within 24 hours of the hemorrhage. A lumbar puncture may reveal blood in the CSF, but carries the risk of herniation from increased ICP. Cerebral angiography studies, including CT angiography, MRA, and digital subtraction angiography (DSA) may be used to determine the source of subarachnoid hemorrhage. Although all of these studies can determine vascular anatomy, DSA is the gold standard if surgery is planned.[10]

Management

Surgery is generally performed 24 to 48 hours after the bleed occurs to prevent a rebleed. Surgical clipping (placement of a titanium clip across the neck of the aneurysm) may be considered if the aneurysm is in an accessible area (Fig. 23-6). Surgical complications include intraoperative aneurysm rupture, incomplete clipping, and accidental clipping of surrounding vessels. Some aneurysms are managed using a technique called coiling. This technique uses soft thrombogenic platinum alloy microcoils, which are introduced into the aneurysm using the femoral artery and fluoroscopic equipment. The coil is advanced through the catheter into the aneurysm sac and detached. The coil occludes the aneurysm and separates it from the cerebral circulation. The risk for hemorrhage or rehemorrhage is decreased with coiling.[12] Complications associated with coiling include embolic stroke, coil migration,

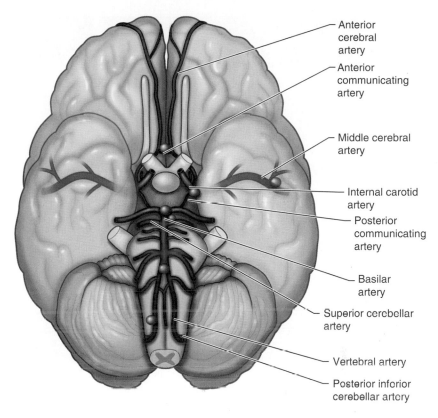

FIGURE 23-5   Circle of Willis with common aneurysm sites (ventral view of the brain).

failure to obliterate the aneurysm, and aneurysm rupture.

Preoperative Care

Before surgical repair, minimal stimulation of the patient is required to prevent rebleeding. Precautionary measures include providing a quiet environment, establishing a bowel regimen to prevent straining (Valsalva maneuver), managing blood pressure, providing sedation, and limiting visitors.[10]

TABLE 23-6	Hunt and Hess Grading Scale for Aneurysms
Grade 0	Unruptured aneurysm
Grade I	Asymptomatic
	Minimal headache
	Slight nuchal rigidity (neck stiffness)
Grade II	Moderate to severe headache
	Nuchal rigidity
	Cranial nerve deficits
Grade III	Lethargy
	Mental confusion
	Mild focal neurological deficit
Grade IV	Stupor
	Moderate to severe motor deficit
	Possible posturing
Grade V	Deep coma
	Posturing
	Declining appearance

Adapted from Mower-Wade D, Cavanaugh MC, Bush C: Protecting a patient with ruptured cerebral aneurysm. Nursing 31(2):52–58, 2001.

Analgesics can be used to relieve headaches. An antipyretic (usually acetaminophen) and hypothermia blankets can be used to manage fever, caused by blood in the subarachnoid space. Antihypertensive medications may be used to manage blood pressure before procedures or surgery. Plasma volume should not be allowed to decrease. Hyponatremia, usually associated with cerebral salt-wasting syndrome rather than SIADH, is managed with sodium replacement and euvolemia.[13]

Postoperative Care

Vasospasm usually occurs 3 to 12 days after a subarachnoid hemorrhage, with peak incidence between days 7 and 10. Vasospasm can cause a large area of brain ischemia or infarction, resulting in severe neurological deficits. Monitoring trends in flow velocity using transcranial Doppler (TCD) allows prompt identification of patients at risk for developing vasospasm. In addition, the results of the neurological examination can be correlated with TCD findings for prompt diagnosis and treatment of vasospasm.

 RED FLAG! *Signs and symptoms of vasospasm, resulting from decreased cerebral blood flow, may include changes in level of consciousness, headache, language impairment, hemiparesis, and seizures.*

Strategies to prevent vasospasm include the administration of nimodipine (a calcium channel blocker) to dilate the small pial vessels, and "triple H" therapy (ie, hypervolemia, hemodilution, and

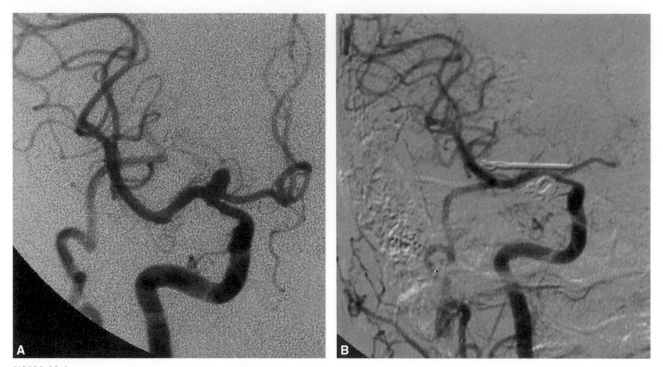

FIGURE 23-6 Aneurysm clipping. (Courtesy of Rafael Tamargo, MD, and Richard Clatterbuck, MD, Johns Hopkins University, Baltimore, MD.)

induced hypertension). "Triple H" therapy is the standard for the prevention and treatment of vasospasm.[14] Hypervolemia causes the cerebral vessels to dilate and the mean arterial pressure (MAP) to increase, thereby improving cerebral perfusion pressure (CPP), decreasing blood viscosity, and increasing regional cerebral blood flow. The patient's hematocrit level is maintained between 30% and 33%. Hypervolemia and hemodilution are accomplished by volume expansion, using both IV colloid and crystalloid solutions. During this therapy, the patient is monitored for pulmonary edema and heart failure. Vasopressors are used to induce hypertension. The objective is to maintain systolic blood pressure at greater than 20 mm Hg over normal or to raise the patient's blood pressure to the point where the neurological deficit improves. When conventional medical therapy is ineffective, acute arterial vasospasm can be managed by intra-arterial antispasmodic administration or by balloon angioplasty, which mechanically dilates and improves cerebral blood flow through the major arterial segments.

Another complication after aneurysmal rupture is hydrocephalus. When there is blood in the subarachnoid space, the red blood cells can occlude the flow of CSF or obstruct reabsorption of CSF through the arachnoid villi. A ventriculoperitoneal shunt may need to be placed to drain CSF into the peritoneal cavity and resolve the hydrocephalus.

Arteriovenous Malformation

Arteriovenous malformations (AVMs) are congenital vascular lesions consisting of a "tangle" of dilated arteries and veins without a capillary system. Because blood is shunted directly from the arterial to the venous circulation without a capillary bed, there is less resistance, and AVMs receive significant blood flow. The arteries and veins enlarge to carry this increased flow, and their walls are characteristically quite thin. Although they are found throughout the central nervous system, approximately 90% of AVMs are located in the cerebrum. Of these, the most common locations are the frontal and temporal lobes, most often supplied by the middle cerebral artery (MCA).[15] AVMs typically enlarge with age; the condition is most often diagnosed in patients in their thirties.

Assessment

Hemorrhage, the most common presenting sign of AVMs, may occur in the subarachnoid, intracerebral, or subdural space. In cases in which the patient has both an AVM and an aneurysm, the aneurysm is more likely to be the cause of hemorrhage.[15] Other presenting signs include seizure, headache, increased ICP, neurological deficits referable to the location of the lesion, bruit, and visual symptoms.

CT and MRI are used to identify an AVM and differentiate it from tumors and other brain lesions. Three-dimensional imaging is useful in establishing the malformation in relation to the surrounding anatomy. Angiography (eg, MRA) is used primarily to evaluate the feeding and draining vessels. fMRI is useful for identifying the AVM in relation to eloquent areas of the brain (ie, the sensory, motor, speech, and visual areas).

TABLE 23-7 Management of Arteriovenous Malformations (AVMs)

Procedure	Indication	Outcome	Potential Complications	Comments
Surgery	Surgically accessible location; smaller lesion	Removal of lesion Decreased risk for bleeding Improved seizure control	Cerebral edema; hemorrhage; neurological deficits	Inpatient hospital stay required Preoperative propranolol believed to minimize postoperative bleeding and edema Maintain mean arterial pressure (MAP) of 70–80 mm Hg perioperatively
Stereotactic radiosurgery	Small lesion (less than or equal to 3 cm) May be used as part of multimodality treatment, or when surgery is not indicated	Reduction in size of lesion	Continued risk for bleeding for 2–3 y	Noninvasive Outpatient, no recovery period Multiple treatments may be required and complete obliteration may take years
Embolization	Useful for larger lesions Used to facilitate other therapies (surgery; radiation) by reducing size of lesion	Reduction in size of lesion Short hospital stay	Stroke, hemorrhage	Not usually curative May need more than one procedure Need to wait days or weeks before surgery or radiation therapy

Management

Management is based on the patient's age, medical condition, and symptoms; the flow associated with the malformation; whether or not there is a history of hemorrhage; and the location of the lesion. Table 23-7 summarizes treatment options.

Stroke

A stroke is a disruption of blood flow to a region of the brain that is sudden in onset and results in permanent damage. Approximately 75% of strokes in the United States are due to vascular obstruction (thrombi or emboli). As in myocardial infarction, a stroke-inducing thrombosis is frequently caused by an atherosclerotic plaque rupture. An embolus may be a result of blood clots (frequently seen in association with atrial fibrillation), fragments of atheromatous plaques, lipids, or air. The remaining 25% of strokes are hemorrhagic, resulting from hypertensive vascular disease (which causes an intracerebral hemorrhage), a ruptured aneurysm, or an AVM.

 RED FLAG! Early recognition and prompt entry into the emergency medical system are essential to reduce death and disability from stroke. Delay in seeking medical care may eliminate the potential for tissue-saving thrombolytic therapy. The "time to needle"—the time from symptom onset (ie, the time the patient was last seen well) to administration of thrombolytic therapy—is 3 to 4.5 hours.[16]

Pathophysiology

When blood flow to any part of the brain is impeded as a result of a thrombus or embolus, oxygen deprivation can lead to ischemia and eventually to infarction (necrosis) of the cerebral tissue. If the neurons are ischemic only and have not yet infarcted, the injury may be reversible. However, necrosis is irreversible. The necrotic zone is surrounded by an ischemic zone called the penumbra. The goal of acute stroke management is to salvage the ischemic penumbra. Without prompt intervention, the entire ischemic penumbra can eventually become an infarcted region.[17] Damage to the brain tissue may also result from localized vasogenic cerebral edema, which forms around the penumbra.

Assessment

A stroke is usually characterized by the sudden onset of focal neurological impairment. Specific manifestations depend on the anatomical location of the lesion. Common signs and symptoms include weakness, numbness, visual changes, dysarthria, dysphagia, or aphasia. It is important to obtain a description of the neurological event; the onset and progression of symptoms; and whether the symptoms are the same as at the time of onset, worsening, resolving, or completely gone. The pattern of symptoms can help determine the diagnosis and identify possible vascular involvement. The National Institutes of Health Stroke Scale (NIHSS) may be used in conjunction with the neurologic assessment to assign a score indicating the severity of the stroke (Table 23-8).[17]

TABLE 23-8 **National Institutes of Health Stroke Scale (NIHSS)**

Instructions	Scale Definition
1a. Level of Consciousness: The investigator must choose a response if a full evaluation is prevented by such obstacles as an endotracheal tube, language barrier, orotracheal trauma/bandages.	0 = **Alert;** keenly responsive. 1 = **Not alert;** but arousable by minor stimulation. 2 = **Not alert;** requires repeated stimulation to attend. 3 = Responds only with reflex motor or autonomic effects or totally unresponsive, flaccid, and areflexic.
1b. LOC Questions: The patient is asked the month and his/her age. The answer must be correct - there is no partial credit for being close.	0 = **Answers** both questions correctly. 1 = **Answers** one question correctly. 2 = **Answers** neither question correctly.
1c. LOC Commands: The patient is asked to open and close the eyes and then to grip and release the non-paretic hand. Substitute another one-step command if the hands cannot be used.	0 = **Performs** both tasks correctly. 1 = **Performs** one task correctly. 2 = **Performs** neither task correctly.
2. Best Gaze: Only horizontal eye movements will be tested. Voluntary or reflexive (oculocephalic) eye movements will be scored, but caloric testing is not done.	0 = **Normal.** 1 = **Partial gaze palsy;** gaze is abnormal in one or both eyes. 2 = **Forced deviation,** or total gaze paresis not overcome by the oculocephalic maneuver.
3. Visual: Visual fields (upper and lower quadrants) are tested by confrontation, using finger counting or visual threat, as appropriate.	0 = **No visual loss.** 1 = **Partial hemianopia.** 2 = **Complete hemianopia.** 3 = **Bilateral hemianopia** (blind including cortical blindness).
4. Facial Palsy: Ask – or use pantomime to encourage – the patient to show teeth or raise eyebrows and close eyes.	0 = **Normal** symmetrical movements. 1 = **Minor paralysis** (flattened nasolabial fold, asymmetry on smiling). 2 = **Partial paralysis** (total or near-total paralysis of lower face). 3 = **Complete paralysis** of one or both sides (absence of facial movement in the upper and lower face).
5. Motor Arm: The limb is placed in the appropriate position: extend the arms (palms down) 90 degrees (if sitting) or 45 degrees (if supine). Drift is scored if the arm falls before 10 seconds. **5a. Left Arm** **5b. Right Arm**	0 = **No drift;** limb holds position for full 10 seconds. 1 = **Drift;** limb holds position, but drifts down before full 10 seconds; does not hit bed or other support. 2 = **Some effort against gravity;** limb cannot get to or maintain (if cued) position, drifts down to bed, but has some effort against gravity. 3 = **No effort against gravity;** limb falls. 4 = **No movement.** UN = **Amputation** or joint fusion.
6. Motor Leg: The limb is placed in the appropriate position: hold the leg at 30 degrees (always tested supine). Drift is scored if the leg falls before 5 seconds. **6a. Left Leg** **6b. Right Leg**	0 = **No drift;** leg holds position for full 5 seconds. 1 = **Drift;** leg falls by the end of the 5-second period but does not hit bed. 2 = **Some effort against gravity;** leg falls to bed by 5 seconds, but has some effort against gravity. 3 = **No effort against gravity;** leg falls to bed immediately. 4 = **No movement.** UN = **Amputation** or joint fusion.
7. Limb Ataxia: The finger-nose-finger and heel-shin tests are performed on both sides with the eyes open.	0 = **Absent.** 1 = **Present in one limb.** 2 = **Present in two limbs.** UN = **Amputation** or joint fusion.
8. Sensory: Sensation or grimace to pinprick when tested, or withdrawal from noxious stimulus in the obtunded or aphasic patient.	0 = **Normal;** no sensory loss. 1 = **Mild-to-moderate sensory loss;** patient feels pinprick is less sharp or is dull on the affected side; or there is a loss of superficial pain with pinprick, but patient is aware of being touched. 2 = **Severe to total sensory loss;** patient is not aware of being touched in the face, arm, and leg.
9. Best Language: The patient is asked to describe what is happening in a picture, to name the items on a naming sheet, and to read from a list of sentences.	0 = **No aphasia;** normal. 1 = **Mild-to-moderate aphasia;** some obvious loss of fluency or facility of comprehension, without significant limitation on ideas expressed or form of expression. 2 = **Severe aphasia;** all communication is through fragmentary expression; great need for inference, questioning, and guessing by the listener. 3 = **Mute, global aphasia;** no usable speech or auditory comprehension.

Instructions	Scale Definition
10. **Dysarthria:** An adequate sample of speech is obtained by asking patient to read or repeat words from a list.	0 = **Normal.** 1 = **Mild-to-moderate dysarthria;** patient slurs some words and can be understood with some difficulty. 2 = **Severe dysarthria;** patient's speech is so slurred as to be unintelligible in the absence of or out of proportion to any dysphasia, or is mute/anarthric. UN = **Intubated** or other physical barrier.
11. **Extinction and Inattention (formerly Neglect):** Sufficient information to identify neglect may be obtained during the prior testing.	0 = **No abnormality.** 1 = **Visual, tactile, auditory, spatial, or personal inattention** or extinction to bilateral simultaneous stimulation in one of the sensory modalities. 2 = **Profound hemi-inattention or extinction to more than one modality;** does not recognize own hand or orients to only one side of space.

Although an area of infarction may not show on the CT scan for 12 to 24 hours, an urgent noncontrast CT scan (obtained within 1 hour of arrival in the emergency department) is performed to rule out intracerebral hemorrhage and facilitate treatment decisions. Diffusion-weighted imaging (DWI) and perfusion-weighted imaging (PWI) are also frequently used to evaluate the patient with acute ischemic stroke. DWI and PWI are MRI-based techniques that help identify the infarct core and penumbra, which is important because the presence of viable tissue directs interventions such as reperfusion. DWI can reveal changes associated with infarcted tissue a few hours after the onset of symptoms (hours before a CT scan or conventional MRI can detect any abnormality). PWI shows the regional abnormalities of cerebral blood flow. Cerebral angiography, traditionally the gold standard for evaluating cerebral vasculature, can demonstrate an arterial occlusion or embolus, but because of the time that it takes to perform cerebral angiography, the window of opportunity to treat a patient with IV thrombolytics may be missed. Alternative studies, such as MRA and CTA, are used to view vasculature and are faster and less invasive. An electrocardiogram (ECG) is obtained to assess for evidence of dysrhythmia (eg, atrial fibrillation).

Management

The management of an ischemic stroke has four primary goals: restoration of cerebral blood flow (reperfusion), prevention of recurrent thrombosis, neuroprotection, and supportive care. If the patient is a candidate for IV thrombolytic therapy, treatment with tissue plasminogen activator (t-PA) begins in the emergency department, and the patient is then moved to the critical care unit for further monitoring. If the patient is not a candidate for thrombolytic therapy, the complexity of the patient's problems determines whether the patient is transferred to the critical care unit, a medical unit, or a stroke specialty unit for ongoing care.

Early Management

The focus of initial treatment is to save as much of the ischemic area as possible. Two emergency treatments are available for stroke management: thrombolytic therapy and interventional radiology.

Thrombolytic Therapy
Thrombolytic agents (eg, t-PA) dissolve clots and permit reperfusion of the brain tissue. The history, neurological examination, NIHSS score, and results of neuroimaging studies assist the physician with the decision to offer thrombolytic therapy. Eligibility criteria for thrombolytic therapy are given in Box 23-4. A major risk of this therapy is intracerebral hemorrhage. If the patient is a candidate for thrombolytic therapy, the systolic blood pressure is maintained at less than 185 mm Hg to the lower risk of hemorrhage. When t-PA is given, 10% of the total dose (0.9 mg/kg, not to exceed 90 mg) is administered as an IV bolus over 1 to 2 minutes, with the remainder infused over 60 minutes. No other antithrombotic or antiplatelet therapy is given for the next 24 hours.

Interventional Radiology
Interventional radiology techniques include intra-arterial thrombolysis (ie, the direct administration of t-PA to the site of the clot via the femoral artery) and the use of mechanical clot removal devices (eg, the **m**echanical **e**mbolus **r**emoval for **c**erebral **i**schemia, or MERCI retriever).

- **Intra-arterial thrombolysis** can be given up to 6 hours after the onset of symptoms. Angiography is required, and the patient must be admitted or transferred to a specialty center equipped to perform the procedure.
- **Mechanical clot removal** entails the use of a device that typically works like a corkscrew to snare and remove the embolus. Mechanical clot removal can be performed up to 8 hours after symptom onset and even longer if obstruction involves the basilar artery. Eligibility criteria for mechanical clot removal are given in Box 23-5. Potential complications include bleeding and vascular dissection or perforation; close monitoring

BOX 23-4 Eligibility Criteria for Intravenous Thrombolytic Therapy

Inclusion Criteria
- Time since symptom onset less than 3 or up to 4.5 hours
- Clinical diagnosis of ischemic stroke with measurable deficit on the National Institutes of Health Stroke Scale (NIHSS)
- Patient older than 18 years

Exclusion Criteria
- Stroke or serious head trauma within past 3 months
- Systolic blood pressure sustained greater than 185 mm Hg or diastolic blood pressure greater than 110 mm Hg, or blood pressure readings that require aggressive treatment
- Conditions that suggest or could precipitate parenchymal bleeding: subarachnoid or intracerebral hemorrhage; recent-onset myocardial infarction; seizures

at onset; major surgery within past 14 days; gastrointestinal or urinary tract hemorrhage within previous 21 days; or arterial puncture of a noncompressible site or lumbar puncture within previous 7 days
- Glucose less than 50 mg/dL or more than 400 mg/dL; international normalized ratio (INR) more than 1.7; platelet count less than 100,000/mm³
- Rapidly improving or deteriorating neurological signs or minor symptoms
- Recent myocardial infarction
- Treatment with IV or subcutaneous heparin within past 48 hours and elevated partial thromboplastin time (PTT)
- Positive pregnancy test result

Adapted from Hock NH: Brain attack: The stroke continuum. Nurs Clin North Am 34(3):718, 1999.

is required for 24 hours following the procedure to detect adverse effects.

Ongoing Management

A collaborative care guide for the patient who has had a stroke is given in Box 23-6. Supportive care measures include the following:

- **Anticoagulation therapy.** Antithrombotic and antiplatelet agents (eg, warfarin) may be administered to prevent future thrombotic or embolic events.
- **Control of hypertension.** Patients with moderate hypertension usually are not treated acutely. If the patient is not a candidate for thrombolytic therapy, the blood pressure is not treated unless it

exceeds 220 mm Hg systolic or 120 mm Hg diastolic because reducing blood pressure reduces the CPP and can cause infarction of the penumbra. When necessary, blood pressure is lowered gradually using short-acting IV antihypertensive agents.
- **Control of ICP.** Elevation of the ICP in a patient who has had a stroke, when it occurs, usually occurs after the first day. Measures to lower ICP are described in Chapter 22.
- **Control of blood glucose level.** Hyperglycemia and hypoglycemia can have potentially deleterious effects in patients who have had a stroke. Glycemic control may be achieved with a continuous insulin infusion or a sliding-scale regimen.

BOX 23-5 Eligibility Criteria for Mechanical Clot Removal

Inclusion Criteria
- Clinical diagnosis of ischemic stroke with aNational Institutes of Health Stroke Scale (NIHSS) score greater than 8
- Occlusion of the internal carotid artery, basilar artery, or vertebral artery on angiography

Exclusion Criteria
- Excessive vessel tortuosity
- Hemorrhagic tendency
- Blood glucose less than 50 mg/dL, elevated international normalized ratio (INR), decreased platelets
- Sustained hypertension
- Large areas of hypodensity on computed tomography (CT)
- Arterial stenosis proximal to the embolus on angiography

Seizures

A seizure is an episode of abnormal and excessive discharge of cerebral neurons. It can result in altered sensory, motor, or behavioral activities and can be associated with changes in the level of consciousness. Specific symptoms depend on the location of the discharge in the brain. The most common sites of seizure origin are the frontal and temporal lobes. The actual period of the seizure (the ictal period) may be followed by a postictal phase of lethargy and disorientation, which varies with the severity of the seizure. Classification of seizure types is summarized in Box 23-7.

Many patients requiring critical care will experience seizures. Patients may experience seizures secondary to conditions such as cerebral tumors, trauma, infection or fever, metabolic disturbances, or anoxia. Critical care nurses may also care for patients with intractable epilepsy who are undergoing testing or surgery to obtain seizure control (Table 23-9).

BOX 23-6 COLLABORATIVE CARE GUIDE for the Patient with a Stroke

OUTCOMES	INTERVENTIONS
Oxygenation/Ventilation Adequate airway is maintained. SpO_2 is maintained within normal limits. Atelectasis is prevented.	• Monitor breath sounds every shift. • Check oxygen saturation every shift. • Instruct patient to cough and deep breathe and use incentive spirometry q2h while awake. • Assist with removal of airway secretions as needed.
Circulation/Perfusion Patient is free of dysrhythmias.	• Monitor vital signs closely. • Manage blood pressure carefully; avoid sharp drops in blood pressure that could result in hypotension and cause an ischemic event secondary to hypotension. • During cardiac monitoring, identify dysrhythmias. • Treat dysrhythmias to maintain adequate perfusion pressure and reduce chance of neurological impairment.
Neurological Adequate CPP is maintained. Effective communication is established.	• Obtain vital signs and perform a neurological assessment to establish a baseline and to monitor for the development of additional deficits. • Use the NIHSS for detection of early changes suggesting cerebral edema or extension of stroke. • Position head of bed at 30 degrees to promote venous drainage. • Assess patient's ability to speak and to follow simple commands. • Arrange for consultation with speech–language pathologist to differentiate language disturbances. • Use communication aids to enhance communication. • Provide a calm, unrushed environment. Listen attentively to the patient. Speak in a normal tone.
Fluids/Electrolytes Electrolytes are within normal limits.	• Monitor laboratory results, especially glucose. • Monitor intake and output.
Mobility/Safety Safety is maintained. Complications of immobility are avoided.	• Initiate DVT precautions (eg, compression stockings, sequential compressive devices, subcutaneous heparin) as ordered. • Perform fall risk assessment. • Consult with physical therapy. • Provide active or passive range-of-motion exercises to all extremities every shift. • Establish splinting routine for affected limbs. • Instruct patient in use of mobility aids and fall prevention strategies. • For visual field cuts, teach scanning techniques.
Skin Integrity Patient is without evidence of skin breakdown.	• Perform skin assessment using the Braden scale. • Provide pressure relief mattress as indicated by Braden scale. • Turn and reposition q2h. • Consult with wound nurse specialist for skin issues and concerns.
Nutrition Patient has adequate caloric intake and does not experience decrease in weight from baseline. Patient is free from aspiration.	• Obtain admission weight. • Perform cranial nerve assessment (including ability to swallow) to identify deficits. • Obtain consultation from speech–language pathologist to determine whether oral intake of food and liquids is safe. • Provide proper diet and assist with feeding as needed. • Monitor calorie intake; implement calorie count, if necessary. • Obtain dietary consultation to obtain recommendation for nutritional supplements.

(continued on page 338)

BOX 23-6 COLLABORATIVE CARE GUIDE for the Patient with a Stroke (continued)

OUTCOMES	INTERVENTIONS
Psychosocial	
Support network is established.	• Assess for family support systems. • Screen for poststroke depression.
Teaching/Discharge Planning	
Risk factors are modified. Secondary preventive measures are taken.	• Provide education about blood pressure management. • Provide information regarding modifiable risk factors and lifestyle changes to reduce the incidence of a secondary stroke.

 RED FLAG! *Status epilepticus (continued seizure activity greater than 30 minutes) is a neurological emergency and requires immediate treatment.*

Pathophysiology

Neurons in the brain possess an electrical charge that reflects a balance between intracellular and extracellular charged ions. The electrical activity of the neuronal membrane is determined by the flow of ions (eg, sodium [Na^+], potassium [K^+], calcium [Ca^{2+}], and chloride [Cl^-]) between these spaces. If the permeability of the cells is altered, their excitability can change, making the neuron more likely to discharge.

Assessment

History taking begins with a description of the event by the patient or witnesses. This description should include

• What the patient was doing at the time of the seizure

• The duration of the seizure
• Unusual symptoms or behaviors before the seizure
• Specific features of the seizure (eg, movements, sensations, sounds, tastes, smells, incontinence)
• Level of consciousness during and after the seizure (recall of the seizure)
• Duration and description of symptoms after the seizure

Also relevant are the patient's sleep patterns, a history of alcohol or drug abuse, the patient's past medical history, a family history of seizure, the presence of possible seizure triggers (eg, menstruation, stress, fevers, metabolic disorders), and the circumstances surrounding seizures that have occurred in the past (ie, age of onset, symptoms, duration, frequency, similarities to present seizure).

In a patient who has not experienced seizures before, CT or MRI may be ordered to assess for a structural lesion. An EEG is obtained to screen for interictal seizure discharges (electrical abnormalities present in between seizures) and to measure cerebral excitability. Often, continuous EEG monitoring, which captures ictal, postictal, and interictal

BOX 23-7 Classification of Seizure Types

Generalized: involves both hemispheres; loss of consciousness; no local onset in the cerebrum
Tonic–clonic (grand-mal)—stiffening; forced expiration (cry); rhythmic jerking
Clonic—symmetrical, bilateral semirhythmic jerking
Tonic—sudden increased tone and forced expiration
Myoclonic—sudden, brief body jerks
Atonic ("drop attacks")—sudden loss of tone; falls
Absence (petit mal)—brief staring, usually without motor involvement
Partial: involves one hemisphere
   Simple partial seizure—no change in level of consciousness; symptoms may be autonomic (eg, respiratory changes, tachycardia, flushing), psychic (eg, déjà vu), or cognitive

• Motor (includes Jacksonian)—frontal lobe
• Somatosensory—parietal lobe
• Visual—occipital lobe

Complex partial seizures—altered level of consciousness; with or without automatisms (eg, lip-smacking, swallowing, aimless walking, verbalizations)—temporal lobe

• Simple partial seizure followed by change in level of consciousness, or
• Starts with change in consciousness

Partial seizure with secondary generalization—continuous EEG monitoring may be necessary to differentiate from generalized seizures

• Simple partial → generalization
• Complex partial → generalization
• Simple partial → complex partial → generalization

Unclassified

TABLE 23-9 Management of Intractable Seizures

Procedure	Indications	Outcome	Potential Complications	Comments
Temporal lobectomy: removal of 6 cm of temporal lobe in the nondominant hemisphere and 4–5 cm in the dominant hemisphere	Intractable anterior temporal lobe seizures; Greater than 5 years' duration; Significant quality-of-life compromise	60%–70% seizure free; 20% greatly improved seizure control	Visual field defects; Dysphasia (usually temporary); Mild memory problems; Depression; Transient psychiatric disturbance; Infection; Bleeding	At 1 y postoperatively, it is expected that seizure status will not change; Medication management continues for 2–3 y postoperatively
Corpus callosotomy: transection of the corpus callosum (or anterior two thirds)	Severe secondarily generalized epilepsy; drop attacks	Reduced number of generalized seizures	Hemiparesis; Transient syndrome of mutism, urinary incontinence, and bilateral leg weakness; Many patients develop learning disabilities	Used when medical options have failed; Seizure-free periods usually temporary and occur in only 5–10% of patients; Wada test or functional MRI (to evaluate side of brain responsible for speech and memory) recommended for left-handed patients
Vagal nerve stimulator: implanted programmable signal generator in the chest with stimulating electrodes to the left vagus nerve	Seizures (often partial) refractory to medication; used when resective surgery is not an option	Reduction in seizure frequency: high stimulation 25%; low stimulation 15%	Changes in voice; Dyspnea; Tingling in neck during stimulation; Rare cases of bradycardia or asystole	Does not generally resolve seizures
Deep brain stimulator: Electrodes placed in deep brain structures (thalamus, hippocampus, internal capsule) and programmed to activate when seizure activity is recorded	Uncontrolled epilepsy	Reduction in seizures	Bleeding; Infection; Neurological deficits	Has been used for tremor in Parkinson's disease; Relatively new use in refractory seizures with unknown long-term outcomes

data, is used in the critical care unit to identify subtle or nonconvulsive seizures in critically ill patients.

Management

Goals of therapy are to maintain airway, breathing, and circulation; stop the seizure; stabilize the patient; and identify and treat the cause. Emergency management of status epilepticus is summarized in Box 23-8.[18]

Spinal Cord Injury

Spinal cord injury is most common in young adults between the ages of 16 and 30 years. Common causes include MVCs, falls, sports, and acts of violence.

Classification

Spinal cord injuries can be classified by mechanism, type of vertebral injury, or level of injury.

Mechanism of Injury

Spinal cord injuries occur as a result of penetrating injury or blunt forces. Typical mechanisms of blunt injury are shown in Fig. 23-7.

- **Hyperflexion injuries** are caused by a sudden deceleration of the head and neck, and are often seen in patients who have sustained trauma from a head-on MVC or diving accident. The cervical region is most often involved, especially at the C5–C6 level.

BOX 23-8 Emergency Treatment of Status Epilepticus

Establish airway (with intubation, if necessary) and administer oxygen.

Stop seizures
- Benzodiazepines (lorazepam, 1 to 2 mg/min over 8 min or diazepam to total of 20 mg). These are short-acting drugs, and simultaneous loading with phenytoin at 50 mg/min or fosphenytoin at equivalent of 150 mg phenytoin/min is necessary; may total 20 mg/kg.
- For persistent seizures, add 5 to 10 mg/kg phenytoin *or* phenobarbital at 50 to 100 mg/min to total of 20 mg/kg.

Monitor electroencephalogram (EEG) and blood pressure
Identify cause. Diagnostic studies may include blood-work (electrolytes; anticonvulsant levels; arterial blood gases; complete blood count; renal and liver function studies; coagulation studies; toxicology studies); CT; lumbar puncture if CNS infection is suspected.

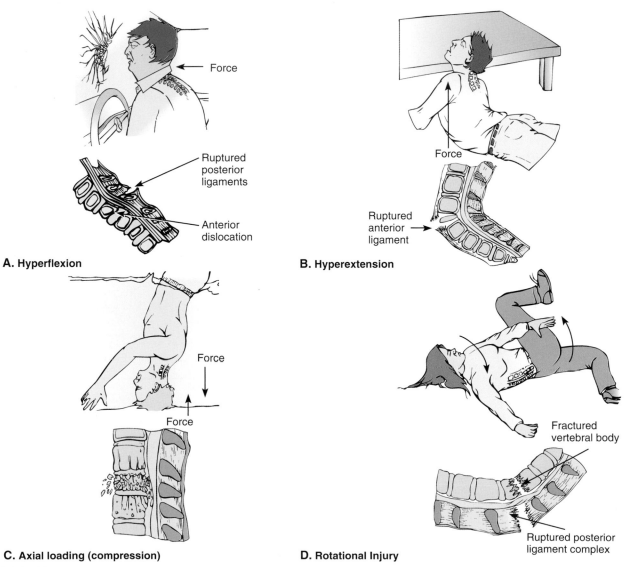

A. Hyperflexion — Force, Ruptured posterior ligaments, Anterior dislocation

B. Hyperextension — Force, Ruptured anterior ligament

C. Axial loading (compression) — Force, Force

D. Rotational Injury — Fractured vertebral body, Ruptured posterior ligament complex

FIGURE 23-7 Mechanisms of spinal cord injury. (From Hickey JV: Clinical Practice of Neurological and Neurosurgical Nursing, 6th ed. Philadelphia, PA: Lippincott Williams & Wilkins, 2009, pp 424–425.)

BOX 23-9 Types of Vertebral Fractures and Dislocations

Fractures

Simple fracture: single fracture; alignment of the vertebrae is intact and neurological deficits do not occur

Compression fracture: fracture caused by axial loading and hyperflexion

Wedge compression fracture: a stable fracture that involves compression of the vertebral body in the cervical area

Teardrop fracture: an unstable fracture that involves a piece of bone breaking off the vertebra; seen in wedge fractures

Comminuted fracture: the vertebra is shattered into several pieces; bone fragments may be driven into spinal cord

Dislocations

Dislocation: one vertebra overrides another

Subluxation: partial or incomplete dislocation

Fracture–dislocation: fracture and dislocation

- **Hyperextension injuries** can be caused by a fall, a rear-end MVC (whiplash), or getting hit in the head (eg, during a boxing match). Hyperextension of the head and neck may cause contusion and ischemia of the spinal cord without vertebral column damage.
- **Axial loading (compression) injuries** typically occur when a person lands on the feet, buttocks, or head after falling, jumping, or diving from a height. Compression of the vertebral column causes a burst fracture that can result in damage to the spinal cord.
- **Rotational injuries** result from forces that cause extreme twisting or lateral flexion of the head and neck. Fracture or dislocation of vertebrae may also occur.

Type of Vertebral Injury

Mechanical forces can result in fracture or dislocation of vertebrae, or both. Box 23-9 presents definitions of types of fractures and dislocations. A fracture may be considered unstable if the longitudinal ligaments are torn.

Level of Injury

Spinal cord injuries can also be classified according to the segment of the spinal cord that is affected:

- Upper cervical (C1–C2) injuries (atlas fractures, atlantoaxial subluxation, odontoid fractures, hangman's fractures)
- Lower cervical (C3–C8) injuries
- Thoracic (T1–T12) injuries
- Lumbar (L1–L5) injuries
- Sacral (S1–S5) injuries

The degree of functional recovery depends on the location and extent of the injury. The level of spinal cord injury is determined by the effect of the injury on sensory and motor function. The dermatome pathways are used to determine the level of sensory loss (Fig. 23-8). Retention of all or some of the motor or sensory function below the level of injury implies that the lesion is incomplete, whereas total loss of voluntary muscle control and sensation below the level of injury suggests that the lesion is complete.

Pathophysiology

Injury to the spinal cord that occurs at the time of impact is referred to as the primary injury. The more mobile areas of the vertebral column (eg, the cervical area) are most frequently involved. Damage to the spinal cord is most often associated with damage to the vertebral column and ligaments. The vertebrae may be fractured, dislocated (subluxed), or compressed. As a result of the injury to the vertebral column, the spinal cord itself may be contused, compressed, or dislocated.

Equally destructive is the injury or damage to the spinal cord that continues for hours after the trauma. Mechanisms of secondary injury include the following:

- During the inflammatory response, immune cells release harmful substances, causing cellular damage.
- Hypoperfusion of the spinal cord from microscopic hemorrhage and edema leads to ischemia.
- The release of catecholamines and vasoactive substances contributes to decreased circulation and perfusion of the spinal cord.
- The release of excess neurotransmitters results in overexcitation of the nerve cells, which allows high levels of calcium to enter the cells, causing cellular death.

Clinical Manifestations

Common clinical manifestations include spinal cord syndromes and autonomic dysfunction.

Spinal Cord Syndromes

Incomplete cord injuries often cause recognizable neurological syndromes that are classified according to the area damaged (Fig. 23-9).

- **Central cord syndrome.** Damage to the spinal cord is centrally located. Hyperextension of the cervical spine often is the mechanism of injury, and the damage is greatest to the cervical tracts supplying the arms. Clinically, the patient may present with greater involvement of the upper extremities over the lower.
- **Brown-Séquard cord syndrome.** Damage is located on one side of the spinal cord. On the same side as the lesion (ipsilaterally), the patient has complete motor paralysis but maintains sensation of pain, temperature, and touch. On the opposite side of the lesion (contralaterally), there is loss of pain, temperature, and touch, but the patient

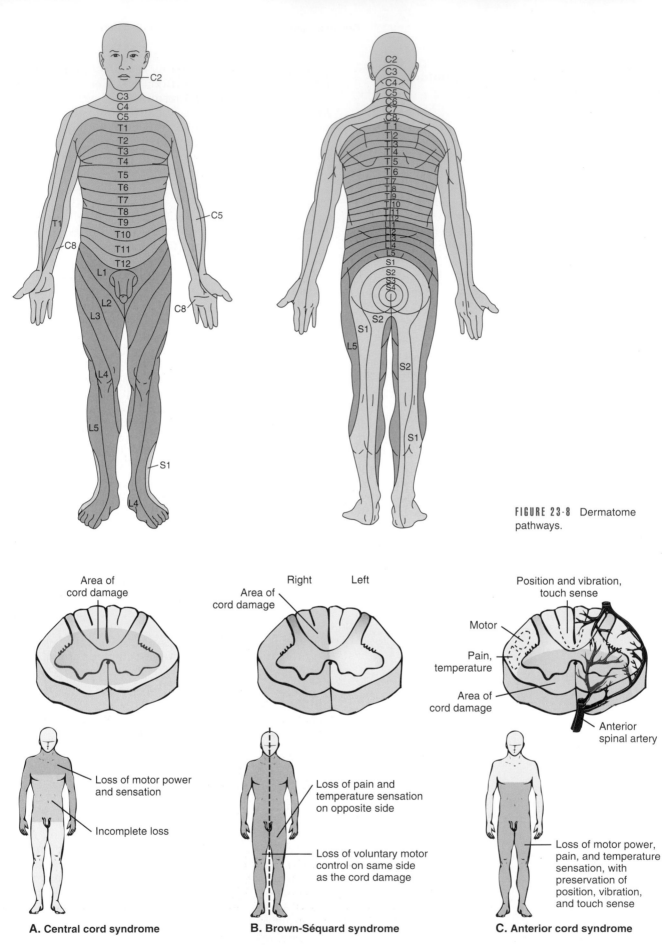

FIGURE 23-8 Dermatome pathways.

Position and vibration, touch sense

Motor

Pain, temperature

Area of cord damage

Anterior spinal artery

Area of cord damage

Loss of motor power and sensation

Incomplete loss

A. Central cord syndrome

Right   Left

Area of cord damage

Loss of pain and temperature sensation on opposite side

Loss of voluntary motor control on same side as the cord damage

B. Brown-Séquard syndrome

Loss of motor power, pain, and temperature sensation, with preservation of position, vibration, and touch sense

C. Anterior cord syndrome

FIGURE 23-9 Spinal cord syndromes. (From Hickey JV: Clinical Practice of Neurological and Neurosurgical Nursing, 6th ed. Philadelphia, PA: Lippincott Williams & Wilkins, 2009, pp 423–425.)

maintains motor function. Clinically, the patient's limb with the best motor strength has the poorest sensation, and vice versa.

- **Anterior cord syndrome.** The anterior aspect of the spinal cord is damaged. Clinically, the patient usually has complete motor paralysis and loss of pain and temperature below the level of injury, with preservation of light touch, proprioception, and vibratory sense.
- **Posterior cord syndrome,** which is rarely seen, is usually the result of a hyperextension injury at the cervical level. Position sense (proprioception), light touch, and vibratory sense are lost below the level of the injury.

Autonomic Dysfunction

The autonomic nervous system carries nerve impulses from the brain and spinal cord to effector organs throughout the body. Sympathetic nerves exit the spinal cord between C7 and L1, and parasympathetic nerves exit between S2 and S4. Therefore, spinal cord injury can result in autonomic nervous system dysfunction. Common manifestations of this dysfunction include spinal shock, neurogenic shock, orthostatic hypotension, and autonomic dysreflexia.

- **Spinal shock** (Fig. 23-10) occurs immediately or within several hours of a spinal cord injury and is caused by primary and secondary injury to the spinal cord. Clinically, the patient exhibits the loss of motor, sensory, reflex, and autonomic function below the level of the injury, with resultant flaccid paralysis. Loss of bowel and bladder function and the body's ability to control temperature (poikilothermia) occur. There is no treatment, and the duration of spinal shock depends on the severity of the insult and the presence of other complications. The return of perianal reflex activity signals the end of the period of spinal shock.
- Spasticity develops after recovery from the period of spinal shock. A physical therapy consult is warranted to develop an exercise, stretching, and positioning program for the patient. Pharmacotherapy (eg, baclofen, dantrolene sodium, diazepam, clonidine) may also be indicated.
- **Neurogenic shock,** a form of distributive shock, is seen in patients with severe cervical and upper thoracic injuries. It is caused by the loss of sympathetic control of the heart and vasculature, resulting in vasodilation and bradycardia. Signs and symptoms include hypotension, severe bradycardia, and

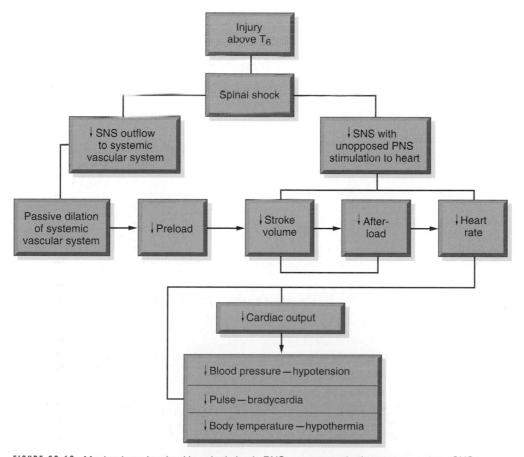

FIGURE 23-10 Mechanisms involved in spinal shock. PNS, parasympathetic nervous system; SNS, sympathetic nervous system. (From Zejdlik C: Management of Spinal Cord Injury. Boston: Jones & Bartlett Publishers, 1992.)

loss of the ability to sweat below the level of injury. The hypotension is managed with IV fluid resuscitation. Symptomatic bradycardia may require temporary external pacing.

- **Orthostatic hypotension** may occur in a patient with a spinal cord injury because the body is unable to compensate for changes in position. The cord injury prevents the vasoconstriction message from the medulla from reaching the blood vessels.
- **Autonomic dysreflexia (hyperreflexia)** is a medical emergency that can occur after the resolution of spinal shock in patients with a spinal cord lesion at T7 or above. The syndrome presents quickly and can precipitate hypertensive crisis and death. In autonomic dysreflexia, a stimulus below the level of injury (Box 23-10) produces a sympathetic discharge that causes reflex vasoconstriction, leading to extreme hypertension and a throbbing headache. The body attempts to reduce the hypertension through superficial vasodilation of vessels above the spinal cord injury, leading to flushing, blurred vision, and nasal congestion. Other signs and symptoms include bradycardia, profuse sweating above the level of the injury, piloerection below the level of injury, pupil dilation, and nausea. Management entails identification and removal of the stimulus. Nursing interventions for managing autonomic dysreflexia are given in Box 23-11.

BOX 23-10　Precipitating Factors in Autonomic Dysreflexia

- Bladder distention, urinary tract infection, bladder or kidney stones
- Bowel distention
- Pressure areas or decubitus ulcers
- Thrombophlebitis
- Acute abdominal problems (eg, ulcers, gastritis)
- Pulmonary emboli
- Menstruation
- Second stage of labor
- Constrictive clothing
- Heterotopic bone
- Pain
- Sexual activity/ejaculation
- Manipulation or instrumentation of bladder or bowel
- Spasticity
- Exposure to hot or cold

Management

Prehospital Management

A spinal cord injury is suspected at the scene of an accident any time the patient has decreased or

---

BOX 23-11　Nursing Management of Autonomic Dysreflexia

Ideally, three members of the healthcare team are available to assist: one to check the blood pressure, one to check the drainage system, and one to notify the physician.

1. Elevate the head of bed.
2. Quickly insert bladder catheter or check bladder drainage system in place to detect possible obstruction.
   - Check to make sure plug or clamp is not in catheter or on tubing.
   - Check for kinks in catheter or drainage tubing.
   - Check inlet to leg bag to make sure it is not corroded.
   - Check to make sure leg bag is not overfull.
   - If none of these are evident, proceed to step 3.
3. Determine whether catheter is plugged by irrigating the bladder slowly with no more than 30 mL of irrigation solution. If symptoms do not subside, proceed to step 4.

 RED FLAG! *Use of greater than 30 ml of irrigation fluid may increase the massive sympathetic outflow already present.*

4. Change the catheter and empty the bladder.
5. If bladder overdistention does not seem to be the cause of the dysreflexia, rule out other potential causes:
   - Check for bowel impaction. Do not attempt to remove impaction, if present. Apply Nupercainal ointment or Xylocaine jelly to the rectum and anal area. As the area is anesthetized, the blood pressure should decrease. After the blood pressure stabilizes, using a generous amount of anesthetizing ointment or jelly, manually remove the impaction.
   - Change the patient's position to relieve pressure.
   - Loosen tight clothing and shoes.
6. Continue monitoring the blood pressure (BP) during this time. If the BP remains elevated and unable to find the source, call the physician immediately. The physician may order an antihypertensive to lower the blood pressure.

absent movement or sensation. An unconscious patient or one with a head injury is treated as though a spinal cord injury has occurred until proved otherwise. Airway patency is assessed, and the cervical spine is immobilized and stabilized. A cervical collar increases the level of stability but does not provide complete immobilization, especially in the case of complete ligamentous disruption.

In-Hospital Management

Early Management

In the emergency department, the primary and secondary surveys are completed. Management priorities include:

- **Assessment and management of the patient's airway and breathing.** Hypoventilation or respiratory failure from inadequate innervation of the respiratory muscles and diaphragm is a common problem after spinal cord injury, particularly in patients with high cervical injuries. In addition, spinal cord edema can act like an ascending lesion and compromise function of the diaphragm. Preexisting pulmonary disease or coexistent chest, laryngeal, tracheal, or esophageal injuries can further compromise respiratory function. If the patient requires ventilatory assistance, elective intubation and mechanical ventilation are followed by a chest radiograph.
- **Assessment and management of the patient's circulatory status.** Hypotension may be due to neurogenic shock or hemorrhagic shock (secondary to associated injuries). Fluid resuscitation is accomplished by the use of crystalloids or blood. Early administration of blood enhances oxygenation and may minimize secondary ischemic injury to the spinal cord.
- **Completion of a thorough neurological assessment, including spine x-rays.** A digital rectal examination is performed to determine whether the injury is incomplete or complete. The lesion is incomplete if the patient can feel the palpating finger or can contract the perianal muscles around the finger voluntarily. Sensation usually accompanies voluntary motor activity, and may be present in the absence of voluntary motor activity. In either case, the prognosis for further motor and sensory return is good. Rectal tone by itself, without the presence of voluntary perianal muscle contraction or rectal sensation, is not evidence of an incomplete cord injury.
- **Assessment for associated injuries.** TBI, intrathoracic injuries, intra-abdominal injuries, retroperitoneal injuries, and fractures of the pelvis or long bones are often seen in association with spinal cord injury.

When the patient is stabilized, frequent assessment of neurological status is necessary to determine the extent of the spinal cord injury and monitor for changes in level of consciousness that may occur secondary to TBI. Most facilities use a specialized flow sheet (eg, the Standard Neurological Classification of Spinal Cord Injury flow sheet) to assess and document the patient's level of functioning. Diagnostic studies may be ordered, including radiographs of the spine, chest, and other structures as clinically indicated; CT and MRI (to evaluate soft tissue and ligament injuries). Flexion–extension views are obtained to assess for ligament involvement in patients who are conscious and can follow commands, even when plain radiographs and CT are negative for bony injury. If the patient is unconscious or unable to tell the examiner if there is pain on flexion, then an MRI is required to rule out ligament injuries. A cervical collar is kept on until the MRI results are obtained or the patient regains consciousness and is able to cooperate with the studies.

The administration of high-dose steroids (eg, methylprednisolone) in the emergency department to reduce swelling and minimize secondary injury is controversial. Some studies have found improvement in function in blunt, incomplete cord injuries. However, steroid use has also been associated with severe pneumonia and sepsis.

Stabilization of the Spine

The goals of ongoing management are to stabilize and realign the spine to prevent further neurological deterioration. This can be accomplished through closed reduction or surgical techniques. Closed reduction of an unstable cervical fracture or subluxation often involves skeletal traction. Short-term cervical traction can be achieved using Gardner–Wells, Vinke, or Crutchfield tongs; long-term cervical traction entails the use of a halo vest. Stable fractures can be immobilized using a Miami J or Aspen collar (cervical fractures), a Minerva brace (cervicothoracic fractures), or a Jewett brace (thoracolumbosacral injuries).

For some patients, surgery may be necessary to stabilize and support the spine. The risks of surgery must be balanced against the possible benefits. Rod placement, laminectomy and fusion, and anterior fusion are techniques used for surgical stabilization. Bone for fusion usually comes from the patient's iliac crest, tibia, or ribs; alternatively, bone can be obtained from a tissue bank. After surgery, the patient receives routine postoperative care. The nurse monitors the patient's motor and sensory status at least every hour for the first 24 hours, and then every 4 hours after that. The physician is notified immediately if any deterioration in neurological status occurs. The nurse also monitors for complications (eg, spinal fluid fistulas, infections, wound dehiscence). Older patients and those with preexisting comorbidities who have open wounds, injuries to the thoracolumbar spine, or complete injuries are at particularly high risk for postoperative infection.[19]

Supportive Care

Supportive care focuses on preventing complications, and initiating prompt interventions to treat any complications that do occur. A collaborative care guide for the patient with a spinal cord injury is given in Box 23-12.

BOX 23-12 COLLABORATIVE CARE GUIDE for the Patient With Spinal Cord Injury

OUTCOMES	INTERVENTIONS
Oxygenation/Ventilation ABGs are within normal limits. Airway patency is maintained. The patient does not aspirate. The patient does not develop pulmonary complications (eg, infection, atelectasis).	• Monitor respiratory rate, arterial oxygen saturation, and pulmonary function test results, and auscultate breath sounds. • Assess need for mechanical ventilation. • Provide for deep breathing, assistive coughing, and incentive spirometer exercises. • Turn frequently; mobilize out of bed to chair when able. • Apply abdominal binder when out of bed. • Consult pulmonology as needed.
Circulation/Perfusion There is no evidence of neurogenic (spinal) shock (T10 injuries and higher). Blood pressure is adequate to maintain vital organ function. There is no development of DVT or pulmonary embolism.	• Monitor for bradycardia, vasodilation, and hypotension. • Assess for dysrhythmias. • Prepare to administer intravascular volume, vasopressors, and positive chronotropic agents. • Begin DVT prophylaxis on admission (eg, external compression device, low-dose heparin or LMWH). • Measure calf and thigh circumference daily and at same location; report increase. • Apply compression hose to lower extremities before mobilizing out of bed.
There is no evidence of orthostatic hypotension.	• Monitor for orthostatic hypotension when raising head of bed and getting out of bed. • Allow patient to "dangle" before mobilizing out of bed. • Consult cardiology as needed.
Neurological There is no evidence of deterioration in neurological status.	• Perform neurological checks and spinal cord function checks q2–4h. • Monitor for deterioration in neurological status and report to the physician.
The vertebral column is maintained in a neutral position and in proper alignment.	• For patients with cervical traction: check the orthopedic frame, traction, and tongs daily to be sure that they are secure. Ensure that traction weights hang freely. • For patients with a halo vest: Ensure that the pins on the halo ring are secure and tight.
Fluids/Electrolytes Serum electrolytes are within normal limits.	• Monitor laboratory studies as indicated by patient's condition. • Assess for dehydration. • Administer mineral/electrolyte replacement as ordered.
Fluid balance is maintained as evidenced by stable weight, absence of edema, normal skin turgor.	• Monitor gastrointestinal and insensible fluid loss. • Make accurate daily fluid intake and output measurements. • Weigh weekly. • Monitor results of laboratory studies, particularly albumin and electrolyte levels.
Mobility/Safety Joint range of motion is maintained and contractures prevented. Muscle tone is maintained. The patient ambulates in a safe manner to the best of his or her ability.	• Position in correct alignment. • Begin range-of-motion exercises early after admission. • Maintain splint, brace, and adaptive device schedule; check for pressure ulcers q4h or more often if indicated. • Consult with physical and occupational therapy.

BOX 23-12 COLLABORATIVE CARE GUIDE for the Patient With Spinal Cord Injury (continued)

OUTCOMES	INTERVENTIONS
Skin Integrity	
Patient is without evidence of skin breakdown.	• Consult with wound care specialist to determine correct type of bed. • Reposition patient at least q2h while in bed. • Position patient to prevent pressure on bony prominences. • Use upright, straight-backed chair when patient is out of bed (not a reclining chair). Use felt pad on chair seat. • Reposition/shift weight q1h when sitting upright. • Use Braden scale to monitor risk for skin breakdown.
Skin integrity is maintained under or around stabilization devices (eg, cervical collar, halo vest).	• Monitor skin underneath stabilization devices and around pins. • Use meticulous skin care underneath stabilization devices and around pins. • Ensure proper fit of vest-like stabilization devices by sliding a finger between the vest and skin.
Nutrition	
Protein, carbohydrate, fat, and calorie intake meet minimal daily requirements. The patient has a fluid intake of up to 3000 mL daily. Aspiration is prevented.	• Consult dietitian. • Encourage fluids, high-fiber diet. • Monitor fluid I&O, calorie count. • Administer parenteral and enteral nutrition as appropriate. • Assist with feeding/feed as needed. Encourage the patient to take small bites and chew well.
Elimination	
Postvoid residuals < 100 mL. Pattern of bowel evacuation every 1–2 d is established.	• Institute bowel and bladder training programs. • Record the frequency and consistency of stool. • If the patient is voiding independently, monitor postvoid residuals.
Comfort/Pain	
Pain < "4" on visual analog scale.	• Assess and differentiate pain from anxiety or stress response. • Administer appropriate analgesic or sedative to relieve pain and monitor patient response. • Use nonpharmacological pain relief techniques (eg, distraction, music, relaxation therapies).
Psychosocial	
Patient adapts to loss of motor and sensory function, and maintains a positive body image.	• Provide emotional support by encouraging expression of concerns, arranging for support services (eg, social services, clergy, neuropsychologist, support groups), and so on.
Integration is made into prior social role.	• Provide patient/family counseling regarding stages of grief, sexual function and management techniques, social services and community resources.
Teaching/Discharge Planning	
Complications associated with loss of bowel or bladder control are prevented.	• Teach patient/family: • Bowel program and training • Dietary habits to maintain bowel function • Bladder training/intermittent catheterization • Prevention of, and signs/symptoms of autonomic dysreflexia
Complications of immobility are prevented.	• Teach patient/family: • Positioning to prevent skin breakdown • Physical therapy exercises • BHT
Patient is discharged to appropriate postacute setting.	• Consult rehabilitation/discharge planner/social services early after admission to initiate placement arrangements.

- **Prevention of respiratory compromise.** Patients with a spinal cord injury, especially injuries above T6, are at risk for respiratory compromise. Respiratory failure is anticipated if the patient's vital capacity is less than 15 to 20 mL/kg and the respiratory rate is greater than 30 breaths/min. If the oxygen saturation value is less than 90% or if the $PaCO_2$ is greater than 45 mm Hg, intubation may be required. Routine bronchial hygiene therapy (BHT) and kinetic therapy using a specialty bed that rotates a minimum of 40 degrees on a continuous basis helps prevent pulmonary complications.

 RED FLAG! *Respiratory complications are the leading cause of death in the acute and chronic phases of spinal cord injury, especially in patients with higher-level injuries.*

- **Prevention of cardiovascular compromise.** The patient is at risk for bradycardia, hypotension, and dysrhythmias because of disruption in the autonomic nervous system. When the blood pressure is not high enough to sustain vital organ perfusion, low-dose dopamine may be administered after adequate fluid resuscitation. Symptomatic bradycardia may require the administration of atropine or the use of a transcutaneous or transvenous pacemaker. Left ventricular dysfunction may occur secondary to the release of β-endorphins; cardiac enzymes should be obtained if there are ECG changes.
- **Pain management.** Pain management is essential in caring for patients with spinal cord injuries. It is not unusual for the patient to report pain, frequently severe pain. The source of the pain may be neuropathic, musculoskeletal, central, or visceral. Abnormal sensation may occur at the level of the lesion in injuries caused by nerve root damage.
- **Thermoregulation.** Ineffective thermoregulation is common in patients with spinal cord injuries above the thoracolumbar area. Interruption of the sympathetic nervous system inhibits thalamic thermoregulatory mechanisms. As a result, the patient cannot sweat to get rid of body heat, and there is an absence of vasoconstriction, resulting in an inability to shiver to increase body heat. Hypothermia is usually managed by using warmed blankets, and the room temperature is adjusted to maintain patient comfort. The goal is to stabilize the patient's temperature above 96.5°F (35.8°C).
- **Mobilization and positioning.** Attention to mobilization and positioning is important to prevent complications of immobility. A turn schedule for the patient is important, even if the patient has not had stabilizing surgery. It may take three staff members to accomplish turning safely, particularly in patients with cervical injuries. One person stabilizes the neck, and the other two flex the hips, knees, and ankles and hold the feet flat on the bed surface while turning the patient's trunk. Foam wedges, pillows, or air-filled rolls are used to maintain alignment.

- **Urinary management.** Initially, an indwelling urinary catheter is placed to prevent the bladder from becoming distended secondary to atony, and to allow for hourly measurement of urinary output. As soon as spinal shock has resolved, the indwelling catheter is removed and bladder training (eg, with intermittent catheterization) begins.
- **Bowel management.** Measures to prevent constipation and begin progress toward bowel continence include maintenance of appropriate intake; daily administration of stool softeners and a suppository; and development of a consistent schedule for bowel elimination. The timing of the program is usually designed to coincide with the peristalsis that occurs after meals to move food through the gastrointestinal tract. Rectal stimulation may be necessary to trigger defecation.
- **Psychological support.** As soon as the patient is medically stable, the nurse begins to focus on the psychosocial issues that are of concern to the patient and family (eg, long-term prognosis, sexual functioning, body image). The nurse answers questions to the best of his or her knowledge; encourages the patient and family to express concerns; and focuses on the patient's abilities without minimizing the patient's disabilities.

CASE STUDY

A coworker finds Mr. S., a 60-year-old man, lying injured on the floor in the service station where he works as a mechanic. It appears that he slipped on the grease on the floor while working on the transmission of a small truck. Paramedics arrive at the scene of the accident within 10 minutes. Mr. S. is able to move his extremities, and he reports neck pain of 6 on a pain scale of 10. He is awake, alert, and oriented to his current location; the date and day of the week; and details of the accident. His pupils are equal and reactive to light. He shows no other signs of injury except for a cut on his forehead. Vital signs are as follows: BP, 170/102 mm Hg; HR, 86 beats/min; and RR, 28 breaths/min (unlabored and regular). The paramedics apply a cervical collar, place Mr. S. on a backboard, and transport him to the medical center by helicopter. He arrives in the emergency department within 45 minutes of the accident.

On initial examination, Mr. S.'s vital signs are as follows: BP, 180/90 mm Hg; HR, 88 beats/min; RR, 24 breaths/min (somewhat shallow respirations); and temperature, 98.6°F (37°C). Mr. S. is sweating and mildly confused. His arm veins are quite distended. According to the paramedics, his motor and sensory function has decreased since his initial evaluation at the scene of the accident. Although he could originally tighten his biceps, now he cannot overcome gravity to raise his arms. Deep tendon reflexes are markedly decreased.

The emergency trauma team starts IV lactated Ringer's solution, inserts an indwelling urinary catheter, and inserts a nasogastric tube, which is connected to low intermittent suction. The trauma physician orders full spine, skull, and chest radiographs. The radiographs reveal that Mr. S. has a dislocated fracture of C5 and C6. The chest film shows a lack of full lung field expansion. Bloodwork results are normal, with the exception of ABGs, which show respiratory acidosis (pH 7.30).

Mr. S. is admitted to the critical care unit, where he is placed in a halo fixation device to realign the cervical vertebrae and stabilize the fracture. Neurogenic shock treatment includes careful IV fluid replacement to avoid overhydration, administration of dopamine if hypotension compromises perfusion of vital organs, and atropine to correct bradycardia if he becomes symptomatic.

Nursing interventions include monitoring neurological signs and vital signs every hour for the first 24 hours and then every 2 hours until Mr. S. is stabilized. The nurses who are caring for Mr. S. pay particular attention to his respiratory status because he is at risk for respiratory failure due to spinal cord edema. They turn him every 2 hours and measure and record the output from the indwelling urinary catheter and nasogastric tube every 4 hours. They make every effort to prevent complications of immobility, both in the critical care and acute care units. After consulting physical and occupational therapy, Mr. S.'s healthcare team initiates a treatment plan. Once past the acute phase of his injury, Mr. S. is transferred to a rehabilitation facility for further recovery and adaptation to his injury.

1. What additional information is needed about Mr. S. to provide him with appropriate care while hospitalized?

2. Based on the information from the case study, list the five priorities of care for Mr. S. Include your rationale for selecting these priorities.

3. What nursing interventions should be implemented based on the priorities of care listed above?

References

1. Marbacher S, et al: Primary reconstruction of open depressed skull fractures with titanium mesh. J Craniofac Surg 19(2):490–495, 2008
2. Thompson H, Mauk K: Care of the patient with mild traumatic brain injury. AANN and ARN Clinical Practice Guidelines Series, 2011
3. Donkin J, Robert V: Mechanisms of cerebral edema in traumatic brain injury: Therapeutic developments. Curr Opin Neurol 23(3):293–299, 2010
4. Ng SC, Poon WS, Chan MT: Cerebral hemisphere asymmetry in cerebrovascular regulation in ventilated traumatic brain injury. Acta Neurochir Suppl 96:21–23, 2006
5. Brain Trauma Foundation: Guidelines for the management of severe traumatic brain injury, J Neurotrauma 24(Suppl 1):s1–s106, 2007
6. Quality Standards Subcommittee of the American Academy of Neurology: Practice parameters: Assessment and management of patients in the persistent vegetative state [summary statement]. Report of the Quality Standards Subcommittee of the American Academy of Neurology. Neurology 45:1015–1018, 1995
7. Lemke DM: Sympathetic storming after severe traumatic brain injury. Crit Care Nurs 27(1):30–37, 2007
8. Bond AE, Draeger CRL, Mandleco B, et al: Needs of family members of patients with severe traumatic brain injury: Implications for evidenced-based practice. Crit Care Nurs 23(4):63–71, 2003
9. World Health Organization: Classification of tumours. In Kleihues P, Cabenne WK (eds): Pathology and Genetics of Tumours of the Nervous System. Lyon, France: IARC Press, 2000
10. Irwin R, Rippe J: Intensive Care Medicine, 6th ed. Lippincott, Williams & Wilkins, 2008, p 2029.
11. Popp J, Deshares E: A Guide to the Primary Care of Neurological Disorders. American Association of Neurosurgeons. 2007, p 303.
12. Raja P, et al: Microsurgical clipping and endovascular coiling of intracranial aneurysms: A critical review of the literature. Neurosurgery 62(6):1187–202, 2008
13. Upadhyay U: Etiology and management of hyponatremia in neurosurgical patients. J Intensive Care Med 2011
14. Dankbaar J, et al: Effect of different components of triple H therapy on cerebral perfusion in patients with aneurysmal subarachnoid hemorrhage: A systemic review. Crit Care 14: R23, 2010
15. Greenberg MS: Vascular malformations. In Handbook of Neurosurgery. New York: Thieme, 2006, pp 835–848
16. Hacke W, et al: Thrombolysis with alteplase 3 to 4.5 hours after acute ischemic stroke. N Engl J Med 359(13):1317–1329, 2008
17. Hickey J (ed): The Clinical Practice of Neurological and Neurosurgical Nursing, 6th ed. Philadelphia, PA: Lippincott Williams & Wilkins, 2009
18. Costello D, Cole A: Treatment of acute seizures and status epilepticus. J Intensive Care Med 22(6):319–347, 2007
19. Dekutoski M, et al: Surgeons perceptions and reported complications in spine surgeries. Spine 35(9S):S9–S21, 2010

Want to know more? A wide variety of resources to enhance your learning and understanding of this chapter are available on thePoint✳. Visit **http://thepoint.lww.com/MortonEss1e** to access chapter review questions and more!

Gastrointestinal System

Patient Assessment: Gastrointestinal System

OBJECTIVES

Based on the content in this chapter, the reader should be able to:

1 Describe the components of the history for gastrointestinal assessment.
2 Explain the use of inspection, auscultation, percussion, and palpation for gastrointestinal assessment.
3 Describe laboratory tests used to evaluate gastrointestinal function.
4 Describe diagnostic studies used to evaluate gastrointestinal function.

When a patient is critically ill, assessment of the gastrointestinal system may reveal signs and symptoms of the patient's primary medical problem or recognize a new complication.

History

Elements of the gastrointestinal history are summarized in Box 24-1. A patient with a gastrointestinal disorder often presents with abdominal pain. The nurse obtains detailed information about the patient's pain (or other symptoms) using the NOPQRST format (see Chapter 12, Box 12-2). To facilitate accurate assessment and documentation of findings, abdominal regions are described in terms of the quadrant method or the nine regions method (Fig. 24-1). Figure 24-2 on page 354 summarizes common causes of pain by location. With many gastrointestinal problems, the pain is referred (Fig. 24-3, p. 354).

Physical Examination

The order of the abdominal examination is inspection, auscultation, percussion, and palpation. Auscultation precedes percussion and palpation because the latter can alter the frequency and quality of bowel sounds. Likewise, if the painful area is palpated first, the patient may tense the abdominal muscles, hindering assessment.

BOX 24-1 Gastrointestinal Health History

History of the Present Illness

Complete analysis of the following signs and symptoms (using the NOPQRST format; see Chapter 12, Box 12-2)

- Abdominal pain
- Anorexia
- Indigestion (heartburn)
- Dysphagia
- Eructation (burping)
- Nausea
- Vomiting
- Hematemesis
- Fever and chills
- Jaundice
- Pruritus
- Diarrhea
- Constipation
- Flatulence
- Bleeding
- Hemorrhoids
- Melena
- Change in appetite
- Recent weight gain or weight loss
- Mouth lesions
- Anal discomfort
- Fecal incontinence
- Change in abdominal girth

Past Health History

- **Relevant childhood illnesses and immunizations:** hepatitis, influenza, pneumococcal, meningococcal
- **Past acute and chronic medical problems, including treatments and hospitalizations:** diabetes, cancer, inflammatory bowel disease, peptic ulcer, gallstones, polyps, pancreatitis, hepatitis, cirrhosis, cystic fibrosis, spinal cord injury
- **Risk factors:** age, heredity, gender, race, tobacco use, physical inactivity, obesity, diabetes mellitus, tattoos, exposure to infectious diseases
- **Past surgeries:** previous gastrointestinal surgeries (mouth, pharyngeal, esophageal, stomach, small intestine, colon, gallbladder, liver, pancreas), abdominal surgeries or trauma
- **Past diagnostic tests and interventions:** upper endoscopy, colonoscopy, upper gastrointestinal series, barium enema

- **Medications, including prescription drugs, over-the-counter drugs, vitamins, herbs, and supplements:** aspirin, steroids, anticoagulants, nonsteroidal anti-inflammatory drugs (NSAIDs), laxatives, stool softeners
- **Allergies and reactions to medications, foods, contrast, latex, or other materials**
- **Transfusions, including type and date**

Family History

- **Health status or cause of death of parents and siblings:** inflammatory bowel disease, malabsorption syndrome, cystic fibrosis, celiac disease, gallbladder disease, any cancers of the gastrointestinal tract

Personal and Social History

- Tobacco, alcohol, and substance use
- Environment: water source
- Diet: food intolerances, coffee intake, special diet
- Dental status: patterns of dental care; presence of dentures, braces, bridges, or crowns
- Bowel habits
- Sleep patterns
- Exercise
- Sources of stress: physical or psychological
- Travel: especially overseas

Review of Other Systems

- **HEENT:** visual changes, headaches, tinnitus, vertigo, epistaxis, sore throat, mouth lesions, swollen glands, lymphadenopathy
- **Respiratory:** shortness of breath, dyspnea, cough, sputum, lung disease, recurrent infections
- **Cardiovascular:** chest pain, palpitations, orthopnea, edema, hypertension, heart failure, dysrhythmia, valvular disease
- **Genitourinary:** incontinence, erectile dysfunction, dysuria, frequency, nocturia
- **Musculoskeletal:** pain, weakness, varicose veins, sensory changes
- **Neurological:** transient ischemic attacks, stroke, cerebrovascular disease, change in level of consciousness, syncope, seizures

Inspection

The nurse inspects the abdomen for symmetry; visible masses; pulsations; tense, shiny skin; discolored areas; rashes; striae (lines resulting from rapid or prolonged skin stretching); ecchymoses; petechiae; lesions; scars; and prominent or dilated veins. Table 24-1 reviews abnormal abdominal findings on inspection.

Auscultation

Auscultation provides information on bowel motility and abdominal organ vasculature (Table 24-2). The diaphragm of the stethoscope is used to systematically assess bowel sounds in all four quadrants. The bell of the stethoscope is used to listen for vascular sounds over the abdominal aorta and the renal, iliac, and femoral arteries (Fig. 24-4, p. 356).

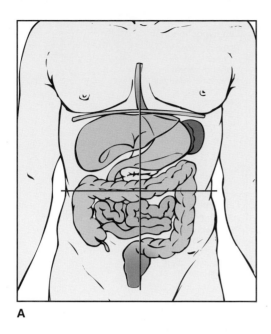

A

Right upper quadrant (RUQ)	Left upper quadrant (LUQ)
Liver and gallbladder Pylorus Duodenum Head of pancreas Hepatic flexure of colon Portions of ascending and transverse colon	Left liver lobe Stomach Body and tail of pancreas Splenic flexure of colon Portions of transverse and descending colon
Right lower quadrant (RLQ)	**Left lower quadrant (LLQ)**
Cecum and appendix Portion of ascending colon	Sigmoid colon Portion of descending colon

B

Right hypochondriac	Epigastric	Left hypochondriac
Right liver lobe Gallbladder	Pyloric end of stomach Duodenum Pancreas Portion of liver	Stomach Tail of pancreas Splenic flexure of colon
Right lumbar	**Umbilical**	**Left lumbar**

Ascending colon
Portions of duodenum
  and jejunum
	Omentum
	Mesentery
	Lower part
	  of duodenum
	Jejunum and ileum
		Descending colon
		Portions of jejunum
		  and ileum

Right inguinal	**Suprapubic or hypogastric**	**Left inguinal**
Cecum Appendix Lower end of ileum	Ileum	Sigmoid colon

FIGURE 24-1 **A:** The quadrant method. **B:** The nine regions method.

RED FLAG! *A bruit (a continuous purring, blowing, or humming sound) heard over the abdominal aorta could be caused by a vascular aneurysm and should be reported immediately if it is a new finding.*

Percussion

Abdominal percussion helps identify air, gas, and fluid in the abdomen and helps determine the size and location of abdominal organs. The nurse percusses the abdomen lightly in all four quadrants of the abdomen, listening for the location and distribution of tympany and dullness.

Palpation

Abdominal palpation is used to establish the presence of abdominal masses and determine the presence, location, and degree of abdominal pain. When disease is present, palpation may result in somatic or visceral pain. Somatic pain, which is localized and accompanied by guarding of the abdominal muscles, reflects inflammation of the skin, fascia, or abdominal surfaces. Visceral pain originates from the organs and is usually dull, diffuse, and generalized.

Light palpation, which is performed first, identifies muscular resistance and areas of tenderness.

Right hypochondriac	Epigastric	Left hypochondriac
Cholecystitis/ cholangitis Hepatitis Metastatic disease to the liver Pleurisy, lower lobe pneumonia, or pneumothorax Congestive hepatomegaly Pyelonephritis Renal colic Duodenal ulcer	Duodenal or gastric ulcer Duodenitis or gastritis Pancreatitis Myocardial infarction or angina Pericarditis Gastroenteritis Mesenteric embolus or thrombus Small bowel obstruction	Pleurisy, lower lobe pneumonia, or pneumothorax Myocardial infarction or angina Pericarditis Pyelonephritis Renal colic Splenic injury
Right lumbar	**Umbilical**	**Left lumbar**
Pancreatitis Pyelonephritis Renal colic Colon obstruction/ gangrene	Appendicitis Small bowel obstruction Rectus sheath hematoma Gastroenteritis Umbilical hernia Abdominal aortic aneurysm Aortic dissection Mesenteric embolus or thrombus	Pancreatitis Pyelonephritis Renal colic Sigmoid diverticulitis Colon obstruction/ gangrene
Right inguinal	**Suprapubic or hypogastric**	**Left inguinal**
Meckel's diverticulum Appendicitis Cecal perforation Groin hernia Colon obstruction/ gangrene Ectopic pregnancy Spigelian hernia Regional enteritis	Rectus sheath hematoma Salpingitis Ectopic pregnancy Tubo-ovarian torsion Mittelschmerz Regional enteritis Endometriosis Abdominal aortic aneurysm	Sigmoid diverticulitis Groin hernia Colon obstruction/ gangrene Ectopic pregnancy Spigelian hernia Regional enteritis

FIGURE 24-2 Common causes of pain by location.

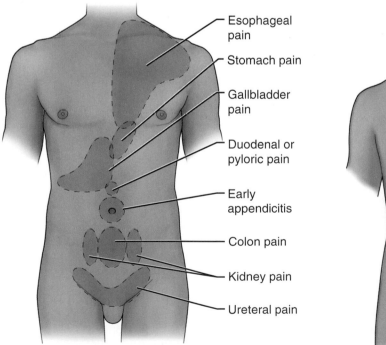

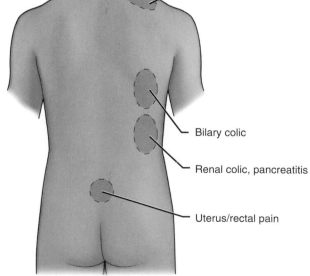

A. Anterior

B. Posterior

FIGURE 24-3 Locations of referred abdominal pain.

TABLE 24-1 Abnormal Abdominal Findings on Inspection

Finding	Characteristic	Possible Cause
Abdominal contour	Concave (scaphoid)	Malnutrition
	Distention	Tumor; excessive fluid (ascites, perforation); gas accumulation; severe malnutrition; peritonitis
Abdominal skin	Bulging	Incisional hernia
	Striae*	Obesity; pregnancy; abdominal tumor; Cushing's syndrome
	Flank ecchymoses (Grey Turner's sign)	Retroperitoneal bleeding; hemorrhagic pancreatitis
	Bluish ecchymosis surrounding umbilicus (Cullen's sign)	Intra-abdominal bleeding; pancreatitis
	Tense, glistening skin	Ascites
	Dilated, tortuous veins	Inferior vena cava obstruction; portal vein hypertension
Umbilicus	Everted	Increased intra-abdominal pressure (from tumor or ascites); ectopic pregnancy
Peristalsis	Strong peristaltic wave	Intestinal obstruction
Aortic pulsations	Obvious and pronounced	Increased intra-abdominal pressure (from tumor or ascites); abdominal aortic aneurysm

*Older striae are white or silver; more recent striae are pink, blue, or purple.

Fingertips are used to depress the abdominal wall 1 cm (0.5 in). Deep palpation is used to locate abdominal organs and large masses. The fingertips are used to depress the abdominal wall firmly to a depth of 7.5 cm (3 in). An enlarged spleen, the edge of the liver, and the pole of the right kidney (but not the left) are usually palpable on deep palpation. The nurse evaluates areas of tenderness detected on light palpation for rebound tenderness (Blumberg's sign) by deeply depressing the area and then releasing the fingertips quickly. If the area hurts more after the fingertips are released, rebound tenderness is present. Rebound tenderness usually indicates peritoneal inflammation (eg, due to infection, abscess, or perforation). Murphy's sign (sharp pain that stops respiration, caused by palpating under the liver border) may be a sign of cholecystitis.

Laboratory Studies

Liver Function Studies

The liver is responsible for many functions, including bile formation and secretion; protein and fat metabolism; detoxification; and the production of enzymes and clotting factors. Table 24-3 summarizes common

TABLE 24-2 Abnormal Abdominal Findings on Auscultation

Sound and Description	Location	Sound	Possible Cause
Bowel sounds	All four quadrants	Hyperactive (high-pitched, rapid, loud, and gurgling)	Gastroenteritis
		High-pitched tinkling and rushes of high-pitched sounds (often accompanied by abdominal cramping)	Obstruction
		Hypoactive (occurring once per minute or less frequently)	Post–bowel surgery; feces-filled colon
		Absent	Peritonitis, paralytic ileus
Systolic bruits (vascular "blowing" sounds resembling cardiac murmurs)	Abdominal aorta	Partial arterial obstruction or turbulent blood flow	Dissecting abdominal aortic aneurysm
	Renal artery		Renal artery stenosis
	Iliac artery		Hepatomegaly
Venous hum (continuous, medium-pitched tone created by blood flow in a large, engorged vascular organ such as the liver)	Epigastric area and umbilicus	Increased collateral circulation between portal and systemic venous systems	Hepatic cirrhosis
Friction rub (harsh, grating sound resembling two pieces of sandpaper rubbing together)	Hepatic	Inflammation of the peritoneal surface of an organ	Liver mass

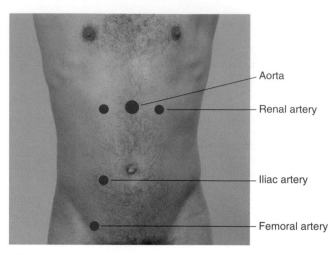

- Aorta
- Renal artery
- Iliac artery
- Femoral artery

FIGURE 24-4   Auscultation sites for vascular sounds. (From Bickley LS: Bates' Guide to Physical Examination, 10th ed. Philadelphia, PA: Lippincott Williams & Wilkins, 2009, p 436.)

laboratory studies used to evaluate liver functions. The clinical significance of any liver chemistry must be evaluated in the context of the patient's history and clinical situation. In addition, a series of values from a laboratory study and combinations of studies provide the most precise picture of the liver's function.

Tests for Evaluating Hepatocellular Injury

When hepatocytes are injured or die, they release aspartate aminotransferase (AST) and alanine aminotransferase (ALT) into the serum. ALT is almost exclusively present in hepatocytes and is the most specific test for hepatocellular damage.[1] AST is also found (to a lesser degree) in the skeletal muscle; therefore, elevations may be related to a skeletal muscle injury or overexertion. Elevations of AST and ALT are often helpful in evaluating acute liver injury and response to treatment, and monitoring those at risk for liver disease because of medical interventions.

TABLE 24-3   Laboratory Studies Used to Evaluate Liver Function

Study	Normal Findings	Clinical Significance
Bile Formation and Secretion		
Serum bilirubin		
Direct (conjugated)	0–5.1 μmol/L	Abnormal in biliary and liver disease; causes clinical jaundice
Indirect (unconjugated)	0–14 μmol/L	Abnormal in hemolysis and in functional disorders of uptake or conjugation
Urine bilirubin	Absent	Abnormal in liver disease
Urobilinogen	Urine: up to 0.09–4.23 μmol/24 h Fecal: up to 0.068–0.34 mmol/24 h	Increased in cirrhosis; biliary obstruction with biliary tract infection; hemorrhage; and hepatotoxicity; decreased in biliary obstruction without biliary tract infection; hepatocellular damage; and renal insufficiency
Protein Studies		
Albumin	35–55 g/L	Decreased in cirrhosis, chronic hepatitis
Globulin	15–30 g/L	Increased in cirrhosis, chronic obstructive jaundice, viral hepatitis
Albumin/globulin ratio	1.5:1 to 2.5:1	Ratio reverses with chronic hepatitis or other chronic liver disease
Total serum protein	60–80 g/L	Decreased in liver disease
Transferrin	220–400 μg/dL	Decreased in cirrhosis, hepatitis, and malignancy; increased in severe iron deficiency anemia
Prothrombin time (PT)	11.0–14.0 s or 100% of control	Prolonged PT in liver disease will not return to normal with vitamin K administration, whereas prolonged PT resulting from malabsorption of fat and fat-soluble vitamins will return to normal with vitamin K administration
Partial thromboplastin time (PTT)	25.0–36.0 s	Increased with severe liver disease or therapy with heparin or other anticoagulants
α-Fetoprotein (AFP)	6–20 ng/mL	Elevated in primary hepatocellular carcinoma
Fat Metabolism		
Cholesterol	less than 200 mg/dL (adults)	Decreased in parenchymal liver disease; increased in biliary obstruction
High-density lipoprotein (HDL)		
Men	35–70 mg/dL	
Women	35–85 mg/dL	
Low-density lipoprotein (LDL)	less than 130 mg/dL	
Very-low-density lipoprotein (VLDL)	25%–50%	

Study	Normal Findings	Clinical Significance
Liver Detoxification		
Serum alkaline phosphatase (AP)	20–90 U/L at 30°C	Level is elevated to more than three times normal in obstructive jaundice, intrahepatic cholestasis, liver metastasis, or granulomas; also elevated in osteoblastic diseases, Paget's disease, and hyperparathyroidism
Ammonia	15–49 µg/dL	An elevation indicates hepatocyte damage (liver converts ammonia to urea)
Enzyme Production		
Aspartate aminotransferase (AST)	8–20 U/L	Any elevation indicates hepatocyte damage
Alanine aminotransferase (ALT)	10–32 U/L	Any elevation indicates hepatocyte damage
Lactate dehydrogenase (LDH)	200–500 U/L	Any elevation indicates hepatocyte damage
γ-Glutamyl transferase (GGT)	0–30 U/L at 30°C	An elevation in GGT along with an elevated AP usually indicates biliary disease; helpful in the diagnosis of chronic liver disease

Tests for Evaluating Liver Synthetic Function

Albumin, total serum protein, and prothrombin time (PT) are measures of liver synthetic function. Individual protein measurements are of greater significance than total protein measurements. Albumin is the predominant protein in the serum; patients with advanced liver disease and cirrhosis tend to have low serum concentrations (hypoalbuminemia). The PT is a measure of the liver's capacity to absorb vitamin K and synthesize clotting factors; a prolonged PT that does not return to normal with vitamin K administration suggests that clotting factor synthesis is impaired.

Tests for Evaluating Excretory Function

Bilirubin is produced by the destruction of mature red blood cells. An elevated serum bilirubin level is roughly proportional to the severity of liver dysfunction. Jaundice is usually present when the serum bilirubin level is greater than 2 to 3 mg/dL. Total bilirubin, as well as unconjugated (indirect) and conjugated (direct) bilirubin levels, should be measured.

The unconjugated form of bilirubin is not water-soluble and is transported to the liver for conjugation and subsequent excretion in the bile. Unconjugated hyperbilirubinemia results from hepatocyte dysfunction in the conjugation process. Conjugated hyperbilirubinemia results from reduced secretion of conjugated bilirubin into the bile and feces or from obstruction of the bile ducts. Obstruction of bile flow may also present with elevated alkaline phosphatase (AP) and γ-glutamyltransferase (GGT) levels.

Pancreatic Function Studies

Table 24-4 lists serum laboratory tests that relate to pancreatic function. Amylase and lipase are digestive enzymes secreted by the pancreas. Serum amylase is found in the pancreas, parotid glands, intestine, liver, and fallopian tubes. Lipase is found primarily in the pancreas. In acute pancreatitis, serum amylase and lipase can be elevated four to six times the normal level, whereas in chronic pancreatitis, serum

TABLE 24-4 Laboratory Studies Used to Evaluate Pancreatic Function

Study	Normal Findings	Clinical Significance
Serum amylase	25–125 U/L	Level is elevated in acute pancreatitis (serum levels peak 4–8 h after onset of condition, then fall to normal within 48–72 h), biliary tract disease, tumors, salivary gland lesions, cerebral trauma, gynecological disorders, and renal failure; low levels usually indicate pancreatic insufficiency
Urine amylase	2 h: 2–34 U 24 h: 24–408 U	Urine values 6–10 h behind serum values; low levels indicate pancreatic insufficiency
Serum lipase	10–40 U/L (adults)	Elevated markedly in acute pancreatitis and pancreatic duct obstruction (remains elevated after amylase returns to baseline); elevations may also be seen with intra-abdominal inflammation and renal insufficiency
Serum glucose	65–110 mg/dL (fasting)	Levels may be increased in chronic liver failure
Serum triglycerides	50–250 mg/dL	Levels increased in alcoholic cirrhosis, diabetes mellitus (untreated), high-carbohydrate diet, hyperlipoproteinemia, and hypertension; levels decreased in malnutrition, vigorous exercise
Serum calcium		
Total	8.2–10.2 mg/dL	High total calcium levels seen in cancer of the liver, pancreas, and other organs
Ionized	4.65–5.28 mg/dL	Useful in tracking the course of disorders such as cancer and acute pancreatitis
Fecal fat	2–5 g/24 h	Amounts greater than 6 g/24 h suggest a decrease in the body's ability to absorb foods; indicative of pancreatic exocrine insufficiency as in chronic pancreatitis

amylase and lipase levels may be normal or very low because the pancreas may no longer be producing the enzymes.

Diagnostic Studies

The nurse caring for the critically ill patient coordinates the preparation for, and possibly the timing of, many diagnostic tests. Table 24-5 summarizes diagnostic studies used for evaluating the gastrointestinal tract. Endoscopy is an important adjunct to radiographic studies because it allows for direct observation and biopsy of portions of the intestinal tract. In some situations, endoscopy also allows for treatment of lesions (eg, removal of polyps, cauterization of vessels, ligation of varices).

TABLE 24-5   **Gastrointestinal Diagnostic Tests**

Test and Purpose	Method of Testing	Nursing Implications
Noninvasive		
Abdominal film		
Used to evaluate organ size, position, intactness, and gas patterns in the stomach, small intestine, and colon	X-rays visualize a single flat plane	• No special preparation needed
Upper gastrointestinal (GI) series (barium swallow)		
Used to visualize the esophagus, stomach, and duodenum; aids in diagnosis of hiatal hernia, ulcers, tumors, foreign bodies, bowel obstruction	Fluoroscopy is used to evaluate the movement of barium through the upper gastrointestinal tract; double-contrast study administers barium first followed by a radiolucent substance (eg, air) to help coat mucosa for better visualization of any type of lesion	• The patient must be NPO for 6 h prior to study
Upper GI series with small bowel follow-through		
Used to visualize the jejunum, ileum, and cecum; aids in the diagnosis of tumors, Crohn's disease, Meckel's diverticulum	Fluoroscopy is used to evaluate the movement of barium through the small bowel	• The patient must be NPO for 6 h prior to study
Barium enema		
Used to visualize the colon; aids in diagnosis of polyps, tumors, fistulas, obstruction, diverticula, and stenosis	Barium is administered via enema to make the colon visible on x-ray	• Bowel cleansing is necessary prior to the procedure
Ultrasonography		
Aids in diagnosis of masses, dilated bile ducts, gallstones, and ascites	High-frequency sound waves are passed over an abdominal organ to obtain an image of the structure	• The patient must be NPO for 6 h prior to study
Hepatobiliary scan		
Used to visualize the biliary system, gallbladder, and duodenum (size, function, vascularity, and blood flow)	Images are obtained as an intravenously injected radioisotope is taken up by the liver and then secreted into the bile	• The patient must be NPO for 6 h prior to study
Tagged red blood cell scan (technetium-labeled red blood cell scintigraphy)		
Aids in the diagnosis of GI bleeding	Red blood cells are labeled with technetium and injected intravenously; images are obtained with a gamma camera that can identify areas of increased radioactivity as a site of slow or intermittent GI hemorrhage	• No special preparation needed
Computed tomography (CT)		
Used to visualize the abdomen, retroperitoneal structures, tumors, cysts, fluid collections, air in a cavity, bleeding	Narrow x-ray beams produce cross-sectional images of organs and tissues; can be performed with or without contrast media	• No special preparation required
Magnetic resonance imaging (MRI)		
Used for evaluating abdominal soft tissue and blood vessels, abscesses, fistulas, tumors, and sources of bleeding	A magnetic field is used to obtain images	• The patient must be able to lie flat, hold his breath for periods of time, and tolerate confinement in the scanner • Metal in the body is a contraindication

Test and Purpose	Method of Testing	Nursing Implications
Magnetic resonance cholangiopancreatography (MRCP) Aids in the diagnosis of disorders affecting the pancreatic ducts and biliary tree	Same as MRI	• Same as MRI
Positron emission tomography (PET) Useful for precisely locating a tumor	Radioactive substances are used to examine the metabolic activity of body structures	• No special preparation needed
Invasive *Esophagogastroduodenoscopy (EGD)* Used to evaluate the upper GI tract	An endoscope is passed through the mouth and advanced to visualize the esophagus, stomach, and duodenum	• The patient must be NPO for 6 h prior to study
Colonoscopy Used to evaluate the large intestine	A flexible fiber-optic endoscope is passed through the rectum and advanced to visualize the large intestine	• Bowel cleansing is necessary prior to the procedure
Endoscopic retrograde cholangiopancreatography (ERCP) Used to visualize the common bile duct, hepatic bile ducts, and pancreatic ducts	A flexible fiber-optic endoscope is inserted into the esophagus, passed through the stomach, and into the duodenum; the common bile duct and the pancreatic duct are cannulated and contrast medium is injected into the ducts to permit visualization and radiographic evaluation	• The patient must be NPO 6 h prior to procedure
Endoscopic ultrasonography Used to evaluate and stage tumors of the GI tract	An ultrasonic transducer built into the distal end of the endoscope allows for high-quality images of the walls of the GI tract	• The patient must be NPO for 6 h prior to study
Enteroclysis Used to visualize entire small intestine; aids in diagnosis of partial bowel obstruction or diverticula	A duodenal tube is used to continuously infuse air in a barium sulfate suspension along with methylcellulose to fill the intestinal loops; transit of contrast filmed at intervals to evaluate progress through the jejunum and ileum	• The patient must be NPO for 6 h prior to study
Gastric lavage Aids in diagnosis of upper GI bleeding, also used to arrest hemorrhage and prepare for further tests	A large gastric tube is used to aspirate or wash out stomach contents	• No special preparation needed
Paracentesis Used to obtain samples of peritoneal fluid for laboratory or cytologic studies, and as a comfort measure (to alleviate accumulations of ascetic fluid)	A long, thin needle is inserted into the abdomen	• No special preparation needed
Peritoneal lavage Used to evaluate blunt or penetrating trauma to the abdomen	The peritoneal cavity is irrigated, and then the irrigating fluid is examined for blood	• No special preparation needed
Biopsy Aids in diagnosis of malignancy		• The patient must be NPO for 6 h prior to study
Percutaneous	A needle is placed through the skin to obtain tissue specimen for pathology evaluation	
Fine-needle aspiration (FNA)	A thin needle is used to obtain cells or minute tissue fragments from a suspect area for examination by light microscopy; usually guided by fluoroscopy, ultrasound, CT, or MRI	

(continued on page 360)

TABLE 24-5 Gastrointestinal Diagnostic Tests (continued)		
Test and Purpose	**Method of Testing**	**Nursing Implications**
Percutaneous transhepatic cholangiography (PTC) Helps to distinguish obstructive jaundice caused by liver disease from jaundice caused by biliary obstruction; during procedure, a percutaneous transhepatic biliary drain may be placed to relieve obstruction	The intrahepatic and extrahepatic biliary ducts are examined fluoroscopically; following percutaneous needle injection of contrast medium into the biliary tree	• The patient must be NPO 6 h prior to study
Angiography Used to visualize defects in the walls of arteries or veins and to evaluate blood flow through the vessels	Radiographic contrast is injected into the vessel under fluoroscopic guidance and x-ray images are obtained	• The patient must be NPO 6 h prior to study

CASE STUDY

Mrs. A. is a 79-year-old woman. Her medical history is significant for coronary artery disease (CAD), hypertension, gastroesophageal reflux disease (GERD), irritable bowel syndrome, and a left modified radical mastectomy and adjuvant therapy for breast cancer 5 years earlier. Mrs. A. sees her primary care physician because she is experiencing abdominal pain and severe itching all over her body. Mrs. A. has taken over-the-counter medications for the pruritus with minimal effect and has multiple self-inflicted scratches on her torso and extremities. In addition, Mrs. A. has also noted yellowing of her sclera that began about 2 weeks ago, a decrease in appetite, a 10-lb weight loss, very dark urine, and clay-colored stools. The physician determines that the abdominal pain Mrs. A. is experiencing begins in the midepigastric area of the abdomen and radiates around both sides to the back.

Laboratory values are significant for the following: total bilirubin, 8.6 μmol/L; ALT, 129 U/L; AST, 120 U/L; AP, 700 U/L; total protein, 4.8 g/L; and albumin, 2.3 g/L. Complete blood count and coagulation studies are within normal limits. CT reveals a 3.5-cm mass in the head of the pancreas, intrahepatic and extrahepatic bile duct dilation with an enlarged gallbladder, no vessel involvement, and no evidence of metastatic lesions.

The physician refers Mrs. A. to an interventional gastroenterologist for endoscopic retrograde cholangiopancreatography (ERCP) and decompression of the biliary tree by placement of an endoscopic stent. This procedure is not successful. Mrs. A. is then seen by interventional radiologists, who perform percutaneous transhepatic cholangiography with placement of an internal–external percutaneous transhepatic biliary drain. This procedure immediately results in the free flow of dark bile into a dependent external bile bag and biliary decompression. Following the procedure, Mrs. A. develops rigor and chills, along with a temperature of 103.5°F (39.7°C). She is transferred from the interventional radiology department directly to the critical care unit.

1. What would be included in an educational plan for Mrs. A. and her family?

2. What directed abdominal assessment would the critical care nurse perform when Mrs. A. is admitted to the critical care unit?

Reference

1. Fischback F, Dunning M (ed): A Manual of Laboratory and Diagnostic Tests, 8th ed. 2009.

Want to know more? A wide variety of resources to enhance your learning and understanding of this chapter are available on **thePoint** ✳. Visit **http://thepoint.lww.com/MortonEss1e** to access chapter review questions and more!

Common Gastrointestinal Disorders

Based on the content in this chapter, the reader should be able to:

1 Describe the pathophysiology, assessment, and management of acute gastrointestinal bleeding in the critically ill patient.
2 Describe the pathophysiology, assessment, and management of acute pancreatitis in the critically ill patient.
3 Describe the pathophysiology, assessment, and management of hepatic failure in the critically ill patient.

Acute Gastrointestinal Bleeding

Acute gastrointestinal bleeding is a common and potentially lethal medical emergency seen in patients admitted to the critical care unit. Prompt recognition and treatment of acute gastrointestinal bleeding is important to improve outcomes.

Upper Gastrointestinal Bleeding

Etiology

Upper gastrointestinal bleeding originates in the esophagus, stomach, or duodenum (Box 25-1). Commonly seen causes of acute upper gastrointestinal bleeding in the critical care unit include the following:

- **Peptic ulcer disease.** Peptic ulcer disease, which includes both gastric and duodenal ulcers, accounts for approximately 60% of cases of acute upper gastrointestinal bleeding.[1] Infection with *Helicobacter pylori*, a gram-negative bacterium that colonizes the protective mucus layer overlying the gastric epithelium, predisposes the mucosa to damage, resulting in chronic gastritis and ulceration.

Aspirin and nonsteroidal anti-inflammatory drugs (NSAIDs) can also cause peptic ulcer disease by directly injuring the mucosal layer. Bleeding from peptic ulcer disease occurs when the ulcer erodes into the wall of a blood vessel.
- **Stress-related erosive syndrome.** Critically ill patients often have one or more risk factors for the development of stress-related erosive syndrome, also known as stress-related mucosal disease (Box 25-2). Decreased perfusion of the stomach mucosa is probably the main mechanism of stress ulcer development. Ulcers may develop in the stomach, duodenum, and esophagus within hours of injury. Stress ulcers are more numerous, shallower, and more diffuse than the ulcers of peptic ulcer disease. Although they tend to be shallow, they may erode into the submucosa and cause massive hemorrhage. Stress ulcer prophylaxis (ie, the administration of medications that inhibit gastric acid secretion, neutralize gastric acid, or protect the gastric mucosa) is important in critically ill patients to lower the incidence of ulcerations and hemorrhage.
- **Esophageal varices.** Increased resistance in the portal venous system can develop as a result

BOX 25-1   Major Causes of Acute Upper Gastrointestinal Bleeding

Esophageal Sources
- Varices
- Esophagitis
- Ulcers
- Tumors
- Mallory–Weiss tears

Gastric Sources
- Peptic ulcers
- Gastritis
- Tumors
- Angiodysplasia
- Dieulafoy's lesions (vascular malformations of unusually large submucosal arteries)

Duodenal Sources
- Peptic ulcers
- Angiodysplasia
- Crohn's disease
- Meckel's diverticulum

of cirrhosis, leading to portal hypertension. In response to portal hypertension, collateral veins develop to bypass the liver and return blood to the systemic circulation. As pressure rises in these veins, they become tortuous and distended, forming varicose veins (varices) in the esophagus, stomach, duodenum, colon, rectum, or anus. Varices are particularly prone to rupture, resulting in massive gastrointestinal hemorrhage.

- **Mallory–Weiss tears.** Mallory–Weiss tears are lacerations of the distal esophagus at the gastroesophageal junction, often associated with heavy alcohol use and a history of forceful vomiting, retching, or violent coughing. Tearing of the underlying venous or arterial bed results in bleeding.

BOX 25-2   Risk Factors for Stress-Related Erosive Syndrome

- Hypotension or shock
- Coagulopathy
- Respiratory failure requiring mechanical ventilation
- Sepsis
- Hepatic failure
- Renal failure
- Multiple or severe trauma
- Burns over 35% of the total body surface area
- Post–organ transplantation status
- Brain or spinal cord injury
- History of peptic ulcer disease or upper gastrointestinal bleeding
- Prolonged stay in critical care unit
- Administration of steroids

Assessment

History

Patients with acute upper gastrointestinal bleeding present with hematemesis (ie, the vomiting of bright red blood or "coffee-ground" material), melena (ie, the passage of foul-smelling, black, tarry, sticky stool), or both. Melena is indicative of upper gastrointestinal bleeding in 90% of cases. It may take several days after bleeding stops for melenic stools to clear, and stools may remain Hemoccult positive for 1 to 2 weeks. Patients with acute upper gastrointestinal bleeding may also present with signs of hypovolemia or hypovolemic shock; the clinical presentation is consistent with the amount of blood loss.

A past medical history is important to obtain because other medical conditions may suggest an underlying cause for the bleeding (eg, patients with renal failure frequently bleed from arteriovenous malformations). A history of a previous episode of upper gastrointestinal bleeding is significant because most upper gastrointestinal bleeds rebleed from the same site.

Physical Examination

The physical examination is directed initially to the assessment of hemodynamic stability with ongoing assessment of vital signs. Tachycardia and orthostatic hypotension indicate hypovolemia secondary to acute blood loss. Orthostatic changes are detected by performing a tilt test (ie, evaluating the patient's blood pressure and heart rate in the supine position and then again after moving the patient to a sitting or standing position). A positive tilt test (ie, a decrease in blood pressure greater than 10 mm Hg with a corresponding increase in heart rate by 15%) implies volume depletion.

Laboratory Studies

Laboratory studies can help determine the extent of bleeding and often provide a clue to the etiology. Common laboratory abnormalities seen in a patient with acute upper gastrointestinal bleeding are listed in Table 25-1. The initial hematocrit and hemoglobin may not accurately reflect initial blood loss because plasma volume is lost in the same proportion as red blood cells. However, fluids administered during resuscitation and redistribution of fluids from the extravascular to the intravascular space eventually produce a hemodilutional effect and result in lowering of the hematocrit.

Diagnostic studies

Endoscopy can be performed urgently at the bedside and is the procedure of choice for the diagnosis of acute upper gastrointestinal bleeding. Endoscopy facilitates identification of the site of the bleed, has prognostic value for assessing the risk for rebleeding (based on the cause of recent bleeding), and has therapeutic capabilities for definitive treatment. When diagnostic endoscopy is unsuccessful, angiography can be used to define the site of bleeding or abnormal vasculature.

TABLE 25-1	Laboratory Abnormalities in a Patient With Acute Upper Gastrointestinal Bleeding	
Laboratory Abnormality	**Cause**	
Decreased hemoglobin and hematocrit	Blood loss, hemodilution resulting from fluid resuscitation	
Mild leukocytosis and hyperglycemia	Immune response to stress	
Elevated blood urea nitrogen (BUN)	Large protein load from breakdown of blood	
Hypernatremia	Hemoconcentration	
Hypokalemia	Potassium loss through emesis, diarrhea	
Prolonged prothrombin time (PT)/partial thromboplastin time (PTT)	Liver disease, concurrent long-term anticoagulant therapy	
Thrombocytopenia	Possible presence of liver disease	
Hypoxemia	Decreased circulating hemoglobin and hypovolemic shock	
Metabolic acidosis	Anaerobic metabolism	

Angiography can detect bleeding rates as low as 1.0 mL/min.[2]

Management

Nursing interventions for a patient with acute upper gastrointestinal bleeding are given in Box 25-3.

 RED FLAG! *Patients with acute upper gastrointestinal bleeding should be given nothing by mouth (NPO) because urgent endoscopy or surgery may be required.*

Initial Management

The initial management of any patient with acute upper gastrointestinal bleeding includes fluid resuscitation to reverse the effects of blood loss and administration of supplemental oxygen to promote oxygen saturation and transport and to prevent ischemia and dysrhythmias. Intubation may be required for actively bleeding patients at high risk for aspiration, those with a diminished mental status, and those in respiratory distress. An indwelling urinary catheter is inserted to monitor urine output and the adequacy of fluid resuscitation.

- **Volume resuscitation.** Patients with acute upper gastrointestinal bleeding require immediate IV access with at least two large-bore (14- to 16-gauge) IV catheters or central access. Because these patients typically require blood replacement in addition to fluids, a type and cross-match is sent early in the course of the blood loss. Isotonic solution, Ringer's lactate or normal saline, is infused to restore circulating volume and to prevent progression to hypovolemic shock. Calcium replacement may be necessary if large numbers of packed red blood cells (PRBCs) are transfused because the citrate in banked blood products can bind calcium

---

BOX 25-3 Nursing Interventions for the Patient With Acute Upper Gastrointestinal Bleeding

- Maintain a patent airway, elevate the head of the bed, and have suction available at the bedside to prevent aspiration of emesis or blood.
- Administer oxygen therapy to treat hypoxia that may result from decreased hemoglobin levels.
- Monitor pulse oximetry.
- Assess and document signs and symptoms of shock (eg, restlessness; diminished peripheral pulses; cool, pale, or moist skin).
- Assess and document vital signs, urine output, hemodynamic values, and arterial oxygen saturation (SaO$_2$).
- Assess and document electrocardiographic monitoring and heart, lung, and bowel sounds.
- Assist with the placement of a central venous pressure (CVP) catheter or a pulmonary artery (PA) catheter.
- Monitor and document central venous pressure (CVP), pulmonary artery pressure, pulmonary artery occlusion pressure (PAOP), cardiac output, and systemic vascular resistance.
- Maintain IV access and administer IV fluids and blood products as ordered.
- Insert a nasogastric tube and lavage as ordered.
- Administer medications as ordered to reduce gastric acid secretion.
- Administer vasopressin or octreotide as ordered.
- Maintain accurate intake and output (including urine, nasogastric drainage, and emesis) every 1 to 2 hours and PRN.
- Monitor electrolytes and report abnormal values.
- Monitor hemoglobin, hematocrit, red blood cell count, prothrombin time (PT), partial thromboplastin time (PTT), and blood urea nitrogen (BUN) and report abnormal values.
- Provide mouth care as needed.
- Explain all procedures to the patient.
- Prepare the patient for diagnostic procedures and therapeutic interventions.
- Monitor the patient for potential complications of endoscopy or colonoscopy (eg, perforation, sepsis, pulmonary aspiration, induced bleeding).
- Teach the patient the importance of seeking medical intervention if signs or symptoms of bleeding recur.
- Encourage smoking cessation and avoidance of alcohol.

and lead to hypocalcemia. If necessary, vasoactive drugs may be used after fluid balance is restored to maintain blood pressure and perfusion to vital body organs.

- **Nasogastric intubation.** A large-bore nasogastric tube may be placed (after an endoscopy identifies the cause of the hemorrhage) to aspirate and lavage gastric contents. The color of gastric aspirate is prognostically significant; slow bleeds (indicated by coffee-ground or black nasogastric drainage) are associated with a lower mortality rate than rapid bleeds (indicated by bright red bloody nasogastric drainage). Lavage may slow or arrest the bleeding and is performed by instilling 250 to 500 mL of room temperature tap water or saline through the nasogastric tube and then removing the lavage fluid with a syringe or by intermittent wall suction until gastric secretions are clear.

RED FLAG! *Lavage may allow better visualization to identify the source of bleeding during endoscopy, but placement of a nasogastric tube prior to endoscopy should be performed with extreme caution because doing so may damage a varix and worsen blood loss.*

RED FLAG! *Lavage is contraindicated if the patient has a visible blood clot on the ulcer bed identified by endoscopy.*

- **Pharmacotherapy.** Proton-pump inhibitors may be administered to patients with acute upper gastrointestinal bleeding to decrease the risk for recurrent bleeding, particularly from ulcers. Decreasing portal pressure with vasopressin, somatostatin, or octreotide (a synthetic analog of somatostatin) may be considered for patients with suspected variceal hemorrhage. These agents decrease portal hypertension by constricting the splanchnic arteries, which reduces portal blood flow. Vasopressin is administered through a central line. Systemic effects of vasopressin include coronary artery constriction, which can result in myocardial ischemia. Concurrent administration of IV or topical nitroglycerin can minimize this effect. Somatostatin and octreotide have the same mechanism of action as vasopressin, with fewer systemic and cardiovascular side effects.

Definitive Management

- **Endoscopy.** In addition to its use in diagnosis, endoscopy is the procedure of choice for the treatment of acute upper gastrointestinal bleeding. Multiple therapeutic options are available, including injection sclerotherapy (injection of an agent such as epinephrine around and into a bleeding vessel), thermal coagulation, the placement of hemostatic clips, and endoscopic variceal ligation (EVL). EVL, the treatment of choice for variceal bleeding, entails endoscopic placement of a rubber band around the base of each varix, causing coagulative necrosis and sloughing of thrombosed varices. Injection sclerotherapy, an alternative to EVL, involves injecting the varices with a sclerosing agent to stop the bleeding. These agents cause local tamponade and vasoconstriction, leading to necrosis and eventual sclerosis (scarring) of the bleeding vessel. Injection sclerotherapy is associated with a higher complication rate than EVL.

- **Angiography.** Most cases of upper gastrointestinal bleeding resolve spontaneously or can be controlled during endoscopy. However, patients with persistent bleeding may require angiography to control the source of bleeding. During angiography, bleeding from an arterial source can be controlled by the infusion of intra-arterial vasopressin or by embolization of the artery.

- **Transjugular intrahepatic portosystemic shunt (TIPS).** In this radiologic procedure, a stent is placed to create a conduit between the hepatic and portal vein, which decreases portal pressure (Fig. 25-1). TIPS may be considered if endoscopic management of esophageal varices fails.

- **Surgery.** Indications for surgical intervention are given in Box 25-4. A bleeding ulcer may be treated by simple suturing (ie, oversew of the ulcer), or by highly selective vagotomy (severing the section of the vagus nerve which innervates parietal glands to decrease gastric acid secretions), antrectomy (removal of the lower portion of the stomach, which contains the most acid-producing cells), or both. Because denervation of the vagus nerve affects gastric motility, pyloroplasty (widening of the opening into the duodenum) is often performed in conjunction with vagotomy to allow for continued gastric emptying. Surgical decompression of portal hypertension may be used for patients with esophageal or gastric varices who are unresponsive to medical and endoscopic therapy. Surgical decompression procedures entail the creation of a bypass to divert some of the blood flow away from the portal vein, around the liver, and into the vena cava, thereby decreasing pressure.

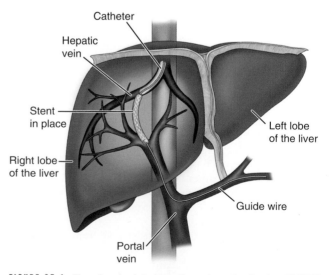

FIGURE 25-1 Transjugular intrahepatic portosystemic shunt (TIPS).

BOX 25-4 **Indications for Surgical Intervention for Acute Upper Gastrointestinal Bleeding**

- Severe hemorrhage unresponsive to initial resuscitation
- Massive bleeding that is immediately life-threatening
- Unavailable or failed endoscopic therapy
- Perforation
- Obstruction
- Suspected malignancy
- Continued bleeding despite aggressive medical therapies

Lower Gastrointestinal Bleeding

Etiology

Lower gastrointestinal bleeding originates in the jejunum, ileum, colon, or rectum, and is less common than upper gastrointestinal bleeding. Common causes of lower gastrointestinal bleeding are listed in Box 25-5. Most patients with acute lower gastrointestinal bleeding who are admitted to the critical care unit have diverticulosis or angiodysplasia.

- **Diverticulosis.** Diverticula (saclike protrusions that usually develop where arteries penetrate the colon wall) are prone to injury. Risk factors for diverticular bleeding include a low-fiber diet, aspirin and NSAID use, advanced age, and constipation. In many cases, diverticular bleeding will stop spontaneously, but up to 25% of patients experience massive bleeding, resulting in the need for surgery.[3]
- **Angiodysplasia** (arteriovenous malformation, angioma) is the term used to describe dilated, tortuous submucosal veins, small arteriovenous communications, or enlarged arteries whose walls lack smooth muscle. Angiodysplasia can occur anywhere in the colon, but it is most common in the cecum and ascending colon. As opposed to bleeding from diverticula, bleeding from angiodysplasia may be venous or arteriovenous and is therefore usually less severe than bleeding from diverticular disease, which is arterial.

BOX 25-5 **Major Causes of Acute Lower Gastrointestinal Bleeding**

- Diverticulosis
- Angiodysplasia
- Malignant tumors
- Polyps
- Ulcerative colitis
- Crohn's disease
- Ischemic colitis
- Infectious colitis
- Hemorrhoids
- Massive upper gastrointestinal hemorrhage

 The Older Patient. *The incidence of angiodysplasia increases with age owing to degeneration of the vessel walls.*

Assessment

Acute lower gastrointestinal bleeding is defined by hemodynamic instability and the sudden onset of hematochezia (stool containing fresh blood that ranges in color from bright red to maroon). Relevant findings in the medical history include abdominal surgery; a previous bleeding episode; anticoagulation therapy; peptic ulcer disease; inflammatory bowel disease; radiation to the abdomen or pelvis; or cardiopulmonary, renal, or liver disease. Initial laboratory studies include a complete blood count, serum electrolytes, blood urea nitrogen (BUN) and creatinine levels, and prothrombin time (PT) and partial thromboplastin time (PTT).

Colonoscopy is the test of choice for evaluation of lower gastrointestinal bleeding. Advantages of colonoscopy include the ability to locate the source of bleeding precisely, the ability to perform biopsies, and the potential for therapeutic intervention. Before colonoscopy, the colon needs to be cleansed with 4 L of polyethylene glycol solution given orally or by nasogastric tube until the fecal waste is clear. If colonoscopy fails to identify a bleeding source, angiography or radionucleotide scanning may be used. Angiography requires active blood loss of 0.5 to 1.0 mL/min to localize a bleeding site because the contrast in the arterial system is present for only a short time.[5] Radionucleotide scanning, which can detect bleeding that occurs at rates as low as 0.04 to 0.05 mL/min, is more sensitive than angiography but less specific than either colonoscopy or a positive angiogram.[1,4] Radionucleotide scanning may be useful before angiography because a positive scan can aid in the localization of the bleed.

An exploratory laparotomy to identify the source of bleedings is indicated for patients with massive or recurrent bleeding and for those patients with high transfusion requirements.

Management

Like patients with acute upper gastrointestinal bleeding, patients with acute lower gastrointestinal bleeding require fluid resuscitation and frequently blood replacement as well. A nasogastric tube is inserted to exclude an upper gastrointestinal source of bleeding (indicated by bloody aspirate). Once it is determined that the source of the bleeding is the lower gastrointestinal tract, colonoscopy is the procedure of choice for definitive treatment. Other therapeutic modalities include angiography and surgery.

- **Colonoscopy.** If a source of bleeding is identified during colonoscopy, therapeutic options include thermal coagulation or injection with epinephrine or other sclerosing agents.
- **Angiography** is reserved for patients with massive, ongoing bleeding when colonoscopy is not an acceptable option, and for those with recurrent

or persistent bleeding from a source not identified on colonoscopy. When an active source is identified, arteriographic intervention with embolization or intra-arterial vasopressin may be used. Embolization is preferred because of the high incidence of complications and rebleeding after stopping the vasopressin infusion.[5]

- **Surgery.** A segmental bowel resection with a primary anastomosis is often necessary for definitive treatment of acute lower gastrointestinal bleeding. In patients who are unstable, a temporary stoma and mucus fistula may be created.

Acute Pancreatitis

Acute pancreatitis is acute inflammation of the pancreas that can also involve surrounding tissues and remote organs. Causes of acute pancreatitis are given in Box 25-6; gallstones and excessive alcohol use account for 70% to 80% of cases.

Acute pancreatitis is self-limiting and mild in 80% to 90% of patients, resolving spontaneously within 5 to 7 days. However, 10% to 20% of patients will develop severe acute pancreatitis, which is associated with local and systemic complications and a significantly higher mortality rate.

Pathophysiology

The acinar cells of the pancreas synthesize and secrete digestive enzymes to assist in the breakdown of starch, fat, and proteins. Normally, these enzymes remain inactive until they enter the duodenum. In acute pancreatitis, pancreatic enzymes become prematurely activated in the pancreas, resulting in autodigestion of the pancreas and the peripancreatic tissue.

Mild acute pancreatitis (called interstitial or edematous pancreatitis) is characterized by areas of fat necrosis in and around pancreatic cells and localized interstitial edema. In severe acute pancreatitis (called hemorrhagic or necrotizing pancreatitis), pancreatic enzymes, vasoactive substances, hormones, and cytokines released from the injured pancreas cause a cascade of events that can lead to local and systemic edema, vascular damage, hemorrhage, and necrosis. Systemic inflammatory response syndrome (SIRS) may develop and can result in distant organ damage and multisystem organ failure. This systemic response is responsible for most of the morbidity and mortality associated with severe acute pancreatitis (Box 25-7). Death during the first 2 weeks of severe acute pancreatitis usually results from pulmonary or renal complications (eg, acute respiratory distress syndrome [ARDS], acute renal failure).

Local complications from acute pancreatitis resulting from inflammation of the peritoneum and fluid accumulation in the peritoneal cavity include pancreatic pseudocyst and pancreatic abscess:

- **Pancreatic pseudocyst** is a collection of inflammatory debris and pancreatic secretions enclosed by epithelial tissue. Signs and symptoms of pancreatic pseudocyst include persistent abdominal pain with nausea and vomiting, a prolonged fever, and elevated serum amylase. A pancreatic pseudocyst can rupture and hemorrhage or become infected, causing sepsis.
- **Pancreatic abscess** is a walled-off collection of purulent material in or around the pancreas that

---

BOX 25-6 Major Causes of Acute Pancreatitis

- Biliary disease (gallstones or microlithiasis, common bile duct obstruction, biliary sludge)
- Chronic alcohol use
- Medications (thiazide diuretics, furosemide, procainamide, tetracycline, sulfonamides, azathioprine, 6-mercaptopurine, angiotensin-converting enzyme inhibitors, valproic acid)
- Hypertriglyceridemia
- Hypercalcemia
- Abdominal trauma (pancreatic injury)
- Endoscopic retrograde cholangiopancreatography (ERCP)
- Infectious processes (mumps, staphylococcal and viral infections)
- Pancreas divisum
- Abdominal surgery
- Gynecologic disorders (eg, ectopic pregnancy, ovarian cyst)
- Total parenteral nutrition (TPN)
- Idiopathic
- Pancreatic tumors

BOX 25-7 Systemic Effects of Acute Pancreatitis

Pulmonary
- Atelectasis
- Acute respiratory distress syndrome (ARDS)
- Pleural effusions

Cardiovascular
- Hypotensive shock
- Septic shock
- Hemorrhagic shock

Renal
- Acute kidney failure

Hematological
- Disseminated intravascular coagulation (DIC)

Metabolic
- Hyperglycemia
- Hypertriglyceridemia
- Hypocalcemia
- Metabolic acidosis

Gastrointestinal
- Gastrointestinal bleeding
- Ileus

usually occurs 6 weeks or more after the onset of acute pancreatitis. Signs and symptoms of pancreatic abscess include an elevated white blood cell (WBC) count, fever, abdominal pain, and vomiting.

 RED FLAG! *Infections after the onset of pancreatitis (eg, due to abscess, pseudocyst, or infection of necrotic tissue), if untreated, are often fatal.*

Assessment

Clinical manifestations of acute pancreatitis are given in Box 25-8. Abdominal pain, the hallmark of acute pancreatitis, is usually midepigastric or periumbilical, with radiation to the back, but it may radiate to the spine, flank, or left shoulder. The pain usually begins abruptly, often after a large meal or large intake of alcohol. It may be steady and severe, or it may increase in intensity over several hours. The pain is usually exacerbated when the patient lies supine and is usually relieved when the patient sits and leans forward or lies in a fetal position. Abdominal pain is often accompanied by nausea, vomiting or both; abdominal distention; tachycardia; hypotension, and a low-grade fever.

 RED FLAG! *A persistent or high fever may indicate complications, such as peritonitis, cholecystitis, or abscess.*

BOX 25-8 Clinical Manifestations of Acute Pancreatitis

History and Physical Examination Findings
- Abdominal pain
- Nausea or vomiting without pain relief
- Tachycardia
- Hypotension
- Low-grade fever
- Diffuse abdominal tenderness and guarding
- Hypoactive or absent bowel sounds
- Abdominal distention
- Grey Turner's sign (flank ecchymosis)
- Cullen's sign (umbilical ecchymosis)
- Jaundice (with biliary disease)

Laboratory Findings
- Elevated serum and urine amylase
- Elevated serum lipase
- Elevated WBC count
- Hypokalemia
- Hypocalcemia
- Elevated bilirubin, aspartate aminotransferase (AST), and prothrombin time (PT) (with liver disease)
- Elevated alkaline phosphatase (AP) level (with biliary disease)
- Hypertriglyceridemia
- Hyperglycemia
- Hypoxemia

BOX 25-9 Ranson's Criteria for Acute Pancreatitis

Evaluate on Admission or on Diagnosis
- Age greater than 55 years
- Leukocyte count greater than 16,000/mL
- Serum glucose greater than 200 mg/dL
- Serum lactate dehydrogenase (LDH) greater than 350 IU/mL
- Serum aspartate aminotransferase (AST) greater than 250 IU/dL

Evaluate During Initial 48 Hours
- Decrease in hematocrit greater than 10%
- Increase in blood urea nitrogen (BUN) greater than 5 mg/dL
- Serum calcium less than 8 mg/dL
- Base deficit greater than 4 mEq/L
- Estimated fluid sequestration greater than 6 L
- Arterial oxygen saturation (PaO_2) less than 60 mm Hg

Laboratory studies ordered in the evaluation of a patient with acute pancreatitis include those used to evaluate pancreatic and liver function and a serum electrolyte panel. Imaging studies ordered to confirm the diagnosis, evaluate severity, and identify potential causes may include computed tomography (CT), abdominal ultrasound, magnetic resonance cholangiopancreatography (MRCP), and endoscopic retrograde cholangiopancreatography (ERCP).

An important aspect of assessment is identifying those patients who are likely to develop severe acute pancreatitis. Early identification permits aggressive treatment and surveillance, which can decrease complications and mortality. Ranson's criteria (Box 25-9) are widely used to assess the severity of acute pancreatitis. Three or more signs identified at the time of admission or during the initial 48 hours are predictive of severe acute pancreatitis, with an associated mortality rate of 10% to 20%.[6] Six or more have a corresponding mortality rate of 39%.[6]

Management

Care of the patient with acute pancreatitis focuses on fluid and electrolyte replacement, pain management, resting the pancreas to prevent the release of pancreatic secretions, and maintaining the patient's nutritional status. A collaborative care guide for the patient with acute pancreatitis is given in Box 25-10.

- **Fluid replacement.** The goal of fluid replacement is to administer enough fluid to obtain a circulating volume sufficient to maintain organ and tissue perfusion and prevent end-stage shock. Patients with severe acute pancreatitis may require 5 to 10 L of fluid replacement within the first 24 hours of hospitalization. Hypovolemia and shock are major causes of death early in the disease process

BOX 25-10 COLLABORATIVE CARE GUIDE for the Patient With Acute Pancreatitis

OUTCOMES	INTERVENTIONS
Oxygenation/Ventilation	
Arterial blood gases (ABGs) are maintained within normal limits.	• Assist the patient to turn, deep-breathe, cough, and use incentive spirometer q4h and PRN. Provide chest physiotherapy. • Assess for hypoventilation, rapid and shallow breathing, and respiratory distress. • Monitor pulse oximetry, end-tidal CO_2, and ABGs. • Administer analgesics if splinting is reducing effective ventilation. • Provide supplemental oxygen as needed.
The patient's lungs are clear.	• Auscultate breath sounds q2–4h and PRN.
The patient has no evidence of atelectasis, pneumonia, or ARDS.	• Suction only when rhonchi are present or secretions are visible in endotracheal tube. • Hyperoxygenate and hyperventilate before and after each suction pass.
Circulation/Perfusion	
Blood pressure, heart rate, and hemodynamic parameters are within normal limits.	• Monitor vital signs q1–2h. • Monitor PA pressures and right atrial pressure q1h and cardiac output, systemic vascular resistance, and peripheral vascular resistance q6–12h if PA catheter is in place. • Maintain patent IV access. • Administer intravascular volume as indicated by real or relative hypovolemia, and evaluate response.
Serum lactate is within normal limits.	• Monitor lactate daily until it is within normal limits. • Administer red blood cells, positive inotropic agents, colloid infusion as ordered to increase oxygen delivery.
The patient does not experience bleeding related to acute gastrointestinal hemorrhage, coagulopathies, or DIC.	• Monitor PT, PTT, complete blood count daily or PRN. • Assess for signs of bleeding. • Observe for Cullen's or Grey Turner's signs. • Administer blood products as indicated.
Fluids/Electrolytes	
The patient is euvolemic.	• Maintain patent IV access. • Monitor daily weights. • Monitor I&O. • Measure abdominal girth q8h at the same location on the abdomen.
There is no evidence of electrolyte imbalance or renal dysfunction.	• Monitor electrolytes daily and PRN. • Assess for signs of lethargy, tremors, tetany, and dysrhythmias. • Replace electrolytes as ordered. • Monitor BUN, creatinine, serum osmolality, and urine electrolytes daily.
Mobility/Safety	
There is no evidence of complications related to bedrest and immobility.	• Initiate deep venous thrombosis (DVT) prophylaxis. • Reposition frequently. • Ambulate to chair when acute phase is past, and hemodynamic stability and hemostasis are achieved.
The patient achieves or maintains ability to conduct activities of daily living (ADLs) and mobilize self.	• Consult physical therapist. • Conduct range-of-motion and strengthening exercises.
There is no evidence of infection and WBCs are within normal limits.	• Monitor for SIRS as evidenced by increased WBC count, increased temperature, tachypnea, tachycardia. • Use strict aseptic technique during procedures. • Maintain invasive catheter tube sterility. • Change invasive catheters; culture blood, line tips, or fluids according to facility protocol.

BOX 25-10 COLLABORATIVE CARE GUIDE (continued)

OUTCOMES	INTERVENTIONS
Skin Integrity	
The patient is without evidence of skin breakdown.	• Assess skin q8h and each time the patient is repositioned. • Turn q2h. • Consider pressure relief/reduction mattress.
Nutrition	
Caloric and nutrient intake meet metabolic requirements per calculation (eg, basal energy expenditure).	• Provide parenteral feeding. • Maintain NPO status. • Consult dietitian or nutritional support service. • Observe fat or lipid restriction as ordered. • Provide small, frequent feedings.
Evidence of metabolic dysfunction is minimal.	• Monitor albumin, prealbumin, transferrin, cholesterol, triglycerides, glucose.
Comfort/Pain Control	
The patient is as comfortable as possible (as evidenced by stable vital signs or cooperation with treatments or procedures).	• Document pain assessment, using numerical pain rating or similar scale when possible. • Administer analgesics and monitor the patient response. • Use nonpharmacological pain management techniques (eg, music, distraction, touch) as adjunct to analgesics.
The patient has minimal nausea.	• Maintain nasogastric tube patency. • Monitor nausea and vomiting. • Administer antiemetic as ordered.
Psychosocial	
The patient demonstrates decreased anxiety.	• Assess the patient's response to anxiety. • Support effective coping behaviors. • Help the patient increase sense of control by providing information, allowing choices, and maintaining as much predictability in routine as possible.
Teaching/Discharge Planning	
The patient and family understand procedures and tests needed for treatment.	• Prepare the patient and family for procedures such as paracentesis, PA catheter insertion, or laboratory studies.
Family understands the severity of the illness, asks appropriate questions, anticipates potential complications.	• Explain the widespread effects of pancreatitis and the potential for complications such as sepsis or ARDS. • Encourage family to ask questions related to pathophysiology, monitoring, treatments, and so on. • Provide appropriate discharge teaching related to dietary limitations, medications, wound care, and so on.

when aggressive fluid resuscitation fails to reverse the shock process.

• **Electrolyte replacement.** Replacement of electrolytes (calcium, magnesium, potassium) is also part of the initial management of patients with acute pancreatitis. Patients with severe hypocalcemia are placed on seizure precautions with respiratory support equipment on hand. Serum magnesium deficiency usually needs to be corrected before calcium and potassium levels can return to normal.

• **Pain management.** Acute pancreatitis is extremely painful. In addition, pain increases pancreatic enzyme secretion. For these reasons, pain control is a nursing priority for patients with acute pancreatitis. Although meperidine has traditionally been

the analgesic of choice because of the potential for sphincter of Oddi spasm that can accompany opioid use, if meperidine is not effective, other analgesics (including morphine) should be used as necessary for pain control.

• **Pancreatic rest.** Gastric distention, food in the stomach, and chyme in the duodenum can all stimulate the pancreas to secrete, further exacerbating the pancreatitis. Interventions include placing the patient on NPO status; placing a nasogastric tube connected to low wall suction to relieve gastric distention; administering proton-pump inhibitors to decrease acid production; and administering octreotide, somatostatin, or sandostatin to decrease pancreatic secretion of digestive enzymes.

- **Nutritional support.** Patients with acute pancreatitis who are on prolonged NPO status with nasogastric suction require nutritional support. Total parenteral nutrition (TPN) has been traditionally used because it provides nutrients without stimulating the pancreas. Increasing evidence suggests that enteral nutrition delivered past the ligament of Treitz to the distal duodenum or jejunum is safe for patients with acute pancreatitis; an added benefit is that enteral nutrition may reduce bacterial translocation by maintaining intestinal barrier function. Supplementation with TPN is appropriate if oral and enteral nutrition cannot provide enough calories to prevent catabolism. Hyperglycemia, which is often seen in acute pancreatitis, is managed by insulin protocol.
- **Surgery.** Surgery for acute pancreatitis is indicated if massive pancreatic necrosis is present in a patient with a worsening clinical status. Pancreatic resection or debridement can be performed to remove dead or infected pancreatic tissue and prevent systemic complications in patients with acute necrotizing pancreatitis. Broad-spectrum antibiotics are administered following surgical debridement of necrotic tissue.

Hepatic Failure

Hepatocytes, the functional cells of the liver, perform many essential functions, including the metabolism of nutrients; the detoxification of medications, toxins, and hormones; the synthesis of clotting factors; and bile formation and secretion. Abnormal liver function is usually not apparent unless a significant acute insult occurs or chronic liver disease is fairly advanced. Hepatic failure occurs when there is a loss of 60% of the hepatocytes, and symptoms are usually detectable after 75% or more of the hepatocytes are injured or killed.

Etiology

Liver failure may be acute or chronic. Common causes of acute liver failure include toxicity (eg, acetaminophen toxicity) and viral hepatitis. Chronic liver failure can develop as a result of long-standing liver disease, such as cirrhosis or chronic hepatitis.

Hepatitis

Hepatitis (ie, diffuse inflammation of the liver) can be noninfectious or infectious in origin (Box 25-11). Acute hepatitis lasts less than 6 months; it either resolves completely with return of normal liver function or progresses to chronic hepatitis. Chronic hepatitis is an inflammatory process that lasts longer than 6 months and may also progress to cirrhosis and possibly liver failure.

Although systemic viral infection can cause hepatitis, hepatitis viruses A, B, C, D, and E infect the liver parenchyma specifically. Infection with hepatitis B, C, or D is most likely to cause acute or chronic liver failure.

- **Hepatitis B virus (HBV).** Acute HBV infection leads to fulminant liver failure in less than 1% of patients. Fulminant liver failure as a result of HBV develops within 4 weeks of the onset of symptoms and is associated with encephalopathy, multiorgan failure, and a mortality rate of 80% if not treated with liver transplantation.[7] Chronic active HBV is seen in 5% to 10% of patients. The degree of liver impairment in chronic active HBV

BOX 25-11 **Causes of Hepatitis**

Infectious Diseases
- Viral hepatitis (A, B, C, D, E)
- Epstein–Barr virus
- Cytomegalovirus
- Herpes simplex virus
- Coxsackievirus B
- Toxoplasmosis
- Adenovirus
- Varicella-zoster virus

Drugs and Toxins
- Alcohol
- Acetaminophen
- Isoniazid
- Salicylates
- Anticonvulsants
- Antimicrobials
- HMG-CoA reductase inhibitors
- α-Methyldopa
- Amiodarone

- Estrogens
- Poisonous mushrooms (eg, *Amanita phalloides*)
- Ecstasy (methylenedioxymethamphetamine)
- Herbal medicines (ginseng, comfrey tea, pennyroyal oil, *Teucrium polium*)

Autoimmune Diseases
- Autoimmune hepatitis
- Primary biliary cirrhosis
- Primary sclerosing cholangitis

Congenital Diseases
- Hemochromatosis (iron overload)
- Wilson's disease (copper deposition)
- α_1-Antitrypsin deficiency

Miscellaneous Causes
- Nonalcoholic fatty liver
- Fatty liver of pregnancy
- Severe right-sided heart failure
- Budd–Chiari syndrome (vascular obstruction)

varies from mild to serious and can progress to cirrhosis.[8]

- **Hepatitis C virus (HCV).** Infection with HCV is the leading cause of liver cirrhosis and liver transplantation in the United States.[9] Chronicity can occur in as many as 55% to 85% of patients who develop acute HCV infection. Of those patients, 5% to 20% develop cirrhosis over the next 20 to 25 years.[9]
- **Hepatitis D virus (HDV).** HDV infection may occur as a superinfection in a patient who has chronic HBV infection, or it may occur simultaneously with an acute HBV infection. HDV can progress to fulminant liver failure or chronic disease.

Cirrhosis

Cirrhosis is a chronic disease characterized by the replacement of normal hepatic tissue with fibrous tissue, which distorts the liver structure, alters blood flow, and impairs hepatocyte function. Common causes of cirrhosis include alcohol abuse and chronic hepatitis. Ongoing insults to the hepatic tissue result in inflammation, fatty deposits, and hepatocyte necrosis, which is followed by the formation of fibrous tissue. These fibrotic changes are irreversible, resulting in impediment of blood flow through the liver (portal hypertension), chronic liver dysfunction, and, eventually, liver failure.

In cirrhosis, inflammation, fibrotic changes, and increased intrahepatic vascular resistance obstruct normal blood flow through the portal vein, leading to portal hypertension (Fig. 25-2). Pressure builds up in the portal system, causing congestion where the portal and systemic venous systems meet (ie, the esophagus, stomach, and rectum), resulting in the development of varices. Congestion as a result of portal hypertension also causes caput medusa (distention

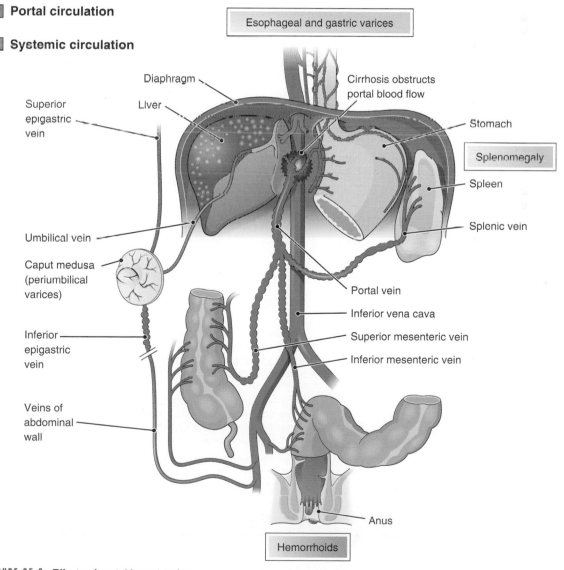

■ Portal circulation

■ Systemic circulation

Esophageal and gastric varices

Diaphragm

Liver

Cirrhosis obstructs portal blood flow

Superior epigastric vein

Stomach

Splenomegaly

Spleen

Splenic vein

Umbilical vein

Caput medusa (periumbilical varices)

Inferior epigastric vein

Portal vein

Inferior vena cava

Superior mesenteric vein

Inferior mesenteric vein

Veins of abdominal wall

Anus

Hemorrhoids

FIGURE 25-2 Effects of portal hypertension.

of the superficial abdominal blood vessels), ascites (abdominal fluid collection), and splenomegaly.

Clinical Manifestations

Because the liver performs so many varied functions, many organ systems are affected in liver failure (Table 25-2). Serious complications of liver failure include hepatic encephalopathy, hepatorenal syndrome, and spontaneous bacterial peritonitis.

Hepatic Encephalopathy

Patients with severe liver disease can develop hepatic encephalopathy (ie, abnormal mental functioning caused by the inability of the liver to remove ammonia and other toxins from the blood). Clinical manifestations of hepatic encephalopathy can be subtle and include changes in memory, personality, concentration, and reaction times. If untreated, more apparent neurologic alterations (eg, cognitive changes, irritability or agitation, reversal of day

TABLE 25-2 **Effects of Impaired Liver Function**

Signs and Symptoms	Cause
Constitutional	
Generalized weakness, malnutrition	Inability to metabolize nutrients
Gastrointestinal	
Right upper quadrant pain (hepatomegaly)	Congestion of liver and portal hypertension
Left upper quadrant pain (splenomegaly)	Congestion of liver and portal hypertension
Loss of appetite	Ascites, fatigue
Abdominal distention (ascites)	Hypoalbuminemia, increased circulating blood volume
Nausea, vomiting/hematemesis	Portal hypertension, variceal hemorrhage
Clay-colored feces (steatorrhea)	Inability to absorb dietary fat
Melena, hematochezia	Portal hypertension, variceal hemorrhage
Pulmonary	
Shortness of breath, dyspnea	Ascites, decreased lung and diaphragmatic expansion
Cardiac	
Tachycardia, hypotension	Sequestration of fluid in the liver and spleen, third-spacing in the peripheral extremities from decreased protein metabolism/low albumin levels
Dysrhythmias	Electrolyte disturbances
Peripheral edema	Impaired protein metabolism
Neurological	
Headache	Impaired metabolism of ammonia and other circulating toxins
Depression/irritability	
Asterixis (a flapping tremor, usually of the hands)	
Genitourinary	
Decreased urinary output	Decreased circulating volume and impaired glomerular filtration rate (GFR)
Frothy, dark amber urine	Excretion of unconjugated bilirubin
Integumentary	
Jaundice	Inability to conjugate bilirubin for excretion
Pruritus, dry skin	Impaired excretion of bilirubin
Bruising, ecchymosis	Impaired ability to synthesize clotting factors, decreased absorption of vitamin K
Spider nevi, caput medusae	Portal hypertension
Palmar erythema	Inability to breakdown aldosterone (hyperdynamic circulation)
Hair loss	Impaired metabolism of circulating hormones
Peripheral edema	Hyperdynamic circulation, low albumin
Endocrine	
Hypoglycemia	Impaired glucose metabolism and storage
Increased weight	Ascites, third-spacing of fluid
Gynecomastia, testicular atrophy (in men)	Inability to metabolize hormones (eg, estrogens)
Immune	
Infection, spontaneous bacterial peritonitis	Impaired Kupffer cell function, splenomegaly

and night schedules, somnolence, terminal coma) develop. Management strategies to reverse hepatic encephalopathy include limiting protein intake to 20 to 40 g/d, administering lactulose (a laxative that acidifies the colon to prevent the absorption of ammonia), and administering neomycin or metronidazole to clear the gut of bacteria that promote nitrogenous production.

Hepatorenal Syndrome

Hepatorenal syndrome is the development of kidney failure in patients with severe liver disease (acute or chronic) in the absence of any other identifiable cause of renal pathology.[11] Ascites, jaundice, hypotension, and oliguria are clinical findings in hepatorenal syndrome; laboratory findings typically include azotemia, elevated serum creatinine, urine sodium less than 10 mEq/L, and hyponatremia. There are two patterns of hepatorenal syndrome:

- **Type 1** is often observed in acute liver failure or alcoholic hepatitis. The onset is rapid, with a creatinine of more than 2.5 mg/dL or a 50% reduction in initial 24-hour creatinine clearance to less than 20 mL/min within 2 weeks. Patients often appear jaundiced and have a significant coagulopathy. Mortality from type 1 hepatorenal syndrome is 80% (at 2 weeks).
- **Type 2** usually occurs in patients with diuretic-resistant ascites. Onset is more insidious, with deterioration in kidney failure over months, but it is also associated with a poor prognosis.[11]

Spontaneous Bacterial Peritonitis

Patients with liver disease may be more susceptible to infection because the hepatic Kupffer cells, which are responsible for phagocytosing foreign material and debris, do not function efficiently. Spontaneous bacterial peritonitis is an acute bacterial infection of ascitic fluid without an identifiable intra-abdominal source of infection. Signs and symptoms of spontaneous bacterial peritonitis include fever, chills, generalized abdominal pain, or tenderness with palpation (but rarely with rebound tenderness). Approximately 30% of patients with spontaneous bacterial peritonitis develop renal failure. If spontaneous bacterial peritonitis is suspected, ascitic fluid samples are sent for analysis and culture. Spontaneous bacterial peritonitis is highly likely if the ascitic fluid leukocyte count is greater than 500 cells/L with more than 50% polymorphonuclear leukocytes.[11] Pending results of the culture, the patient is treated with broad-spectrum antibiotics.

Management

A collaborative care guide for the patient with cirrhosis and impending liver failure is given in Box 25-12. Management goals include prevention of additional stress on liver function and early recognition and treatment of complications. Interventions include monitoring nutritional markers and providing nutrition; monitoring fluid balance, urinary output, electrolytes, and chemistry studies; monitoring pharmacotherapy (ie, drug types and dosages); and monitoring bleeding times, platelet function, hematocrit, and clinical manifestations of bleeding (eg, bleeding gums, epistaxis, ecchymosis, petechiae, hematemesis, hematuria, melena).[10]

Ascites is managed through bedrest, a low-sodium diet (no more than 2000 mg/d), fluid restriction, and diuretic therapy.[12] Diuresis with spironolactone (an aldosterone antagonist) is first-line diuretic therapy for ascites; spironolactone may also be used in combination with furosemide.[12] Ascites absorption has an upper limit of 700 to 900 mL/d during diuresis therapy. If diuresis exceeds this limit, it may be at the expense of the intravascular volume and may potentiate hemodynamic instability. Monitoring for electrolyte imbalance, particularly hypokalemia, is essential.

Paracentesis is also used to treat ascites in patients unresponsive to salt restriction and maximal diuretic therapy. Ascitic fluid (up to 4 to 6 L/d) is withdrawn from the abdomen through percutaneous needle aspiration. Close monitoring of vital signs is important during paracentesis because a sudden loss of intravascular pressure may precipitate hypotension, decreased renal perfusion, and tachycardia. Volume expanders (eg, albumin) are recommended if 5 L or more of ascitic fluid is withdrawn during a single paracentesis procedure.[17] As with any invasive procedure, there is an increased risk for infection, particularly when the patient has refractory ascites due to continued deterioration of liver function and requires repeated large-volume paracentesis. For these patients, paracentesis does not improve the overall poor prognosis, and liver transplantation must be considered.

A TIPS procedure (see Fig. 25-1, p. 364) may be used to manage ascites and acute variceal hemorrhage nonsurgically. Absolute contraindications to a TIPS procedure include heart failure, severe tricuspid regurgitation, multiple hepatic cysts, uncontrolled systemic infection or sepsis, unrelieved biliary obstruction, and severe pulmonary hypertension (mean pressures greater than 45 mm Hg).[13] Complications include shunt occlusion, shunt stenosis, and hepatic encephalopathy.[14] Hepatic encephalopathy increases after a TIPS procedure because the shunt diverts some of the portal blood flow away from the liver parenchyma.

BOX 25-12 COLLABORATIVE CARE GUIDE for the Patient With Cirrhosis and Impending Liver Failure

OUTCOMES	INTERVENTIONS
Oxygenation/Ventilation	
ABGs are maintained within normal limits.	• Monitor pulse oximetry and ABGs, respiratory rate and pattern, and ability to clear secretions. • Validate significant changes in pulse oximetry with arterial blood saturation measurement.
The patient has no evidence of pulmonary edema or atelectasis.	• Assist the patient to turn, cough, deep-breathe, and use incentive spirometer q2h.
Breath sounds are clear bilaterally.	• Provide chest percussion with postural drainage if indicated q4h. • Monitor effect of ascites on respiratory effort and lung compliance. • Position on side and with head of bed elevated to improve diaphragmatic movement.
Circulation/Perfusion	
The patient achieves or maintains stable blood pressure and oxygen delivery.	• Monitor vital signs, including cardiac output, systemic vascular resistance, oxygen delivery, and oxygen consumption.
Serum lactate is within normal limits.	• Monitor lactate daily until it is within normal limits. • Administer red blood cells, positive inotropic agents, colloid infusion as ordered to increase oxygen delivery.
The patient does not experience bleeding related to coagulopathies, varices, hepatorenal syndrome.	• Monitor PT, PTT, complete blood count daily. • Assess for signs of bleeding (eg, blood in gastric contents, stools, or urine); observe for petechiae, bruising. • Administer blood products as indicated. • Assist with insertion and manage the esophageal tamponade balloon tube. • Perform gastric lavage as needed.
Fluids/Electrolytes	
The patient is euvolemic.	• Obtain daily weights.
The patient does not gain weight due to fluid retention.	• Monitor I&O. • Monitor electrolyte values. • Measure abdominal girth daily at the same location on the abdomen. • Monitor signs of volume overload (eg, cardiac gallop, pulmonary crackles, shortness of breath, jugular venous distention, peripheral edema). • Administer diuretics as ordered.
Mobility/Safety	
The patient is alert and oriented.	• Assess serum ammonia level. • Administer lactulose as ordered.
Ammonia level is within normal limits.	• Monitor level of consciousness, orientation, thought processing. • Assess for asterixis. • Take precautions to prevent falls.
The patient achieves or maintains ability to conduct ADLs and mobilize self.	• Consult physical therapist. • Conduct range-of-motion and strengthening exercises.
There is no evidence of infection and WBC count is within normal limits.	• Monitor for SIRS as evidenced by increased WBC count, increased temperature, tachypnea, tachycardia. • Use aseptic technique during procedures. • Maintain invasive catheter tube sterility. • Change invasive catheters; culture blood, line tips, or fluids according to facility protocol.

BOX 25-12 COLLABORATIVE CARE GUIDE (continued)

OUTCOMES	INTERVENTIONS
Skin Integrity	
The patient is without evidence of skin breakdown.	• Assess skin q8h and each time the patient is repositioned. • Turn q2h. Assist or teach the patient to shift weight or reposition. • Consider pressure relief/reduction mattress.
Nutrition	
Nutritional intake meets calculated metabolic need (eg, basal energy expenditure equation).	• Consult dietitian for metabolic needs assessment and recommendations. • Provide nutrition by oral, enteral, or parenteral feeding. • Sodium, protein, fat, or fluid restriction may be necessary. • Provide small, frequent feedings.
Evidence of metabolic dysfunction is minimal.	• Monitor albumin, prealbumin, transferrin, BUN, cholesterol, triglycerides, bilirubin, AST, alanine aminotransferase (ALT). • Administer cleansing enemas and cathartics if ordered.
Comfort/Pain Control	
The patient is as comfortable as possible (as evidenced by stable vital signs or cooperation with treatments or procedures).	• Assess pain and discomfort from ascites, bleeding, pruritus. • Document pain assessment, using numerical pain rating or similar scale when possible.
The patient has minimal pruritus.	• Administer analgesics cautiously and monitor the patient response. • Bathe with cool water, blot dry. • Lubricate skin. • Administer antipruritic medication; apply to skin PRN as ordered.
Psychosocial	
The patient demonstrates decreased anxiety.	• Assess the patient's response to illness. Provide time to listen. • Assess effect of critical care environment on the patient. • Minimize sensory overload. • Provide adequate time for uninterrupted sleep. • Encourage flexible visiting hours for family. • Plan for consistent caregiver.
Teaching/Discharge Planning	
The patient and family understand procedures and tests needed for treatment of hepatic dysfunction.	• Prepare the patient and family for procedures such as paracentesis or laboratory studies. • Teach the patient and family information regarding sodium, protein, and fluid restrictions. Provide written materials.
The patient and family are prepared for home care.	• Teach signs and symptoms of progressing hepatic failure (eg, change in mentation, skin coloration, ascites). • Teach signs and symptoms of occult bleeding and respiratory infection. • Teach home medication regimen. • Teach comfort measures.

CASE STUDY

Mr. R., a 66-year-old retired welder, presents to the emergency room with severe midepigastric pain and protracted vomiting. He tells the nurse that the pain worsens when he lies down on his back, but pulling his knees into his chest lessens it somewhat. When asked about alcohol consumption, Mr. R. tells the nurse that he consumes about two six-packs of beer daily. On admission, his vital signs are as follows: BP, 94/60 mm Hg; HR, 124 beats/min; RR, 32 breaths/min; temp, 101.5°F. The results of initial laboratory studies are Hgb, 14.2 g/dL; Hct, 45%; white blood cells (WBCs), 19,000 cells/mm³; glucose, 325 mg/dL; lactate dehydrogenase (LDH), 560 IU/mL; and aspartate aminotransferase (AST), 330 IU/dL.

Mr. R. is admitted to the critical care unit with the diagnosis of pancreatitis. An IV line is placed and fluid resuscitation is initiated. In addition, a nasogastric tube is inserted and Mr. R. is placed on NPO status. Within 24 hours, Mr. R.'s pulmonary status has deteriorated, necessitating intubation and mechanical ventilation. A chest x-ray shows "white out" with bilateral fluffy white infiltrates.

1. Evaluate the severity of Mr. R.'s condition using Ranson's criteria.

2. What systemic complication did Mr. R. develop after admission? What is the mechanism that leads to systemic complications in severe acute pancreatitis?

3. What nursing interventions are employed to "rest" the pancreas?

References

1. Albeldaui M: Managing acute upper gastrointestinal bleeding, preventing recurrences. Cleveland Clinic J Med 77(2):131–142, 2010
2. Laing C, et al.: Acute gastrointestinal bleeding: Emerging role of multidetector CT angiography and review of current imaging technique. Radiographics 27:1055–1070, 2007
3. Wilkins T, et al.: Diverticular bleeding. Am Fam Physician 80(9): 977–983, 2009
4. Hammond KL, Beck DE, Hicks TC, et al.: Implications of negative technetium 99m-labeled red blood cell scintigraphy in patients presenting with lower gastrointestinal bleeding. Am J Surg 193(3):404–408, 2007
5. Gillespie C, et al.: Mesenteric embolization for lower gastrointestinal bleeding. Dis Colon Rectum 53(9): 1258–1264, 2010
6. Carroll J: Acute pancreatitis: Diagnosis, prognosis and treatment. Am Fam Physician 75(10): 1513–1520, 2007
7. Perrillo R, Nair S: Hepatitis B and D. In Feldman M, Friedman LS, Sleisenger MH (eds): Sleisenger & Fordtran's Gastrointestinal and Liver Disease, 8th ed. Philadelphia, PA: WB Saunders, 2006, pp 1647–1681
8. Lok A, McMahan B: Chronic hepatitis B. Hepatology 45: 507–539, 2007
9. Doyle M, et al.: Liver transplant for hepatitis C virus. Arch Surg 143(7): 679–685, 2008
10. Sherman M, et al.: Management of chronic hepatitis C: Consensus guidelines. Can J Gastroenterol 21(suppl C): 25C–34C, 2007
11. Munoz S: The hepatorenal syndrome. Med Clin N Am 92(4):813–837, 2008
12. Runyon B: Management of adult patient with ascites due to cirrhosis: An update. AASLD Practice Guidelines. Hepatology 49(6): 2087–2107, 2009
13. Colombato L: The role of transjugular intrahepatic portosystemic shunt (TIPS) in the management of portal hypertension. J Clin Gastroenterol 41(suppl 3):S344–S351, 2007
14. Masson S, et al.: Hepatic encephalopathy after transjugular intrahepatic portosystemic shunt insertion: A decade of experience. QJM 101(6):493–501, 2008

Want to know more? A wide variety of resources to enhance your learning and understanding of this chapter are available on the**Point** ✳. Visit **http://thepoint.lww.com/MortonEss1e** to access chapter review questions and more!

Endocrine System

Patient Assessment: Endocrine System

OBJECTIVES

Based on the content in this chapter, the reader should be able to:

1 Describe the assessment of hypothalamus and pituitary gland function in the critically ill patient.
2 Describe the assessment of thyroid gland function in the critically ill patient.
3 Describe the assessment of endocrine pancreas function in the critically ill patient.
4 Describe the assessment of adrenal gland function in the critically ill patient.

Many patients admitted to the critical care unit will have a known endocrine disorder that is either a concomitant problem or the cause for admission. However, many patients have endocrine disorders that are not recognized before the onset of an acute illness. For this reason, endocrine function is considered in the assessment of all critically ill patients.

Endocrine disorders can affect all body systems and are usually caused by the overproduction or underproduction of hormones. Because the endocrine system is complex and its effects on the body are widespread, assessment entails a systematic review of many physiological functions. General manifestations of endocrine disorders include changes in vital signs, energy level, fluid and electrolyte levels, and the ability to carry out activities of daily living (ADLs). Other parameters to be observed include heat or cold intolerance, changes in weight, fat redistribution, changes in sexual functioning, and altered sleep patterns. Elements of the endocrine history are summarized in Box 26-1. Common laboratory studies used to assess endocrine gland function are summarized in Table 26-1.

Hypothalamus and Pituitary Gland

The pituitary gland is often called the "master gland" of the endocrine system because, under the control of the hypothalamus, it secretes hormones that affect the functioning of other endocrine glands (eg, thyroid-stimulating hormone [TSH] and adrenocorticotropic

BOX 26-1 Endocrine Health History

History of the Present Illness

Complete analysis of the following signs and symptoms (using the NOPQRST format; see Chapter 12, Box 12-2):

- Excessive urination
- Excessive thirst
- Dehydration
- Edema
- Constipation
- Diarrhea
- Cold or heat intolerance
- Fatigue or lethargy
- Cognitive changes
- Depression
- Menstrual cycle irregularities
- Weight gain or loss
- Changes in appetite

Past Health History

Relevant childhood illnesses and immunizations: mental retardation, iodine deficiency

- **Past acute and chronic medical problems, including treatments and hospitalizations:** diabetic emergencies, hypertension, hypercholesterolemia, tachydysrhythmias, heart failure, myocardial infarction, Graves' disease, Hashimoto's thyroiditis, head injury, cerebral vascular accident, pancreatitis, unexplained infections, adenoid or neck/chest radiation
- **Risk factors:** age, heredity, gender, race, tobacco use, alcohol use, elevated cholesterol, obesity, sedentary lifestyle, growth spurt cycles, pregnancy, gestational diabetes, delivery of an infant weighing more than 9 lb, anemia
- **Past surgeries:** neurosurgical procedures, thyroidectomy, parathyroidectomy, adrenalectomy

- **Medications, including prescription drugs, over-the-counter drugs, vitamins, herbs and supplements:** amiodarone, phenytoin, carbamazepine, chlorpropamide, corticosteroids, opioids, lithium, aspirin, iodides, heparin, levothyroxine (Synthroid), neoplastic drugs, estrogen, methadone, androgens, β-adrenergic blockers, nonsteroidal anti-inflammatory drugs (NSAIDs), potassium, diuretics
- **Allergies and reactions to medication, foods, contrast, latex, or other materials**
- **Transfusions, including type and date**

Family History

- **Health status or cause of death of parents and siblings:** thyroid disease, diabetes, lipid disorders, cerebral aneurysm, cancer, autoimmune disorders

Personal and Social History

- Tobacco, alcohol, and substance use
- Diet
- Sleep patterns: insomnia
- Exercise

Review of Other Systems

- **HEENT:** headaches, dizziness, weakness, visual changes
- **Cardiovascular:** tachycardia, atrial fibrillation, bradycardia
- **Genitourinary:** sexual dysfunction, infertility, abnormal vaginal bleeding, chronic vaginitis, excessive or inadequate urine output
- **Neurological:** tremulousness, cognitive changes, neuropathy
- **Immune:** recurrent or chronic infections
- **Integument:** poor wound healing, bruising, striae, petechiae, hirsutism

---

hormone [ACTH]). In addition, the pituitary gland secretes antidiuretic hormone (ADH, vasopressin), which controls water excretion by the kidney.

History and Physical Examination

Disorders of the hypothalamus or pituitary gland that alter the production or release of ADH result in fluid and electrolyte imbalances; therefore, physical examination of the patient involves the careful assessment of skin turgor, buccal membrane moisture, vital signs, and weight. The nurse strictly monitors intake and output in patients experiencing fluid balance alterations. The color, concentration, and volume of the urine are noted with each measurement.

Laboratory Studies

Laboratory studies are used to diagnose and determine the degree of fluid imbalance caused by alterations in ADH secretion, and to distinguish between two common disorders of ADH secretion, diabetes insipidus (DI) and syndrome of inappropriate antidiuretic hormone (SIADH) (Table 26-2). In addition to urine specific gravity, serum osmolality, and urine osmolality (see Chapter 18), serum ADH radioimmunoassay may be ordered to measure ADH levels in the blood.

Diagnostic Studies

Imaging studies, such as computed tomography (CT) and magnetic resonance imaging (MRI), may be ordered to detect lesions in the pituitary–hypothalamic area (eg, brain tumors, aneurysms, edema resulting from surgical exploration or traumatic injuries, necrotic lesions).

Thyroid Gland

The thyroid hormones triiodothyronine (T_3) and thyroxine (T_4) are regulated by the hypothalamus and the pituitary gland in a negative feedback system (Fig. 26-1).

TABLE 26-1 Laboratory Studies Used to Assess Endocrine Disorders

Test	Normal Adult Values	Abnormal Values
Serum antidiuretic hormone (ADH)	1–13.3 pg/mL	High in syndrome of inappropriate antidiuretic hormone (SIADH) Low in diabetes insipidus (DI)
Urine specific gravity	1.010–1.025 with normal hydration and volume	Low in DI High in SIADH High in diabetes mellitus with dehydration
Total T$_4$	4–12 µg/dL	High in hyperthyroidism Low in hypothyroidism
Free T$_4$	0.8–2.7 ng/mL	High in hyperthyroidism Low in hypothyroidism
Free T$_4$ index	4.6–12 ng/mL	High in hyperthyroidism Low in hypothyroidism
Free T$_3$	260–480 pg/dL	Low in hypothyroidism
Thyroid-stimulating hormone (TSH)	260–480 pg/dL	High in primary hypothyroidism Low in anterior pituitary hypofunction (secondary hypothyroidism) and in hyperthyroidism
Urine ketones	Negative	Positive in diabetic ketoacidosis (DKA)
Serum ketones	2–4 mg/dL	High in DKA
Glucagon	Normal fasting values: 50–200 pg/mL	High in diabetes mellitus, DKA, HHS
Fasting blood glucose	65–110 mg/dL	High in diabetes mellitus
Insulin level	0–24 fU/mL	High in insulinoma Low in diabetes mellitus
C-peptide level	0.5–2.0 ng/mL	Low in diabetes mellitus
Cortisol	8 a.m. 5–23 µg/dL 4 p.m. 3–16 µg/dL	High in hypersecretion (eg, Cushing's disease) High in stress, trauma, and surgery Low in hyposecretion of ACTH by pituitary and in adrenal insufficiency
Cortisol stimulation	Should increase to 18 µg/dL	Low or absent in adrenal insufficiency and hypopituitarism

HHS, hyperosmolar hyperglycemic syndrome; T$_3$, triiodothyronine; T$_4$, thyroxine.

History and Physical Examination

Manifestations of thyroid hormone disorders are widespread because thyroid hormones affect nearly every cell and tissue in the body. Signs and symptoms associated with over- or undersecretion of thyroid hormone are illustrated in Figure 26-2.

Physical examination begins with inspection of the neck area for enlargement and symmetry of the gland. The patient is then asked to swallow while the nurse observes the thyroid rising. Next, the thyroid gland is palpated for size, shape, symmetry,

TABLE 26-2 Comparison of Laboratory Values in Diabetes Insipidus (DI) and Syndrome of Inappropriate Antidiuretic Hormone (SIADH)

Laboratory Test	DI	SIADH
Antidiuretic hormone (ADH)	Decreased	Increased
Serum osmolality	Increased	Decreased
Serum sodium	Increased	Decreased
Urinary output	Increased	Decreased
Urine specific gravity	Decreased	Increased
Urine osmolality	Decreased	Increased

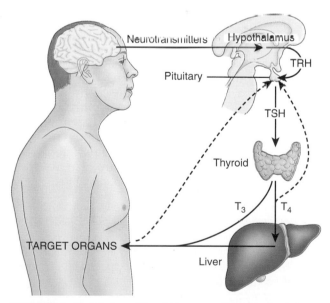

FIGURE 26-1 Regulation of thyroid hormone. Thyroid-stimulating hormone (TSH), which stimulates the production and release of the thyroid hormones triiodothyronine (T$_3$) and thyroxine (T$_4$), is released by the anterior pituitary gland in response to thyrotropin-releasing hormone (TRH), secreted by the hypothalamus. Low circulating levels of T$_3$ and T$_4$ stimulate the secretion of TRH (solid lines), and high circulating levels of T$_3$ and T$_4$ inhibit the secretion of TRH (dashed lines). (From Smeltzer SC, Bare BG, Hinkle JL, et al.: Brunner & Suddarth's Textbook of Medical–Surgical Nursing, 12th ed. Philadelphia, PA: Lippincott Williams & Wilkins, 2010, p 1254)

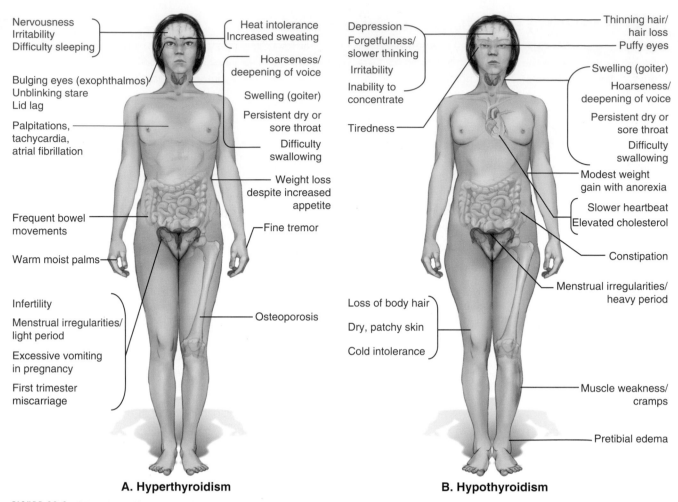

A. Hyperthyroidism

Nervousness
Irritability
Difficulty sleeping

Heat intolerance
Increased sweating

Bulging eyes (exophthalmos)
Unblinking stare
Lid lag

Hoarseness/
deepening of voice

Swelling (goiter)

Persistent dry or
sore throat

Palpitations,
tachycardia,
atrial fibrillation

Difficulty
swallowing

Weight loss
despite increased
appetite

Frequent bowel
movements

Fine tremor

Warm moist palms

Infertility

Menstrual irregularities/
light period

Osteoporosis

Excessive vomiting
in pregnancy

First trimester
miscarriage

B. Hypothyroidism

Depression
Forgetfulness/
slower thinking
Irritability
Inability to
concentrate

Thinning hair/
hair loss

Puffy eyes

Swelling (goiter)

Hoarseness/
deepening of voice

Tiredness

Persistent dry or
sore throat

Difficulty
swallowing

Modest weight
gain with anorexia

Slower heartbeat
Elevated cholesterol

Constipation

Menstrual irregularities/
heavy period

Loss of body hair

Dry, patchy skin

Cold intolerance

Muscle weakness/
cramps

Pretibial edema

FIGURE 26-2 Clinical manifestations of hyperthyroidism (**A**) and hypothyroidism (**B**).

and presence of tenderness. Thyromegaly (goiter) or thyroid nodules can be detected by palpation. Occasionally, a thyroid bruit (caused by excessive or turbulent blood flow associated with a hypermetabolic state) can be detected by listening over the gland with the bell of the stethoscope. Vital sign changes, skin changes (including edema), neurological changes, and weight changes are also assessed as part of the physical examination.

The Older Patient. There is a higher prevalence of hypothyroidism in the elderly population. Often, older patients present with atypical initial symptoms, such as depression, apathy, and immobilization.[1] Hyperthyroidism in the elderly is much less common. When hyperthyroidism is present, it is likely to go undetected because common findings (eg, weight loss, fatigue, palpitations and tachycardia, mental confusion, anxiety) are often erroneously attributed to "old age." Due to delayed detection of the condition, an older adult with hyperthyroidism may present with new-onset atrial fibrillation (the consequence of worsening heart failure or unstable angina) or thyrotoxic crisis (a severe and life-threatening form of hyperthyroidism).

Laboratory Studies

The following laboratory studies may be ordered to evaluate thyroid gland function:

- **Thyroid-stimulating hormone test (thyrotropin assay).** This highly sensitive test measures circulating TSH from the anterior pituitary. Measuring TSH helps determine whether hypothyroidism is primary (ie, caused by dysfunction of the thyroid gland) or secondary (ie, caused by hypofunction of the anterior pituitary gland). In patients with hyperthyroidism, the TSH level is extremely low because high circulating levels of thyroid hormones inhibit the secretion of TSH by the anterior pituitary.
- **Thyroid hormone levels.** Less than 1% of the secreted T_3 and T_4 remains free and physiologically active in the plasma. The remainder is bound to plasma proteins manufactured by the liver. Total T_4 measures both the free T_4 and the portion carried by thyroxine-binding globulin (TBG). Free T_4 measures the circulating, unbound levels of T_4. Because any factor that affects protein levels or protein binding can affect the total T_4 levels,

free T_4 is often more accurate than total T_4. The T_4 index is a mathematical calculation used to correct the total T_4 for the amount of TBG that is present, thereby increasing the accuracy of the total T_4 measurement. Free T_3 levels may also be ordered.

 RED FLAG! *Many critically ill patients have alterations in protein levels owing to malnutrition, hepatic dysfunction, medications, or advanced age. These alterations affect TSH and total T_4 levels, necessitating careful analysis of the results of these tests.*

Diagnostic Studies

The radioactive iodine uptake test measures the rate of iodine uptake by the thyroid gland following oral administration of a radioactive iodine tracer. A probe is placed over the thyroid gland to evaluate the uptake of the radioactive iodine. Normally, the radioactive iodine is evenly distributed in the thyroid gland, and the scan shows a normal size, position, and shape.

A thyroid scan, which entails measuring uptake of the radioactive iodine tracer at specific times, may be performed in conjunction with the radioactive iodine uptake test. The patient must be NPO for 8 hours prior to the procedure and thyroid hormone replacement therapy is typically stopped 7 days prior to prevent interference with test results.

CT or MRI can identify enlargement of the thyroid gland but is unable to determine the functioning of the thyroid gland or identify small masses (eg, cysts). Ultrasonography can detect masses, cysts, and enlargement of the gland.

Endocrine Pancreas

Disorders of the endocrine pancreas (eg, diabetes mellitus) are characterized by chronic hyperglycemia and result in major shifts of fluids and electrolytes and blood glucose levels. Patients with diabetes mellitus are frequently admitted to the critical care unit for treatment of acute complications of diabetes, such as diabetic ketoacidosis (DKA), hyperosmolar hyperglycemic syndrome (HHS), and hypoglycemia.

History and Physical Examination

When an acute complication of diabetes is suspected, an effort is made to establish the diagnosis quickly so that life-preserving therapy can be started. Initial data collection includes an abbreviated history (obtained from the family or friends when the patient is unconscious), a search for a diabetic identification card, and rapid assessment for clinical clues of volume depletion. After asking about the diabetic regimen, medications, and recent changes in health, the nurse performs a review of systems. During the interview, the nurse observes the patient's cognition and responsiveness.

The physical examination includes blood pressure, heart and respiratory rate, breathing pattern, heart sounds and rhythm, breath sounds, capillary refill, color and warmth of extremities, temperature, assessment of hydration status (eg, skin turgor), and assessment of level of consciousness.

Laboratory Studies

Laboratory studies to evaluate glucose regulation include the following:

- **Fasting blood glucose level.** In critically ill patients, measuring glucose levels from blood samples drawn from venous lines, central lines, or arterial lines is preferred over fingerstick glucose testing. Fingerstick testing requires adequate tissue perfusion for accuracy and in many critically ill patients, tissue perfusion is impaired. Blood glucose levels are measured at least 8 hours after the last food intake to evaluate carbohydrate metabolism. Two-hour postprandial glucose testing is helpful as well, especially in people with known diabetes mellitus.
- **Glycosylated hemoglobin (HbA$_{1c}$ or A1C) testing** offers information about the average amount of glucose present in the patient's bloodstream for the past 3 to 4 months, by measuring the amount of glucose attached to hemoglobin in the erythrocytes. (The average lifespan of an erythrocyte is 100 to 120 days.)
- **Insulin level.** This test measures the amount of circulating serum insulin in the fasting state.
- **C-peptide level.** C-peptide is a byproduct of insulin production. Low values (or no insulin C-peptide) indicate that the person's pancreas is producing little or no insulin, as in type 1 diabetes.[2]
- **Glucagon level.** Glucagon, a hormone produced in the α-cells in the islets of Langerhans, controls the production, storage, and release of glucose. Normally, insulin opposes the action of glucagon. A deficiency of glucagon occurs when pancreatic tissue is lost because of chronic pancreatitis or pancreatic tumors. Increased glucagon levels occur in diabetes, acute pancreatitis, chronic renal failure, cirrhosis, and in the presence of catecholamine secretion (as occurs with infection, high stress levels, or pheochromocytoma).
- **Serum ketones.** Elevated serum ketone levels suggest that the body is metabolizing fat for energy in lieu of dietary carbohydrates, a condition seen in critically ill patients with type 1 diabetes.
- **Urine ketones.** Ketones are not normally found in the urine; when they are, they are associated with diabetes and other disorders of altered carbohydrate metabolism.

Adrenal Gland

The adrenal gland is anatomically and functionally divided into two distinct parts—the outer cortex and the inner medulla (Fig. 26-3). Disorders of

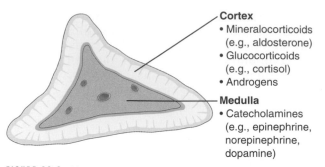

FIGURE 26-3 Hormones secreted by the adrenal gland.

- **Cortex**
  - Mineralocorticoids (e.g., aldosterone)
  - Glucocorticoids (e.g., cortisol)
  - Androgens
- **Medulla**
  - Catecholamines (e.g., epinephrine, norepinephrine, dopamine)

The Older Patient. An expected result of aging is decreased secretion of cortisol and aldosterone, which can result in a diminished response to acute illness or trauma. The older patient may have a decreased ability to maintain appropriate fluid and electrolyte balance and may mount diminished responses to stressors such as critical illness or trauma.

the adrenal gland have widespread effects on the body because the adrenal hormones regulate major body system functions, including fluid and electrolyte balance, sympathetic nervous system responses, inflammation, and metabolism.

Cortisol is a steroid hormone that is released in response to stress. Cortisol secretion is regulated by a negative feedback system through the hypothalamic–pituitary axis. The hypothalamus releases corticotropin-releasing hormone (CRH), which in turn stimulates the release of ACTH (adrenocorticotropin) from the anterior pituitary. ACTH then stimulates the adrenal cortex to secrete cortisol. Critically ill patients often experience adrenal cortical insufficiency or cortisol resistance.

History and Physical Examination

A summary of the clinical manifestations of adrenal cortical insufficiency and excess is given in Table 26-3.

Laboratory Studies

Laboratory studies for evaluation of adrenal gland function include the following:

- **Cortisol levels.** Cortisol levels are elevated in people with adrenal hyperfunction and decreased in those with adrenal hypofunction. Adrenal hyperfunction may be caused by excess secretion of ACTH by the pituitary gland; hypofunction may be the result of anterior pituitary hyposecretion, hepatitis, or cirrhosis. Cortisol secretion is diurnal; it is normally higher in the early morning and lower in the evening. This variation is lost in

TABLE 26-3 **Manifestations of Adrenal Cortical Insufficiency and Excess**

Parameter	Adrenal Cortical Insufficiency	Adrenal Cortical Excess
Electrolytes	Hyponatremia[a] Hyperkalemia[a]	Hypokalemia
Fluids	Dehydration[a] (eg, elevated BUN)	Edema
Blood pressure	Hypotension Shock[a] Orthostatic hypotension	Hypertension
Musculoskeletal	Muscle weakness[a] Fatigue[a]	Muscle wasting Fatigue
Hair and skin	Skin pigmentation	Easy bruisability Hirsutism, acne, and striae (abdomen and thighs)
Inflammatory response	Low resistance to trauma, infection, and stress	Decrease in eosinophils, lymphocytopenia
Gastrointestinal	Nausea, vomiting[a] Abdominal pain[a]	Possible gastrointestinal bleeding
Glucose metabolism	Hypoglycemia[a]	Impaired glucose tolerance Glycosuria Elevated blood sugar
Emotional	Depression and irritability	Emotional lability to psychosis
Other	Menstrual irregularity Decreased axillary and pubic hair in women	Oligomenorrhea Impotence in the male Centripetal obesity (moon face and buffalo hump)

[a]Occurs with acute adrenal insufficiency.

BUN, blood urea nitrogen.

From Porth CM: Pathophysiology: Concepts of Altered Health States, 5th ed. Philadelphia, PA: Lippincott Williams & Wilkins, 1998, p 80

patients with adrenal hyperfunction and in people under stress.

- **Cortisol stimulation.** To perform this test, a baseline cortisol blood level is drawn, and then blood samples are taken 30 and 60 minutes after cosyntropin (a synthetic ACTH preparation) is administered. The adrenal glands normally respond to the cosyntropin by synthesizing and secreting cortisol. The response to cosyntropin is decreased or absent in people with adrenal insufficiency. The cortisol stimulation test may be contraindicated in the presence of infections, inflammatory diseases, and cardiac disease. Long-term steroid therapy affects results.

CASE STUDY

Mr. J., a 58-year-old black man, arrives in the emergency department after his wife discovers him unarousable at their home. She tells the nurse that he has been very fatigued and lethargic for the past several days, and she has noticed that he has been drinking a lot of juice lately. In addition, she reports that he has been getting up frequently at night to urinate and has complained of blurred vision. He takes medication for high blood pressure and high cholesterol, but his wife is not sure of the exact names. Mr. J. is a nonsmoker, and he drinks a glass of wine every other week at home. He is not allergic to any medications. Both of his parents had diabetes, and two of his brothers have diabetes as well. Currently, he works at a computer firm and is relatively sedentary.

The nurse notes that Mr. J. is a lethargic but oriented, overweight male with flushed, slightly diaphoretic skin. His skin turgor is poor, with a sluggish capillary refill time. His vital signs are as follows: BP, 95/50 mm Hg; HR, 118 beats/min; and RR, 24 breaths/min. He is afebrile. He has postural hypotension. Laboratory test results show a glucose level of 610 mg/dL, mildly positive serum ketones, and normal white blood cells. An ECG shows sinus tachycardia (rate, 115 to 120 beats/min).

The staff starts an IV line for the administration of normal saline and an insulin infusion. Mr. J. is then transferred to the critical care unit, where he is placed on continuous ECG monitoring to assess for signs of hypokalemia. Frequent electrolyte profiles are sent and monitored for abnormalities. Hypokalemia is detected, necessitating potassium replacement therapy. Mr. J.'s serum glucose level is monitored closely and is lowered slowly (75 to 100 mg/dL/h). After 6 hours of insulin administration, Mr. J.'s glucose level is decreased to 230 mg/dL. At this time, his IV fluids are changed to D5½ NS. Over the next 3 hours, Mr. J.'s glucose level stabilizes between 130 and 150 mg/dL.

1. What is the constellation of symptoms that Mr. J. displayed at home that are associated with the insidious development of diabetes mellitus?

2. What specific risk factors for type 2 diabetes mellitus does Mr. J. have?

3. Why was Mr. J. initially administered normal saline and then changed to D5½ NS?

References

1. Klubo-Gwiezdzinska J, Wartofsky L: Thyrotropin blood levels, subclinical hypothyroidism and the elderly patient. Arch Intern Med 169(21):1949–1951, 2009
2. American Diabetes Association: Position statement: Diagnosis and classification of diabetes mellitus. Diabetes Care 30(1):S42–S47, 2007

Want to know more? A wide variety of resources to enhance your learning and understanding of this chapter are available on thePoint . Visit **http://thepoint.lww.com/MortonEss1e** to access chapter review questions and more!

Common Endocrine Disorders

Based on the content in this chapter, the reader should be able to:

1 Describe the pathophysiology, assessment, and management of the two major disorders of antidiuretic hormone (ADH) secretion: syndrome of inappropriate antidiuretic hormone (SIADH) and diabetes insipidus (DI).
2 Describe the pathophysiology, assessment, and management of two major crises of thyroid function: thyrotoxic crisis and myxedema coma.
3 Describe the pathophysiology, assessment, and management of three diabetic emergencies: diabetic ketoacidosis (DKA), hyperosmolar hyperglycemic syndrome (HHS), and hypoglycemia.
4 Describe the pathophysiology, assessment, and management of adrenal crisis.

Disorders of Antidiuretic Hormone Secretion

Antidiuretic hormone (ADH) is synthesized in the hypothalamus and stored in the posterior pituitary. It is released in response to specific conditions (eg, hyperosmolar states) and results in the reabsorption of water in the renal tubules. There are two major disorders related to ADH secretion. Syndrome of inappropriate antidiuretic hormone secretion (SIADH) is characterized by excess levels of ADH. Diabetes insipidus (DI) involves a deficiency of ADH. Both of these disorders can produce severe fluid and electrolyte imbalances and adverse neurological changes.

Syndrome of Inappropriate Antidiuretic Hormone Secretion

In SIADH, secretion of ADH is increased, despite the fact that, initially, the osmolality level is normal.

The increased ADH causes the kidneys to reabsorb more water, resulting in an increase in total-body water. As excess water is reabsorbed, the osmolality decreases, and the patient becomes hyponatremic. The normal feedback system regulating the release and inhibition of ADH fails, and ADH secretion continues despite the decreased osmolality of the plasma. Common causes of SIADH are summarized in Box 27-1.

Assessment

Water retention, dilutional hyponatremia, and, eventually, water intoxication secondary to sustained ADH effect characterize SIADH. Signs and symptoms are predominantly neurological and gastrointestinal (Box 27-2). When the serum sodium level decreases to less than 125 mEq/L, more pronounced manifestations of cerebral edema (eg, headache, nausea and vomiting, restlessness, muscular irritability, seizures) may be seen. Seizure precautions may be necessary.

BOX 27·1 Common Causes of Syndrome of Inappropriate Antidiuretic Hormone (SIADH)

Malignancies
- Pulmonary carcinoma (oat cell carcinoma)
- Pancreatic adenocarcinoma
- Prostate or thymus cancer
- Leukemia

Central Nervous System (CNS) Causes
- Traumatic brain injury (TBI)
- Hemorrhage (subdural hematoma, subarachnoid hemorrhage)
- Brain abscess
- CNS infection
- Hydrocephalus
- Brain tumor

Pulmonary Causes
- Mechanical ventilation
- Chronic obstructive pulmonary disease (COPD)
- Respiratory failure
- Lung abscess, infection

Medications
- Nicotine
- Morphine
- Chlorpropamide, hypoglycemics, insulin
- Antineoplastic agents
- Tricyclic antidepressants
- Anesthetics
- Clofibrate
- Diuretics

Other Causes
- HIV/AIDS
- Senile atrophy
- Pain
- Fear
- Myocardial infarction
- Idiopathic causes

The Older Patient. *Older patients are more susceptible to hyponatremia because of their lower body water content.*

Laboratory studies used in the evaluation of SIADH include serum ADH, serum sodium, serum and urine osmolality, and urine specific gravity. Findings include elevated serum ADH, low serum sodium, low serum osmolality, elevated urine osmolality, and elevated urine specific gravity.

Management

There are three goals in the management of SIADH: treat the underlying disease (when possible), alleviate excessive water retention, and manage the hyponatremia.

BOX 27·2 Signs and Symptoms of Syndrome of Inappropriate Antidiuretic Hormone Secretion (SIADH)

Neurological
- Personality changes
- Headache
- Decreased mentation
- Lethargy
- Decreased tendon reflexes
- Disorientation/confusion
- Seizures and coma

Gastrointestinal
- Abdominal cramps
- Nausea
- Vomiting
- Diarrhea
- Anorexia

Fluid restriction is usually successful for correcting hyponatremia when sodium levels are between 125 and 135 mEq/L or the patient is asymptomatic. A diuretic may also be administered to remove excess volume. The nurse monitors intake and output hourly. As a general guideline, water intake should not exceed urinary output until the serum sodium concentration normalizes and symptoms abate.

In severely symptomatic patients with acute hyponatremia, administration of 3% hypertonic saline is used to correct hyponatremia. A slow infusion rate (0.1 mg/kg/min) prevents rapid volume overload, osmolality shifts, and the development of complications such as pulmonary edema and central pontine myelinolysis. Usually, 300 mL given IV over 4 to 6 hours is appropriate, with frequent monitoring of sodium levels.

RED FLAG! *Central pontine myelinolysis (CPM) (characterized by brain dehydration, cerebral bleeding, and demyelination) can result when correction of hyponatremia by hypertonic saline infusion is too rapid. Central pontine myelinolysis can have long-term residual effects and may be fatal. Signs and symptoms include seizures, movement disorders, akinetic mutism, quadriparesis, and unresponsiveness. This complication can be avoided by ensuring that sodium levels do not increase at a rate of more than 1 to 2 mEq/L/h.*

Medications that interfere with the ADH–renal tubule interaction may be administered. Conivaptan is an ADH inhibitor that blocks vasopressin receptors in the renal collecting ducts to decrease water reabsorption. Other medications that block the effects of ADH at the tubules include demeclocycline, phenytoin, lithium, and fludrocortisone.

Diabetes Insipidus

Diabetes insipidus (DI) is caused by insufficient secretion of ADH. In the absence or reduction of ADH, the kidneys lose the ability to reabsorb water, leading to significant diuresis (up to 20 L of urine per day) and hypovolemia. Serum osmolality becomes concentrated, serum sodium levels increase, and urine output continues to be high regardless of the amount of fluid intake. Patients who are not alert and cannot detect thirst can quickly become dehydrated.

DI may be nephrogenic or central. Nephrogenic DI (characterized by failure of the kidney to respond to ADH) is a very rare genetic disorder. Central DI, which can develop after any event that causes edema or direct damage to the pituitary–hypothalamic area (eg, traumatic brain injury, brain surgery, brain tumor, stroke), is more common. It may be transient, temporary, partial, or permanent, depending on the underlying cause. For example, after trauma or surgery, edema in the pituitary–hypothalamic area may induce temporary DI that resolves as the edema abates. In cases of severe trauma or hemorrhage, the structures may be completely damaged and the patient may develop permanent DI.

Major complications of DI include hypovolemic shock, cardiovascular collapse, hypernatremia, and tissue hypoxia. Seizures and encephalopathy can result from fluid and electrolyte imbalance. Prognosis is excellent as long as the patient receives prompt and aggressive treatment.

Assessment

Polyuria, polydipsia, and dehydration are the hallmarks of DI. Signs of dehydration include dry skin, dry mucous membranes, confusion, sunken eyes, constipation, poor skin turgor, lethargy, muscle weakness, muscle pain, pallor, and possibly weight loss. Findings on evaluation of vital signs may include severe tachycardia, hypotension, low central venous pressure (CVP), and a possible rise in body temperature. Laboratory findings include reduced levels of ADH, high serum osmolality, hypernatremia, and low urine osmolality and urine specific gravity.

Management

The objective of therapy is to prevent dehydration and electrolyte imbalance, while treating the underlying cause and preventing complications. Central diabetes insipidus responds well to exogenous vasopressin administration (Table 27-1). Nursing management focuses on monitoring fluid and electrolyte balance. The nurse monitors hourly intake and output and laboratory test results (serum and urine electrolytes and osmolality, urine specific gravity). Fluid replacement, often with a hypotonic solution to replace the free water, is determined by the free water deficit:

$$\text{Free water deficit} = 0.6 \times ([\text{serum Na}/140] - 1)$$

Measurement of serum electrolytes every 6 to 8 hours is recommended to ensure adequate fluid replacement.

Thyroid Gland Dysfunction

Patients with extreme forms of hyperthyroidism (thyrotoxic crisis) or hypothyroidism (myxedema coma) require admission to the critical care unit.

Thyrotoxic Crisis

Thyrotoxic crisis (thyroid storm) is a critically severe form of hyperthyroidism. The condition may develop spontaneously, but it occurs most

---

TABLE 27-1 **Medications Commonly Administered for Diabetes Insipidus**

Drug	Dosage	Route of Administration	Duration of Drug	Adverse Effects
Desmopressin (DDAVP)	5–20 µg each day	Nasal spray (cannot be given if nasal passage is blocked)	8–24 h	Headache, chest pain, nausea, diarrhea, edema
Aqueous pitressin	2–4 U every 4–6 h	Intramuscularly, subcutaneously, intranasally, intravenously	1–8 h	Headache, chest pain, nausea, diarrhea, edema
Pitressin tannate in oil	2.5–5 U	Intramuscularly	36–48 h	Headache, chest pain, nausea, diarrhea, edema
Lysine vasopressin nasal spray	5–20 U three to seven times daily; titrate to output	Intranasally	2–6 h	—
Chlorpropamide	100–250 mg/d	By mouth	60–72 h	Hypoglycemia, headache, tinnitus, alcohol intolerance, gastrointestinal disturbances, diarrhea
Clofibrate	250–500 mg	By mouth	6–8 h	Gastrointestinal disturbances

commonly in people who have undiagnosed or partially treated severe hyperthyroidism. Many patients who experience thyrotoxic crisis have Graves' disease (the most common type of hyperthyroidism) or toxic multinodular adenoma. Untreated thyrotoxic crisis can cause myocardial infarction, heart failure, cardiovascular collapse, coma, and death.

 The Older Patient. *Delayed diagnosis of hyperthyroidism in elderly patients can occur, because hyperthyroidism in this population often presents with atypical or masked symptoms. Undiagnosed hyperthyroidism puts the older adult at risk for developing thyrotoxic crisis.*

The cause of thyrotoxic crisis is poorly understood. Precipitating factors are varied, and can be categorized according to whether the patient has a known preexisting condition (eg, hyperthyroidism) or not (Box 27-3). Physiological mechanisms thought to induce thyrotoxic crises include the sudden release of large quantities of thyroid hormone and low tissue tolerance to triiodothyronine (T_3) and thyroxine (T_4). Stimulation of the sympathetic nervous system brought on by the abrupt release of large quantities of thyroid hormone is thought to produce the hypermetabolic manifestations seen during thyrotoxic crisis.

Assessment

Signs and symptoms of hyperthyroidism affect all body systems (see Chapter 26, Fig. 26-2) and include sweating, heat intolerance, hyperactivity, nervousness, tremors, palpitations, and tachycardia. Extremes of these manifestations, specifically a temperature greater than 104°F (40°C) in the absence of an infection, may be present in thyrotoxic crisis. Central nervous system (CNS) abnormalities include agitation, restlessness, delirium, seizures, and coma. Cardiovascular and pulmonary complications can develop rapidly and lead to death.

Laboratory studies may show elevated total T_4, free T_3, and free T_4 levels. The thyroid-stimulating hormone (TSH) level is extremely low because the levels of circulating hormones T_3 and T_4 are so elevated. Serum electrolytes, liver function tests, and complete blood counts may help identify the precipitating cause.

A radioactive iodine uptake test typically shows increased uptake in the thyroid gland. Electrocardiography and cardiac monitoring may show atrial fibrillation, supraventricular tachycardia, sinus bradycardia, heart block, conduction disturbances, and ventricular dysrhythmias.

Management

Management goals for thyrotoxic crisis are fourfold: (1) treating the precipitating factor or factors, (2) controlling excessive thyroid hormone release, (3) inhibiting thyroid hormone biosynthesis, and (4) treating the peripheral effects of thyroid hormone.[1]

Antithyroid drugs (Table 27-2) are used to control the synthesis and release of thyroid hormone. If the thyrotoxic crisis was precipitated by the excessive ingestion of thyroid replacement hormones, removal of the excess hormone can be accomplished by plasmapheresis, dialysis, hemoperfusion adsorption, or the administration of cholestyramine.

BOX 27-3 Precipitating Factors Associated With Thyroid Crisis

In the Presence of a Known Preexisting Condition
- Trauma
- Infection
- Stress
- Coexistent medical illness (eg, myocardial infarction, pulmonary disease)
- Pregnancy
- Exposure to cold
- Alcohol
- Medications
  - Nonsteroidal anti-inflammatory drugs (NSAIDs)
  - Chronic steroid therapy
  - β-Adrenergic blockers
  - Narcotics
  - Anesthetics
  - Tricyclic antidepressants
  - Glucocorticoid therapy
  - Insulin therapy
  - Thiazide diuretics
  - Phenytoin
  - Chemotherapy agents
  - Contrast media dye
  - Thyroid medication
  - Amiodarone

In the Presence of an Unknown Preexisting Condition
- Pituitary tumors
- Thyroid tumors
- Radiation therapy of the head and neck
- Autoimmune disease
- Neurosurgical procedures
- Metastatic malignancies (eg, lung, breast)
- Surgery
- Long-term illness
- Shock
- Postpartum stress
- Trauma

TABLE 27-2   Medications Used to Treat Hyperthyroidism

Medication	Mechanism of Action	Nursing Considerations
Thioamides Propylthiouracil (PTU) Methimazole	Blocks synthesis of hormones (conversion of T_4 to T_3)	Monitor cardiac parameters. Observe for conversion to hypothyroidism. Watch for rash, nausea, vomiting, agranulocytosis, lupus syndrome.
Iodides Sodium iodide Potassium iodide Saturated solution of potassium iodide (SSKI)	Suppresses release of thyroid hormone	Given 1 h after PTU or methimazole. Watch for edema, hemorrhage, gastrointestinal upset. Discontinue for rash. Watch for signs of toxic iodinism. Mix with juice or milk. Give by straw to prevent staining of teeth.
Glucocorticoids Dexamethasone	Suppresses thyroid hormone release	Monitor intake and output. Monitor glucose. May cause hypertension, nausea, vomiting, anorexia, infection
β-Adrenergic blockers	Blocks catecholamines Treats symptoms	Monitor cardiac status. Hold for bradycardia or decreased cardiac output. Use with caution in patients with heart failure.

Management also focuses on monitoring and treating the multisystemic effects of the hypermetabolic state. Cardiovascular function, fluid and electrolyte balance, neurological status, and vital signs require close attention.

- For patients with cardiovascular complications, measures are taken to decrease myocardial oxygen consumption, decrease the heart rate (ideally to below 100 beats/min), manage dysrhythmias, and increase cardiac output. Digoxin, diltiazem, diuretics, or a combination of these agents may be administered, along with oxygen therapy.
- Acetaminophen is recommended for fever control; aspirin is not appropriate because it increases free T_3 and T_4 levels. Tepid baths or a cooling blanket may be necessary. It is important to avoid cooling to the point of shivering, as this may have a rebound effect of raising body temperature.
- IV fluids are necessary to replace the fluids lost due to the excessive hyperthermia, tachypnea, diaphoresis, and diarrhea that often accompany thyrotoxic crisis.
- If the patient's level of consciousness decreases, the patient's ability to maintain the airway must be assessed.
- Maintaining a calm environment helps to manage the extreme agitation and restlessness experienced by the patient with thyrotoxic crisis.

Myxedema Coma

Myxedema coma is a rare but life-threatening hypometabolic state characterized by severe depression of the sensorium. It is usually seen in older patients during the winter months. The most common precipitating factor is pulmonary infection; other factors include trauma, stress, medications (eg, narcotics or barbiturates), surgery, and metabolic disturbances. In addition to coma, complications of myxedema coma include pericardial and pleural effusions, megacolon with paralytic ileus, and seizures. Death can result if severe hypoxia and hypercapnia are not reversed.

Assessment

In myxedema coma, the depressed level of consciousness is one of coma or near coma. Other clinical manifestations include swelling (particularly of the hands, feet, periorbital region, and larynx), hypothermia, hypoventilation, hypoxemia, and bradycardia. Patients with myxedema coma do not shiver, although some may have body temperatures below 80°F (26.6°C).

Laboratory studies commonly reveal a decrease in levels of T_4 and free T_4, and markedly elevated TSH levels. Arterial blood gases (ABGs) usually show a decreased arterial oxygen tension (PaO_2) and increased arterial carbon dioxide tension ($PaCO_2$). A chest radiograph detects pleural effusion. Electrocardiographic changes include bradycardia, a prolonged PR interval, decreased amplitude of the P wave and QRS complex, and development of heart blocks.

Management

Mechanical ventilation is used to control hypoventilation, hypercapnia, and respiratory arrest. Normal or hypertonic saline and glucose are administered IV to correct dilutional hyponatremia and hypoglycemia. Vasopressor therapy may be needed in addition to fluid replacement to correct hypotension.

Pharmacological therapy includes the administration of thyroid hormone and corticosteroids. Initial drug therapy is 300 to 500 µg T_4 IV to saturate all protein-binding sites and establish a relatively normal T_4 level. Subsequent doses may range from 75 to 100 µg daily. Alternatively, T_3 can be administered. Guidelines for T_3 replacement are 25 µg IV every 8 hours for the first 24 to 48 hours. Hormone replacement should occur slowly, with continuous monitoring of the patient during treatment to avoid sudden increased metabolic demand and resultant myocardial infarction.

Additional interventions include rewarming of the patient, treating abdominal distention and fecal impaction, and preventing complications related to aspiration, immobility, skin breakdown, and infection in the comatose patient.

Diabetic Emergencies

Acute, life-threatening complications that can occur in patients with diabetes mellitus include diabetic ketoacidosis (DKA), hyperosmolar hyperglycemic syndrome (HHS), and hypoglycemia. Patients with type 1 diabetes are most likely to experience DKA and patients with type 2 diabetes HHS.

Diabetic Ketoacidosis

DKA is a critical illness resulting from severe insulin deficiency that leads to the disordered metabolism of proteins, carbohydrates, and fats. Clinical manifestations include severe hyperglycemia and hyperosmolality, metabolic acidosis, and fluid and electrolyte imbalances. DKA seldom occurs in patients with type 2 diabetes because these patients still secrete just enough insulin to avoid ketoacidosis; however, it is possible for patients with type 2 diabetes to manifest DKA as a result of catabolic stress associated with severe critical illness. The most common precipitating cause of DKA is infection (especially urinary tract infection and pneumonia).[2] Other precipitating factors include severe illness (eg, stroke, myocardial infarction, pancreatitis); alcohol or drug abuse; trauma; or discontinuation of insulin therapy (eg, due to lack of knowledge or lack of financial resources).

DKA is associated with a 2% to 5% mortality rate.[3] The cause of death is rarely a direct result of the metabolic acidosis or the hyperglycemia; instead, death is more often related to the underlying illness that precipitated the metabolic decompensation.

Pathophysiology

Three major physiological disturbances exist in DKA: (1) hyperosmolality due to hyperglycemia, (2) metabolic acidosis due to accumulation of ketoacids, and (3) volume depletion due to osmotic diuresis (Fig. 27-1).

Hyperglycemia and Hyperosmolality
The first major consequence of DKA is hyperosmolality due to hyperglycemia. As the serum glucose increases, the serum osmolality increases incrementally. The hyperglycemia seen in DKA is the result of insulin deficiency and excessive hepatic (gluconeogenesis) and renal (glycogenolysis) glucose production, as well as reduced glucose utilization in peripheral tissues. When the blood glucose level exceeds the normal threshold of about 180 mg/dL, glucose begins to escape into the urine (glycosuria) because the reabsorption capacity of the tubules is exceeded. Glycosuria promotes an osmotic diuresis that leads to hypovolemia and a decreased glomerular filtration rate (GFR), which in turn reduces glucose losses and permits the blood glucose level to rise even higher. This serum hyperosmolality and dehydration accounts for the lethargy, stupor, and ultimately, coma that occurs as DKA worsens.

Ketoacidosis
The second major consequence of severe insulin deficiency is uncontrolled ketogenesis. Lipase causes the breakdown of triglycerides into glycerol and free fatty acids; free fatty acids are released as precursors of ketoacids. In the liver, they are oxidized to form ketones. Insulin normally controls the ketones, but in cases of insulin deficiency, ketones accumulate, causing ketoacidosis.

The anion gap is frequently measured to determine the presence of ketones, which are unmeasured anions. The anion gap is determined by subtracting the total measured anions (chloride plus bicarbonate) from the total measured cations (sodium plus potassium). The normal value is 12 to 15 mEq/L. A high anion gap indicates metabolic acidosis and is used as an indirect measure of the ketoacids present. As the ketoacids continue to accumulate, the anion gap increases. As the ketoacidosis is corrected with insulin administration, the anion gap will decrease until it reaches a normal level.

Lactic acidosis, resulting from poor tissue perfusion and hypovolemia, also contributes to the metabolic acidosis seen in DKA. The excess carbon dioxide and ketones are removed by hyperventilation. Kussmaul's respirations (deep, rapid breathing) associated with "fruity"-smelling breath are characteristic physical findings in DKA that are the result of the body's attempt to eliminate ketones and correct the metabolic acidosis.[3]

Volume Depletion
As described earlier, glycosuria promotes an osmotic diuresis. Additionally, high ketone levels cause osmotic diuresis because ketoacids are excreted in the urine largely as sodium, potassium, and ammonium salts. This osmotic diuresis can result in the loss of 5 to 8 L of fluid (15% of total body water in

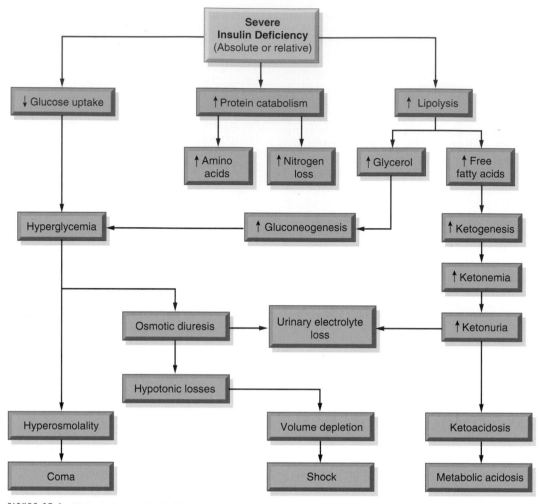

FIGURE 27-1 Diabetic ketoacidosis (DKA) is characterized by three major pathophysiological disruptions: coma, shock, and metabolic acidosis.

a 70-kg adult). The body perceives the urinary loss of large quantities of sodium and water as a serious threat to the maintenance of circulation, and a variety of compensatory mechanisms are called into play to prevent vascular collapse and shock. One such compensatory mechanism is a shift of body fluids into the vascular space from the extravascular compartments. The higher the blood glucose level, the more water is drawn out of the cells and into the vascular space. Hyperosmolality provides a temporary mechanism for preventing vascular collapse; however, vascular volume continues to decrease as DKA progresses.

As vascular volume decreases, glomerular filtration also decreases. The excretion of potassium by the kidney occurs through the exchange of potassium for sodium. Adequate sodium must be present at the exchange site in the kidney for the rate of potassium excretion to keep pace with the need for excretion. When renal perfusion decreases, sodium levels may not be adequate for this exchange. As a result, despite a total-body depletion of potassium, the serum potassium level may initially be above normal, even to dangerously high levels. Once treatment

begins with fluid and insulin, the potassium levels decrease quickly and will need to be replaced. Other consequences of diminished vascular volume include decreased tissue perfusion, hypotension, and the development of shock and acute renal failure.

Assessment

Initial assessment includes an immediate bedside determination of glucose level, followed by laboratory analysis of a blood sample to confirm the diagnosis. A more complete assessment follows, which includes a detailed history and physical examination, a search for precipitating causes, and more complete laboratory tests (eg, blood glucose, blood chemistries, osmolality, anion gap, pH, ABGs, urine acetone, urine glucose). Physical examination and laboratory findings in DKA are summarized in Box 27-4.

Management

Treatment goals include the following:

- Improve circulatory volume and tissue perfusion
- Correct electrolyte imbalances

BOX 27-4 Clinical Manifestations of Diabetic Ketoacidosis (DKA)

- Polyuria and polydipsia
- Hyperventilation (Kussmaul's respirations) and "fruity" breath
- Lethargy, stupor, coma
- Abdominal cramping, anorexia, nausea and vomiting
- Acute weight loss
- Hyperglycemia
- Glycosuria
- Volume depletion
- Hyperosmolality
- Increased anion gap (greater than 15 mEq/L)
- Decreased bicarbonate (less than 10 mEq/L)
- Decreased pH (less than 7.45)

- Decrease serum glucose and serum osmolality levels
- Correct ketoacidosis
- Determine precipitating events

A collaborative care guide for the patient with DKA is given in Box 27-5.

Fluid Replacement

The immediate threat to life in a critically ill keto-acidotic patient is volume depletion. The goal is to reverse the severity of the extracellular volume depletion and restore renal perfusion as soon as possible. The first liter of 0.9% (normal) saline may be infused in 1 hour in patients with normal cardiac function. This replaces only a fraction of the extracellular loss in the average patient, which can range from 6 to 8 L.

Volume losses continue throughout the first hours of treatment until the glycosuria and osmotic diuresis are controlled. Fluid replacement continues at roughly 1 L/h until hemodynamic stability is attained. Hypotonic solutions (eg, 0.45% normal saline) can be administered at a rate of 150 to 250 mL/h after the intravascular volume has been restored, or if the serum sodium level is greater than 155 mg/dL. Other plasma expanders, such as albumin and plasma concentrates, may be necessary if low blood pressure and other clinical signs of vascular collapse do not respond to saline alone.

 RED FLAG! *Rapid infusion of saline in a patient with DKA can lower serum osmolality, which lowers the osmotic pressure of the plasma. This allows fluid to leak out of the vascular space, contributing to the development of pulmonary or cerebral edema, particularly in older adults. Patients must be observed carefully during the first 24 to 36 hours for signs of pulmonary or cerebral edema.*

Insulin Therapy

Insulin is the cornerstone of management of DKA. It decreases the ketones and manages ketoacidosis, inhibits hepatic gluconeogenesis, restores cellular protein synthesis, and increases peripheral glucose utilization. Guidelines for insulin administration are given in Box 27-6 on page 394.

Initially, insulin administration involves giving an IV bolus of regular insulin at 0.15 U/kg body weight. This is followed by a continuous infusion of regular insulin at a dose of 0.1 U/kg/h (5 to 10 U/h) to produce a steady decline in glucose concentrations at a rate of 65 to 125 mg/h. When the plasma glucose level reaches 250 mg/dL, the insulin infusion is decreased to half the current dose and dextrose (5% or 10%) is added to the IV fluids. As the insulin infusion is stopped, sliding scale insulin therapy is initiated to maintain normal glycemic control.

 RED FLAG! *Blood sugar should not fall too fast or too far. Sudden and rapid lowering of the blood sugar level with insulin allows water to shift very rapidly into the cells, causing cerebral edema and vascular collapse. To prevent these complications, insulin doses are administered at a rate that will promote a slow, steady decline, and early volume replacement includes sodium, water, and glucose along with insulin therapy.*

Potassium and Phosphate Replacement

Potassium is not given until the laboratory report is available because the initial plasma potassium level in patients with DKA can range from very low to very high. If the initial serum potassium level is low, IV potassium is usually started right away. This is particularly important because insulin drives potassium into cells (lowering the serum potassium level) and fluid administration dilutes the serum potassium concentrations even further. If the initial potassium level is normal or high, IV potassium is usually withheld until the level begins to drop and urine flow is established. Potassium is usually replaced at concentrations of 20 to 40 mEq/L, depending on the serum potassium level. Frequent potassium levels are obtained and patient is monitored for the development of dysrhythmias.

Phosphate levels usually also drop during therapy, potentially worsening tissue hypoxia by increasing red blood cell affinity for oxygen. Thus, less oxygen is released at the tissue level. Phosphate replacement is usually combined with potassium replacement in the form of potassium phosphate salts.

Bicarbonate Replacement

Bicarbonate replacement in patients with DKA is controversial because evidence-based research has failed to demonstrate its benefit in patients with an arterial pH between 6.9 and 7.1. Patients with mild or moderate metabolic acidosis due to ketones who are treated with 0.9% sodium, water, and insulin eventually excrete and metabolize the ketones, thus increasing pH. However, some experts recommend bicarbonate replacement with severe acidosis as indicated by an arterial pH of 7.0 or less. It is also necessary to give bicarbonate

BOX 27-5 COLLABORATIVE CARE GUIDE for the Patient With Diabetic Ketoacidosis (DKA)

OUTCOMES	INTERVENTIONS
Oxygenation/Ventilation	
ABGs are maintained within normal limits.	• Provide chest physiotherapy, turning and deep breathing, coughing, incentive spirometry q4h and PRN.
There is no evidence of acute respiratory failure.	• Continuously monitor patient's respiratory rate, depth, and pattern. Observe for Kussmaul's respirations, rapid and shallow breathing, and other signs of respiratory distress. • Monitor ABGs, pulse oximetry and, if intubated, end tidal CO_2. • Provide supplemental oxygen. • Prepare for intubation and mechanical ventilation.
The patient's lungs are clear.	• Auscultate breath sounds q2h and PRN.
There is no evidence of atelectasis or pneumonia.	• Take daily chest x-ray. • Provide chest physiotherapy q4h. • Mobilize out of bed as soon as patient is stabilized.
Circulation/Perfusion	
Blood pressure and heart rate are within normal limits. If PA catheter is in place, hemodynamic parameters are within normal limits.	• Monitor vital signs q1h and PRN. • Assess for dehydration/hypovolemia: tachycardia, decreased CVP and PAOP. • Assess for hypervolemia: neck vein distention, pulmonary crackles and edema, increased CVP and PAOP. • Administer vasopressor agents if hypotension is related to vasodilation.
Patient is free of dysrhythmias.	• Monitor ECG continuously. • Evaluate and treat the cause of dysrhythmias (eg, acidosis, hypoxia, hypokalemia/ hyperkalemia).
Fluids/Electrolytes	
There is evidence of rehydration without complications: • balanced intake and output • normal skin turgor • hemodynamic stability • intact sensorium	• Infuse normal saline or lactated Ringer's, then 0.45% normal saline. • Monitor serum osmolality, urine output, neurological status, and vital signs closely during rehydration. Observe for complications of DKA (eg, shock, renal failure, decreased LOC, and seizures). • Assess BUN, creatinine, urine for glucose and ketones.
Serum electrolyte levels and acid–base balance are normal.	• Assess and replace electrolytes as indicated. • Closely monitor potassium fluctuations as serum glucose is decreased and acidosis reversed. • Assess arterial pH and bicarbonate level q2–4h during rehydration and insulin administration.
Serum glucose returns to normal range.	• Monitor serum glucose q30–60min, then q1–4h after level <300 mg/dL. • Administer IV insulin bolus then continuous low dose infusion. • Infuse $D_5$1/2 normal saline or D_5W after glucose is <250 mg/dL.
Mobility/Safety	
The patient is free of injury related to altered sensorium or seizures.	• Place on seizure and fall precautions. • Assess neurological status q1h, then q2–4h after initial rehydration phase.
The patient maintains muscle tone and joint range of motion.	• Provide range-of-motion exercises q4h. • Reposition in bed q2h. • Mobilize to chair when condition stable. • Consult physical therapist.

BOX 27-5 COLLABORATIVE CARE GUIDE (continued)

OUTCOMES	INTERVENTIONS
Skin Integrity Patient is without evidence of skin breakdown.	• Assess risk for skin breakdown using the Braden Scale. • Initially assess skin and circulation q1–2h for 12 h. • If risk for skin breakdown low, assess skin q8h and each time patient is repositioned. • Turn q2h. • Consider pressure relief/reduction mattress if at risk for skin breakdown.
Nutrition Nutritional intake meets calculated metabolic need (eg, basal energy expenditure equation).	• Provide parenteral feeding if patient is NPO. • Provide clear, then full, liquid diet, and assess patient response. • Progress to diabetic diet (ADA). • Consult dietitian or nutritional support service regarding special nutritional needs.
There is no evidence of metabolic dysfunction.	• Monitor albumin, prealbumin, transferrin, cholesterol, triglycerides, glucose, and protein levels.
Comfort/Pain Control Patient is as comfortable as possible (as evidenced by stable vital signs or cooperation with treatments or procedures).	• Document pain assessment, using numerical pain rating or similar scale when possible. • If analgesics are needed, administer cautiously due to risk of respiratory and neurological complications. • Consider nonpharmacological pain management techniques (eg, distraction, touch).
The patient experiences relief from nausea, vomiting, and abdominal pain or tenderness.	• Maintain nasogastric tube patency. • Assess bowel sounds q1–2h. • Administer antiemetic as ordered. • Provide ice chips and frequent oral hygiene.
Psychosocial Patient demonstrates decreased anxiety.	• Provide nonjudgmental atmosphere in which patient can discuss concerns and fears. • Provide patients who are intubated with a method to communicate. • Provide patients with decreased LOC with sensory input. • Provide for adequate rest and sleep.
Teaching/Discharge Planning Patient and family understand the tests needed for treatment.	• Prepare patient and family for procedures such as EEG, ECG, and multiple laboratory studies.
Patient and family understand the severity of the illness, ask appropriate questions, and anticipate potential complications.	• Explain the widespread effects of diabetes and the potential for complications of DKA such as seizures, renal failure, or vascular collapse. • Encourage patient and family to ask questions related to complications, pathophysiology, monitoring, treatments, and so on.
Patient and family are prepared for home care.	• Teach information needed to manage diabetes: diabetic diet, skin care, glucose monitoring, insulin administration, signs and symptoms of hypoglycemia and hyperglycemia, and appropriate actions. • Discuss sick-day management and factors that can precipitate DKA. • Initiate contacts with diabetic support groups, social services, and home health agency.

BOX 27-6   Guidelines for Insulin Administration in Diabetic Ketoacidosis (DKA)

- Administer insulin IV through an IV infusion pump to minimize the trauma of repeated injections.
- Flush tubing well with insulin mixture before infusing to patient to prevent tubing from absorbing too much insulin.
- When the serum glucose level reaches 250 mg/dL, the IV fluids should be changed to a glucose-based solution.
- Changes in blood glucose levels and the patient's clinical status should clearly indicate a beneficial response to insulin and fluid replacement. If the blood glucose level does not decrease and blood pressure and urine output do not stabilize, insulin or fluid replacement may not be adequate.

when there is cardiac decompensation. The bicarbonate deficit is replaced slowly over several hours intravenously to raise the level to 10- to 12-mEq/L, at minimum.

Promoting Comfort

Gastric motility is greatly impaired in DKA. Gastric distention with dark, hemopositive fluid and vomiting is common. Insertion of a nasogastric tube to decompress the stomach can increase comfort and decrease the risk for aspiration. The patient should not eat or drink in this phase of the illness; ice chips may help decrease thirst. Later, when distention lessens and motility returns, oral intake can be resumed.

Hyperosmolar Hyperglycemic Syndrome

HHS, characterized by marked hyperglycemia and hyperosmolality without ketoacidosis, may develop in patients with type 2 diabetes when they become critically ill. HHS has a higher mortality rate than any other complication of diabetes (20% to 40%), a result of the high serum osmolality levels and the comorbidities that often accompany the disorder.

 The Older Patient. Frail elderly people are at high risk for developing HHS; acute illness increases their risk even more.

Pathophysiology

Table 27-3 compares HHS and DKA. It is speculated that patients who develop HHS may have just enough insulin to prevent ketosis but not enough to control the glucose level. Pathophysiologically, the mechanisms of disease are the same as for DKA—a reduction in circulating insulin or insulin resistance occurs, coupled with hyperglycemia and the extreme hyperosmolar syndrome. However, because insulin is still being produced, excessive ketone production does not occur. The acidosis that patients with HHS may develop is attributed to lactic acidosis from poor tissue perfusion, rather than ketoacidosis.

HHS develops slowly over days to weeks, and patients often experience polydipsia, polyuria, and progressive decline in level of consciousness. Marked dehydration occurs with the typical fluid loss associated with HHS (about 9 L). As dehydration worsens, serum glucose and serum osmolality increase, and a life-threatening cycle of hyperglycemia, hyperosmolality, osmotic diuresis, and profound dehydration

TABLE 27-3   Comparison of Signs and Symptoms of Diabetic Ketoacidosis (DKA) and Hyperglycemic Hyperosmolar Syndrome (HHS)

	DKA	HHS
Onset	Gradual or sudden, usually less than 2 d	Gradual, usually more than 5 d
Previous history of diabetes mellitus	85% (15% have new onset)	60%
Type of diabetes mellitus	Type 1	Type 2
Age of patient	Usually younger than 40 y	Usually older than 60 y
Mortality risk	1%–15%	20%–40%
Drug history	Insulin	Steroids, thiazides, oral agents
Physical signs	Polydipsia, polyuria, dehydration, Kussmaul's respirations, mental status changes, "fruity breath," febrile at times, ketoacidosis, nausea and vomiting	Dehydration, obtundation, hypothermia, toxic appearance, nonketotic
Glucose level	Mean, 600 mg/dL Range, 250–1200 mg/dL	Mean, 1100 mg/dL Range, 400–4000 mg/dL
Ketones	Present	Absent
Osmolality (mean)	320 mOsm/L	400 mOsm/L
Arterial pH (mean)	7.07	7.26
Bicarbonate	Markedly low (less than 10 mEq/L)	Normal or greater than 15 mEq/L
Anion gap	Greater than 12 mEq/L	Less than 12 mEq/L, variable

Adapted from American Diabetes Association: Position statement: Hyperglycemic crisis in patients with diabetes mellitus. Diabetes Care 27(suppl 1):S94–S104, 2004.

ensues. Worsening dehydration leads to CNS dysfunction, manifested as confusion and lethargy.

Factors that can precipitate HHS include

- Infection (30% to 60% of patients; urinary tract infections and pneumonia are most common)
- Acute illness (eg, stroke, myocardial infarction, pancreatitis) with stress response
- Excessive carbohydrate intake or exposure (eg, through dietary supplements, total enteral support with tube feedings, peritoneal dialysis)
- Medications (corticosteroids, thiazide diuretics, sedatives, sympathomimetics)

 The Older Patient. *The possibility of HHS should be considered when an older patient with diabetes presents with the new onset of an acute, serious infection or illness (eg, myocardial infarction, pancreatitis, pneumonia).*

Assessment

Often family members or long-term care personnel report that the patient has become a bit drowsy, taken in less food and fluid over several days, and slept more until he or she became difficult to awaken. The clinical manifestations of HHS are reviewed in Table 27-3, as are the laboratory values, which differ from those of DKA in terms of glucose and osmolality levels, presence of ketones, and serum pH.

Management

Therapy for HHS is directed at correcting the volume depletion, controlling hyperglycemia, and identifying the underlying cause of the HHS and treating it. The amount of volume depletion is usually greater in HHS than in DKA. Rapid rehydration is more cautiously carried out in an elderly patient with comorbidities. Isotonic saline is administered initially to correct the fluid imbalance, and some patients may require as many as 9 to 12 L of fluid overall. The nurse must be vigilant for signs of fluid overload during rehydration; critically ill patients (especially those who are elderly and have cardiac or renal disease) may require hemodynamic monitoring during fluid resuscitation. The nurse also monitors fluid intake, urine output, blood pressure, central pressures, pulse, breath sounds, neurological status, and laboratory test results.

 The Older Patient. *Older patients who develop HHS are at risk for intravascular thrombosis and focal seizures because of the hemoconcentration of the blood and the hyperosmolar state. Use of seizure precautions is necessary at all times.*

Patients receive low doses of insulin along with the fluid replacement. It is necessary to give low-dose insulin by continuous infusion (0.1 U/kg/h) because these patients are vulnerable to the sudden loss of circulating blood volume that occurs with higher doses of insulin and a rapid blood sugar reduction. As the glucose level returns close to normal (250 to 300 mg/dL), the insulin infusion is decreased and dextrose is added to the IV fluids to prevent a sudden drop in the blood glucose level. At this point, insulin therapy can be changed to the subcutaneous route.

Investigation of the underlying cause of HHS is warranted, and treatment, if possible, is necessary. Removal of exogenous sources of glucose (tube feedings, medications) is appropriate while treating patients in the hyperglycemic state. Critical care management continues until the patient's hyperglycemic state has stabilized, his or her neurological condition and vital signs return to normal, and the precipitating cause has resolved.

Hypoglycemia

Insulin-induced hypoglycemia, the most common diabetes-related emergency, is a well-recognized complication among patients with type 1 diabetes.[4] Mild hypoglycemia causes unpleasant symptoms and discomfort; however, severe hypoglycemia can lead to serious complications (eg, seizures, coma) and death if not reversed. The more profound the hypoglycemia and the longer it lasts, the greater the chance of transient or even permanent cerebral damage after blood glucose levels are restored.

Pathophysiology

Because the neurons in the brain cannot store glucose, the brain depends on the glucose supplied by the circulation for energy. The term neuroglycopenia refers to hypoglycemia sufficient to cause brain dysfunction that results in personality changes and intellectual deterioration. The brain recognizes an energy deficiency when the serum glucose level falls abruptly to about 45 mg/dL; however, the exact level at which symptoms occur varies widely from person to person, and it is not uncommon for levels as low as 30 to 35 mg/dL to occur (eg, during glucose tolerance tests) without causing symptoms in people with long-term diabetes. As the blood glucose level falls below normal, impairment of higher cerebral functions (eg, trouble thinking or concentrating) is followed by the release of epinephrine by the autonomic nervous system, producing symptoms such as tachycardia and sweating. As hypoglycemia persists and worsens, consciousness is progressively impaired, leading to stupor, seizure, or coma.

Assessment

Clinical manifestations of hypoglycemia are given in Box 27-7. Blood glucose measurement, before the administration of glucose if possible, verifies the diagnosis.

A major focus of assessment is determining the precipitating cause of the hypoglycemic reaction so that measures can be taken to prevent future reactions. Common causes of hypoglycemic reactions are listed in Box 27-8. Frequently, the precipitating event is clear (eg, a skipped meal or an unusually strenuous bout of exercise). Problems with insulin

BOX 27-7 Clinical Manifestations of Hypoglycemia

- Personality and behavioral changes
- Difficulties with motor function (eg, trouble walking, slurred speech)
- Cortical changes (eg, aphasia, vertigo, localized weakness, focal seizures)
- Autonomic neurological responses (eg, tachycardia, pallor, sweating, anxiety, tremor, headache)
- Impaired consciousness (eg, stupor, seizure, coma)

dosage or administration may also be an issue. The nurse investigates every detail of insulin therapy thoroughly, especially any recent change in any part of the regimen. Prescription errors, mismatched syringe and insulin units, use of new injection sites, or an atypical (eg, early or late) response to insulin therapy may emerge as the cause of the reaction. Oral hypoglycemic agents can also produce severe and long-lasting hypoglycemia, especially in patients who are older and undernourished, with impaired renal or hepatic function. Finally, the administration or withdrawal of other medications (see Box 27-8) must also be considered as the precipitating event for recurrent insulin reactions.

Management

Treatment of insulin reactions is always glucose. The amount of glucose needed to reverse an insulin reaction acutely is not large. In an average-sized adult, less

BOX 27-8 Common Causes of Hypoglycemia

- Insulin shock
- Insulinoma
- Inborn errors of metabolism
- Stress
- Weight loss
- Postgastrectomy status
- Alcohol
- Glucocorticoid deficiency
- Fasting hypoglycemia
- Profound malnutrition
- Prolonged exercise
- Severe liver disease
- Severe sepsis
- Drug effects
  - Ethanol
  - Salicylates
  - Quinine
  - Haloperidol
  - Insulin
  - Sulfonylureas
  - Sulfonamides
  - Allopurinol
  - Clofibrate
  - β-Adrenergic blockers

than 15 g (3 tsp) of glucose can raise the blood glucose level from 20 to 120 mg/dL. If the patient can swallow, the most convenient form of delivery is a glucose- or sucrose-containing drink because it is absorbed into the intestines. If the patient is too groggy, stuporous, or uncooperative to drink, the glucose is administered as an IV bolus (25 g of 50% dextrose given over several minutes). If this route or dosage is unavailable, 1 mg of glucagon is given subcutaneously or intramuscularly. The response to oral glucose takes 5 to 15 minutes, whereas the response to IV glucose should occur within 1 or 2 minutes at most.

Adrenal Crisis

Adrenal crisis (acute adrenal insufficiency) is a life-threatening complication that can develop in critically ill patients when the additional stress of injury or illness quickly depletes cortisol stores or causes cortisol resistance, rendering the body unable to meet metabolic needs. Adrenal crisis can also result from worsening of primary or secondary adrenal insufficiency or bilateral adrenal hemorrhage.

Assessment

Because adrenal insufficiency affects both glucocorticoids and mineralocorticoids, many body functions are affected, including glucose metabolism, fluid and electrolyte balance, cognitive state, and cardiopulmonary status. Signs and symptoms of an impending adrenal crisis are summarized in Box 27-9. Laboratory values in acute adrenal

BOX 27-9 Signs and Symptoms of Impending Adrenal Crisis

Aldosterone Deficiency
- Hyperkalemia
- Hyponatremia
- Hypovolemia
- Elevated blood urea nitrogen (BUN)

Cortisol Deficiency
- Hypoglycemia
- Decreased gastric motility
- Decreased vascular tone
- Hypercalcemia

Generalized Signs and Symptoms
- Anorexia
- Nausea and vomiting
- Abdominal cramping
- Diarrhea
- Tachycardia
- Orthostatic hypotension
- Headache
- Lethargy, fatigue, weakness
- Hyperkalemic electrocardiographic changes
- Hyperpigmentation

insufficiency show hyponatremia, hyperkalemia, decreased serum bicarbonate levels, hypoglycemia, anemia, leukocytosis, and elevated blood urea nitrogen (BUN). Metabolic acidosis may occur because of the dehydration.

Management

The immediate goal of therapy is to administer the needed corticosteroid replacement and restore fluid and electrolyte balance. The corticosteroid of choice for critically ill patients is hydrocortisone (50 mg every 6 to 8 hours) because it most resembles endogenous cortisol. Fluid resuscitation is started with normal saline. The rate of fluid and electrolyte replacement is dictated by the degree of volume depletion, serum electrolyte levels, and clinical response to therapy. Associated medical or surgical problems may indicate the need for invasive blood pressure and hemodynamic monitoring.

CASE STUDY

Mr. B., a 19-year-old college student, was brought to the emergency department by his roommate because he had been experiencing fatigue, weakness, nausea, and vomiting for 4 days. Mr. B., diagnosed with diabetes mellitus at 8 years of age, follows a maintenance insulin regimen of 22 U of longer-acting insulin glargine at bedtime and a sliding scale of NovoLog premeals. Four days prior to coming to the hospital, Mr. B. had developed flulike symptoms, including a cough, fatigue, fever and chills, nausea, and intermittent vomiting. During this period, he omitted his evening insulin and then took no further insulin for several days because he was not eating anything.

On admission, Mr. B.'s vital signs are as follows: rectal temp, 100.6°F (38.1°C); HR, 128 beats/min; RR, 32 breaths/min and deep; and BP, 90/52 mm Hg. He is oriented but lethargic, with coarse rales at both lung bases. Admission laboratory work reveals the following: hematocrit, 48.6%; white blood cells (WBCs), 36,400/mm³; glucose, 710 mg/dL; Na⁺, 128 mEq/L; K⁺, 5.7 mEq/L; chloride, 90 mEq/L; bicarbonate, 4 mEq/L; blood urea nitrogen (BUN), 43 mg/100 mL; creatinine, 2.3 mg/dL; serum ketones, 4+; and urine glucose and ketones, 4+. Arterial blood gas (ABG) values are as follows: arterial blood pH, 7.06; PaO_2, 112 mm Hg; $PaCO_2$, 13 mm Hg; and bicarbonate, 2.5 mEq/L. The admission chest film is negative for pneumonia.

Emergency department physicians diagnose Mr. B. with diabetic ketoacidosis (DKA), and the initial therapy consists of several liters of IV normal saline and 20 U regular insulin by IV push, followed by an infusion of insulin at 5 U/h during the first 9 hours. Mr. B.'s mental status improves rapidly. The flow sheet below summarizes the biochemical changes over the first 15 hours.

Time	Sugar	pH	Na	K	Cl	HCO₃	BUN/ Creatinine
1:00 PM	710	7.06	128	5.7	90	4	43/2.3
3:00 PM	492		132	4.8	101	6	41/1.7
5:15 PM	375	7.25	137	4.1	106	8	45/1.4
10:00 PM	303		139	4.7	114	15	27/1.2
4:00 AM	304		143	4.3	113	22	22/1.1

By the time of discharge 4 days later, Mr. B. is eating well, and it is evident that his blood glucose is controlled on his usual doses of insulin glargine.

1. Mr. B. receives diagnoses of ketosis and acidosis. What are the indicators of ketosis and acidosis?

2. Mr. B. experiences volume depletion and electrolyte imbalances. Why does this occur and what are the clues?

3. How could Mr. B.'s complication of diabetes be prevented?

References

1. Reid JR, Wheeler SF: Hyperthyroidism: Diagnosis and treatment. Am Fam Physician 72(4):623–631, 2005
2. Eisebarth G, Polonsky K, Buse J: Type I diabetes mellitus. In Kronenberg: Williams Textbook of Endocrinology, 11th ed. Philadelphia, PA: Saunders Elsevier, 2008:Chapter 31
3. Savage M: Management of diabetic ketoacidosis. Clin Med 11(2):154–156, 2011
4. Brackenridge A, Wallbank H, Lawrenson RA, et al.: Emergency management of diabetes and hypoglycemia. Emerg Med J 23(3):183–185, 2006

Want to know more? A wide variety of resources to enhance your learning and understanding of this chapter are available on the**Point** ✳. Visit **http://thepoint.lww.com/MortonEss1e** to access chapter review questions and more!

Hematological and Immune Systems

NINE

Patient Assessment: Hematological and Immune Systems

OBJECTIVES

Based on the content in this chapter, the reader should be able to:

1 Describe those areas of a patient's history and physical assessment pertinent to assessing hematological and immune functions.
2 Summarize the laboratory tests used to evaluate hematological and immune functions.
3 Summarize diagnostic studies used to evaluate hematological and immune functions.
4 Describe key aspects of the assessment of the immunocompromised patient.

General Assessment

History

The patient history is essential when evaluating potential hematological or immune disorders. Elements of the hematological and immunological history are summarized in Box 28-1.

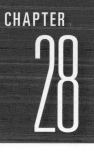

The Older Patient. *When obtaining the health history of an older adult, be aware that risk factors associated with hematological disorders include decreased iron intake resulting from poor dentition (difficulty chewing meat) or a fixed income (inability to afford sources of iron such as meat or supplements); low-grade gastrointestinal bleeding from undiagnosed colon cancer, hemorrhoids or polyps, or the use of nonsteroidal anti-inflammatory drugs (NSAIDs) for the treatment of arthritis; poor absorption of vitamin B_{12} as a result of atrophic gastritis; declining immune function; and anticoagulation therapy (eg, to treat atrial fibrillation).*

Physical Examination

Because a hematological or immunological disorder can affect all body systems, a thorough head-to-toe physical examination is necessary. However, particular attention is paid to the skin, liver, spleen, and lymph nodes, which often manifest many of the

BOX 28-1 Hematological and Immunological Health History

History of the Present Illness

Complete analysis of the following signs and symptoms (using the NOPQRST format; see Chapter 12, Box 12-2)
- Unusual bruising or bleeding
- Frequent infections
- Fatigue or malaise
- Headache
- Dizziness
- Gait disturbance
- Pain
- Enlarged lymph nodes
- Fevers or night sweats
- Weakness
- Limb pain or limp
- Seizure
- Weight loss
- Vomiting
- Heat intolerance
- Poor wound healing
- Nevi

Past Health History

- **Relevant childhood illnesses and immunizations:** mononucleosis, malabsorption, hepatitis, pernicious anemia
- **Past acute and chronic medical problems, including treatments and hospitalizations:** anemia, cancer, infections, autoimmune disorders, inherited hematologic disorders, cirrhosis, HIV, major trauma, sepsis
- **Risk factors:** recent exposure to benzenes, pesticides, mustard gas, antineoplastic agents
- **Past surgeries:** splenectomy, cardiothoracic surgery, total gastrectomy
- **Past diagnostic tests and interventions:** bone marrow aspiration, radiation therapy, chemotherapy, blood transfusions, administration of blood products (cryoprecipitate)

- **Medications, including prescription drugs, over-the-counter drugs, vitamins, herbs, and supplements:** chemotherapeutic agents, antibiotics, antihypertensives, diuretics, glucocorticoids, nonsteroidal anti-inflammatory drugs (NSAIDs), aspirin, heparin, warfarin, antiplatelet agents
- **Allergies and reactions to medications, foods, dye, latex or other materials**
- **Transfusions, including type and date**

Family History

- **Health status or cause of death of parents and siblings:** cancer, anemia, inherited hematologic disorders

Personal and Social History

- Tobacco, alcohol, and substance use
- Environment: exposure to chemicals
- Diet: insufficient intake of foods rich in iron, folic acid, vitamin B_{12}
- Sleep patterns: disruptive sleep patterns
- Exercise

Review of Other Systems

HEENT: oral infections, gum bleeding, epistaxis, mouth sores, sore throat, jaundiced sclera, conjunctival pallor, retinal hemorrhages
Cardiovascular: palpitations, tachycardia, new-onset chest pain
Respiratory: recent upper or lower respiratory tract infection, hemoptysis
Gastrointestinal: blood in emesis or stools, "tarry" stools, unintentional weight loss
Musculoskeletal: weakness, bone pain, back pain, arthralgia
Neurological: mental status changes, pain to touch
Genitourinary: blood in urine, urinary tract infection, heavy menstruation, vaginal bleeding

---

physical signs of hematological or immunological dysfunction.

- **Inspection.** Inspection of the skin, conjunctiva, and nail beds may reveal pallor or cyanosis (signs of tissue hypoxia), jaundice (a sign of excessive hemolysis), or purpuric lesions (a sign of a clotting disorder). Nail abnormalities (eg, clubbing, spoon-shaped nails, longitudinal striations) may also be a sign of tissue hypoxia. Lesions of the oral mucosa (eg, white patches or plaques) may be a sign of immunocompromise. It is also important to inspect the lymph nodes from head to toe, noting any that are visibly enlarged.
- **Auscultation.** Auscultation of the liver and spleen may reveal a friction rub, which could indicate peritoneal inflammation. Splenic friction rubs may indicate infarction.

- **Percussion.** Percussion is used to establish the size of the liver and spleen, both of which sound dull on percussion. Hepatomegaly or splenomegaly can indicate a number of hematological or immunological conditions.
- **Palpation.** Palpation is used to assess the lymph nodes; enlargement, tenderness, texture (hard, soft, or firm), and whether they are fixed or movable should be noted. The nurse also palpates the spleen to confirm splenomegaly.

Laboratory Studies

Laboratory test results are usually the most sensitive and specific determinants of hematological and immune problems. A complete blood count (CBC) provides an overall indication of bone marrow production of red blood cells (RBCs), white blood cells (WBCs), and platelets, and indicates the patient's hemoglobin level, hematocrit level, RBC indices, and WBC differential.

Tests to Evaluate Red Blood Cells

RBC indices (Table 28-1) are laboratory values that describe RBC structure (size) and hemoglobin content. A peripheral smear (Table 28-2) can also be used to evaluate RBC structure. A reticulocyte count, which counts the number of immature RBCs recently released from the bone marrow, aids in evaluating RBC production. The reticulocyte count is expressed as a percentage of the total RBC count. Tests to evaluate iron (Table 28-3) are also often ordered in the assessment of RBC disorders.

Tests to Evaluate White Blood Cells

White Blood Cell Count and Differential

Because WBCs detect and destroy pathogens, an elevated WBC count usually indicates infection and tends to correlate with the severity of the infection. The WBC count measures circulating leukocytes and should always be assessed in conjunction with the WBC differential and the patient's clinical condition. The WBC differential is relative and describes the percentages of the WBC subtypes (neutrophils, eosinophils, basophils, monocytes, and lymphocytes). WBC subtypes can also be measured using absolute numbers. It is important to consider both the absolute and relative values of the WBC subtypes when assessing the differential. For example, 60% segmented neutrophils may seem to be within normal limits, but if total WBCs are 18,000 cells/mm³,

the absolute value (18,000 × 0.60) is 10,800 cells/mm, well above normal. Table 28-4 indicates normal relative and absolute values for the WBC count and differential.

There are numerous potential abnormalities in the WBC differential. A left shift refers to an increase in the number of bands (immature WBCs), which usually indicates an infectious process. The presence of blasts in the peripheral blood is always an aberrant finding and suggests the presence of leukemia or a myeloproliferative disorder.

T- and B-Lymphocyte Tests

Identification of types of circulating lymphocytes and their subtypes can be useful in characterizing hematological malignancies and identifying immunological and autoimmune diseases.[1] Lymphocytes are classified as T cells and B cells. T cells are important in the body's ability to distinguish between self and nonself. T-cell subtypes can be measured and assist with certain diagnoses (eg, AIDS). When an antigen stimulates B cells, they differentiate into plasma cells and produce antibodies. Autoimmune diseases occur when the body produces antibodies directed against its own tissues. The antibodies against various tissues can be evaluated through serum and urine tests.

Tests to Evaluate Coagulation

Platelet Count

Platelet count (obtained from the CBC) is used to evaluate primary hemostasis (ie, the aggregation of platelets at the site of vessel injury). A platelet count of less than 150,000/mm is abnormal, but

TABLE 28-1 Red Blood Cell (RBC) Indices

Test	Normal Value	Significance	Clinical Implications
Mean corpuscular volume (MCV)	82–98 mm³	Expresses the volume occupied by a single RBC.	Low value indicates RBCs are smaller than normal (microcytic). High value indicates RBCs are larger than normal (macrocytic). MCV results are the basis of the classification system used to evaluate anemias.
Mean corpuscular hemoglobin (MCH)	26–34 pg/cell	Indicates the average weight of hemoglobin in each RBC.	Low value is associated with microcytic anemia. High value is associated with macrocytic anemia.
Mean corpuscular hemoglobin concentration (MCHC)	32–36 g/dL	An expression of the average concentration of hemoglobin in the RBCs; it is a calculated value that represents the ratio of the weight of the hemoglobin to the volume of the RBC.	Low value is associated with anemia and iron deficiency. High value is associated with hereditary spherocytosis.
Red cell distribution width (RDW)	11.5–14.5	Indicates the degree of abnormal variation in the size of the RBCs.	Low values have no known cause; high values are associated with iron deficiency, vitamin B_{12} or folate deficiency. Used to differentiate anemias from one another and from thalassemia.

TABLE 28-2 Peripheral Smear RBC Abnormalities

Abnormality	Potential Diagnoses	Further Testing
Nucleated (immature) RBCs	Acute hemorrhage, hypoxia, megaloblastic anemia, hemolytic anemia, bone marrow malignancy, granulomas, asplenia	Vitamin B_{12} and folate levels; assessment for bleeding; O_2 saturation, arterial blood gases for hypoxia
Spherocytes, elliptocytes	Hemolytic anemia from hereditary spherocytosis, hereditary elliptocytosis	Reticulocyte count, serum bilirubin, serum lactate dehydrogenase, direct Coombs', osmotic fragility
Rouleaux formations	Multiple myeloma	Serum protein electrophoresis, urine for Bence Jones proteins
Target cells, sickle cells, red cell cytoplasmic inclusions	Sickle cell anemia, thalassemia	Hemoglobin studies (hemoglobin electrophoresis, hemoglobin F and A_2)
Schistocytes	Thrombotic thrombocytopenic purpura, mechanical hemolysis (prosthetic heart valve)	Reticulocyte count, serum lactate dehydrogenase, serum bilirubin, coagulation studies, cardiac auscultation

RBC, red blood cell.

TABLE 28-3 Laboratory Studies to Measure Iron Levels

Test	Normal Value	Significance	Clinical Implications
Serum iron	Men: 70–175 µg/dL Women: 50–150 µg/dL	Indicates the amount of iron in the serum.	Helpful in differentiating anemias Serum iron value not useful on its own; must be evaluated in context of other laboratory studies used to evaluate iron levels
Serum ferritin	Men: 18–270 ng/mL Women: 18–160 ng/mL	Reflects the body's iron stores and is the most reliable indicator of total body iron status.	Decreased value usually indicates iron-deficiency anemia; increased value occurs in iron excess
Total iron-binding capacity (TIBC)	250–450 mg/dL	Indicates the maximum amount of iron that can be bound to transferrin.	Useful for differentiating anemia from chronic inflammatory disorders

TABLE 28-4 White Blood Cell (WBC) Count and Differential: Laboratory Abnormalities

Test	Normal Value: Relative	Normal Value: Absolute (cells/mm³)	Significance	Possible Causes of Abnormal Results
WBC count		4500–10,000	Measures number of WBCs	Infection, inflammation, leukemia, trauma, stress, steroids, hemorrhage, dehydration
Granulocytes	50%–70%		Type of WBC categorized by presence of granules in cytoplasm	See specific granulocyte subtypes below
Segmented neutrophils	3%–5%	2500–7000	Mature neutrophil with nuclei segmented into lobes	*Increased:* bacterial infection, inflammatory disorder, tissue destruction, malignancy, drug-induced hemolysis, diabetic ketoacidosis, myeloproliferative disorders, idiopathic, smoking, obesity *Decreased:* compromised immune system, depressed bone marrow, heart-lung bypass, hemodialysis, overwhelming infection, tuberculosis, typhoid
Band neutrophils	1%–3%	135–500	Immature neutrophil with nuclei that have smooth edges, unsegmented	*Increased:* acute stress, active bacterial infection *Decreased:* compromised immune system
Eosinophils	0.4%–1%	100–300	Also known as acidophils (acid loving); combat infections caused by parasites; play a role in allergic reactions; cause bronchoconstriction in asthma	*Increased:* parasitic infection, asthma, allergies, dermatoses (hives and eczema), adrenal insufficiency *Decreased* (note: a low eosinophil count is not a cause for concern); Cushing's disease; administration of glucocorticosteroids; various pharmaceuticals
Basophils	4%–6%	40–100	Similar mechanism to mast cells in allergic response; triggered by immunoglobulin E binding to antigens; releases proinflammatory mediators	*Increased:* hyperlipidemia, viral infections (smallpox, chickenpox), inflammatory conditions (ulcerative colitis, chronic sinusitis, asthma), Hodgkin's lymphoma, increased estrogen, hypothyroidism, myeloproliferative disorders, *Decreased:* stress, hyperthyroidism, pregnancy
Monocytes	25%–35%	200–600	Monocytes become macrophages after migration into tissue; macrophages perform phagocytosis	*Increased:* viral infection, parasitic infection, myeloproliferative disorders, inflammatory bowel disease, sarcoidosis, cirrhosis, drug reactions *Decreased:* administration of glucocorticoids, aplastic anemia, lymphocytic anemia
Lymphocytes		1700–3500	Primary source of viral defense and antibody production	*Increased:* viral infections, pertussis, tuberculosis, acute lymphoblastic leukemia, cytomegalovirus infection, mononucleosis, post transfusion, splenomegaly, hyperthyroidism, connective tissue disorder *Decreased:* AIDS, bone marrow suppression, aplastic anemia, steroid use, neurological disorders (multiple sclerosis, myasthenia gravis, Guillain–Barré syndrome)

spontaneous bleeding from thrombocytopenia alone usually does not happen unless the platelet count falls below 20,000/mm. However, prolonged bleeding from surgery or trauma may occur with platelet counts of 40,000 to 50,000/mm. Severe, spontaneous hemorrhage may result when platelet counts reach 5000 to 10,000/mm. Platelet disorders may result from thrombocytopenia (eg, due to decreased bone marrow production, splenic sequestration, or peripheral destruction of platelets by the body's own

BOX 28-2 Common Causes of Platelet Disorders in Critically Ill Patients

Thrombocytopenia
- Heparin
- Sepsis
- AIDS
- Disseminated intravascular coagulation (DIC)
- Thrombotic thrombocytopenic purpura (TTP)

Abnormal Platelet Function
- Renal insufficiency
- Cardiopulmonary bypass
- Medications (eg, aspirin, clopidogrel, dextran)

immune system) or from abnormal platelet function (Box 28-2).

A platelet count greater than 400,000/mm indicates increased platelet production or decreased platelet destruction. These platelets may function abnormally, causing aberrant bleeding and clotting. Primary thrombocytosis may result from bone marrow disease. Reactive thrombocytosis may be caused by chronic inflammation, infection, malnutrition, acute stress, malignancy, splenectomy, or the postoperative state.

Peripheral Smear
A peripheral blood smear may reveal megathrombocytes (large platelets), which may be present during premature platelet destruction.

Platelet Function Assay
The platelet function assay (PFA) evaluates the adhesion and aggregation qualities of the platelets. This test is helpful in the evaluation of platelet function in patients with menorrhagia, drug-induced platelet dysfunction, and high-risk pregnancy.[2]

Bleeding Time
The bleeding time test assesses the length of time required for a clot to form at the site of vessel injury. Prolonged bleeding time in a patient with a normal platelet count may indicate a disorder of platelet function.

Prothrombin Time and Activated Partial Thromboplastin Time
Screening for coagulation abnormalities includes evaluating the prothrombin time (PT) and the activated partial thromboplastin time (APTT). Prolongation of either of these tests indicates coagulation factor deficiencies or inhibition. PT, which measures the amount of time it takes for a fibrin clot to form in a plasma sample following the addition of a thromboplastin reagent, is used to identify abnormalities in the extrinsic and common pathways. Because interpretation of PT is highly variable depending on the laboratory, the World Health Organization introduced the international normalized ratio (INR) to provide a common standard for interpretation of PT.

The APTT measures how well the coagulation sequences of the intrinsic and common pathways are functioning.

Clotting factor deficiencies or inhibition of clotting factors can lead to bleeding disorders, characterized by recurrent oozing of blood and hematoma formation. Bleeding disorders caused by clotting factor abnormalities may be congenital (eg, von Willebrand's disease, hemophilia A, hemophilia B) or acquired (eg, as a result of vitamin K deficiency, severe trauma, hemorrhage, massive transfusion, overwhelming infection, severe liver disease, or disseminated intravascular coagulation [DIC]). Laboratory testing for an acquired disorder of hemostasis varies, based on the suspected etiology of the disorder. In general, testing includes PT, APTT, thrombin time, fibrinogen levels, and fibrin degradation product (FDP) or D-dimer levels (Table 28-5). Bleeding time and liver enzyme and liver function tests are also ordered.

Inappropriate activation of clotting factors can lead to a hypercoagulable state, which increases the tendency for thrombosis. Risk factors for hypercoagulability are given in Box 28-3.

Tests to Evaluate Immune System Functioning
Common laboratory tests to assess immune system functioning are reviewed in Table 28-6.

Diagnostic Studies

Diagnostic studies used in the evaluation of hematological and immunological disorders include the following.

- **Bone marrow aspiration and biopsy.** Biopsy provides information about the precursors of the blood's components to determine whether hematological abnormalities are a production defect. Bone marrow examination is useful in detecting infiltrative processes (eg, malignancy), which can affect blood cell production.
- **Computed tomography (CT)** evaluation of the lymph nodes of the chest, abdomen, and pelvis may be used to determine the presence of masses in suspected malignancy, especially lymphoma. Liver disease (an important factor in coagulopathy) and splenomegaly may also be evaluated using CT.
- **Positron emission tomography (PET)** is used in patients with lymphoma and non-Hodgkin's lymphoma to diagnose and stage cancer, evaluate response to therapy, and assess for recurrence.
- **Intradermal skin testing** is used to evaluate cell-mediated immunity. In this study, various antigens are injected just below the skin's surface to check for delayed-type hypersensitivity. Cutaneous anergy (ie, failure to react to the injected antigens) implies a defect in cellular immunity, such as may be seen in AIDS, leukemia, or lymphoma.

TABLE 28-5 **Laboratory Studies for the Evaluation of Clotting**

Laboratory Test	Description	Clinical Significance
PT	Screens for dysfunction in the extrinsic and common pathways Measures the patient's response to warfarin therapy.	Used to monitor response to anticoagulation therapy with warfarin Prolonged PT indicates: • Liver disease • Vitamin K deficiency • Clotting factor deficiency • DIC Certain drugs can cause prolonged PT, including: • Warfarin • Allopurinol • Aspirin • β-lactam antibiotics • Chlorpropamide • Digoxin • Diphenhydramine • Phenytoin sodium
APTT	Screens for dysfunction in the intrinsic and common pathways Measures the patient response to heparin therapy	Prolonged APTT indicates • Disorders of any coagulation factors *except* VII and XII • Associated clinical conditions: ○ DIC ○ von Willebrand's disease ○ Liver disease • Certain drugs can affect APTT, including: ○ Heparin ○ Chlorpromazine ○ Codeine ○ Phenothiazines ○ Salicylates
Thrombin time	Measuring clotting time of a plasma sample to which thrombin has been added; thrombin converts fibrinogen to fibrin in final coagulation phase	Increased thrombin clotting time may indicate: • DIC • Liver disease • Clotting factor deficiencies • Shock • Hematological malignancies Decreased thrombin clotting time may indicate: • Thrombocytosis
Fibrinogen level	Measures fibrinogen level to determine primary hemostasis status	Elevated fibrinogen level indicates conditions of: • Tissue damage • Inflammation Decreased fibrinogen level may indicate: • DIC • Severe liver disease • TTP • Trauma
Fibrin degradation product (FDP) level	Measures FDP level to determine fibrinolytic activity (FDPs are the byproducts of fibrin)	Increased FDP level may indicate: • DIC • VTE
D-Dimer	Measures FDP levels (more specific than FDPs)	Elevated D-dimer may indicate: • Pulmonary embolism • Venous and arterial thrombotic conditions (eg, DVT)

APTT, activated partial thromboplastin time; DIC, disseminated intravascular coagulation; DVT, deep venous thrombosis; PT, prothrombin time

Assessment of Immunocompetence

Immunocompetence refers to the body's ability to protect itself against disease. Physical and psychological stress from overwhelming illness or trauma in the critically ill patient can depress functioning of the immune system. Invasive procedures, indwelling catheters, IV lines, mechanical ventilation, nutritional compromise, and the critical care environment itself can predispose

BOX 28-3 Risk Factors for Hypercoagulability

Physiological
- Pregnancy/postpartum status
- Venous stasis
- Age greater than 40 years
- Immobilization
- Previous venous thromboembolism

Pathological
- Malignancy
- Liver disease
- Disseminated intravascular coagulation (DIC)
- Polycythemia
- Lupus anticoagulant

- Vascular injury
- Sepsis
- Heart failure
- Myocardial infarction
- Inherited abnormalities

Environmental
- Smoking
- Stress
- Heat

Iatrogenic
- Surgery/postsurgical status
- Estrogen therapy

patients to infection, sepsis, and septic shock. Key nursing responsibilities for the critically ill patient include assessing the patient's risk factors for infection (Fig. 28-1) and reducing susceptibility to infection.

 The Older Patient. Older patients experience a decline in immune system function and frequently have comorbidities, such as diabetes, chronic

obstructive pulmonary disorder (COPD), and renal disease, making them more susceptible to infections.

 RED FLAG! Patients who are severely immunosuppressed may not display the typical signs of infection. Fever and redness or pus at infection sites may be diminished because of the decreased numbers of WBCs required to produce these physical signs.

TABLE 28-6 Laboratory Studies for the Evaluation of Immune Function

Laboratory Test	Clinical Significance/ Normal Values	Use
C-reactive protein (CRP)	Levels less than 10 mg/L indicate the patient no longer has clinically active inflammation; high or increasing levels are consistent with infection, inflammation, or both	Evaluation of various inflammatory conditions, including rheumatoid arthritis and systemic lupus erythematosus
Antinuclear antibody (ANA)	Low titers are negative	Screening and diagnosis of autoimmune disorders
Human leukocyte antigen (HLA) typing	HLA is a protein marker found on most of the body's cells; typing involves either serologic or DNA methods	Determination of tissue compatibility for organ transplantation; also used to determine paternity and to diagnose HLA-related disorders
	Results are reported as phenotype for each of the six HLA loci tested	
	Antibody screen test is reported as the percentage of panel reactive antibodies (PRAs); percent PRA is number of wells reactive with the patient's serum expressed as a percentage	
	Cross-match is reported as compatible or incompatible	
Erythrocyte sedimentation rate (ESR)	Men: 1–13 mm/h Women: 1–20 mm/h	Evaluation of inflammatory state; females tend to have a higher ESR; ESR increases with age
Immunoglobulins (Igs)	IgA: 160–260 mg/dL IgG: 950–1550 mg/dL IgM: 50–300 mg/dL IgD: 0–9 mg/dL IgE: 0.002–0.2 mg/dL	Assessment of immunodeficiency state and certain cancers, including multiple myeloma and macroglobulinemia; also used to assess response to immunizations
Complement system	C3: 75–150 mg/dL C4: 13–40 mg/dL	Diagnosis of systemic lupus erythematosus and other immunological disorders

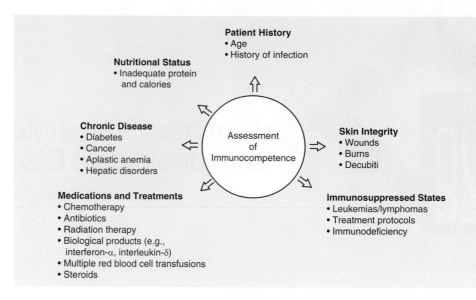

FIGURE 28-1 Risk factors for impaired immunocompetence.

CASE STUDY

Mr. N., a 63-year-old white man, is admitted to the coronary care unit with complaints of "crushing" chest pain with radiation to the left arm and concomitant shortness of breath for the past 2 days. The chest pain has been unrelieved by rest and sublingual nitroglycerine tablets. He also complains of being "exhausted for no good reason" and that he "can't seem to catch his breath." Mr. N. reports having had tarry black stools for the past 4 weeks and bright red blood in his stool the morning of admission. His past medical history is significant for coronary artery disease (CAD), type 2 diabetes mellitus, hyperlipidemia, gastric ulcer disease, and an appendectomy in 1975. He stopped taking his "stomach medications" (omeprazole) several months ago. He has a 70-pack-year history of smoking and reports drinking 2 to 4 oz of alcohol per day.

Objective assessment findings include the following: HR, 112 beats/min; BP, 90/60 mm Hg; RR, 24 breaths/min and shallow; pallor of the oral mucosa; and a low pitch, low intensity S_4 heart sound on auscultation. A 12-lead ECG demonstrates T-wave inversion in leads II, III, and aVF, indicating ischemia in the inferior wall of the heart.

A complete blood count (CBC) with all indices is drawn, and the following results are reported: hemoglobin, 9.4 g/100 mL; hematocrit, 28%; mean corpuscular volume (MCV), 72 mm³, mean corpuscular hemoglobin (MCH), 20 pg/cell; mean corpuscular hemoglobin concentration (MCHC), 22%; reticulocyte count, 5%; serum iron, 43 μg/dL; serum ferritin, 15 ng/mL; total iron-binding capacity (TIBC), 450 mg/dL; and serum transferrin, 150 mg/dL. An increase in the white blood cell (WBC) count is also noticed.

1. What is Mr. N.'s primary health problem?

2. Identify at least three subjective findings consistent with this primary health problem.

3. Identify at least six objective findings consistent with this primary health problem and discuss how these findings are implicated in the problem.

4. What is the significance of the elevated WBC count?

References

1. Bagby G: Leukopenia and leukocytosis. In Goldman L, Ausiello D (eds): Cecil Medicine, 23rd ed. Philadelphia, PA: Saunders Elsevier, 2007, Chapter 173
2. Tantry U, Gurbel P: Assessment of oral antithrombotic therapy by platelet function testing. Nature Rev Cardiol. 2011

Want to know more? A wide variety of resources to enhance your learning and understanding of this chapter are available on thePoint . Visit **http://thepoint.lww.com/MortonEss1e** to access chapter review questions and more!

CHAPTER 29

Common Hematological and Immunological Disorders

Based on the content in this chapter, the reader should be able to:

1 Describe the pathophysiology, assessment, and management of disseminated intravascular coagulation (DIC).
2 Describe common forms of thrombocytopenia in the critically ill patient and explain their assessment and management.
3 Describe common forms of anemia in the critically ill patient and explain their assessment and management.
4 Discuss nursing care of the critically ill patient with sickle cell disease.
5 Describe nursing care of the critically ill patient with neutropenia.
6 Describe nursing care of the critically ill patient with a lymphoproliferative disorder.
7 Describe nursing care of the critically ill patient with HIV infection.

Disseminated Intravascular Coagulation

Disseminated intravascular coagulation (DIC) is an acquired coagulopathy characterized by inappropriate triggering of the coagulation cascade, leading to consumption of clotting factors and, ultimately, bleeding. All critically ill patients are at risk for developing DIC because many are in a state of physiological disequilibrium characterized by bacteremia, hypovolemia, hypotension, hypoxia, and acidosis, all of which have procoagulant effects. In addition, the patient's critical illness itself could result in the development of DIC. Increased awareness of DIC as a potentially catastrophic complication in the critically ill patient facilitates earlier recognition and intervention.

 RED FLAG! *Care of the patient at risk for DIC requires constant assessment of all body systems for signs and symptoms of inappropriate clotting and bleeding.*

Pathophysiology

Many conditions can serve as the initial triggering event (Box 29-1). Instead of a localized response to tissue damage or vascular injury, there is systemic coagulation activity with widespread intravascular clotting. Because of the rapidity and amount of intravascular thrombin formation, clotting factors are used up at a rate exceeding factor replenishment. The result is unregulated clot formation in the microvasculature with platelet and fibrinogen consumption. Activation of coagulation mechanisms also activates the fibrinolytic system. The

BOX 29-1 Selected Disease States Associated With Disseminated Intravascular Coagulation (DIC)

- Infection (bacterial endotoxins, viremias)
- Burns
- Heat stroke
- Brain injury
- Crush injuries and necrotic tissue
- Obstetrical complications (eg, amniotic fluid embolism, missed abortion, eclampsia, retained placenta, abruptio placentae)
- Intravascular hemolysis (eg, hemolytic transfusion reactions, massive blood replacement therapy)
- Acute liver disease

- Prolonged low cardiac output states (eg, cardiac failure, prolonged cardiopulmonary bypass, hemorrhagic shock, cardiopulmonary arrest)
- Vasculitis
- Immunological disorders (eg, immune complex disorders, allograft reaction, incompatible blood transfusion)
- Surgery
- Pancreatitis
- Malignancies (eg, leukemias, solid tumors)
- Chemoradiation therapy

breakdown of fibrin and fibrinogen results in the byproduct, fibrin degradation products (FDPs), which interfere with platelet function and the formation of the fibrin clot. Thus, the patient experiences simultaneous thrombosis and bleeding and is at risk for hemodynamic instability due to activation of the inflammatory system (Fig. 29-1).

A patient with DIC is vulnerable to a wide variety of complications resulting from the thrombotic and hemorrhagic disease processes. Thrombosis may result in ischemia or infarction in any organ, with concomitant loss of function. With ongoing fibrinolysis and depletion of clotting factors and platelets, bleeding into subcutaneous tissues, skin, and

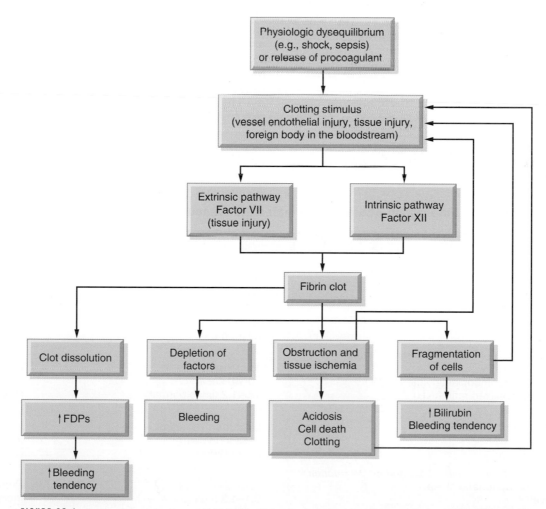

FIGURE 29-1 Cycle of thrombosis and bleeding in disseminated intravascular coagulation (DIC). FDPs, fibrin degradation products.

mucous membranes, or more serious organ hemorrhage, may result.

Assessment

DIC may be acute in presentation, evidenced by severe clinical deterioration, or chronic, evidenced by mildly abnormal laboratory values and minimal, varied clinical symptoms. Acute DIC, which is most common in the critical care setting, is characterized by clot formation (resulting in emboli and perfusion defects) and consumption of clotting factors and unchecked clot dissolution (resulting in bleeding).

- **Clotting** may be manifested clinically as cyanosis, gangrene, mental status changes, altered level of consciousness, cerebrovascular infarct, pulmonary embolus, bowel ischemia and infarction, and kidney insufficiency or failure. Thrombosis may involve both arteries and veins. Total occlusion of microvessels in the digits or earlobes can result in demarcation cyanosis.
- **Bleeding** is a manifestation of later disease. The patient may bleed from the nose, gums, lungs, gastrointestinal tract, urinary tract, surgical sites, injection sites, and intravascular access sites. Other clinical findings associated with bleeding may include peripheral cyanosis, petechial rashes, and purpura fulminans (cutaneous hemorrhage and necrosis associated with infections and sepsis).

Regardless of the inciting event, there are four basic diagnostic components of DIC: excessive rate of clot formation, increased rate of clot dissolution, consumption of essential clotting factors, and end-organ damage resulting from the excessive clotting process.[1] Laboratory studies used to assess these areas are summarized in Table 29-1.

Management

A collaborative care guide for the patient with DIC is given in Box 29-2. Definitive therapy for DIC requires elimination of the causative agent; however, some causes cannot be easily eliminated. Supportive care includes maintaining adequate fluid volume status, taking measures to minimize bleeding, improving perfusion to organs and tissues, controlling pain, and providing psychosocial support.

Patients with significant hemorrhage require replacement therapy and repletion of clotting factors. Fresh frozen plasma contains components of both the coagulation and fibrinolytic systems and may be given to attempt to correct the coagulopathy. Platelet transfusions are usually given only to patients with active bleeding or a platelet count of less than 20,000–50,000/mm³, but is controversial due to the potential to cause more clotting following administration. Cryoprecipitate may be given to patients with plasma fibrinogen levels below 100 mg/dL. The usual adult dose is 5 to 10 U, with each unit raising the fibrinogen level by 5 to 10 mg/dL. Administration of antithrombin III, which balances clot production, shortens the duration of DIC and can be replaced using heat-treated pooled plasma concentrates. Red blood cell (RBC) transfusions, although not useful for repleting coagulation factors, may be given to increase hemoglobin and oxygen-carrying capacity. The use of heparin to minimize clotting (thereby slowing the progression of DIC) is controversial because heparin also increases the patient's risk for bleeding. Few clinical studies have shown heparin to be effective in patients with acute DIC.

TABLE 29-1 Laboratory Findings in Acute Disseminated Intravascular Coagulation (DIC)

Test	Normal Value	Value in DIC
Massive Intravascular Clotting		
Platelet count	150,000–400,000/mm³	Decreased
Fibrinogen level	200–400 mg/100 mL	Decreased
Thrombin time	7.0–12.0 sec	Prolonged
Protein C level	4 µg/mL	Decreased
Protein S level	23 µg/mL	Decreased
Secondary Depletion of Essential Clotting Factors		
Prothrombin time (PT)	11–15 sec	Prolonged
Activated partial thromboplastin time (APTT)	30–40 sec	Prolonged
International normalized ratio (INR)	1.0–1.2 times normal	Prolonged
Excessive/Accelerated Fibrinolysis		
Fibrin degradation products (FDPs)	Less than 10 mg/mL	Increased
D-dimer assay	Less than 50 µg/dL	Increased
Antithrombin III level	89%–120%	Decreased
Clinical Effects of Microvascular Clotting/Cell Destruction		
Schistocytes on peripheral smear		Present
Bilirubin level	0.1–1.2 mg/dL	Increased
Blood urea nitrogen (BUN)	8–20 mg/dL	Increased

BOX 29-2 COLLABORATIVE CARE GUIDE for the Patient With Disseminated Intravascular Coagulation (DIC)

OUTCOMES	INTERVENTIONS
Oxygenation/Ventilation Arterial blood gases (ABGs) are within normal limits.	• Monitor pulse oximetry and ABGs. • Validate significant changes in pulse oximetry with co-oximetry arterial saturation measurement. • Transfuse as necessary to increase oxygen-carrying capacity. • Encourage use of incentive spirometer, cough and deep breathing q2h. Turn patient q2h.
Breath sounds are clear bilaterally.	• Suction oropharynx and trachea carefully when necessary. • Encourage use of incentive spirometer, cough and deep breathing q2h. Turn patient q2h.
Circulation/Perfusion Patient achieves and maintains adequate clinical perfusion.	• Monitor tissue perfusion: color, temperature, pulse, capillary refill, level of consciousness, urine output, and PaO_2. • Monitor vital signs q1–4h based on clinical condition. • Monitor cardiac output, stroke volume, systemic vascular resistance, and pulmonary artery pressures q4h if pulmonary artery catheter is in place.
Serum lactate is within normal limits.	• Monitor lactate daily until it is within normal limits. • Administer RBCs, positive inotropic agents, IV infusions as ordered to increase oxygen delivery. • Assess patient for potential sources of lactate (eg, ischemic bowel, ischemic distal digits) or decreased ability to clear lactate (liver dysfunction).
Hematological Patient does not experience bleeding related to coagulopathies.	• Monitor PT, PTT, CBC, FDP, D-dimer, and fibrinogen levels daily; more frequently if monitoring for acute changes or response to therapy. • Assess q4h for signs of hematological involvement, including thrombotic and hemorrhagic manifestations. • Quantify degree of bleeding (weigh dressings, count pads, measure drainage; test stool, urine, drains, and emesis for heme). • Assess individual organs for signs and symptoms of bleeding: crackles, decreased SaO_2 with pulmonary bleeding; visual changes (diplopia, blurred vision, visual field deficit) with retinal thrombosis/hemorrhage; back pain, flank pain, abdominal pain consistent with visceral organ bleeding. • Administer blood and coagulation factors as indicated. • Maintain strict adherence to bleeding precautions. • Avoid invasive procedures and treatments. • Avoid medications that inhibit coagulation or promote thrombosis. • Apply pressure to puncture sites for 3–5 min, then use pressure dressing.
Fluids/Electrolytes Patient is euvolemic.	• Take daily weights. • Monitor I&O; replace/diurese as required. • Maintain IV access and fluid replacement therapy.
Mineral and electrolyte levels are within normal limits.	• Monitor and replace Mg and PO_4 daily and PRN.
Mobility/Safety There is no evidence of bruising due to preventable injury.	• Institute bleeding precautions, including padded side rails, no sharp objects at or around bedside, assistance out of bed, and padded self-protective devices (if necessary). • Assess for bleeding/bruising q2h or more frequently.

(continued on page 412)

OUTCOMES	INTERVENTIONS
Skin Integrity Patient is without evidence of skin breakdown.	• Assess skin q8h and each time patient is repositioned for pressure areas, petechiae, and ecchymosis. • Turn q2–4h. • Consider pressure relief/reduction mattress, and avoid shearing forces. • Perform range-of-motion exercises every shift. • Use Braden scale to assess risk for skin breakdown.
Nutrition Nutritional intake meets calculated metabolic need (eg, basal energy expenditure equation).	• Consult dietitian for metabolic needs assessment and recommendations. • Provide parenteral feeding if NPO. • Assess for gastrointestinal bleeding and report.
Comfort/Pain Control Patient is as comfortable as possible (as evidenced by stable vital signs or cooperation with treatments or procedures).	• Document pain assessment, using numerical pain rating or similar scale when possible. • Correlate pain ratings with sites of potential ischemia/infarction/hemorrhage, and notify physician. • Provide warm compresses to promote vasodilation and decrease ischemic pain as indicated (with physician approval). • Provide analgesia and sedation as indicated by assessment. • Monitor patient response to medication.
Psychosocial Patient demonstrates decreased anxiety.	• Educate patient and family regarding disease process and actions taken to correct disorder. • Provide areas of control to patient and family as possible (eg, performance of ADLs, visitors). • Provide explanations and reassurance before procedures. • Consult social services or clergy as appropriate. • Provide for adequate rest and sleep.
Teaching/Discharge Planning Patient and family understand procedures and tests needed for treatment.	• Prepare the patient and family for procedures, such as blood transfusions and laboratory studies. • Educate the patient and family regarding clinical parameters and patient presentation required for safe discharge from unit/hospital.

Thrombocytopenia

Thrombocytopenia occurs when there is decreased production, increased destruction of platelets, or increased sequestration of platelets in the spleen (Box 29-3). Three of the most common types of thrombocytopenia in critically ill patients are heparin-induced thrombocytopenia (HIT), thrombotic thrombocytopenic purpura (TTP), and immune thrombocytopenic purpura (ITP):

• **Heparin-induced thrombocytopenia (HIT).** Although many medications can induce thrombocytopenia, heparin is the most common medication used in the critical care unit that is associated with thrombocytopenia. Anticoagulation with continuous IV heparin carries the greatest risk, but any type of heparin therapy can cause thrombocytopenia. HIT typically appears 4 to 14 days after initiation of heparin therapy, but it can occur as early as 10 hours after administration if the patient has been exposed to heparin within the previous 100 days, or several days after withdrawal of all forms of heparin. The hallmark of HIT is a decrease in platelet count to less than 50% of the baseline or to less than 150,000/mm³, or the occurrence of an unexplained thromboembolic event. (HIT is characterized by thrombosis, rather than bleeding.) Any unexpected and substantial percentage decline in platelet count that occurs during heparin treatment raises suspicion for HIT. Terminating heparin therapy resolves the thrombocytopenia, confirming the diagnosis.

 RED FLAG! *HIT is associated with life- and limb-threatening consequences, including deep venous thrombosis (DVT), arterial occlusion, ischemic stroke, limb gangrene, myocardial infarction, and pulmonary embolism.*

BOX 29-3 Causes of Thrombocytopenia

Decreased production of platelets
- Marrow infiltration (eg, malignancy, myelofibrosis, granulomatous disease)
- Marrow failure (eg, medication, chemotherapy, aplastic anemia, severe iron deficiency)
- Infection (eg, HIV, Epstein-Barr virus, tuberculosis)
- Alcohol use
- Nutritional deficiency

Increased destruction of platelets
- Disseminated intravascular coagulation (DIC)
- Sepsis
- Intravascular prosthetic devices
- Vasculitis
- Thrombotic thrombocytopenic purpura (TTP)
- Immune mediated

Sequestration of platelets
- Splenic enlargement (eg, tumor infiltration, infection)
- Splenic congestion (eg, portal hypertension, hepatic disease)

- **Thrombotic thrombocytopenic purpura (TTP)** is an acute disorder with a mortality rate of 30% to 40%. Patients with TTP have absent or decreased levels of platelet-aggregating factor inhibitor, which is normally present in plasma. As a result, platelets become sensitized and clump in blood vessels, causing occlusion. Initiation of the disease process may be related to endothelial damage, autoimmune disorders, viral or bacterial infection, toxic agents, or genetic predisposition. Five classic findings suggest TTP (Table 29-2). Not every patient exhibits all five findings; however, thrombocytopenia and hemolytic anemia must be present for the diagnosis to be considered. Following treatment, patients with TTP may be "cured," relapse years later, or have a chronic relapsing course.

 RED FLAG! *TTP is an emergency because of its extremely high mortality rate. Early recognition and prompt initiation of treatment are imperative to improve patient survival.*

- **Immune thrombocytopenic purpura (ITP)** is an immune-mediated disorder of platelet destruction. Acute ITP typically occurs in childhood. Chronic ITP usually occurs in adults, more often in women than men. In chronic ITP, the platelet membrane is coated with an autoantibody (usually IgG), and the sensitized platelets are destroyed in the spleen and liver. In at least 50% of patients with ITP, no known causative agent is identified; other patients may have underlying autoimmune, rheumatic, or lymphoproliferative diseases or HIV infection. ITP is diagnosed when other disorders of platelet destruction are ruled out.

Assessment

The history, physical examination, and initial laboratory data help identify potential causes of thrombocytopenia. Elements of the history that may be significant include symptoms of associated disorders (eg, symptoms of infection, malignancy, or liver disease); a patient or family history of bleeding; a history of platelet transfusion, and the patient's medication and alcohol history. The physical examination includes a thorough examination of the skin and oropharynx for petechiae and bruising, and evaluation of the stool for guaiac. Fever is frequently present in TTP.

Management

The initial step in management of thrombocytopenia is to hold any drugs that may be suspected to induce thrombocytopenia. Patients with mild to moderate thrombocytopenia without bleeding require no treatment. Platelet transfusions are indicated when the platelet count is below 20,000–50,0000/mm^3 or when the patient has spontaneous bleeding or the potential for increased bleeding risk. In sequestration- or destruction-mediated thrombocytopenia, the

TABLE 29-2 Clinical Manifestations of Thrombotic Thrombocytopenic Purpura (TTP)

Abnormality	Underlying Cause	Clinical Manifestations
Thrombocytopenia	Increased consumption of platelets	Bleeding, ecchymosis, purpura at various sites
Microangiopathic hemolytic anemia	Rupture of red blood cells (RBCs) as they pass through partially occluded vessels	Schistocytes, reticulocytosis, elevated serum lactate dehydrogenase and bilirubin, jaundice, pallor, weakness
Neurological abnormalities	Interrupted blood flow to the brain	Headache, mental changes, confusion, transient ischemic attacks, strokes, seizures, coma
Renal dysfunction	Obstruction of intraglomerular capillaries and infarction of renal cortex	Proteinuria, microscopic hematuria, elevated blood urea nitrogen (BUN) and creatinine, renal failure
Fever	Possibly due to hemolysis or vascular infarction of the hypothalamus	Persistent elevation of temperature during acute phase

response to platelet transfusion is typically very poor because transfused platelets are destroyed very quickly by the same mechanism that causes the disease. For these patients, platelet transfusion is used only for life-threatening bleeding and immediately prior to performing any invasive procedures. All patients who receive blood products must be monitored for allergic reactions, anaphylaxis, and volume overload.

 RED FLAG! *Platelet transfusion is contraindicated in patients with TTP because the transfused platelets may aggregate, resulting in myocardial infarction, stroke, coma, or death.*

Acutely ill patients with TTP require immediate infusions of fresh frozen plasma until plasmapheresis can be performed. In plasmapheresis, 2 to 3 L of the patient's plasma is removed and replaced with an equal amount of fresh plasma. Plasmapheresis is repeated daily until the platelet count is greater than 150,000/mm³; this may take 5 to 10 days or more. Antiplatelet agents and prednisone may be used, although the effectiveness of these therapies is controversial.

Patients with ITP are treated initially with corticosteroids to induce immunosuppression. It usually takes a few days of corticosteroid therapy before the platelet count begins to rise. When the platelet count is critically low (less than 5000/mm³) or the patient shows signs of serious bleeding, IV immunoglobulin (IVIG) therapy is given in addition to steroids. Patients with chronic ITP who fail to respond to steroids or are steroid dependent may require splenectomy. Patients who undergo splenectomy require pneumococcal, meningococcal, and *Haemophilus influenzae* type B vaccines.

Thrombocytopenia (bleeding) precautions are taken for patients with all types of thrombocytopenia and include the following:

- Avoidance of medications that inhibit platelet function (eg, aspirin, antiplatelet agents, nonsteroidal anti-inflammatory drugs [NSAIDs])
- Avoidance of trauma (this may preclude the placement of central venous catheters and other invasive procedures)
- Evaluation of continued blood loss and assessment of daily laboratory data for adequacy of the platelet count and other parameters of hemostasis

Anemia

Anemia is prevalent in critically ill patients; the causes are multifactorial and include preexisting disease, blood loss from multiple sources, and suppressed erythropoiesis. For some patients, acute anemia requiring intensive monitoring and intervention is the primary reason for admission to the critical care unit; others have anemia as a concurrent problem or develop anemia during their hospitalization. Nearly 67% of patients admitted to critical

care units have hemoglobin levels of 12.0 g/dL or less, and nearly 95% of patients have below-normal hemoglobin levels by their third day on the unit.[2,3] Phlebotomy for diagnostic tests has been reported to account for approximately 30% to 50% of anemia cases in the critical care unit.[4] It is estimated that for every 100 mL of blood drawn, there is an associated decrease in hemoglobin of 0.7 g/dL and in hematocrit of 1.9%.[4] The impact is significant, especially in patients who remain on the unit for several weeks.

 The Older Patient. Anemia is common in the elderly, and its prevalence increases with age. As with other cells, the body's capacity for RBC replacement decreases with age. Although most elderly people are able to maintain their hemoglobin and hematocrit levels within a normal range under normal circumstances, situations such as bleeding may exceed the body's capacity for RBC replacement. In older adults, anemia can be associated with neurologic and cognitive disorders, cardiovascular complications, and increased risk for mortality.

The clinical consequences of anemia depend on the degree of the anemia. In general they include

- Impaired tissue oxygenation
- Impaired organ function
- Increased susceptibility to bleeding
- Increased risk for postoperative mortality
- Increased probability of transfusion
- Decreased survival

Types of Anemia

Typically, anemias are classified by cause: blood loss anemia; increased destruction of RBCs (hemolytic anemia); or decreased production of RBCs (deficiency, or hypoproliferative anemias):

- **Blood loss anemia** is probably the most common anemia requiring admission to the critical care unit. Blood loss as the underlying cause must always be ruled out in any patient with acute anemia. The condition may be chronic and caused by cancer, ulcers, or gastritis. Management focuses on identifying and treating the underlying source of blood loss.
- **Hemolytic anemias** result from the destruction of RBCs. They may be congenital or acquired and can vary greatly in severity. The most common types of congenital hemolytic anemias are caused by enzyme defects or RBC membrane defects. Acquired hemolytic anemias are summarized in Table 29-3.
- **Deficiency anemias** result from inadequate production of RBCs. Common causes of deficiency anemias are summarized in Table 29-4.

 The Older Patient. In the elderly, anemia is usually the result of bleeding, infection, malignancy, or chronic disease. Combined deficiencies are common in older adults.

TABLE 29-3 Acquired Hemolytic Anemias

Type of Acquired Hemolytic Anemia	Underlying Mechanism	Interventions
Microangiopathic	Vasculitis causes fragmentation of red blood cells (RBCs)	Removal of causative factor; iron and folate supplements; transfusion
Associated with infectious disease (eg, malaria)	Indirect: infection causes splenomegaly Direct: infectious agent invades and destroys RBC membrane	Treatment of underlying infection; transfusion
Associated with liver disease	Abnormally shaped RBCs and congestive splenomegaly lead to RBC destruction	Splenectomy; transfusion
Autoimmune		
• Warm antibody	Approximately 50% of cases are idiopathic; known causative factors include collagen diseases, lymphoproliferative disorders, and medication reactions	Glucocorticoids; splenectomy; immunosuppressive agents; transfusion; IV immunoglobulin (IVIG); discontinuation of medication
• Cold reactive	Exposure to cold triggers the attachment of complement-fixing immunoglobulin M (IgM) antibodies to RBCs, causing agglutination and hemolysis	Avoidance of exposure to cold; transfusion; plasma exchange, use of blood warmer
Associated with abnormal cardiac valves	RBCs are damaged as they pass through abnormal valve	Valve repair or replacement; iron and folate supplements
Associated with hypothermia or use of cold cardioplegia	Membrane damage shortens life span of RBCs	Keep patient warm or rewarm patient

Assessment

Clinical manifestations of anemia include pallor, hypotension, weakness, depressed mood, impaired cognitive function, and easy fatigability. Tachycardia, chest pain (new-onset, or worsening of existing angina), dyspnea, and dizziness may result from decreased perfusion secondary to the anemia. Patients with hemolytic anemia may have splenomegaly, jaundice, and dark urine due to the excretion of bilirubin. Laboratory evaluation for anemia includes a complete blood count (CBC) with RBC indices, a reticulocyte count, iron studies, and a peripheral smear analysis.

Management

Management focuses on identifying and correcting the underlying cause of the anemia. Supportive measures may include nutritional supplementation, blood transfusion, and the administration of erythropoietin-stimulating proteins. Key nursing interventions for the patient with anemia are given in Box 29-4.

• **Nutritional supplementation.** Parenteral iron (IV injection is preferred) may be administered when the patient is unable to take oral medications, or in the presence of malabsorption or severe renal failure. Close patient observation is necessary

TABLE 29-4 Deficiency Anemias

Type of Deficiency Anemia	Underlying Mechanism	Interventions
Iron deficiency anemia	Chronic blood loss, inadequate iron intake or absorption	Iron supplements; correction of underlying cause
Megaloblastic anemia	Impaired DNA synthesis causes cells to continue to grow without dividing; causes include deficiencies of vitamin B_{12}, folate, or both	Vitamin B_{12} replacement; folic acid supplement
Anemia of chronic disease	Chronic disease (eg, renal failure, infections, malignancy, rheumatoid arthritis) is associated with suppressed RBC production, decreased RBC survival time, and low serum erythropoietin levels	Transfusion; recombinant human erythropoietin (rHuEPO); correction of underlying disorder
Aplastic anemia	The bone marrow's ability to generate all types of blood cells is impaired; causes include medications, chemical exposures, viruses, and immunologic and congenital disorders	Transfusion; immunosuppression; bone marrow transplantation

BOX 29-4 Nursing Interventions for the Patient With Anemia

- Implement interventions to increase oxygen delivery (eg, oxygen therapy) and decrease metabolic needs and oxygen demand (eg, promoting a restful environment).
- Ensure adequate pain control and provide comfort measures to minimize agitation.
- Implement strategies to reduce phlebotomy blood loss, including
  - Eliminating standing orders for laboratory tests
  - Organizing blood draws to eliminate duplicate testing
  - Consolidating multiple collections
  - Using smaller collection tubes
  - Using devices that return waste blood to the patient
  - Using continuous noninvasive monitoring techniques for arterial blood gas (ABG) monitoring

because severe anaphylactic reactions may occur with iron therapy. Vitamin C is often given to aid in the absorption of iron. Folic acid and vitamin B$_{12}$, if needed, should be considered.

- **Blood transfusion.** Transfusion of packed RBCs is reserved for management of active bleeding or for the patient who is experiencing serious symptoms from anemia. Blood transfusion is associated with myriad complications (Box 29-5), and the risks versus the benefits of blood transfusion in critically ill patients continues to be an area of study. Although a widely accepted practice is to consider transfusion when a patient's hemoglobin levels drop to 6 to 8 g/dL, a better practice is to transfuse when the risks of decreased oxygen-carrying capacity outweigh the risks of transfusion. For example, some patients (eg, cardiac patients, patients with sepsis, patients with higher APACHE II scores) may require transfusions at a higher hemoglobin level.

BOX 29-5 Complications of Blood Transfusion

- Volume overload
- Transfusion-related acute lung injury (TRALI)
- Febrile reactions
- Hemolytic reactions (resulting from transfusion of ABO-incompatible blood)
- Bloodborne infection (from contaminated donor blood)
- Increased risk for healthcare-associated infections (HAIs), increasing risk for sepsis and multisystem organ dysfunction syndrome (MODS)
- Immunologic dysfunction (triggered by an immune system response to donor leukocytes), which may lead to exacerbation of infections, earlier recurrence of malignancy, and postsurgical complications (eg, impaired wound healing, increased likelihood of mortality)

If transfusion therapy is prescribed, the nurse plays an important role in identifying the correct patient and ensuring ABO compatibility to prevent adverse and potentially fatal outcomes. Transfusion of critically ill patients with leuko-reduced blood (ie, blood from which the white blood cells [WBCs] have been removed by filtration) lowers the risk of some of complications associated with blood transfusion (eg, febrile reactions, immune reactions).

- **Erythropoietin-stimulating proteins.** Administration of erythropoietin-stimulating proteins to increase hemoglobin levels may reduce the need for transfusion in many patients; however, RBC replacement is much more gradual with the use of these agents. Complications of recombinant human erythropoietin (rHuEPO) therapy (eg, hypertension, seizures, arteriovenous shunt thromboses, increased blood viscosity) are infrequent and are seen mostly in patients on renal dialysis. Contraindications for rHuEPO therapy include uncontrolled hypertension and hypersensitivity to albumin.

Sickle Cell Disease

Sickle cell disease is a chronic hereditary hemolytic anemia that occurs almost exclusively in people of African descent. The sickle cell gene causes hemoglobin abnormalities. When oxygen and pH levels decrease, RBCs containing the abnormal hemoglobin become elongated, sickle shaped, and rigid. These abnormal cells are unable to pass through small blood vessels, causing inflammation, obstruction of the vessels, and decreased delivery of oxygen that perpetuates the cycle with more sickling and results in microinfarcts of the heart, skeleton, spleen, and central nervous system (CNS). The cells are destroyed when the body recognizes their abnormal structure. Patients with sickle cell disease are prone to experiencing sudden, painful vasoocclusive crises, characterized by severe deep pain in the long bones, joints, and abdomen that may be accompanied by fever, malaise, and leukocytosis.

Complications of sickle cell disease that may necessitate admission to the critical care unit include

- Splenic failure (resulting from repeated splenic infarcts)
- Overwhelming infection (eg, sepsis)
- Stroke
- Cardiac chamber enlargement and heart failure
- Pulmonary hypertension
- Renal failure
- Acute chest syndrome (caused by pulmonary infarction from fat embolism)
- Acute respiratory distress syndrome (ARDS)

Treatment includes aggressive IV fluid hydration to decrease blood viscosity and maintain renal perfusion. Oxygen administration may be needed to maintain adequate tissue perfusion and prevent further sickling of the RBCs. Around-the-clock dosing with a strong opioid is necessary to relieve the intense pain that accompanies vasoocclusive crisis. Infection is treated early with broad-spectrum antibiotics until the causative agent can be identified. Anemia is usually well tolerated and RBC transfusion is not frequently required.

Neutropenia

The most common type of WBC deficiency is neutropenia (ie, a neutrophil count of less than 1500 cells/mm³). Severe neutropenia, in which the neutrophil count is less than 200 cells/mm³, is called agranulocytosis. Neutropenia has a variety of causes (Table 29-5). Because neutrophils are essential to the defense against bacterial infections, patients with neutropenia are susceptible to overwhelming infection and life-threatening sepsis. Infections frequently originate in the respiratory tract as a result of bacteria or fungi that colonize the airways. The risk for infection is related to the severity of the neutropenia.

 RED FLAG! In patients with neutropenia, untreated infections can be rapidly fatal, particularly if the neutrophil count is less than 250/mm³.

Assessment

Patients with neutropenia may present with fever, shaking, chills, and systemic infection. However, in patients with severe neutropenia, the usual signs of the inflammatory response to infection may be absent. Skin infections and mouth ulcers are common because neutrophils normally provide the first line of defense against organisms that inhabit the skin and gastrointestinal tract. Physical examination may reveal splenomegaly. Laboratory studies include viral serology for hepatitis and HIV, and antinuclear antibody (ANA) to screen for autoimmune disorders. Bone marrow aspiration and biopsy may be needed if the neutropenia is severe or the cause is not apparent.

In neutropenic patients, it is important to assess the degree of immunosuppression. One way to do this is by calculating the absolute neutrophil count (ANC). The ANC is calculated by adding the segmented neutrophils and band neutrophils (from the WBC differential) and then multiplying the result by the total WBC count. For example:

Segs = 42%, Bands = 10%, Total WBC count = 4100 cells/mm³
42 + 10 = 52%
0.52 × 4100 = 2132 cells/mm³ (ANC)

Usually neutropenic precautions are instituted for patients with an ANC of less than 1000 cells/mm³.

Management

Neutropenia is treated by identifying and managing the underlying cause. If the neutropenia is severe, a hematopoietic growth factor that stimulates bone marrow production of new neutrophils and enhances the activity of already circulating neutrophils may be administered. Patients with severe neutropenia or those with recurrent or serious infections may also benefit from steroids or IVIG treatment. Transfusions are used cautiously in patients who may require bone marrow transplantation. Infections are treated aggressively to prevent progression to septic shock and death.

Meticulous attention to sterile technique, prevention of infections, infection control procedures, and vigilant surveillance of invasive lines and equipment are mainstays of care. Attention must be paid during daily oral care to ensure that superinfection with *Candida* or herpesvirus has not developed. Antibacterial mouthwashes decrease the risk for infection. Assessment for early indications of infection (eg, fever, chills, tachycardia, tachypnea) may allow for prompt and aggressive initiation of antibiotics to reduce morbidity and mortality. Diarrhea may be a side effect of neutropenia. *Clostridium difficile* infection must be considered and treated if present.

Lymphoproliferative Disorders

Lymphoproliferative disorders (disorders in which lymphoid tissue increases by reproducing) may originate in the bone marrow or in the lymph nodes and thymus. Because blood cells circulate throughout the body, these neoplasms are systemically disseminated

TABLE 29-5 Causes of Neutropenia

Cause	Mechanism
Accelerated removal of white blood cells (WBCs) from the circulation (eg, due to inflammation and infection)	Removal of neutrophils from the circulation exceeds production
Pharmacotherapy	
• Cytotoxic drugs used in cancer therapy	Depressed bone marrow function with decreased production of all blood cells
• Phenothiazines, propylthiouracil, and others	Toxic effect on bone marrow precursors
• Aminopyrine, certain sulfonamides, phenylbutazone, and others	Immune-mediated destruction
Neoplasms involving bone marrow (eg, leukemias and lymphomas)	Overgrowth of neoplastic cells, which crowd out granulopoietic precursors
Idiopathic (occurs in the absence of other disease or provoking influence)	Autoimmune reaction

from the onset. Nursing care of the critically ill patient with a lymphoproliferative disorder includes vigilant assessment for and prevention of infection, and delivery of therapy specific to the patient's disease- and treatment-associated complications.

Lymphomas

Lymphomas are lymphoproliferative disorders of the lymph nodes and thymus.

- **Hodgkin's lymphoma** begins as a malignancy in a single lymph node and spreads to surrounding lymph nodes.
- **Non-Hodgkin's lymphoma** is a diverse group of malignancies that originate in the lymphoid cells. Non-Hodgkin's lymphoma can occur as a discreet mass (eg, involvement of a single lymph node) or as widespread disease that affects multiple organ systems, including the bone marrow.

Patients with advanced lymphoma are usually admitted to the critical care unit for management of complications that arise from the disease or its treatment. These complications include

- Severe dyspnea, superior vena cava syndrome (compression of the superior vena cava by the tumor), or both, resulting from extensive thoracic disease
- Obstruction of the bowel or the ureters resulting from abdominal disease
- Pancytopenia resulting from bone marrow involvement
- Impaired immune function and frequent, severe infections resulting from extensive involvement of the lymphatic system
- Headaches, visual disturbances, motor dysfunction, and increased intracranial pressure (ICP) resulting from CNS involvement

Leukemias

Leukemias are lymphoproliferative disorders of the bone marrow. Leukemias are characterized by rapid proliferation of hematopoietic stem cells, resulting in the accumulation of abnormal (leukemic) cells in the bone marrow and decreased production of normal blood cells. Leukemias commonly are classified according to their predominant cell type (lymphoblastic or myelogenous) and whether the condition is acute or chronic:

- **Acute lymphoblastic anemia.** Immature lymphocytes proliferate, replacing the normal cells of the bone marrow and infiltrating other tissues (eg, the liver, spleen, and lymph nodes).
- **Acute myelogenous leukemia** causes abnormal production of erythrocytes, neutrophils, megakaryocytes, and macrophages. The malignant cells proliferate but do not differentiate into mature, functional cells. The blood, bone marrow, or both contain more than 30% immature blast cells.

Patients with leukemia are most often admitted to the critical care unit because of complications of the leukemia or its treatment, including pancytopenia, DIC, leukostasis, and tumor lysis syndrome.

- **Leukostasis** is a condition in which the high number of blasts increases blood viscosity, leading to aggregation (clumping) of blasts in the capillaries. Manifestations include headache, confusion, CNS infarcts, acute respiratory insufficiency, and pulmonary infiltrates. Leukostasis requires immediate treatment with leukapheresis (removal of WBCs from the circulation) and hydroxyurea to lower the blast count rapidly. Chemotherapy is initiated to stop leukemic cell production in the bone marrow.
- **Tumor lysis syndrome** is a metabolic imbalance caused by rapid cancer cell death. Most patients experience this complication 1 to 5 days after initiation of chemotherapy or radiation therapy. Rapid cancer cell death causes the release of intracellular contents (potassium, phosphorus, and nucleic acids) into the circulating serum. Normally, the kidneys filter these metabolic waste products and excrete them, but if production is more rapid than excretion or if there is renal insufficiency, electrolytes and uric acid accumulate in the serum, resulting in hyperkalemia, hyperphosphatemia, and hyperuricemia. Hyperphosphatemia causes the kidneys to excrete calcium, resulting in hypocalcemia. Hyperuricemia causes deposition of uric acid crystals in the urinary tract and may lead to renal failure.[5,6] Treatment entails lowering serum potassium, phosphorus, and uric acid levels; correcting acidosis; and providing aggressive IV hydration to promote diuresis and prevent renal failure. If renal failure develops, continuous renal replacement therapy (CRRT) is needed.

HIV Infection

Impaired cellular immunity is the underlying pathophysiological condition of HIV infection. Patients with HIV infection exhibit impaired activation of both cellular and humoral immunity, but HIV primarily infects the CD4+ T cells of the immune system, which play a major role in the overall immune response (Fig. 29-2). Approximately 30% of the

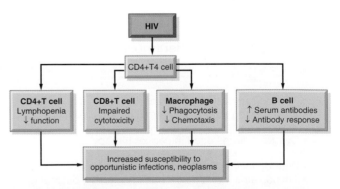

FIGURE 29-2 Infection of the CD4+ T cell with HIV results in profound lymphopenia and decreased functional abilities and loss of stimulus for T- and B-cell activation. In addition, the cytotoxic activity of the CD8+ T cell is impaired, and the functional abilities of the macrophages are affected.

Symptoms of HIV infection

AIDS-related illnesses and opportunistic infections

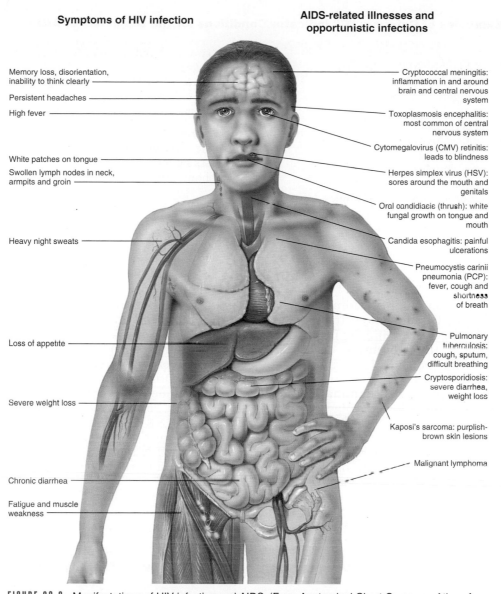

Memory loss, disorientation, inability to think clearly

Persistent headaches

High fever

White patches on tongue

Swollen lymph nodes in neck, armpits and groin

Heavy night sweats

Loss of appetite

Severe weight loss

Chronic diarrhea

Fatigue and muscle weakness

Cryptococcal meningitis: inflammation in and around brain and central nervous system

Toxoplasmosis encephalitis: most common of central nervous system

Cytomegalovirus (CMV) retinitis: leads to blindness

Herpes simplex virus (HSV): sores around the mouth and genitals

Oral candidiasis (thrush): white fungal growth on tongue and mouth

Candida esophagitis: painful ulcerations

Pneumocystis carinii pneumonia (PCP): fever, cough and shortness of breath

Pulmonary tuberculosis: cough, sputum, difficult breathing

Cryptosporidiosis: severe diarrhea, weight loss

Kaposi's sarcoma: purplish-brown skin lesions

Malignant lymphoma

FIGURE 29-3 Manifestations of HIV infection and AIDS. (From Anatomical Chart Company: Atlas of Pathophysiology, 3rd ed. Springhouse, PA: Springhouse, 2010, p 267.)

viral burden in a person who is HIV positive is regenerated daily.

HIV infection exists on a continuum, from asymptomatic infection with HIV, to a variety of infections and symptoms of decreasing immunocompetence (Fig. 29-3), to unquestionable AIDS. Clinical categories and CD4+ T cell counts are used to determine where on the disease continuum a patient fits. When a patient has one of the category C clinical indicator conditions (Box 29-6) or a CD4+ T cell count of less than 200 cells/mm³ the diagnosis of AIDS is made.

Although people with HIV infection may be admitted to the critical care unit for a completely unrelated problem (eg, trauma), usually they are admitted because of complications of an

opportunistic infection. Single infections may develop in critically ill patients with AIDS, but patients often have multiple infections simultaneously. *Pneumocystis* pneumonia (PCP) is the most common opportunistic infection in patients with HIV infection requiring admission to the critical care unit; usually, these patients are experiencing impending or actual respiratory failure. Symptoms of respiratory compromise often are more severe than diagnostic studies (eg, chest radiographs, blood gas values) indicate. Therefore, early aggressive therapy for PCP using IV trimethoprim and sulfamethoxazole and corticosteroids is the treatment of choice. Even with urgent, aggressive treatment, many patients require mechanical ventilation for progressive hypoventilation.

BOX 29-6 Examples of Category "C" Indicator Conditions for the Diagnosis of AIDS

Infections
- Candidiasis (bronchial, tracheal, pulmonary, esophageal)
- Disseminated coccidioidomycosis
- Cryptococcosis
- Chronic intestinal cryptosporidiosis
- Disseminated cytomegalovirus
- HIV-related encephalopathy
- Disseminated herpes simplex
- Disseminated histoplasmosis
- Disseminated *Mycobacterium avium* complex or *Mycobacterium kansasii*
- Miliary or extrapulmonary *Mycobacterium tuberculosis*
- *Pneumocystis jiroveci* pneumonia
- Recurrent *Salmonella* septicemia
- Toxoplasmosis of the brain

Neoplasms
- Invasive cervical cancer
- Kaposi's sarcoma
- Lymphoma (Burkitt's, immunoblastic, or brain)

Opportunistic infections are the leading cause of death in patients with HIV infection; therefore, a primary management goal in critically ill patients with HIV infection is the prevention or resolution of opportunistic and healthcare-associated infections (HAIs). Adherence to infection control practices to prevent bacterial contamination and complications is essential when caring for critically ill patients with HIV infection. Potent combination therapy with antiretroviral agents, known as highly active antiretroviral therapy (HAART), also has a significant impact on the outcomes of patients with opportunistic infections. The use

of HAART commonly results in an increase in CD4+ T cell count and may return it to the normal range; this is known as immune reconstitution.[6] Administration of HAART also can rapidly reduce viral load, thereby decreasing the incidence of complications. Drug groups used in HAART therapy include the nucleoside reverse transcriptase inhibitors (NRTIs), nonnucleoside reverse transcriptase inhibitors (NNRTIs), and protease inhibitors (PIs). Side effects of these medications that the critical care nurse needs to be aware of when caring for a patient receiving HAART therapy are summarized in Box 29-7.

BOX 29-7 Side Effects of Agents Used in Highly Active Antiretroviral Therapy (HAART)

Nucleoside Reverse Transcriptase Inhibitors (NRTIs)
- Hypersensitivity reactions (may be fatal); symptoms may include fever, rash, nausea and vomiting, malaise, loss of appetite, sore throat, cough, and shortness of breath
- Pancreatitis
- Peripheral neuropathy
- Lactic acidosis
- Hepatic steatosis (potentially life threatening; symptoms include headache and hyperlipidemia)

Non-Nucleoside Reverse Transcriptase Inhibitors (NNRTIs)
- Rash; including the severe skin disorder Stevens-Johnson syndrome
- Headaches
- Increased transaminase levels
- Hepatitis

Protease Inhibitors (PIs)
- Gastrointestinal disturbances (diarrhea, nausea, vomiting)
- Hyperlipidemia
- Fat maldistribution
- Hyperglycemia
- Increased transaminase levels
- Headache
- Possible increased risk for bleeding in patients with hemophilia

CASE STUDY

Mr. C. is a 64-year-old African American male with a known history of coronary artery disease (CAD) and an inferior wall myocardial infarction last month. He presents to the emergency department complaining of chest pain unrelieved by sublingual nitroglycerin. His home medications include aspirin, a statin, and a β-adrenergic blocker. An initial 12-lead ECG and cardiac enzymes are normal. After initiation of oxygen and an IV nitroglycerin drip, his pain is relieved. However, because of his recent myocardial infarction, he is admitted to the telemetry unit with orders for serial cardiac enzymes and an 12-lead ECG in the morning. Medication orders include continuing the aspirin and statin, increasing the dose of β-adrenergic blockers, and adding heparin (1 mg/kg subcutaneously every 12 hours).

The next afternoon, Mr. C. has had no further chest pain, his cardiac enzymes have remained normal, and his 12-lead ECG is unchanged. All the results from his morning laboratory work are within normal limits, with the exception of a mildly low platelet count of 140,000/mm³. The cardiologist believes that Mr. C. can be discharged home on the increased β-blocker dose with a follow-up in the office next week.

Mr. C. is dressing to go home when he calls the nurse to his room because he is experiencing chest pain and shortness of breath. The nurse calls for a "stat" 12-lead ECG and places him on 2 L of oxygen via nasal cannula. His vital signs are as follows: HR, 110 beats/min; RR, 32 breaths/min; and BP, 90/64 mm Hg. Chest auscultation reveals clear lungs and a tachycardic but regular heart rhythm. The stat 12-lead ECG remains unchanged from the 12-lead ECG he had earlier in the morning. The nurse calls the cardiologist, who requests that Mr. C. be transferred to the critical care unit.

In the critical care unit, Mr. C. becomes more tachypneic, his oxygen saturation is 85% on 2 L of oxygen, and his BP is now 80/40 mm Hg. His lungs remain clear. He is placed on 100% oxygen administered via a nonrebreather mask. His cardiologist arrives on the unit and orders a 500-mL IV fluid bolus of normal saline. Following a second fluid bolus and with the oxygen therapy, Mr. C.'s BP increases to 96/60 mm Hg, and his oxygen saturation is 95%. He remains dyspneic. He is sent for a stat CT scan of the chest.

While Mr. C.'s CT scan is being done, the nurse has a chance to review his chart. The nurse notices that Mr. C.'s platelet count on admission was 285,000/mm³, but this morning it was 140,000/mm³. About that time, the CT department calls to report that Mr. C. has a pulmonary embolism. The nurse reports both of these findings to the cardiologist. A stat complete blood count (CBC) is ordered and the results are as follows: hemoglobin, 11.2 g/dL; hematocrit, 32.8%; and platelets, 63,000/mm³.

In reviewing Mr. C.'s past medical record, the nurse notes that Mr. C. was administered heparin during his previous hospitalization for acute myocardial infarction. The nurse raises the possibility with the doctor that Mr. C. is experiencing heparin-induced thrombocytopenia (HIT). The heparin is immediately stopped, and Mr. C. is started on argatroban, a direct thrombin inhibitor, instead. Even though Mr. C. has no lower extremity edema or discomfort, a lower extremity venous ultrasound is performed to rule out deep venous thrombosis (DVT).

After 2 days of therapy, Mr. C.'s oxygen saturation is 99% on 2 L of oxygen. His platelet count is substantially higher, although it is still less than 150,000/mm³. He is transferred out of the critical care unit and remains on the direct thrombin inhibitor. The next morning, his platelet count has increased to 159,000/mm³. Mr. C. is started on warfarin, 5 mg each evening. On day 5 of warfarin therapy, Mr. C.'s international normalized ratio (INR) is 2.2. On day 6 of warfarin therapy, his INR is 2.5, and his platelet count is 324,000/mm³. The direct thrombin inhibitor is stopped. Mr. C. no longer requires supplemental oxygen and he is ambulatory on the unit without shortness of breath.

Mr. C. is discharged home on his prior medications of aspirin, statin, and the increased dose of the β-adrenergic blocker. He is given a prescription for warfarin, 5 mg daily, and an appointment to have his INR checked in 3 days. In addition to teaching Mr. C. and his wife about warfarin therapy and anticoagulation, the nurse instructs them to inform healthcare providers that he is not to be given heparin because of this episode of HIT. The nurse suggests that Mr. C. obtain a medical alert bracelet with this information.

1. Mr. C.'s critical care nurse discovered that he received heparin during his previous admission for an acute myocardial infarction. What is the importance of this history?

2. Mr. C. is treated for HIT before the diagnosis is confirmed by laboratory testing. Why?

3. Despite his thrombocytopenia, Mr. C. is started on anticoagulation. What is the rationale?

References

1. Saitoch G, et al: Natural history of dissimenated intravascular coagulation diagnosis based on the newly diagnostic criteria for critically ill patient: Results of a multicenter, prospective survey. Crit Care Med 36(1):145–150, 2008
2. DeBellis R: Anemia in critical care patients: Incidence, etiology, impact, management and use treatment guidelines and protocols. Am J Health Syst Pharm 64(3 suppl 2):514–521, 2007
3. Corwin HL, Gettinger A, Pearl RG, et al: The CRIT study: Anemia and blood transfusion in the critically ill—current clinical practice in the United States. Crit Care Med 32(1):39–52, 2004
4. Shander A, Spence RK, Amin A: The hospitalists' perspective: Evidence-based strategies for inpatient anemia. Medscape. Available at http://www.medscape.com/viewprogram/5481. Released June 30, 2006
5. Del Toro G, Morris E, Cairo MS: Tumor lysis syndrome: Pathophysiology, definition, and alternative treatment approaches. Clin Adv Hematol Oncol 3:54–61, 2005
6. Tiu RY, Mountonakis SE, Dunbar AJ, et al.: Tumor lysis syndrome. Semin Thromb Hematol 33(4):397–404, 2007

Want to know more? A wide variety of resources to enhance your learning and understanding of this chapter are available on the **Point** ✴. Visit **http://thepoint.lww.com/MortonEss1e** to access chapter review questions and more!

Integumentary System

Patient Assessment: Integumentary System

Based on the content in this chapter, the reader should be able to:

1 Describe the components of the history for integumentary assessment.
2 Explain the use of inspection and palpation for general integumentary assessment.
3 Describe wound assessment techniques.
4 Describe the assessment of pressure ulcers.

The skin of a critically ill person is exposed to insults ranging from pressure ulceration to hypersensitivity drug reactions and opportunistic infections.

History

Elements of the integumentary health history are summarized in Box 30-1.

Physical Examination

Physical examination includes assessment of the general condition of the integument and assessment of wounds or pressure ulcers if present.

General Assessment

Inspection and palpation are the primary assessment techniques used to evaluate the integument.

Inspection

Inspection of the general appearance of the skin includes the following:

- Assessment of color
- Determination of the presence of lesions or rashes
- Assessment of the condition of the hair and nails

Skin Color
Skin color is expected to be uniform over the body, except in areas with greater degrees of vascularity. In people with light skin, the genitalia, upper chest,

BOX 30-1 Integumentary Health History

History of the Present Illness

Complete analysis of the following signs and symptoms (using the NOPQRST format; see Chapter 12, Box 12-2):

- Changes in skin color, pigmentation, temperature, or texture
- Changes in a mole
- Excess dryness or moisture
- Skin itching
- Excess bruising
- Delay in healing
- Skin rash or lesions
- Hair loss or increased growth
- Changes in hair texture
- Changes in nails

Past Health History

- **Relevant childhood illnesses and immunizations:** impetigo, scabies or lice exposure, measles, chicken-pox, scarlet fever
- **Past acute and chronic medical problems, including treatments and hospitalizations:** diabetes, peripheral vascular disease, stroke, Lyme disease, Parkinson's disease, immobility, malnutrition, trauma, skin cancers, radiation treatments, HIV/AIDS, autoimmune disease
- **Risk factors:** age, sun exposure, tanning bed use
- **Past surgeries:** skin biopsy
- **Past diagnostic tests and interventions:** allergy testing
- **Medications, including prescription drugs, over-the-counter drugs, vitamins, herbs, and supplements:** aspirin, antibiotics, barbiturates, sulfonamides, thiazide diuretics, oral hypoglycemic agents, tetracycline, antimalarials, antineoplastic agents, hormones, metals, topical steroids
- **Allergies and reactions to medications, foods, contrast, latex or other materials**
- **Transfusions, including type and date**

Family History

- **Health status or cause of death of parents and siblings:** skin cancer, autoimmune diseases

Personal and Social History

- Tobacco, alcohol, and substance use
- Environment: exposure to insects and pests, exposure to plants, exposure to dyes or toxic chemicals, exposure to environmental temperature extremes
- Occupation/leisure activities: farmers, roofers, creosote or coal workers, furniture repair and refinishing, gardening
- Diet: change in diet, recent weight loss or gain, loss of appetite
- Sleep patterns: sleeplessness, anxiety
- Ability for self-care and hygiene
- Recent travel

Review of Systems

- **Cardiovascular:** swelling of extremities, cold extremities, varicose veins
- **Musculoskeletal:** immobility, weakness
- **Neurological:** loss or decrease in sensation, numbness, pain or neuropathy
- **Endocrine:** altered glucose levels

---

and cheeks may appear pink or have a reddish tone. These same areas may appear darker in people with dark skin.

Skin color abnormalities (eg, pallor, cyanosis, jaundice, erythema) manifest differently depending on the person's normal skin tone (Table 30-1).

Lesions

Skin lesions are variously described by their color, shape, cause, or general appearance. See Table 30-2 on pages 425–426 and Table 30-3 on page 427. They are considered abnormal conditions and arise from many factors. It is important to note

TABLE 30-1 Skin Color Abnormalities

Skin Color Abnormality	Underlying Cause	Manifestation in Light-Skinned People	Manifestation in Dark-Skinned People
Pallor	Decreased blood flow	Excessively pale skin	Yellowish-brown or ashen color to the skin
Cyanosis	Increased deoxyhemoglobin in the cutaneous circulation (hypoxia)	Grayish-blue color of the palms and soles of the feet, the nail beds, the lips, the earlobes, and the mucous membranes	Ashen-gray color of the conjunctiva, oral mucous membranes, and nail beds
Jaundice	Increased red blood cell (RBC) hemolysis, liver disease	Yellow color of the sclera, lips, and hard palate	Yellow-green color of the sclera and palms and soles of the feet
Erythema	Inflammation, cellulitis	Reddish tone	Deeper brown or purple tone

TABLE 30-2 **Primary Skin Lesions**

Type	Description	Examples	Illustration
Macule	Less than 1 cm in diameter, flat, nonpalpable, circumscribed, discolored	Brown: freckle, junctional nevus, lentigo, melasma Blue: Mongolian spot, ochronosis Red: Drug eruption, viral exanthema, secondary syphilis Hypopigmented: vitiligo, idiopathic guttate hypomelanosis	Macule
Patch	Less than 1 cm in diameter, flat, nonpalpable, irregular shape, discolored	Brown: larger freckle, junctional nevus, lentigo, melasma Blue: Mongolian spot, ochronosis Red: Drug eruption viral exanthema, secondary syphilis Hypopigmented: vitiligo, idiopathic guttate hypomelanosis	Patch
Papule	Less than 1 cm in diameter, raised, palpable, firm	Flesh, white or yellow: flat wart, milium, sebaceous hyperplasia, skin tag Blue or violaceous: venous lake, lichen planus, melanoma Brown: seborrheic keratosis, melanoma, dermatofibroma, nevi Red: acne, cherry angioma, early folliculitis, psoriasis, urticaria, and eczema	Papule
Nodule	Greater than 1 cm, raised, solid	Wart, xanthoma, prurigo nodularis, neurofibromatosis	Nodule
Plaque	Greater than 1 cm, raised, superficial, flat topped, rough	Psoriasis, discoid lupus, tinea corporis, eczema, seborrheic dermatitis	Plaque
Tumor	Large nodule	Metastatic carcinoma, sporotrichosis	Tumor

(continued on page 426)

TABLE 30-2 Primary Skin Lesions (continued)

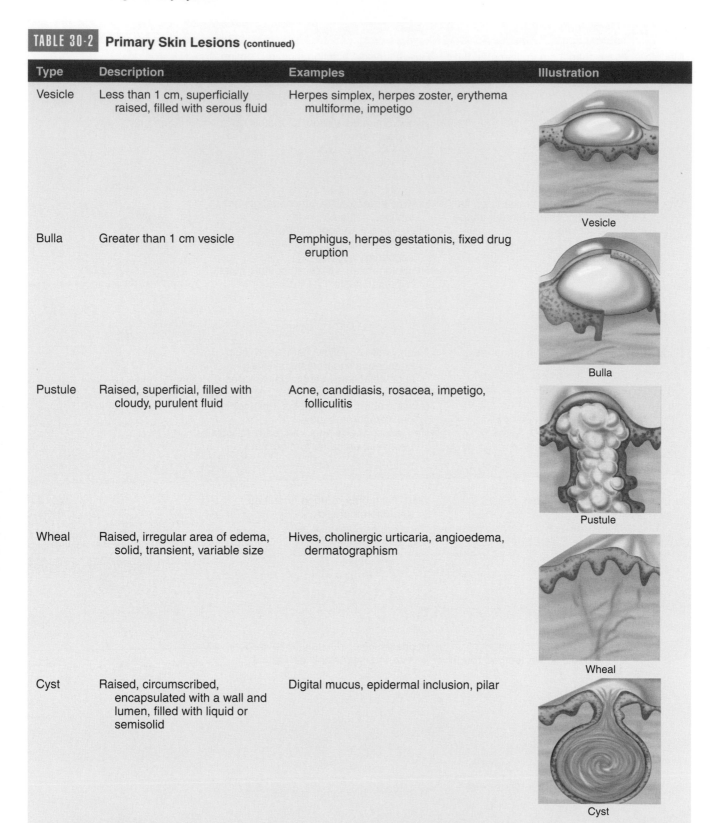

Type	Description	Examples	Illustration
Vesicle	Less than 1 cm, superficially raised, filled with serous fluid	Herpes simplex, herpes zoster, erythema multiforme, impetigo	Vesicle
Bulla	Greater than 1 cm vesicle	Pemphigus, herpes gestationis, fixed drug eruption	Bulla
Pustule	Raised, superficial, filled with cloudy, purulent fluid	Acne, candidiasis, rosacea, impetigo, folliculitis	Pustule
Wheal	Raised, irregular area of edema, solid, transient, variable size	Hives, cholinergic urticaria, angioedema, dermatographism	Wheal
Cyst	Raised, circumscribed, encapsulated with a wall and lumen, filled with liquid or semisolid	Digital mucus, epidermal inclusion, pilar	Cyst

From Rhoads J: Advanced Health Assessment and Diagnostic Reasoning. Philadelphia, PA: Lippincott Williams & Wilkins, 2006, pp 81–83.

TABLE 30-3 Secondary Skin Lesions

Type	Description
Crust	Dried exudates over a damaged epithelium; may be associated with vesicles, bullae, or pustules. Large adherent crust is a scab.
Erosion	Loss of superficial epidermis; does not extend to the dermis; may be associated with vesicles, bullae, or pustules.
Fissure	Crack in the epidermis usually extending into the dermis.
Keloid	Hypertrophied scar tissue; secondary to collagen formation during healing; elevated irregular and red; more common in African Americans.
Lichenification	Thickening and roughening of the skin; accentuated skin markings; may be secondary to repeated rubbing irritation and scratching.
Scale	Skin debris on the surface of the epidermis secondary to desquamated, dead epithelium. Color and texture vary.
Scar	Skin mark left after healing of wound or lesion that represents replacement by connective tissue of the injured tissue. Young scars are red or purple. Mature scars are white or glistening.
Ulceration	Loss of epidermis, extending into dermis or deeper. Bleeding and scarring are possible.

the following when assessing any abnormal skin lesions:

- Anatomical location
- Distribution
- Color
- Size
- Pattern
- The appearance of the lesion's borders or edges
- Whether the lesion is flat, raised, or sunken

Vascular lesions can be either a normal variation (eg, a nevus flammeus or port-wine stain, considered a birthmark) or an abnormal finding. Abnormal vascular lesions include the following.

- **Petechiae** are small (1- to 3-mm) purple or red lesions that result from tiny hemorrhages in the dermal or submucosal layers. They are easily seen on light-skinned people and more difficult to see on those with dark skin (Fig. 30-1A). They may be seen on the oral mucosa and in the conjunctiva. They do not disappear when pressure is applied to them.[1]
- **Purpura** are very similar to petechiae, only larger. Purpura may appear brownish red.
- **Ecchymoses** are bruises. They may appear as purple to yellowish green rounded or irregular lesions and are more easily seen in people with light skin (see Fig. 30-1B).
- **Spider angiomas** are fiery red lesions that are most often located on the face, neck, arms, or upper trunk (see Fig. 30-1C). Spider angiomas are seldom seen below the waist. They resemble a spider, with a central body that is sometimes raised and surrounded by erythema, and radiating "legs."[2] These lesions are most often associated with liver disease and vitamin B deficiency.
- **Urticaria** is a reddened or white, raised, nonpitting plaque that often occurs as a result of an allergic reaction, often to a food or drug. The lesion often changes shape and size during the course of the reaction. Urticaria usually resolves completely over days to several weeks as the excess local fluid is reabsorbed.

Rashes

Rashes are often caused by infection or drug therapy. In the critical care setting, antibiotics and corticosteroids place patients at risk for fungal and yeast infections, which are most often the result of an opportunistic infection by normal flora. Candidiasis presents in the groin and under the breasts of female patients with "erythema, a whitish pseudomembrane, and peripheral papules and pustules."[3] Oral candidiasis (thrush) manifests as a whitish coating of the oral mucosa, especially the tongue. This painful condition may produce fissures on the tongue and often restricts a patient's oral intake.

 RED FLAG! *A rash that develops along with a change in pharmacotherapy may be a sign of an allergic hypersensitivity reaction.*

Condition of the Hair and Nails

The nurse assesses the patient's scalp, hair, and body hair for the presence of infection or infestation.

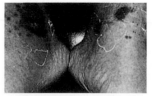

A. Petechiae/purpura

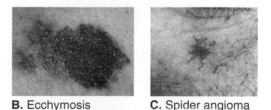

B. Ecchymosis   **C.** Spider angioma

FIGURE 30-1 Abnormal vascular lesions. (**A,** from Kelley WN: Textbook of Internal Medicine. Philadelphia, PA: JB Lippincott, 1989. **B,** from Bickley LS: Bates' Guide to Physical Examination and History Taking, 9th ed. Philadelphia, PA: Lippincott Williams & Wilkins, 2003, p 141. **C,** from Marks R: Skin Disease in Old Age. Philadelphia, PA: JB Lippincott, 1987.)

which may be evidenced by flaking, sores, lice, louse eggs, or ringworm. Inspection of the nails and nail beds can reveal information about the patient's general state of health. Nail beds that are bluish or purplish may indicate cyanosis; nail beds that are pale may indicate reduced arterial blood flow. Clubbing, which suggests chronic oxygen deficiency, is present when the angle of the nail is 180 degrees or greater (Fig. 30-2). Terry's nails, which may be seen in chronic disease states such as cirrhosis, heart failure, and type 2 diabetes mellitus, are whitish with a distal band of dark reddish-brown color, and the lunulae may not be visible (Fig. 30-3).[2]

Palpation

The nurse palpates the skin to assess for moisture, temperature, mobility and turgor, and edema.

- **Moisture.** The level of moisture may reflect underlying conditions. Common terms for describing the moistness of the skin include dry (may be seen in hypothyroidism), diaphoretic (may be seen with fever or increased metabolism), and clammy (may be seen with low cardiac output).
- **Temperature.** The general skin temperature (ie, cool, warm, or hot) is assessed using the dorsal surface of the hand. The nurse assesses the temperature bilaterally and compares for symmetry.

TABLE 30-4 Pitting Edema Scale

Scale	Description	Depth of Indentation	Return to Baseline
4+	Severe	8 mm	2–5 min
3+	Moderate	6 mm	1–2 min
2+	Mild	4 mm	10–15 sec
1+	Trace	2 mm	Disappears rapidly

From Rhoads J: Advanced Health Assessment and Diagnostic Reasoning. Philadelphia, PA: Lippincott Williams & Wilkins, 2006, p 253.

- **Mobility and turgor** may yield information about the patient's fluid volume balance. Skin mobility may be decreased in a patient with increased edema, and skin turgor is decreased in a patient with dehydration.[2]
- **Edema,** classified as either nonpitting or pitting, may result from several underlying conditions. Nonpitting edema, which does not depress when palpated, is often seen in the presence of local inflammation. Pitting edema retains the depression made when it is palpated and usually occurs in dependent body parts. Pitting edema can be further classified by the depth of the depression and, occasionally, by the amount of time it takes the depression to rebound (Table 30-4).

Wound Assessment

A wound is a break in skin integrity. Wounds may be acute (caused by surgery or trauma) or chronic (eg, as a result of diabetes, pressure, malnutrition, peripheral vascular disease, immune deficiencies, or infection).[4] An acute wound may become a chronic wound at any time.

Acute and chronic wounds may be defined as partial- or full-thickness wounds. Partial-thickness

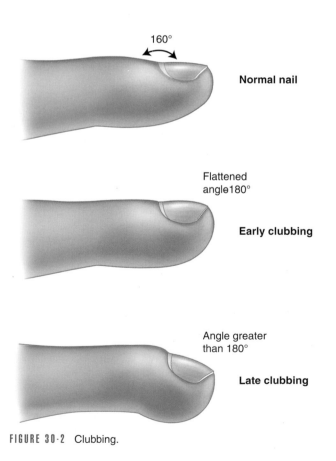

160°

Normal nail

Flattened angle180°

Early clubbing

Angle greater than 180°

Late clubbing

FIGURE 30-2 Clubbing.

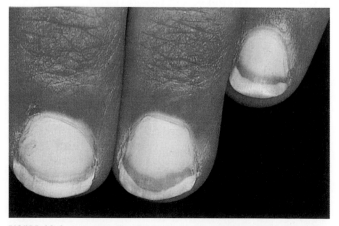

FIGURE 30-3 Terry's nails. (From Bickley LS: Bates' Guide to Physical Examination and History Taking, 10th ed. Philadelphia, PA: Lippincott Williams & Wilkins, 2009, p 193.)

BOX 30-2 Wound Assessment

Location: Document the location, using anatomical positions.

Size: Document the size, in centimeters or millimeters. Terminology such as "the size of a half dollar" should be avoided, because it leads to inconsistent and inaccurate documentation. Measure the length from the 1200 to 1800 position. Measure the width from the 0900 to 0300 position (see Fig. 30-4).

Depth: Use a sterile swab to determine the depth (see Fig. 30-5).

Undermining or tunneling: Document the presence or absence of undermining, which occurs when there is loss of tissue along the wound margins (the "lip of tissue"),[7] or tunneling, a tunnel opening somewhere in the wound bed (see Fig. 30-6).

Tissue type: Describe the wound bed. The tissue in the wound bed should be beefy red (as opposed to pale). Note the presence or absence of granulation tissue (shiny red, grainy, or bumpy tissue). Assess for necrotic tissue, which presents as black or brown tissue. Slough, which is yellow and stringy in appearance, may also be present in the wound bed. If the wound bed is not visible, document the presence and condition of the eschar (scab), sutures, staples, or other wound closure.

Drainage: Note the presence or absence of drainage. If drainage is present, describe its odor, color, amount, and consistency.

Wound margins: Describe the wound margins. Note whether the surrounding tissue is clean, dry, reddened, edematous, pale, intact, or blistered.

Drains and tubes: Note the type of drain or tubing, and its location (using anatomical or clock positions).

Condition of dressing: Describe the amount and type of drainage on the dressing, as well as the ease with which the dressing was removed.

Pain: Evaluate on a 0 to 10 scale (or other institution-approved assessment scale). Provide pain relief as needed before, during, and after wound assessment or dressing change.

---

wounds involve the epidermis and may involve the dermis. A partial-thickness wound is shallow and is usually moist and painful (because loss of the epidermis exposes the nerve endings). Full-thickness wounds involve loss of the epidermis, dermis, and subcutaneous tissue, and they may involve muscle, tendons, ligaments, and bone. A full-thickness wound involves a large amount of tissue loss and appears as a crater or crevice.

The nurse completely assesses and accurately documents all wound characteristics (Box 30-2). Photography may be used for wound documentation. Figures 30-4 through 30-6 illustrate techniques for wound measurement.

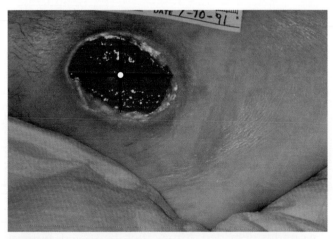

FIGURE 30-4 Linear measurements of the wound are taken at the greatest length and width perpendicular to each other. (From Baranoski S, Ayello EA: Wound Care and Essentials Practice Principles, 2nd ed. Philadelphia, PA: Lippincott Williams & Wilkins, 2008, p 84.)

Pressure Ulcer Assessment

Pressure ulcers are wounds caused by pressure, shearing, and friction. The nurse assesses both the patient's risk for developing pressure ulcers, and for the presence and stage of pressure ulcers.

Determining Risk for Pressure Ulcers

Identifying those people most at risk for pressure ulcer development is a focus of assessment.[5] Characteristics of high-risk patients are summarized in Box 30-3. The Braden Scale for Predicting Pressure Sore Risk, recommended in the U.S. Agency for Health Care Policy and Research guidelines and widely used in hospital settings, requires daily assessment of six parameters. The scale provides a numerical score ranging from a very high risk score of 6 to a very limited risk or minimal risk score of 23 (Fig. 30-7). Adults with a score below 16 are considered at risk, and specific interventions are recommended to prevent the development of ulcers.

 The Older Patient. *Older adults with a Braden Scale score of less than 18 are considered at risk for pressure ulcer development.*

The development of pressure ulcers can be a preventable complication. A schedule for turning and positioning the patient (eg, every 2 hours) is an effective, easily implemented intervention for relief of pressure. Specialty beds that are designed to reduce pressure by inflating, deflating, alternating pressures, or laterally rotating are often used in the critical care setting. Although these beds do relieve some pressure, they do not eliminate all pressure;

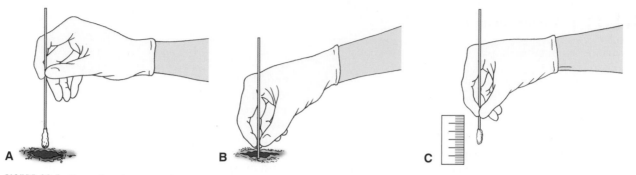

FIGURE 30-5 Procedure for measuring wound depth. **A:** Put on gloves. Gently insert the swab into the deepest portion of the wound that you can see. **B:** Grasp the swab with your thumb and forefinger at the point corresponding to the wound margin. **C:** Carefully withdraw the swab while maintaining the position of your thumb and forefinger. Measure from the tip of the swab to that position. (From Thomas Hess C: Clinical Guide: Wound Care, 5th ed. Philadelphia, PA: Lippincott Williams & Wilkins, 2005, p 21.)

therefore, regular turning of the patient from side to side is still required.

Assessing for the Presence and Stage of Pressure Ulcers

When assessing the skin, the nurse must be vigilant for signs of skin breakdown. Pressure applied by the weight of the body reduces arterial and capillary

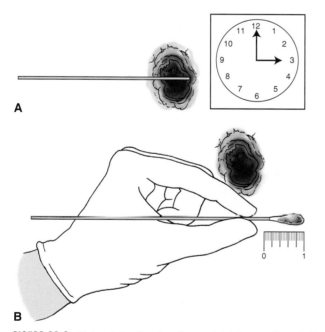

FIGURE 30-6 Determining the direction and depth tunneling. **A:** To assess the direction of tunneling, put on gloves and insert the swab into the sites where tunneling occurs. Progressing in a clockwise direction, document the deepest sites where the wound tunnels. (Twelve o'clock points in the direction of the patient's head, so in this example, tunneling occurs at three o'clock.) **B:** To assess the depth of tunneling, insert the swab into the tunneling areas, and grasp the swab where it meets the wound margin. Remove the swab, place it next to a measuring guide, and document the measurement centimeters. (From Thomas Hess C: Clinical Guide: Wound Care, 5th ed. Philadelphia, PA: Lippincott Williams & Wilkins, 2005, p 23.)

blood flow, leading to ischemia and skin breakdown. Common pressure points where breakdown can occur include the occiput, scapula, sacrum, buttocks, ischium, and heels. Pressure ulceration of the toes can occur as a result of the pressure of the bed linens on the feet. Dressing devices, wound appliances, and tubes (eg, endotracheal tubes, tracheostomy tubes, nasogastric tubes) can place pressure on underlying skin, resulting in pressure sores. In a patient with a tracheostomy tube, the back of the neck must be assessed because the endotracheal tube holder may be applied too tightly. In a patient with a nasogastric tube, the tape securing the tube must be removed regularly and the condition of the tip of the nose and nares assessed for changes resulting from pressure from the tube.

When a pressure ulcer is present, the nurse observes for and documents the stage (Fig. 30-8). When staging a pressure ulcer, the nurse keeps the following points in mind:

- Bruising in the surrounding tissue of a Stage II wound should increase suspicion for a deeper ulcer.
- Reverse staging is inappropriate (eg, "Stage IV wound is now Stage III"). Lost muscle or subcutaneous tissue cannot be replaced, and the tissue that fills in the wound bed is not the same as the tissue that has been lost. Therefore, it is more appropriate to document "healing stage IV wound."
- Pressure ulcers covered with debris or eschar (dry scab or slough resulting from a burn) are considered unstageable, because eschar prevents assessment of the wound bed. Documentation is "unstageable, wound covered by eschar." If the wound is debrided, it may then be staged, but not all pressure ulcers should be debrided for that purpose.

BOX 30-3 Patients at High Risk for Pressure Ulcers

- Patients with decreased level of consciousness or sensation
  - Brain or spinal cord injury
  - Peripheral neuropathy (eg, from diabetes)
  - Stroke
- Patients with sedation or frequent analgesic dosing
- Patients with poor circulation
  - Hypotension
  - Heart failure
  - Peripheral vascular insufficiency

- Elderly patients
- Patients who are malnourished or dehydrated
- Patients experiencing incontinence and diaphoresis
- Patients with impaired mobility
  - Neuromuscular disease
  - Spinal cord injuries

Braden Scale
FOR PREDICTING PRESSURE SORE RISK

Patient's Name _____ Evaluator's Name _____ Date of Assessment ____

SENSORY PERCEPTION Ability to respond meaningfully to pressure-related discomfort	1. Completely Limited: Unresponsive (does not moan, flinch, or grasp) to painful stimuli, due to diminished level of consciousness or sedation. OR limited ability to feel pain over most of body surface.	2. Very Limited: Responds only to painful stimuli. Cannot communicate discomfort except by moaning or restlessness. OR has a sensory impairment which limits the ability to feel pain or discomfort over 1/2 of body	3. Slightly Limited: Responds to verbal commands, but cannot always communicate discomfort or need to be turned. OR has some sensory impairment which limits ability to feel pain or discomfort in 1 or 2 extremities.	4. No Impairment: Responds to verbal commands. Has no sensory deficit which would limit ability to feel or voice pain or discomfort.	
MOISTURE Degree to which skin is exposed to moisture	1. Constantly Moist: Skin is kept moist almost constantly by perspiration, urine, etc. Dampness is detected every time patient is moved or turned.	2. Very Moist: Skin is often, but not always, moist. Linen must be changed at least once a shift.	3. Occasionally Moist: Skin is occasionally moist, requiring an extra linen change approximately once a day.	4. Rarely Moist: Skin is usually dry, linen only requires changing at routine intervals.	
ACTIVITY Degree of physical activity	1. Bedfast: Confined to bed	2. Chairfast: Ability to walk severely limited or nonexistent. Cannot bear own weight and/or must be assisted into chair or wheelchair.	3. Walks Occasionally: Walks occasionally during day, but for very short distances, with or without assistance. Spends majority of each shift in bed or chair.	4. Walks Frequently: Walks outside the room at least twice a day and inside room at least once every 2 hours during waking hours.	
MOBILITY Ability to change and control body position	1. Completely Immobile: Does not make even slight changes in body or extremity position without assistance.	2. Very Limited: Makes occasional slight changes in body or extremity position but unable to make frequent or significant changes independently.	3. Slightly Limited: Makes frequent though slight changes in body or extremity position independently.	4. No Limitations: Makes major and frequent changes in position without assistance.	
NUTRITION Usual food intake pattern	1. Very Poor: Never eats a complete meal. Rarely eats more than 1/3 of any food offered. Eats 2 servings or less of protein (meat or dairy products) per day. Takes fluids poorly. Does not take a liquid dietary supplement. OR is NPO and/or maintained on clear liquids or IVs for more than 5 days.	2. Probably Inadequate: Rarely eats a complete meal and generally eats only about 1/2 of any food offered. Protein intake includes only 3 servings of meat or dairy products per day. Occasionally will take a dietary supplement. OR receives less than optimum amount of liquid diet or tube feeding.	3. Adequate: Eats over half of most meals. Eats a total of 4 servings of protein (meat, dairy products) each day. Occasionally will refuse a meal, but will usually take a supplement if offered. OR is on a tube feeding or TPN regimen which probably meets most of nutritional needs.	4. Excellent: Eats most of every meal. Never refuses a meal. Usually eats a total of 4 or more servings of meat and dairy products. Occasionally eats between meals. Does not require supplementation.	
FRICTION AND SHEAR	1. Problem: Requires moderate to maximum assistance in moving. Complete lifting without sliding against sheets is impossible. Frequently slides down in bed or chair, requiring frequent repositioning with maximum assistance. Spasticity, contractures or agitation leads to almost constant friction.	2. Potential Problem: Moves feebly or requires minimum assistance. During a move skin probably slides to some extent against sheets, chair, restraints, or other devices. Maintains relatively good position in chair or bed most of the time but occasionally slides down.	3. No Apparent Problem: Moves in bed and in chair independently and has sufficient muscle strength to lift up completely during move. Maintains good position in bed or chair at all times.		

Braden Scale Scores
1 = Highly Impaired
3 or 4 = Moderate to Low Impairment
Total Points Possible: 23
Risk Predicting Score: 16 or Less

NPO: Nothing by Mouth

IV: Intravenously
TPN: Total parenteral nutrition

Total Score ____

FIGURE 30-7   The Braden scale is a widely used screening tool to identify people at risk for pressure ulcers. (Courtesy of Barbara Braden and Nancy Bergstrom. Copyright, 1988. Reprinted with permission.)

Stage I. Skin is unbroken but appears red; no blanching when pressed.

Stage II. Skin is broken, and there is superficial skin loss involving the epidermis alone or also the dermis. The lesion is a shallow ulcer with a reddish base, resembling a vesicle, erosion, or blister. Nonpressure-related causes of erosion, ulceration, or blistering (e.g., skin tears, tape burns, maceration) are excluded.

Stage I

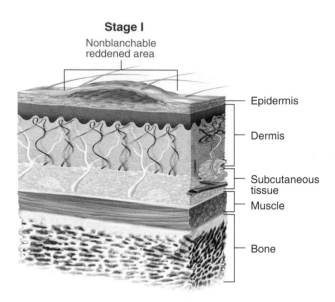

Stage II

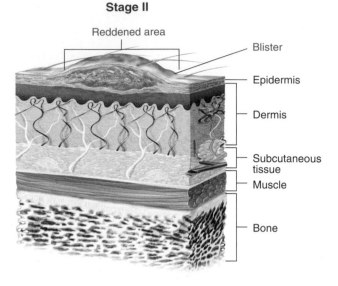

Stage III. Pressure area involves epidermis, dermis, and subcutaneous tissue. The ulcer resembles a crater. Hidden areas of damage may extend through the subcutaneous tissue beyond the borders of the external lesions but not through underlying fascia.

Stage IV. Pressure area involves epidermis, dermis, subcutaneous tissue, bone, and other support tissue. The ulcer resembles a massive crater with hidden areas of damage in adjacent tissue.

Stage III

Stage IV

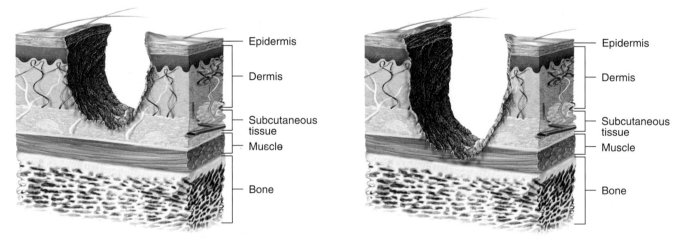

FIGURE 30-8 Pressure ulcers staging. (From Weber J, Kelley J: Health Assessment in Nursing, 4th ed. Philadelphia, PA: Lippincott Williams & Wilkins, 2010, p 194.)

CASE STUDY

Mrs. H., a 62-year-old widow, has been in the critical care unit for the past 2 weeks after being diagnosed with respiratory failure and pneumonia. Her medical history includes obesity, type 2 diabetes mellitus, and chronic obstructive pulmonary disease (COPD). She has been intubated and is on mechanical ventilation. She has received continuous enteral feedings through a nasogastric tube, numerous antibiotics, and dopamine for blood pressure support during her first 3 days in the critical care unit. She has a triple-lumen central venous access catheter.

Mrs. H. is scheduled for a tracheostomy tomorrow, and she will also have a percutaneous gastric feeding tube inserted at that time. She has an indwelling urinary catheter, as well as an incontinence fecal bag, which is draining liquid stool. Over the past 5 days, she has received a benzodiazepine for sedation at least once per day. Physical therapy consultation was made on day 3, and two caregivers assist her with a pivot to a chair twice each day. Her family visits daily and helps her communicate with a pencil and paper tablet.

1. What factors place Mrs. H. at increased risk for developing pressure ulcers?

2. What are Mrs. H.'s risk factors related to compromised integument that may lead to infection?

References

1. Johannsen L: Skin assessment. Dermatol Nurs 17(2): 165–166, 2005
2. Bickley LS, Szilagyi PG: The skin. In Bickley LS (ed): Guide to Physical Examination and History Taking, 9th ed. Philadelphia, PA: Lippincott Williams & Wilkins, 2007
3. Kaufman C: Candidiasis. In Goldman L, Ausiello D (ed): Cecil Medicine, 23rd ed. Philadelphia, PA. Suanders Elsevier, 2007, Chapter 359
4. Baranoski S, Ayello EA: Wound Care Essentials: Practice Principles, 2nd ed. Philadelphia, PA: Lippincott Williams & Wilkins, 2008
5. Lyder C, Ayello E: Pressure ulcers: A patient safety issues. In Hughes R (ed): Patient Safety and Quality: An Evidence-Based Handbook for Nurses. AHQR publication, 2008, Chapter 12

Want to know more? A wide variety of resources to enhance your learning and understanding of this chapter are available on the**Point** . Visit **http://thepoint.lww.com/MortonEss1e** to access chapter review questions and more!

Patient Management: Integumentary System

OBJECTIVES

Based on the content in this chapter, the reader should be able to:

1 Explain the normal healing process.
2 Describe nursing care for a critically ill patient with a wound.
3 Describe the proper technique for obtaining a surface culture.

Wound Healing

Phases of Wound Healing

Optimal wound healing occurs in a moist environment. The wound-healing process comprises three phases (Fig. 31-1):

- The *inflammatory phase* begins immediately after the wound occurs. It includes vasoconstriction (to control bleeding and hold the wound together), platelet aggregation and fibrin deposition at the site (to form a clot), and phagocytosis (to destroy bacteria and remove the wound's cellular debris, providing a clean wound bed for healing). Clinical findings during the inflammatory phase include erythema, edema, and pain.
- The *proliferation phase* involves the development of collagen, new blood vessels, and connective tissue to create granulation tissue. The wound edges contract, decreasing the overall size of the wound. The wound is beefy red and shiny, with a grainy or bumpy appearance. Epithelialization results in a scar.
- The *maturation phase* involves remodeling of the collagen fibers to increase the tensile strength of the scar tissue. It has been estimated that only 70% to 80% of the skin's original strength is attained when the wound is healed.

Methods of Wound Healing

Wounds can heal through primary, secondary, or tertiary intention (Fig. 31-2):

- **Primary intention** is used with surgical wounds or lacerations. The edges of the wound are drawn together (approximated) by sutures, staples, or glue, shortening the time required for the wound to heal to about 4 to 14 days overall. Primary intention is associated with a decreased risk for infection and minimal scarring.
- **Secondary intention** occurs when the wound edges cannot be approximated to each other due to significant tissue loss. The potential for infection and scarring is increased because of the inability to approximate the edges. Secondary intention may occur in acute or chronic wounds.
- **Tertiary intention (delayed primary intention).** The wound is not closed for a period (eg, 3 to 5 days) to allow infection, edema, or both, to resolve. The wound is packed or irrigated to remove exudate and cellular debris; then the wound edges are approximated, and the wound is closed as it is in primary intention. Scarring is usually greater than that seen with primary intention but less than that seen with secondary intention.

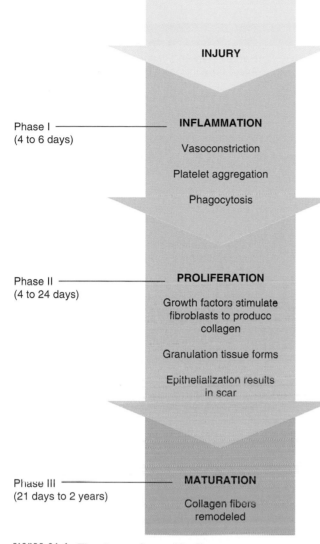

FIGURE 31-1 The stages of wound healing.

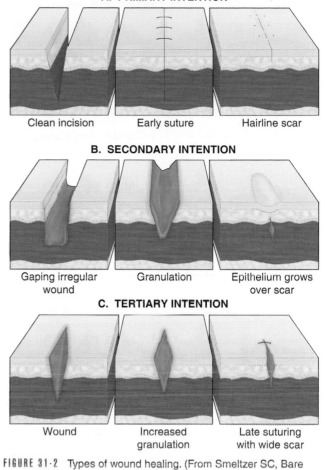

FIGURE 31-2 Types of wound healing. (From Smeltzer SC, Bare BG, Hinkle JL, et al.: Brunner & Suddarth's Textbook of Medical—Surgical Nursing, 12th ed. Philadelphia, PA: Lippincott Williams & Wilkins, 2010, p 474.)

Wound Care

Critically ill patients often have multiple risk factors for impaired wound healing (Table 31-1). Care of specific wounds common in critically ill patients is summarized in Table 31-2. General interventions taken by the healthcare team to promote wound healing include cleansing, closure, drain care, dressing, and debridement.

 RED FLAG! In all areas of wound care, the nurse needs to focus on pain assessment and control. The choice of pain medication and the delivery method used (eg, continuous drip, epidural, patient-controlled analgesia pump, local anesthesia) depends on the patient's status.

Wound Cleansing

Cleansing of the wound and the periwound area aims to remove bacteria and cellular debris without damaging the wound bed or granulating tissue. Normal saline or an approved commercial cleanser is used to cleanse the wound. Open wounds are cleansed starting in the middle and moving outward in a circular motion to include the periwound area. Incisions are cleansed from top to bottom, again starting in the middle and moving outward.

RED FLAG! Povidone-iodine (Betadine), acetic acid, sodium hypochlorite (Dakin's solution), and hydrogen peroxide destroy granulation tissue and prolong the healing process, and should not be used routinely to cleanse wounds.

Wound Closure

The goal of all wound care is ultimately the closure of the wound and restoration of skin integrity.

Vacuum-Assisted Wound Closure (Negative Pressure Therapy)

Vacuum-assisted wound closure (VAC) is a system that assists wound closure by providing localized negative pressure to the wound bed and wound

TABLE 31-1 Factors Affecting Wound Healing

Factors	Rationale	Nursing Interventions
Advanced age	With age, the skin becomes less resilient and the amount of subcutaneous tissue decreases.	Handle skin and tissues gently. Avoid tape if possible.
Hemorrhage	Accumulation of blood and dead cells creates a growth medium for organisms.	Monitor vital signs. Observe site for evidence of bleeding and infection.
Hypovolemia	Insufficient blood volume leads to vasoconstriction and reduced oxygen and nutrients available for wound healing.	Monitor for volume deficit (circulatory impairment). Correct by fluid replacement as prescribed.
Edema	Reduces blood supply by exerting increased interstitial pressure on vessels.	Elevate edematous area; apply cool compresses.
Inadequate dressing technique		
Too small	Permits bacterial invasion and contamination.	Follow guidelines for proper dressing technique.
Too tight	Reduces blood supply carrying nutrients and oxygen.	
Nutritional deficits	Patients who are on nothing by mouth (NPO) status for longer than 24–48 h are at risk for slowed healing owing to the lack of an adequate supply of protein, carbohydrates, and other nutrients. Protein-calorie depletion may occur. Insulin secretion may be inhibited, causing blood glucose to rise.	Monitor laboratory test results; document intake and output and daily weights; obtain a nutritional assessment by a dietitian; institute total parenteral or peripheral parenteral nutrition or enteral feedings and calorie counts. Correct deficits and administer vitamin supplements as prescribed. Monitor blood glucose levels.
Foreign bodies	Foreign bodies retard healing.	Keep wounds free of dressing threads and powder from gloves.
Oxygen deficit (eg, as a result of inadequate lung or cardiovascular function or vasoconstriction) leading to insufficient tissue oxygenation	Adequate oxygenation is necessary to promote healing.	Encourage deep breathing, turning, and controlled coughing.
Drainage accumulation	Accumulated secretions hamper healing process.	Monitor closed drainage systems for proper functioning. Institute measures to remove accumulated secretions.
Medications		
Corticosteroids	May mask presence of infection by impairing normal inflammatory response.	Be aware of action and effect of medications the patient is receiving.
Anticoagulants	May cause hemorrhage.	
Broad-spectrum and specific antibiotics	Effective if administered immediately before surgery for specific pathology or bacterial contamination. If administered after wound is closed, it is ineffective because of intravascular coagulation.	
Patient overactivity	Prevents approximation of wound edges.	Use measures to keep wound edges approximated: taping, bandaging, splints. Encourage rest.
Systemic disorders (eg, hemorrhagic shock, acidosis, hypoxia, renal failure, hepatic disease, sepsis)	Depress cell functions that directly affect wound healing.	Administer prescribed treatments to address underlying cause.

Factors	Rationale	Nursing Interventions
Immunosuppressed state	The patient is more vulnerable to bacterial and viral invasion; defense mechanisms are impaired.	Provide maximum protection to prevent infection. Restrict visitors with colds; institute mandatory hand hygiene by all staff.
Wound stressors (eg, vomiting, Valsalva maneuver, heavy coughing, straining)	Produce tension on wounds, particularly of the torso.	Encourage frequent turning and ambulation and administer antiemetic medications as prescribed. Assist the patient in splinting incision.

Modified from Smeltzer SC, Bare BG, Hinkle JL, et al.: Brunner & Suddarth's Textbook of Medical—Surgical Nursing, 12th ed. Philadelphia, PA: Lippincott Williams & Wilkins, 2010, p 475.

margins. Tubing, similar to that of suction tubing, is placed into a special foam dressing. The foam dressing is shaped in wedges that are cut to fit the wound. The foam wedges and tubing are then covered with an occlusive transparent dressing and the tube is connected to the vacuum unit at low suction levels (Fig. 31-3). The occlusive dressing promotes a moist environment for healing, and the negative pressure removes excessive wound drainage, assisting in pulling the wound margins together and stimulating granulation tissue.[1] The dressing has the appearance of being "vacuum-packed" when it is secure and occlusive. If the dressing is not collapsed, there is a leak in the system, and the dressing must be replaced securely to maintain negative pressure.

 RED FLAG! *The foam wedge dressing must not be placed in direct contact with exposed blood vessels, organs, or nerves.*

The VAC system decreases length of wound healing, the frequency of dressing changes (thus

TABLE 31-2 Care of Specific Wounds

Wound Type	Description	Wound Care
Venous stasis ulcer	• Usually found on the medial aspect of the lower leg • Irregular wound margins, ruddy appearance • Presents as a shallow crater with mild to heavy drainage	• Compression therapy using an Unna boot or a multiple-wrap dressing to provide continuous compression • Elevation of the affected leg above heart level to decrease edema
Arterial (ischemic) ulcer	• Usually found on the distal leg and dorsal aspect of the foot and toes • Round, regular, smooth wound margins • "Punched-out" appearance, pale wound bed • May be shallow or deep • Affected leg may be cool to the touch, cyanotic, and pale with minimal hair distribution	• Occlusive dressing • Vascular deficit must be addressed surgically
Diabetic foot ulcer	• Primarily found on the plantar aspect of the foot, heels, and metatarsals • Frequently not recognized early, due to neuropathy	• A dressing that provides a moist environment is used to promote wound healing • Debridement • Assessment for infection, osteomyelitis, and delayed wound healing • Special shoes to offload the patient's weight
Skin tear	• Partial-thickness, acute wound • Occurs when the skin is thin and fragile • May be due to removal of tape or transparent occlusive dressings	• Gentle cleansing with normal saline (or other institution-approved cleanser) • Application of hydrogel and a nonadherent dressing • Kling or Coban is used to hold the dressing in place without tape
Pressure ulcer	Appearance depends on stage; see Chapter 30	• Stage I and II pressure ulcers: hydrocolloid dressings • Stage III and IV pressure ulcers: absorptive hydrofiber dressings or calcium alginates covered with hydrocolloid or occlusive transparent dressings; foam dressings; vacuum-assisted wound closure (VAC)

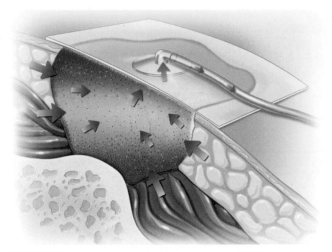

FIGURE 31-3   A vacuum-assisted wound closure (VAC) device assists wound closure by providing localized negative pressure to the wound bed and wound margins. (Courtesy of KCI Licensing, Inc., 2007.)

decreasing patient discomfort and nursing labor), the length of stay, complications, and hospital readmissions, while it promotes the salvage of limbs.[2] The VAC system can be used in both acute and chronic wounds.[1] Indications and contraindications are summarized in Box 31-1. Nursing responsibilities include wound assessment and documentation; placing the patient on the VAC system, changing the canister; and maintaining the system.

Sutures, Staples, and Wound Adhesives

Sutures or staples must be cleaned with sterile normal saline or a wound cleanser. Immediately

---

BOX 31-1   **Indications and Contraindications for Vacuum-Assisted Wound Closure (VAC)**

Indications
- Chronic wounds (eg, diabetic and nonhealing Stage III and IV pressure ulcers)
- Flaps and grafts
- Dehisced incisions (ie, split open along natural or suture lines)
- Acute and traumatic wounds
- Burns

Use with Caution
- Active bleeding
- Anticoagulant therapy
- History of uncontrolled bleeding
- In an infected wound (use only with appropriate antibiotic therapy)

Contraindications
- Untreated osteomyelitis
- Necrotic tissue with eschar
- Malignancies of the wound
- Nonenteric and unexplored fistulas

---

after surgery, the wound needs to be covered with a dry sterile dressing. After the initial postoperative period, the staples or sutures are frequently left open to air.

Wound adhesives may be used on surgical or traumatic wounds to approximate the wound margins after sutures are used to close the underlying tissue. The wound adhesive appears like a shiny, clear coating over the incision. Incisions in which wound adhesives are used are gently rinsed with a wound cleaner and left uncovered. Steri-Strips should not be used in conjunction with wound adhesives.

 RED FLAG! *Wound adhesives must not be placed in the wound bed. Doing so may lead to delayed wound healing or infection.*

Wound Drain Care

Often, a drain is inserted in the wound to prevent the pooling of exudate in the wound bed, which can decrease healing and increase the potential of infection or tunneling. The most common types of drains are Hemovac drains, Penrose drains, and Jackson-Pratt drains. Basic care of all drains and tube sites includes cleansing with sterile normal saline and applying a dressing to stabilize the tube and prevent contamination of the site with drainage. Drain and tube insertion sites are typically not left open to air because of the risk for infection. Antibiotic ointment may be applied. Impregnated gauzes for packing and various solutions (eg, Betadine, Dakin's solution) may be used in the event that the wound is infected; however, they should not be used as a routine wound treatment for a prolonged time because they destroy granulating tissue and inhibit the normal healing process.

Some wounds may have high volumes of exudate. When this is the case, the wound may be "pouched" or "bagged" to contain the drainage, protect the surrounding tissue from breakdown, and allow for accurate measurement of wound output. The same supplies used for ostomy pouching may be used for pouching a wound[3] (Fig. 31-4), or a product designed specifically for pouching high-volume draining wounds may be used. The nurse assesses the wound margins for skin breakdown and applies protective ointments or uses protective skin wipes as needed.

Wound Dressings

Wound dressings are used to protect the wound from infection and promote a moist environment. The dressing of choice depends on the wound.

Wet-to-Dry Dressings

Wet-to-dry dressings are frequently used in clinical practice; however, evidence has shown that they are actually detrimental to the wound.[4] A wet-to-dry dressing may be used for debridement of the wound, but when it is removed, indiscriminate debridement of both necrotic and granulating tissue occurs.

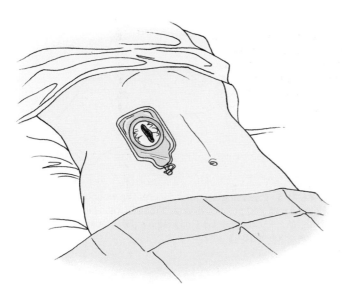

FIGURE 31-4 "Pouching" a high-volume draining wound. (From Thomas Hess C: Clinical Guide: Wound Care, 5th ed. Philadelphia, PA. Lippincott Williams & Wilkins, 2005, p 100.)

This constant debriding of the wound increases the patient's discomfort, promotes infection (due to frequent dressing changes), slows the healing process, and may enlarge the wound.

Wounds need a moist environment to heal without impediment. If a wet-to-dry dressing is used for nondebridement purposes, the optimal method is wet to moist, changing the dressing every 4 hours, and covering the wet-to-dry dressing with a transparent dressing to promote and maintain a moist wound environment. If the dressing is not being used for the purpose of debridement, the nurse may moisten the dressing prior to removal to prevent it from adhering to the wound.

Absorptive Dressings

Absorptive dressings include calcium alginates, foam dressings, and hydrocolloids:

- **Calcium alginates** are made from brown seaweed. They come in ropelike or flat pieces that must be "fluffed" and packed into the wound bed. Calcium alginates have an absorptive quality and can hold up to 20 times or more their weight in wound drainage. As the calcium alginate absorbs the wound drainage, it changes to a gel that is easily removed from the wound. Calcium alginates may be covered with a hydrocolloid or a transparent dressing.
- **Foam dressings** have the advantage of being highly absorptive. They are available in various shapes and sizes and are placed over the wounds. Minimal trauma occurs to the wound bed and surrounding tissue. Foam dressings, like calcium alginates, provide a moist wound environment.
- **Hydrocolloids** are occlusive, self-adhesive, and absorptive, although their absorptive capacity is not as great as that of calcium alginates or foam

dressings. They are used most frequently in the treatment of stage I and stage II pressure ulcers. Hydrocolloids need to be changed less frequently than calcium alginates and foam dressings (ie, only every 3 to 5 days).

 RED FLAG! *Absorptive dressings must always be used with caution if the wound is infected.*

Hydrogels

Hydrogels, which are water- or glycerin-based, are most frequently used for dry wounds. They help maintain a moist wound environment, promoting granulation, epithelialization, and autolytic debridement.

Silver Dressings

Silver (Ag) dressings are impregnated with silver, which has a bactericidal effect. The potential for bacteria to develop a resistance to silver is negligible. Silver dressings work well in conjunction with other medical and pharmacotherapeutic treatments. In some cases, a silver gel (eg, SilvaSorb gel) is combined with a hydrogel and applied into the wound.

Bilayered Dressings

Bilayered dressings are engineered dressings that are applied as "grafts" to noninfective, chronic wounds that fail to progress with other forms of treatment. Depending on the type and brand, these dressings may be composed of fibroblast, collagen, and growth factors. They act by giving the wound a "jump start." They are frequently used on venous stasis ulcers and diabetic foot ulcers or on exposed bone, tendon, or joint tissue.

Wound Debridement

Debridement is the removal of necrotic (dead) or devitalized tissue. Necrotic or devitalized tissue presents as dark brown, black, yellow, pale, cyanotic, or crusty eschar. To promote optimal wound healing, this tissue needs to be removed from the wound. Debridement may be autolytic, chemical, or mechanical. Occasionally, a combination of debridement methods may be used throughout the healing process.

- In **autolytic debridement,** the body uses its own ability to lyse and dissolve necrotic tissue. Hydrocolloid dressings are frequently used to promote autolytic debridement. This type of debridement is not optimal in wounds that have large amounts of necrotic tissue.
- In **chemical debridement,** proteolytic enzymes or collagen-based drugs are applied topically to the wound. Chemical debridement requires caution because some enzyme agents are nonselective and may destroy healthy tissue in addition to necrotic and devitalized tissue.
- In **mechanical debridement,** necrotic or devitalized tissue is removed using wet-to-dry dressings,

whirlpools, or sharps (ie, a scalpel or scissors). Whirlpool debridement is not as effective as other methods, increases the potential for infection, and can macerate wound margins. Sharps debridement is a surgical procedure that may require anesthesia, IV conscious sedation, a local anesthetic, or a combination of the three. Wet to dry dressings are nonselective and will debride both healthy and unhealthy tissue.

Wound Cultures

All wounds are considered contaminated and have the potential to become infected; however, routine wound cultures are not recommended unless there are signs and symptoms of infection (Box 31-2). Several methods may be used to culture a wound, including fluid biopsy, wound (tissue) biopsy, and surface culture (culture swab). Wounds that contain necrotic tissue or tunneling need both aerobic and anaerobic cultures.

A surface culture is usually done first. The wound is cleansed or irrigated with sterile normal saline before swabbing the wound. After the wound is cleansed, the swab is gently rolled or rotated, starting at the 12-o'clock position and moving in a zig-zag pattern from side to side down the wound to the 6-o'clock position (Fig. 31-5).[3]

 RED FLAG! Exudate and necrotic tissue are not cultured—doing so provides invalid results.

A colony count of 100,000 organisms/mL indicates an infection that needs to be treated with the appropriate antibiotic.[5] At colony counts of greater than 100,000 organisms/mL, normal wound healing is inhibited, and the wound becomes a chronic wound.[3] Wounds that do not respond to antibiotic treatment need to be recultured by wound biopsy.

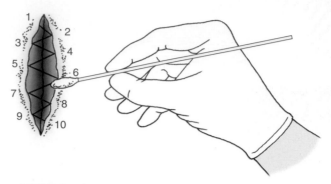

FIGURE 31-5   Collecting a wound culture. The wound edges are swabbed using 10-point coverage. (From Thomas Hess C: Clinical Guide: Wound Care, 5th ed. Philadelphia, PA: Lippincott Williams & Wilkins, 2005, p 104.)

CASE STUDY

Mr. K. is a 34-year-old male who was involved in a motor vehicle injury. He sustained multiple injuries, including splenic laceration grade II, liver laceration grade III, and a right open femur fracture with a large traumatic wound. He underwent exploratory abdominal surgery for repair of the liver and splenic lacerations. His abdominal incision was left open to minimize the risk for abdominal compartment syndrome, and a vacuum-assisted wound closure (VAC) system was placed on the abdominal wound. Mr. K.'s right leg wound was cleaned intraoperatively, and postoperatively, it is draining copious amounts of serosanguinous fluid.

1. What type of dressing would be required for the open, draining wound?

2. Would the nurse expect to routinely culture the wound bed?

3. What are the nurse's responsibilities with regard to the VAC system?

BOX 31-2   Signs and Symptoms of Wound Infection

- Fever
- Erythema
- Edema
- Induration
- Foul odor
- Purulent or increased amount of exudates
- Abscess
- Cellulitis
- Discoloration of granulation tissue
- Friable granulation tissue (bleeds easily)
- Increased or unexpected pain or tenderness
- Elevated white blood cell (WBC) count

References

1. V.A.C.® Therapy Clinical Guidelines. KCI Licensing, Inc., 2007
2. Niezgoda JA, Page JC, Kaplan M: The economic value of negative pressure wound therapy. Ostomy Wound Manage 51(2A):445–475, 2005
3. Thomas Hess C: Clinical Guide: Wound Care, 5th ed. Philadelphia, PA: Lippincott Williams & Wilkins, 2005
4. Cowan L, Stechmiller J: Prevalence of wet to dry dressing in wound care. Adv Skin Wound Care 22(12):567–573, 2009
5. Fischbach FT, Dunning MB III: Nurse's Quick Reference to Common Laboratory and Diagnostic Tests, 4th ed. Philadelphia, PA: Lippincott Williams & Wilkins, 2006

Want to know more? A wide variety of resources to enhance your learning and understanding of this chapter are available on the**Point** ※. Visit **http://thepoint.lww.com/MortonEss1e** to access chapter review questions and more!

Burns

Based on the content in this chapter, the reader should be able to:

1 Describe the classification of burn injuries.
2 Describe the pathophysiology of a burn injury.
3 Describe injuries that can occur in conjunction with a burn injury.
4 Describe the initial priorities for assessment and care of a patient with a burn injury.
5 Describe the ongoing assessment and care of a patient with a burn injury.

Classification of Burn Injuries

Burn injuries are described in terms of causative agent, depth, and severity.

Causative Agent

A burn injury usually results from energy transfer from a heat source to the body. The heat source may be thermal, chemical, or electrical. Exposure to ionizing radiation can also cause burns.

Thermal Burns

Thermal burns may be caused by contact with flames, a hot object, or steam.

Chemical Burns

Chemical burns may be caused by exposure to acids or alkali (eg, hydrofluoric acid, formic acid, anhydrous ammonia, cement, phenol), white phosphorus, certain elemental metals, nitrates, hydrocarbons, or tar. With chemical burns, contact time is directly related to the severity of injury. For all chemical burns, hydrotherapy to limit the effects of the chemical should be initiated immediately and continued until the pain is resolved; this may take 2 to 3 hours or longer. If exposure has occurred to the eyes, the eyes should be flushed continuously until a full evaluation can be completed by an ophthalmologist.

RED FLAG! Attempts to neutralize an acid or alkali delay initiation of hydrotherapy and may cause further burn injury by producing additional chemical reactions.

Electrical Burns

The effects of electricity on the body are determined by the type of current, the amount of current, the pathway of the current, the duration of contact, the area of contact, the resistance of the body, and the voltage.

Low-voltage injuries are those caused by 1000 V or less. Low-voltage current travels the path of least resistance; therefore, tissue, nerves, and muscle are easily damaged, whereas bone is not. These injuries often occur at home (eg, damaged extension cords) and involve the hands and oral cavities. A low-voltage burn of the hand usually consists of a small, deep burn that may involve vessels, tendons, and nerves.

Although these burns involve a small area, they may be severe enough to require amputation.

High-voltage current is concentrated at its entrance to the body, then diverges centrally, and finally converges before exiting. The most severe damage to tissue occurs at the sites of contact and exit. High-voltage electric entry wounds are charred and leathery in appearance, whereas exit wounds are more likely to "blow out" as the charge exits.

Depth

Many factors alter the response of body tissues to heat. The depth of the burn depends on the temperature of the causative agent, the duration of exposure to the causative agent, and the areas of the body that are exposed to that agent. Damage to the skin is frequently described according to the depth of injury (Box 32-1).

BOX 32-1 Classification of Burns by Depth of Injury

Depth	Tissues Involved	Usual Cause	Characteristics	Pain	Healing
Superficial (first-degree)	Epidermis, minimal epithelial damage	Sunburn or brief exposure to hot liquid, flash, flame	Dry, Blisters after 24 hours, Pinkish red, Blanches with pressure	Painful, Pruritus during healing	3 to 6 days, No scarring
Superficial partial-thickness (second-degree)	Epidermis, superficial dermis	Flash, hot liquids	Moist, Pinkish or mottled red, Blisters, Some blanching	Pain, Hyperesthetic	10 to 14 days, Minimal scarring
Deep partial-thickness (second-degree)	Epidermis, part of dermis: epidermal-lined hair and sweat glands intact	Flash, hot liquids, hot solids, flame, and intense radiant injury	Dry, pale, waxy, No blanching	Sensitive to pressure	30 days to months, Late hypertrophic scarring; marked contracture formation, May require skin grafting
Full-thickness (third-degree)	Epidermis and dermis; may involve subcutaneous fat, muscle, and bone	Sustained flame, electrical, chemical, and steam	Leathery, cracked avascular, white, cherry red, brown, or black, No blanching	Little pain; deep pressure	Cannot self-regenerate; needs grafting

Severity

To assess the severity of the burn, several factors must be considered:

- The percentage of total-body surface area (TBSA) burned (Fig. 32-1)
- The depth of the burn
- The causative agent and length of exposure
- The anatomical location of the burn
- The person's age
- The person's medical history
- The presence of concomitant injury
- The presence of inhalation injury

The injury severity grading system, developed by the American Burn Association (ABA), provides a consistent way of determining and describing the severity of a burn injury (Box 32-2). Minor injuries are treated in the emergency department with outpatient follow-up every 48 hours until the risk for infection is reduced and wound healing is under way. Patients with moderate, uncomplicated burn injuries or major burn injuries are referred to a regional burn center and, if needed, transferred for specialized care. The ABA's criteria for transfer to a burn center are given in Box 32-3.

Pathophysiology

Burn injuries have both local (Box 32-4) and systemic effects. Major changes at the cellular level are responsible for the tremendous systemic response noted in a patient with burns. Disruption of the cell membrane results in increased vascular permeability, loss of plasma proteins, and a decrease in circulating volume. Increased vascular permeability leads to the formation of interstitial edema, which usually peaks within 24 to 48 hours of injury. Patients with burn injuries often develop acute respiratory distress syndrome (ARDS) following the development of pulmonary interstitial edema.[1] The systemic release of vasoactive substances initiates the systemic inflammatory response syndrome (SIRS). The potent mediators and cytokines deplete the intravascular volume, decreasing blood flow to the kidneys and the gastrointestinal tract. If left uncorrected, hypovolemic shock, metabolic acidosis, and hyperkalemia may occur.

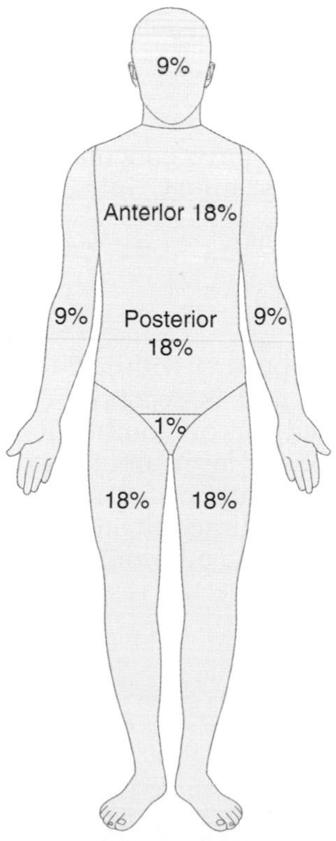

AREA	PERCENT OF BURN					SEVERITY OF BURN		TOTAL PERCENT
	0-1 Year	1-4 Years	5-9 Years	10-15 Years	Adult	2°	3°	
Head	19	17	13	10	7			
Neck	2	2	2	2	2			
Ant. Trunk	13	13	13	13	13			
Post. Trunk	13	13	13	13	13			
R. Buttock	2½	2½	2½	2½	2½			
L. Buttock	2½	2½	2½	2½	2½			
Genitalia	1	1	1	1	I			
R. U. Arm	4	4	4	4	4			
L. U. Arm	4	4	4	4	4			
R. L. Arm	3	3	3	3	3			
L. L. Arm	3	3	3	3	3			
R. Hand	2½	2½	2½	2½	2½			
L. Hand	2½	2½	2½	2½	2½			
R. Thigh	5½	6½	8½	8½	9½			
L. Thigh	5½	6½	8½	8½	9½			
R. Leg	5	5	5½	6	7			
L. Leg	5	5	5½	6	7			
R. Foot	3½	3½	3½	3½	3½			
L. Foot	3½	3½	3½	3½	3½			
Total	Blue areas indicate 2° Red areas indicate 3°					Total		

A. Rule of Nines **B.** Lund and Browder chart

FIGURE 32-1 Methods of calculating the percentage of the body surface area. **A:** The "rule of nines" method divides the body into parts in multiples of 9% and is useful for quick assessment. **B:** The Lund and Browder method provides more accurate assessment because surface measurements are assigned to each body part by patient age. However, because this method of measuring burn size is time-consuming, it should be done after resuscitation efforts are well established.

BOX 32-2 Classification of Severity of Burn Injury

Minor Burn Injury
- Second-degree burn of less than 15% total-body surface area (TBSA) burn in adults or less than 10% TBSA in children
- Third-degree burn of less than 2% TBSA not involving special care areas (eyes, ears, face, hands, feet, perineum, joints)
- Excludes all patients with electrical injury, inhalation injury, or concurrent trauma; all poor-risk patients (ie, extremes of age, concomitant disease)

Moderate, Uncomplicated Burn Injury
- Second-degree burns of 15% to 25% TBSA in adults or 10% to 20% in children

- Third-degree burns of less than 10% TBSA not involving special care areas
- Excludes all patients with electrical injury, inhalation injury, or concurrent trauma; all poor-risk patients (ie, extremes of age, concomitant disease)

Major Burn Injury
- Second-degree burns of greater than 25% TBSA in adults or 20% in children
- All third-degree burns of greater than or equal to 10% TBSA
- All burns involving eyes, ears, face, hands, feet, perineum, joints
- All patients with inhalation injury, electrical injury, or concurrent trauma; all poor-risk patients

---

The end results of the local and systemic responses are dramatic if the burn covers more than 20% of the TBSA. The person with a major burn injury experiences a form of hypovolemic shock known as burn shock (Fig. 32-2). As a result of increased capillary permeability, fluid (comprised of water, sodium and other electrolytes, and plasma proteins) leaks from the vascular compartment, resulting in edema in the burned tissue and throughout the body. This "leak" causes a decrease in cardiac output, hemoconcentration of red blood cells (RBCs), and diminished perfusion to major organs. In some instances, with burns exceeding 60% of the TBSA, depressed cardiac output does not respond to aggressive volume resuscitation due to a myocardial depressant factor. The loss of fluid throughout the body's intravascular space results in thickened, sluggish flow of the remaining circulatory blood volume. The antigen–antibody reaction to burned tissue adds to circulatory congestion by causing agglutination (clumping) of cells.

BOX 32-3 Criteria for Referral to a Burn Center

- Partial-thickness burns greater than 15% of total-body surface area (TBSA)
- Burns that involve the face, hands, feet, genitalia, perineum, or major joints
- Third-degree burns in any age group
- Electrical burns, including lightning injury
- Chemical burns
- Inhalation injury
- Burn injury in patients with preexisting medical disorders that could complicate management, prolong recovery, or affect mortality
- Concomitant trauma, in which the burn injury poses the greatest risk for morbidity or mortality
- Children with burns in hospitals without qualified personnel or equipment for the care of children
- Patients with burns who will require special social, emotional, or long-term rehabilitative intervention

---

The pathophysiological response after burn injury is biphasic. In the early postinjury (ebb) phase, generalized organ hypofunction develops from decreased cardiac output. In patients receiving adequate fluid resuscitation, the cardiac output usually returns to normal late in the first 24 hours after the burn injury. As plasma volume is replenished during the second 24 hours, the cardiac output increases to hypermetabolic levels (hyperfunction phase) and slowly returns to more normal levels as the burn wounds are closed.[2]

Concomitant Problems

Many patients with burn injury have concomitant problems, including pulmonary injury, infection, and trauma.

Pulmonary Injury

Pulmonary damage usually appears within 24 to 48 hours of the burn injury and is secondary to the inhalation of superheated air or combustible products. In an incident involving large amounts of steam, the risk for injury is far greater because water has a heat-carrying capacity 4000 times greater than air and can be inhaled deep into the pulmonary system. Pulmonary injury may also be the result of a systemic process related to SIRS.

Inhalation Injury

Inhalation injury is the leading cause of death in the first 24 hours after burn injury. Three stages of inhalation injury have been described:

- Acute pulmonary insufficiency occurs in the first 36 hours after injury.
- Pulmonary edema occurs between 6 and 72 hours after injury.
- Bronchopneumonia occurs 3 to 10 days after injury.

BOX 32-4   Localized Tissue Response to Burn Injury

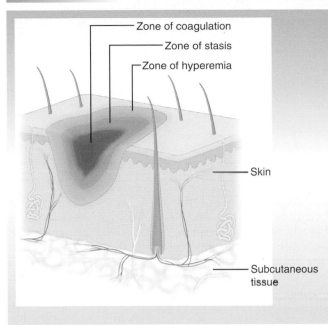

- **Zone of coagulation:** Area where the most damage has been sustained; temperatures have reached 113°F (45°C). The tissues are black, gray, khaki, or white and have undergone protein coagulation and cell death. This area has lost the ability to recover and requires surgical intervention.
- **Zone of stasis:** Contains cells that are at the most risk for becoming necrotic in the initial 24 to 72 hours, depending on the conditions and resuscitation.
- **Zone of hyperemia:** The area of increased blood flow needed for tissue recovery (*active hyperemia*) and the removal of metabolic waste products (*reactive hyperemia*). This area heals rapidly and has no cell death.

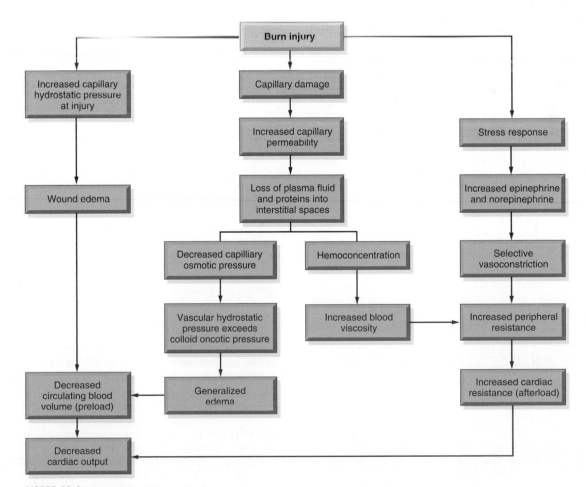

FIGURE 32-2   Fluid shifts in burn shock.

BOX 32-5 History and Physical Examination Findings Suggestive of Inhalation Injury

- History of incident occurring in a confined area
- Singed nasal hairs
- Burns of the oral or pharyngeal mucous membranes
- Burns in the perioral area or neck
- Carbonaceous sputum
- Change in voice (hoarseness)
- Stridor
- Dyspnea
- Tachypnea

TABLE 32-1 Signs and Symptoms of Carbon Monoxide Poisoning

Carboxyhemoglobin Saturation (%)	Clinical Presentation
10	No symptoms
20	Headache, vomiting, dyspnea on exertion
30	Confusion, lethargy, changes on electrocardiogram (ECG)
40–60	Coma
More than 60	Death

Inhalation of superheated air may cause blisters and edema in the supraglottic area around the vocal cords, leading to airway obstruction. Early intubation may prevent airway obstruction. Tracheobronchial and parenchymal lung injuries are usually a result of incomplete combustion of chemicals and result in a chemical pneumonitis. Edema in the trachea and alveoli may develop any time from the first few hours up to 7 days after the injury. Usually edema occurs within 24 hours of injury; however, changes may not become apparent until the second 24-hour period following injury. The alveoli may collapse, leading to atelectasis and the rapid development of ARDS.

History and physical assessment findings that suggest the potential for inhalation injury are given in Box 32-5. Serial arterial blood gas (ABG) measurements show a decreasing arterial oxygen tension (PaO_2). Subtle changes in the patient's sensorium may also indicate hypoxia. Usually, the admission chest x-ray appears normal because changes are not evident until 24 to 48 hours after the burn. A sputum specimen is obtained for culture and sensitivity studies. Laryngoscopy and bronchoscopy may be of value in determining the presence of extramucosal carbonaceous material (the most reliable sign of inhalation injury) and the state of the mucosa (blistering, edema, erythema).

Carbon Monoxide Toxicity

Patients who are found in closed areas in the presence of combusted gases (eg, from a faulty furnace or vehicle exhaust) are at greatest risk for carbon monoxide exposure. Carbon monoxide (a nonirritating, odorless, colorless gas that is formed as a result of incomplete combustion of any carbon fuel) competes with oxygen for uptake by hemoglobin, thereby acting as an asphyxiant. Because hemoglobin has 200 to 300 times the affinity for carbon monoxide that it has for oxygen, carbon monoxide readily displaces the oxygen, leading to the formation of carboxyhemoglobin and a reduction in systemic arterial oxygen content. The signs and symptoms of carbon monoxide poisoning depend on the amount of carboxyhemoglobin that is present in the patient's blood (Table 32-1).

When carbon monoxide poisoning is suspected, 100% high-flow oxygen is administered. Carbon monoxide has a half-life of 4 hours if the patient breathes room air and 45 minutes if the patient is breathing 100% oxygen. Serial ABGs are the most accurate way to assess responsiveness to oxygen therapy because unlike pulse oximetry, they distinguish between oxygen and carbon monoxide in hemoglobin.

Infection

Severe burn injury results in loss of the mechanical barrier to the environment (ie, the skin) and compromises the immune system. For this reason, infection is the most common cause of death in patients with burns after the first 7 days.

 RED FLAG! *Actions of the healthcare team can affect patient survival positively or negatively. Catheters must be handled with sterile or clean technique, depending upon type of catheter, and hands must be washed before and after handling the patient, the patient's bed, or equipment. When dressings are removed and wounds exposed, sterile gloves must be worn.*

Diagnosis of invasive infection in the patient with burns is difficult because most patients with burns have elevated core temperatures and white blood cell (WBC) counts. In a patient with burns, a more useful sign of infection is the appearance of glucose in the urine, particularly if this appears paradoxically when the blood glucose level is within normal limits. Hyperglycemia and increased difficulty in controlling the blood glucose level in a person with diabetes are signs of threatening sepsis. Manifestations of multisystem organ dysfunction syndrome (MODS; see Chapter 33) are almost certain signs of septic shock.

A biopsy of the burn wound permits a quantitative assay of the number of colony-forming units (CFUs) of bacteria per gram of tissue, and allows isolation and identification of the invading organism. Burn wound sepsis is likely if the colony count is greater than 105 CFU/g.

Trauma

Concomitant traumatic injuries (eg, fractures, head trauma) pose significant risk for the burn patient. The burn wounds may mask some of the classic signs of underlying injuries (eg, ecchymosis, swelling).

BOX 32·6 Primary Survey of a Patient with Burn Injury

Airway
- Assess immediately for signs of inhalation injury, which indicate need to secure the airway.

Breathing and Ventilation
- Assess for circumferential full-thickness burns of the chest that may impair ventilation.

Circulation
- Pay special attention to the distal pulses of any extremity with circumferential burns. Doppler ultrasonography can be used to assess for pulses.
- If possible, perform IV cannulation by inserting two large-bore catheters into skin that is unburned. A central venous catheter should be inserted when indicated.
- Assess for risk factors for impaired circulation, including decreased sensation, progressive worsening of pain, paresthesias, decreased capillary refill, and pallor of extremity.

Disability
- Assess for level of consciousness. Typically, the patient with burns is alert and oriented. If the patient is not alert and oriented, assess for associated injuries such as inhalation injury, head trauma, substance abuse, or preexisting medical conditions using the AVPU (**A**lert, responds to **V**erbal stimuli, responds to **P**ainful stimuli, **U**nresponsive) method.

Exposure
- Remove all of the patient's clothes to complete the primary and secondary surveys.
- After examination, cover the patient with a clean, dry sheet and warm blankets to prevent evaporative cooling. If possible, IV fluids are warmed to 98.6°F (37°C) to 104°F (40°C) before administering.

Knowledge of the circumstances surrounding the burn injury (eg, car accident, explosion) can help guide the assessment for concomitant traumatic injuries. For example, patients with electrical injuries must be evaluated for fractures secondary to the violent muscular contraction that occurs after exposure, with special focus on the cervical spine and long bones.

Assessment and Management

The initial assessment of the patient with burns is like that of any trauma patient (see Chapter 34). Because proper stabilization of the patient is crucial for successful transfer to a burn center, the primary and secondary surveys are completed before transfer. Box 32-6 discusses the primary survey specific to burn patients. The secondary survey, which takes place after resuscitative measures have been initiated, includes a detailed history and physical examination of the patient and a complete history of the accident (Box 32-7). While taking the history, the nurse notes preexisting conditions. During the physical examination, burn depth and size are assessed. Laboratory and diagnostic studies that are indicated for patients with burns include the following:

- Complete blood count (CBC)
- Comprehensive chemistry panel, including blood urea nitrogen (BUN)

BOX 32·7 Secondary Survey of a Patient with Burn Injury: History of Preceding Events

Thermal Burns
- How did the burn occur?
- Did the burn occur inside or outside?
- Did the clothes catch fire?
- How long did it take to extinguish the fire?
- Were there any explosions?
- Was the patient found in a smoke-filled room?
- How did the patient escape?
- Did the patient jump out of a window?
- Were there other people injured or killed at the scene?
- Was the patient unconscious at the scene?
- Was there a motor vehicle crash?
- Was the car severely damaged?
- Was there a car fire?
- Are the purported circumstances of the injury consistent with the burn characteristics (is there possibility of abuse)?

For Scald Injuries
- How did the burn occur?
- What was the temperature of the liquid?

- What was the liquid; how much liquid was involved?
- What was the burn cooled with?
- Who was present when the burn took place?
- Where did the burn take place? Is there possibility of abuse?

Chemical Burns
- What was the agent?
- How did the exposure occur?
- What was the duration of contact?
- Did contamination take place?

Electrical Burns
- What kind of electricity was involved?
- Did the patient lose consciousness?
- Did the patient fall?
- What was the estimated voltage?
- Was cardiopulmonary resuscitation (CPR) administered at the scene?

- Creatinine level
- Urinalysis
- ABGs with a carboxyhemoglobin
- Electrocardiogram (ECG)
- Chest radiograph

After the primary and secondary surveys are complete, the burned area is usually covered with a dry sheet. Ice can be applied to small superficial burns. If the patient has a high-voltage electrical burn or cardiac changes are noted, continuous cardiac monitoring is established. If the patient has a chemical burn, the area is immediately flushed with large amounts of water to remove the chemical, and all contaminated clothing is removed and bagged. If the patient is going to be transferred to a burn center, initiation of fluid resuscitation, insertion of a nasogastric tube, and insertion of an indwelling urinary catheter may be carried out during the secondary survey.

Resuscitative Phase

The resuscitative phase begins immediately after the burn has occurred. Resuscitative measures are ongoing and constantly evaluated.

Providing Hemodynamic Support

Therapy is aimed at supporting the patient through the period of hypovolemic shock ("burn shock") until capillary integrity is restored. Fluid resuscitation is the primary intervention in the resuscitative phase in the critical care unit. Goals for fluid resuscitation are as follows:

- Correct fluid, electrolyte, and protein deficits.
- Replace continuing losses and maintain fluid balance.
- Prevent excessive edema formation.
- Maintain a urine output in adults of 30 to 50 mL/h.

Numerous formulas have been developed for fluid resuscitation in the patient with burns, including the Baxter (Parkland) formula, the Brooke formula, the modified Brooke formula, the ABA consensus formula, the dextran formula, and the Evans formula. These formulas differ primarily in recommended volume administration and salt content. In general, lost crystalloid and colloid solutions must be replaced rigorously. Free water, given as 5% dextrose in water (D_5W) with or without added electrolytes, is regulated so that insensible fluid loss is covered with the goal of keeping the patient's sodium concentration at 140 mEq/L. The ABA recommends the use of the ABA consensus formula:

- **First 24 hours:** Lactated Ringer's solution (2 to 4 mL/kg/% TBSA in adults; 3 to 4 mL/kg/%TBSA in children); half given over first 8 hours, remaining half given over next 16 hours
- **Second 24 hours:** Colloid-containing fluid (0.3 to 0.5 mL/kg/%TBSA), plus electrolyte-free fluid (in adults) or half-normal saline (in children) to maintain adequate urine output

---

BOX 32-8 Indications of Adequate Fluid Replacement

Blood pressure: Normal to high ranges
Pulse rate: less than 120 beats/min
Central venous pressure (CVP): 8 to 12 cm H_2O
Pulmonary capillary wedge pressure (PCWP): 12 to 18 mm Hg
Urine output: 30 to 70 mL/h
Lungs: Clear
Sensorium: Clear
Gastrointestinal tract: Absence of nausea and adynamic ileus

Fluid resuscitation formulas are guidelines, and individual patients may require more or less than 2 to 4 mL/kg per percentage TBSA during the first 24 hours. Patients who often require more fluid than the formula predicted include those with electrical injuries, inhalation injuries, delayed resuscitation, prior dehydration at time of injury, and concomitant trauma.

 RED FLAG! Large amounts of fluids are given over a short period of time during fluid resuscitation immediately after the burn, putting the patient at risk for fluid overload and pulmonary edema. Care must be taken to avoid these complications, although it is difficult when it is necessary to infuse large amounts of fluids so rapidly.

After the first 24 hours following injury, replacing the massive evaporative water loss is a major consideration in fluid management. In patients with previously normal renal function, the onset of spontaneous diuresis is a hallmark indicating the end of the resuscitative phase. Infusion rates can be decreased by 25% for 1 hour if the urine output is satisfactory and can be maintained for 2 hours; the reduction may then be repeated. Urinary outputs must be maintained within normal limits of 30 to 70 mL/h (0.5 mL/kg/h) in the adult. Other indications of adequate fluid replacement are listed in Box 32-8.

Patients are usually weighed daily. A gain of 15% of admission weight may be expected with the large amounts of fluids that are being administered. Intake and output must be monitored meticulously. Inadequate fluid resuscitation places the patient at risk for the development of rhabdomyolysis (the release of myoglobin and hemoglobin from damaged cells) and acute renal insufficiency.

Providing Pulmonary Support

Patients with concomitant pulmonary injuries will require pulmonary support to address complications such as upper airway edema, tracheobronchial injury, bronchospasm, and bronchopneumonia.

- **Upper airway edema.** In patients with inhalation injury, upper airway edema peaks 24 to 48 hours after injury. If the injury is mild or moderately severe, placing the patient in a high Fowler's position and administering humidified oxygen and aerosolized racemic epinephrine may be sufficient to limit further edema formation. Severe upper airway obstruction usually requires endotracheal intubation to protect the airway until the edema subsides.

- **Tracheobronchial injury.** In patients with mild tracheobronchial injury, atelectasis may be prevented by frequent bronchial hygiene therapy (BHT). In patients with more severe injury, more frequent suctioning may be necessary, and bronchoscopic removal of debris may be appropriate. These patients usually require endotracheal intubation and mechanical ventilatory support.
- **Bronchospasm.** Patients with bronchospasm are treated with aerosolized or intravenously administered bronchodilators.
- **Bronchopneumonia.** Bronchopneumonia may develop at any time and may be hematogenous (miliary) or airborne. Airborne bronchopneumonia is most common, with onset occurring soon after injury. It is often associated with a lower airway injury or aspiration. Hematogenous bronchopneumonia begins as a bacterial abscess secondary to another septic source, usually the burn wound. The time of onset usually is 2 weeks after injury. Empiric antibiotic therapy is initiated and then modified according to culture and sensitivity test results.

Escharotomy

Edema formation in the tissues under the tight, unyielding eschar of a circumferential burn of a deep partial thickness or full-thickness injury produces significant vascular compromise in the affected limb (compartment syndrome). Doppler ultrasonography is the most reliable means of assessing arterial blood flow; loss or decrease of the ultrasonic signal is an indication for escharotomy. The nurse performs hourly assessments of the radial, ulnar, and palmar arch pulses (in the upper extremity) or the posterior tibial and dorsalis pedis pulses (in the lower extremity). If needed, an escharotomy is performed as a bedside procedure. Local anesthesia is rarely necessary because full-thickness injuries are insensate; opioids and benzodiazepines are used for patient comfort.

Reparative Phase

Once the patient is stabilized, measures are taken to promote healing and prevent infection. Box 32-9 provides a collaborative care guide for the patient with burns.

Ensuring Optimal Nutrition

Appropriate nutrition plays a significant role in improving outcome for patients with severe burn injuries. Early enteral feeding (within the first 24 hours of injury) may reduce the translocation of bacteria from the intestinal lumen, thereby reducing the patient's risk for developing septicemia.[3,4] Enteral feeding also prevents hypercatabolism. One approach is to slowly infuse tube feedings through the nasogastric tube or enteral feeding tube at a rate of 10 to 20 mL/h. Although this rate does not meet the nutritional needs of an adult patient, it is enough to protect the gut mucosa. The rate is steadily increased to meet the estimated calculated caloric requirements according to the patient's tolerance of enteral feeding. Patients with minor burns may be able to satisfy their caloric and fluid needs through oral intake only.

Judging the amount of protein necessary for recovery from burn injuries is difficult. Massive and unquantified loss of protein from the burn wound exudates precludes nitrogen balance studies based on urine excretion alone. Dietary protein should be started at an administration rate of 1.2 g/kg/d and should be increased if there is no subsequent increase in serum protein markers. It is important to avoid overfeeding of protein because doing so predisposes the patient to sepsis, and amounts of protein greater than 3 g/kg/d in adults are usually not tolerated because of azotemia.

Providing Musculoskeletal Support

Physical and occupational therapy begins on day 1 of a burn injury. Independent of the patient's general condition, injured upper and lower extremities can be elevated to allow adequate venous drainage and reduce edema. Patients with burn injuries are also at risk for the development of contractures:

- The burn wound will shorten by contraction until it meets an opposing force. Across a flexor surface, this may result in a contracture.
- Although tightly flexed positions are preferred by patients for comfort, they result in severe contractures.

Range-of-motion exercises prevent tendon shortening and restriction of joint motion by burn scar contractures. Range-of-motion exercises (passive initially, progressing to active) are initiated immediately and continued throughout the hospitalization and rehabilitation period. The range-of-motion exercises are carried out with each dressing change or more often if indicated. Positioning the body with the extremities extended is also important. Special splints are used to maintain arm, legs, and hands in extended, yet functional, positions. Later, when the wounds have healed sufficiently, the person is custom-fitted for a special pressure garment that helps prevent hypertrophic scarring. The garment must be worn almost 24 hours a day for approximately 1 year.

Managing Pain and Anxiety

The pain associated with burns is managed aggressively. All opioids are given intravenously because

(text continues on page 452)

BOX 32-9 COLLABORATIVE CARE GUIDE for the Patient With a Burn

OUTCOMES	INTERVENTIONS
Oxygenation/Ventilation	
A patent airway is maintained.	• Auscultate breath sounds q2–4h and PRN.
Lungs are clear to auscultation.	• Assess for inhalation injury, and anticipate intubation. • Assess quantity and color of tracheal secretions. • Suction endotracheal airway when appropriate. • Hyperoxygenate and hyperventilate before and after each suction pass.
Peak, mean, and plateau pressures are within normal limits for a patient on a ventilator.	• Monitor airway pressures q1–2h. • Monitor lung compliance q8h. • Administer bronchodilators and mucolytics. • Perform chest physiotherapy q4h. • Monitor airway pressures and lung compliance for improvement after interventions.
The patient is without evidence of atelectasis or infiltrates.	• Turn side to side q2h. • Consider kinetic therapy or prone positioning. • Obtain chest x-ray daily.
ABGs are within normal limits.	• Monitor carboxyhemoglobin and carbon monoxide levels. • Monitor ABGs using cooximeter analysis of arterial saturation. (Pulse oximeter and calculated SaO_2 are inaccurate measures in the presence of carbon monoxide.) • Provide humidified oxygen. • Consider hyperbaric therapy.
Circulation/Perfusion	
Blood pressure, heart rate, CVP, and pulmonary artery pressures are within normal limits.	• Assess vital signs q1h. • Assess hemodynamic pressures q1h if the patient has pulmonary artery catheter. • Administer intravascular volume as ordered to maintain preload (see below).
Temperature is within normal limits.	• Monitor temperature q1h. • Maintain a warm environment, and use warming lights or blankets to prevent hypothermia. • Treat fever with antipyretics and cooling blankets.
Perfusion to extremities is maintained; pulses are intact.	• Monitor perfusion using pulse oximetry, Doppler, palpation q1h. • Elevate burned extremities. • Prepare for escharotomy or fasciotomy.
Fluids/Electrolytes	
Restore and maintain fluid balance. Urine output 30 to 70 mL/h or 0.5 mL/kg. CVP, 8 to 12 mm Hg; pulmonary artery occlusion pressure (PAOP), 12 to 18 mm Hg; blood pressure, within normal limits; heart rate, less than 120 beats/min.	• Assess intake and output q1h. • Give lactated Ringer's 4 mL/kg/% burn, divided into first 24 hours postburn. • Monitor for spontaneous diuresis, and reduce IV infusion rate as indicated. • Take daily weight.
Electrolyte, mineral, and renal function values are within normal limits.	• Monitor and replace minerals and electrolytes. • Monitor BUN, creatinine, myoglobin, and urine electrolytes and glucose. • Monitor neurological status. • Monitor and treat dysrhythmias.

BOX 32-9 COLLABORATIVE CARE GUIDE (continued)

OUTCOMES	INTERVENTIONS
Mobility/Safety	
The patient is free of joint contractures.	• Provide passive and active range-of-motion exercises q1–2h. • Apply positioning splints as needed.
The patient is without evidence of complications related to immobility.	• Turn and reposition q2h. • Consider kinetic therapy. • Consider deep venous thrombosis (DVT) prophylaxis.
There is no evidence of infection.	• Maintain strict sterile technique, and monitor technique of others. • Maintain sterility of invasive catheters and tubes. • Per hospital protocol, change dressings and invasive catheters. Culture wounds, blood, urine, as necessary. • Monitor SIRS criteria: increased WBC count, increased temperature, tachypnea, tachycardia.
Skin Integrity	
Unburned skin is without evidence of skin breakdown.	• Assess skin q4h and each time the patient is repositioned. • Turn q2h. • Consider pressure relief/reduction mattress.
Burns begin healing without complications.	• Treat burns per facility protocol; apply topical medications and debride as indicated. • Monitor skin graft viability. • Protect grafted areas (eg, bed cradle, dressings). • Consider air-fluidized bed to enhance healing and relieve pressure from burned surface.
Nutrition	
Nutritional intake meets calculated metabolic need (eg, basal energy expenditure equation).	• Provide parenteral or enteral nutrition within 24 hours of injury. • Consult dietitian for metabolic needs assessment and recommendations. • Monitor protein and calorie intake. • Monitor albumin, prealbumin, transferrin, cholesterol, triglycerides, glucose.
Comfort/Pain Control	
The patient will indicate/exhibit adequate relief of discomfort/pain.	• Assess pain and discomfort using objective pain scale q4h, PRN, and following administration of pain medication. • Administer analgesics before procedures, and monitor the patient response. • Use nonpharmacological pain management techniques.
Psychosocial	
The patient demonstrates decreased anxiety.	• Assess vital signs during treatments, discussions, and so forth. • Administer sedatives before treatments/procedures. • Consult social services, clergy, and so forth as appropriate. • Provide for adequate rest and sleep. • Encourage discussion regarding long-term effects of burns, available resources, and coping strategies.
Teaching/Discharge Planning	
The patient and family understand procedures and tests needed for treatment.	• Prepare the patient and family for procedures such as debridement, escharotomy, fasciotomy, intubation, and mechanical ventilation.

absorption of the drug is unpredictable when administered intramuscularly. Patient-controlled analgesia (PCA) is ideal for patients who are awake and sufficiently oriented to use the pump. Patients are also given anxiolytics for anxiety related to appearance, procedures, and fear.

Providing Wound Care

Cleansing

Wound-cleansing protocols vary according to facility. Most commonly, protocols state that at each dressing change, the burn wounds are to be cleansed with water and chlorhexidine and observed for signs of infection and rate of healing. Many burn centers employ hydrotherapy because the warm, flowing water helps to loosen exudates and clean the wound. Range-of-motion exercises are also provided as part of hydrotherapy. Because hydrotherapy is usually painful, patients should receive an analgesic 20 to 30 minutes before the procedure and small, frequent doses throughout as needed. Limiting the duration of the procedure to 20 minutes is important for the patient's pain tolerance and to prevent hypothermia.

Application of Topical Antimicrobial Agents

Common antimicrobial agents used in the treatment of burn injuries are summarized in Table 32-2. No single agent is totally effective against all burn wound infections. The choice of agent depends on the wound depth, location, condition, and on the presence of specific organisms.

Water-soluble topical agents are preferred because they do not hold in heat and macerate the wound. With the application of any topical agent, it is important to use sterile technique. Antimicrobial creams should be applied to the thickness recommended by the manufacturer and reapplied at the necessary frequency to maintain consistent coverage.

 RED FLAG! *The application of topical antimicrobial agents inhibits the rate of wound epithelialization and may increase the metabolic rate. Electrolyte imbalances (eg, sodium leaching by silver nitrate) and acid–base abnormalities may occur.*

Debridement

Eschar covers the burn wound until it is excised or has separated spontaneously. It is desirable to debride the eschar and perform skin graft closure before the eschar becomes infected. However, systemic complications such as hypovolemia or sepsis may delay this course of action.

Small burn wounds may be allowed to separate on their own if there is no evidence of infection. Larger burn wounds may require mechanical or chemical debridement. Mechanical debridement is accomplished surgically by applying wet-to-dry dressings or mechanically scrubbing. In surgical debridement, the wound is excised to viable bleeding points while minimizing the loss of viable tissue. Surgical excision should be done as soon as the patient is hemodynamically stable, usually within 72 hours. After excision is complete, hemostasis is achieved by spraying topical thrombin on the wound or applying sponges soaked in a 1:10,000 epinephrine solution. After removal of necrotic tissue, the exposed underlying structures are dressed with a temporary or permanent covering to provide protection and prevent infection.

TABLE 32-2   Topical Antimicrobial Agents Used in the Treatment of Burns

Medication	Advantages	Disadvantages	Nursing Implications
Mafenide acetate	Broad-spectrum, penetrates eschar within 3 h of application	Painful application, acid–base imbalances (metabolic acidosis)	Apply twice a day, leave open to air Administer Bicitra to correct acidosis
Silver nitrate	Painless application, broad-spectrum, rare sensitivity	No eschar penetration, discolors wound and environmental surfaces, must be kept moist	Wet-to-wet dressing with nonadherant layer, followed by a gauze layer every 24 h
Silver sulfadiazene	Painless application, broad-spectrum, easy application	May cause transient leukopenia, minimal eschar penetration	Apply a moderate layer and wrap in a gauze dressing every 12 h Monitor serial complete blood counts (CBCs)
Bacitracin	Painless application, nonirritating	No eschar penetration, antimicrobial spectrum not as wide as other agents	Apply a thin layer and nonadherant dressing; if used on face, leave open to air
Mupirocin	Antimicrobial spectrum broader than bacitracin	Expensive	Apply a thin layer and nonadherant dressing; if used on face, leave open to air
Neomycin	Painless application	Antimicrobial spectrum not as wide as other agents	Apply a thin layer and nonadherant dressing; if used on face, leave open to air

Chemical debridement is the application of a proteolytic substance to burn wounds to shorten the time of eschar separation. The wound is cleaned and debrided of any loose necrotic material; the agent is applied directly to the wound bed and covered with a layer of fine-mesh gauze; a topical antimicrobial agent is applied; and the entire area is covered with saline-soaked gauze. The dressing is changed two to four times per day. Chemical debridement has the advantage of eliminating the need for surgical excision. However, because hypovolemia may occur as a result of excessive fluid loss through the wound, burns of more than 20% TBSA should not be treated in this manner.

Grafts

The ideal substitute for lost skin is an autograft of similar color, texture, and thickness from a close location on the body. Sheets of the patient's epidermis and a partial layer of the dermis are harvested from unburned locations. These grafts, referred to as split-thickness skin grafts, can be applied to the wound as a sheet graft or a mesh graft. In a sheet graft, the harvested skin is applied to the surgically excised area. In a mesh graft, the harvested skin is slit and then placed on the burn site. The slits allow the skin to expand, providing for greater coverage and facilitating draping over uneven surfaces.

Grafts must be inspected frequently to ensure that fluid is not collecting underneath them. Fluid accumulation is prevented by rolling a cotton-tipped applicator over the graft to express any trapped fluid. Small incisions may be made in a sheet graft to allow for improved drainage. After adherence has begun, usually after 24 hours, the fluid may be removed with a very small-gauge needle (26-gauge) to avoid disrupting the adherence of the graft.

Dressings are used after surgery to immobilize the grafted area and prevent shearing and dislodging of the graft. Postoperative dressings also provide compression to minimize hematoma and seroma formation, but they may be a source of vascular compression in the extremities. Pulse checks distal to the dressings are documented every 4 hours for 24 hours after surgery. The dressings are usually left in place until the third postoperative day. Until that time, the dressings are moistened every 6 hours with a solution containing normal saline and polymyxin. On postoperative day 3, the dressings are removed and the physician evaluates the success of the grafting. The grafted area is then covered with a nonadherent dressing and a gauze layer, which are secured with a gauze roll. All components of the dressing are moistened with the antibiotic solution.

The donor site is covered during surgery with a single layer of fine-mesh gauze. The gauze is kept dry and in place until separation from the donor site begins. Positioning to prevent pressure on the site and to allow for drying is important, as is daily inspection to detect early signs of infection or cellulitis.

Itching is common as healing occurs. Massaging a mild, nonirritating lotion into the healed skin provides lubrication, aids in range of motion, and promotes circulation.

Providing Psychological Support

Providing psychological support for the patient and the family is an important task of the critical care nurse. On admission, the patient most often is awake, alert, anxious, and overwhelmed by the suddenness and magnitude of injuries. Family members are also often afraid and anxious. The physical appearance of the patient and the high-technology atmosphere of the burn unit are overwhelming. Preparing the family for the initial visit by explaining what to expect and escorting them to the bedside is extremely important.

Weekly meetings of the healthcare team and the family to discuss the patient's care plan, progress, and prognosis can be useful. Critically ill patients with burns are likely to experience a series of small gains combined with intermittent setbacks, and this pattern does not stop until the burn wounds are closed, which can be 2 to 3 months after injury. Although the patient tends to concentrate on the present, the family members look to the future and want to know what to expect. The nurse provides the family with information about the patient's condition and treatments using an honest and open approach.

Rehabilitative Phase

Patients with extensive burns require many months for recovery and rehabilitation. Physical and psychological rehabilitation measures are begun in the critical care unit and continued throughout the recovery period.

CASE STUDY

Mr. M., 29 years old, was in an industrial fire caused by an indoor explosion at his job. He was able to get out of the building unassisted. An ambulance transported Mr. M. to the emergency department of the nearest hospital, where he arrived 45 minutes after the fire. Mr. M.'s burn is estimated to cover 60% of his total-body surface area (TBSA).

Mr. M. is well nourished and in relatively good health. He does not use tobacco products or recreational drugs, but he does drink about one case of beer per week. He has no significant medical or surgical history. There is no hypertension, cardiac or renal disease, diabetes, or cancer in his family history. The nurse taking Mr. M.'s history notes that his voice is hoarse.

Physical assessment reveals burns to the face with singed nasal and facial hairs. The presence of carbonaceous sputum is noted in the mouth. Mr. M. is also found to have circumferential burns of the upper extremities (bilaterally), the anterior torso, portions of the posterior torso, and scattered areas of the lower extremities (bilaterally). Mr. M. states that his usual weight is 154 lb (70 kg).

For airway protection, Mr. M. is intubated, and a nasogastric tube is inserted. IV catheters are placed in the bilateral upper extremities, and an indwelling urinary catheter is inserted. Tetanus immunization is given prophylactically. IV analgesics are given in small, frequent doses as indicated for pain.

The regional burn center is contacted and transport arranged. Mr. M. is wrapped in clean, dry dressings and wool blankets and airlifted. A copy of all documentation is sent with him. When Mr. M. arrives 3 hours after the accident, the healthcare team at the burn center confirms his airway and assesses his pulses with a focus on the upper extremities secondary to the circumferential burns. Pulses are present in all distal extremities but slightly diminished bilaterally in the upper extremities.

Mr. M.'s initial vital signs are: HR, 144 beats/min; BP, 108/58 mm Hg; RR (assisted via the ventilator with a set rate), 12 breaths/min; and temp, 96.8°F (36.0°C). Breath sounds are auscultated with coarse rhonchi. The cardiac monitor demonstrates sinus tachycardia without ectopy. An arterial line and central line are placed in the left femoral artery and vein, respectively. Admission laboratory studies are sent. A chest x-ray is taken. Due to his circumferential burns, distal pulses are assessed at least every hour. The upper-extremity pulses are difficult to palpate and are confirmed with Doppler ultrasound. Bronchoscopy is performed, revealing carbonaceous material in the bilateral upper airways with reddening throughout; the bilateral lower airways appear to be uninjured. A continuous infusion of fentanyl and midazolam is given for analgesic relief and sedation, with additional dosing as indicated.

When resuscitation is well under way, the Lund–Browder chart is used to calculate the burn wound size; it is found to be 44% TBSA. Full-thickness (third-degree) burns account for 36% of the injuries; the texture is leathery, and the surface dry with thrombosed vessels. The remaining partial-thickness burns are reddened, moist, and weeping serous fluid where thin-walled blisters have ruptured. Mr. M. reports that these are very painful to palpation.

Mr. M.'s initial fluid requirements are calculated using the concensus formula, and determined to be 3080 mL (385 mL/h) over the first 8 hours (from the time of the burn injury), followed by 3080 (193 mL/h) over the next 16 hours. It is now 3 hours since the time of the burn. Mr. M. had received 750 mL at the transferring facility and 350 mL while in transport, which means that he needs an additional 1980 mL of fluid to satisfy the requirements for the first

8 hours from the time of the burn. This amount is divided over the remaining 5 hours to determine that Mr. M. should receive 396 mL/h. Since the placement of the urinary catheter, Mr. M's urine output has been 180 mL (an average of 60 mL/h). Although this is currently adequate, it will be closely monitored because it has been trending down.

Mr. M. is taken to the shower room, and all wounds are manually debrided. The following topical agents are applied: silver sulfadiazine cream to all partial-thickness and full-thickness burns, bacitracin ophthalmic around the eyes and bacitracin ointment to the rest of the face, and mafenide acetate (Sulfamylon) cream to the ears. A pressure relief mattress is ordered to decrease Mr. M.'s risk for skin breakdown, with particular concern for the occiput, sacrum, and heels. The head of the bed is elevated to 30 degrees, and the bilateral upper extremities are placed in airplane slings to elevate the hands and abduct the axilla.

Selected initial laboratory results are as follows: Na$^+$, 143 mEq/L; K$^+$, 3.5 mEq/L; chloride, 107 mEq/L; blood urea nitrogen (BUN), 19.0 mg/dL; creatinine, 0.9 mg/dL; white blood cell (WBC) count, 18,100 cells/mm^3; and hematocrit, 47.6%. Urine outputs for hours 6 and 7 from the time of the burn are 23 and 17 mL, respectively, and the IV rate of fluid administration is increased by 20% to 475 mL/h.

Nine hours after the burn, Mr. M.'s forearms are tight and edematous, and pulses in the upper extremities are no longer present per Doppler. Fluid resuscitation appears controlled; Mr. M. is not hypotensive, with a blood pressure of 112/63 mm Hg. His heart rate has decreased so that it is within the expected range (128 beats/min), and his urinary output is adequate (43 mL last hour). Escharotomies are performed to the medial and lateral aspects of both arms and the dorsum of the hands. Pulses are immediately palpable at the conclusion of this procedure. A small-bore feeding tube is placed, and a nutrient-dense tube feeding is started and increased slowly as tolerated.

Albumin 5% is added to Mr. M.'s fluid resuscitation during the second 24 hours at 39 mL/h (0.3 mL/70 kg/44% TBSA for 30% to 49% TBSA burn). The burn wounds are to be cleansed twice a day with 4% chlorhexidine gluconate soap. Alternating solutions are applied to all burn wounds except the face, with mafenide acetate in the morning and silver sulfadiazine in the evening. Mafenide acetate is always applied to the ears, with bacitracin to the face and bacitracin ophthalmic around the eyes. Nursing and rehabilitative personnel provide passive range of motion to all major joints frequently, with particular attentiveness to the hands.

Mr. M. is taken to the operating room on postburn day 3 for a full excision and grafting. The sheet graft is observed hourly for the first 24 hours postoperatively; blebs are rolled to ensure that grafts adhere. After this time, small hematomas are aspirated using a tuberculin syringe. Donor sites are elevated on leg nets to expose to the air. Heat lamps are used at low settings to assist with drying.

Mr. M. is weaned from the ventilator postoperatively and extubated the morning of postburn day 5. Aggressive bronchial hygiene therapy (BHT) is initiated to reduce the risk for pneumonia. Mr. M. is started on vancomycin for burn wound cellulitis, which is stopped after 5 days when resolved. Mr. M. is assisted to the bedside chair on postoperative day 5 (postburn day 8), and diet is advanced as tolerated. He is assisted to the standing table on postoperative day 9 (postburn day 12). When Mr. M. is tolerating 50% of his daily caloric needs orally, enteral feeds are changed to only night feeds and stopped when he is tolerating more than 75%. He begins ambulating on postoperative day 11 (postburn day 14) and is transferred to the ward.

1. Discuss the clinical rationale for performing prophylactic intubation of Mr. M. before transport, versus waiting to see if he develops respiratory compromise.

2. How is a neurovascular assessment performed in a patient who is intubated?

3. How does the use of alcohol relate to potential complications for the fluid resuscitation of Mr. M.?

4. Discuss the pathophysiological effect of circumferential burns on Mr. M's peripheral perfusion.

5. Discuss why only the partial-thickness (second-degree) and full-thickness (third-degree) burns are considered, and not the superficial (first-degree) burns, when calculating the TBSA for fluid replacement.

6. Discuss the potential complications of under-resuscitation and over-resuscitation of patients with burns.

References

1. Boots R, et al.: Respiratory complications in burns: An evolving spectrum of injury. Clin Pulm Med 16(3): 132–138, 2009
2. Warden GD: Fluid resuscitation and early management. In Herndon DN (ed): Total Burn Care, 3rd ed. Philadelphia, PA: Saunders, 2007, pp 107–118
3. LaBorde PJ: Management of patients with burn injury. In Smeltzer SC, Bare BG (eds): Brunner and Suddarth's Textbook of Medical-Surgical Nursing, 10th ed. Philadelphia, PA: Lippincott Williams & Wilkins, 2004, pp 1703–1745
4. Hedman TL, Quick CD, Richard RL, et al: Rehabilitation of burn casualties. In Pasquina PF, Copper RA (ed): Care of the Combat Amputee. District of Columbia: Borden Institute, 2009, pp 277–379

Want to know more? A wide variety of resources to enhance your learning and understanding of this chapter are available on the**Point** ✳. Visit **http://thepoint.lww.com/MortonEss1e** to access chapter review questions and more!

ELEVEN

Multisystem Dysfunction

Shock and Multisystem Organ Dysfunction Syndrome

OBJECTIVES

Based on the content in this chapter, the reader should be able to:

1 Describe common pathophysiological processes involved in the generalized shock response.
2 Describe the pathophysiology, assessment, and management of the major types of shock.
3 Describe the relationship between sepsis, systemic inflammatory response syndrome (SIRS), severe sepsis, septic shock, and multisystem organ dysfunction syndrome (MODS).

Shock

Clinical conditions that result in cellular hypoperfusion are often referred to as shock states. Although shock states have different causes and different presentations, they all share some similar features, such as hypoperfusion, hypercoagulability, and activation of the inflammatory response. In hypoperfused states, the lack of sufficient oxygen causes the cells to convert to anaerobic metabolism. Anaerobic metabolism is not an efficient method of energy production, and the adenosine triphosphate (ATP) produced is insufficient to meet cellular demands.

Anaerobic metabolism also produces lactic acid as a by-product, leading to metabolic acidosis. If oxygen continues to be insufficient to meet cellular demands for energy, cell death ensues. As more cells die, tissues and organs become progressively dysfunctional and eventually end-organ failure ensues.

Shock is believed to progress through three increasingly severe stages. Although the stages are not always easily identified, they identify shock as a progressive, rather than a static, process. Timely reversal of the shock state prevents development of multiple end-organ failure and death—hence the phrase "time is tissue."

• **Stage 1.** During states of shock, the body activates compensatory mechanisms (Fig. 33-1) in an effort to maintain circulatory volume, blood pressure, and cardiac output. During this initial, nonprogressive stage, compensatory mechanisms are effective in maintaining relatively normal vital signs and cerebral perfusion, and the shock state often goes unrecognized. If the cause of the shock is successfully treated at this time, the patient may make a full recovery.

 The Older Patient. *Normal physiologic changes that occur with aging may limit the body's ability to respond effectively to shock states.*

• **Stage 2.** In the intermediate, progressive phase, compensatory mechanisms begin to fail, metabolic and circulatory derangements become more pronounced, and the inflammatory and immune responses may become fully activated. Signs of dysfunction in one or more organs may become apparent. Interventions that target both the cause of the shock and the resulting metabolic,

circulatory, and inflammatory responses are necessary to save the patient's life.
• **Stage 3.** In the final, irreversible stage, cellular and tissue injury are so severe that the patient's life is not sustainable even if metabolic, circulatory, and inflammatory derangements are corrected. At this point, full-blown multisystem organ dysfunction syndrome (MODS) may become evident.

🛑 **RED FLAG!** *The patient's clinical presentation depends on the cause of the shock state and the degree of compensation, but altered level of consciousness, tachypnea, tachycardia, hypotension, decreased urine output, and metabolic acidosis are commonly seen in all states of hypoperfusion.*

When treating patients in shock states, the goals are to reestablish adequate organ perfusion and oxygenation and to lessen the inflammatory response as quickly as possible. Early recognition of the shock state and ongoing assessments to evaluate the effectiveness of interventions and identify progression of

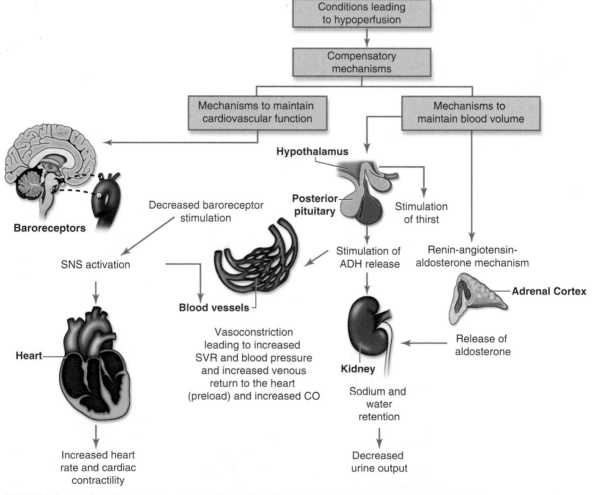

FIGURE 33-1 Compensatory mechanisms. During states of low perfusion (low blood pressure), compensatory mechanisms are initiated and result in increases in heart rate, systemic vascular resistance (SVR), preload, and cardiac contractility in an effort to restore appropriate circulatory volume. ADH, antidiuretic hormone; CO, cardiac output; SNS, sympathetic nervous system.

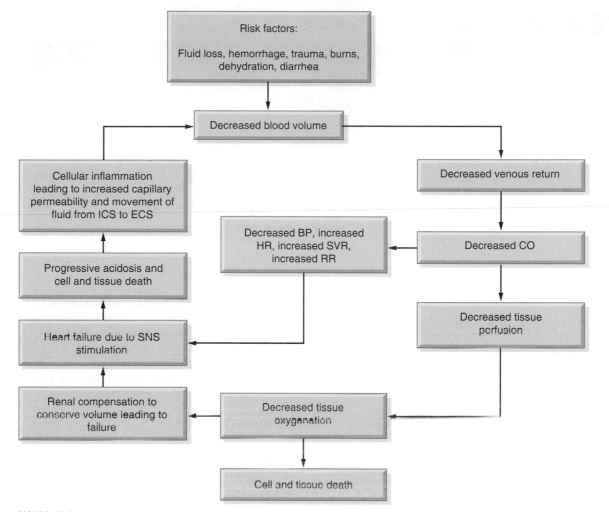

FIGURE 33-2 Pathophysiology of hypovolemic shock. BP, blood pressure; CO, cardiac output; ECS, extracellular space; HR, heart rate; ICS, intracellular space; RR, respiratory rate; SNS, sympathetic nervous system; SVR, systemic vascular resistance.

the shock state are key. Assessments such as gastric pH, sublingual end-tidal carbon dioxide ($ETCO_2$), and central venous oxygen saturation measurements may facilitate earlier recognition of hypoperfusion.

Shock can be classified as hypovolemic, cardiogenic, or distributive.

Hypovolemic Shock

Hypovolemic shock is a result of inadequate circulating blood volume, which may be caused by sudden blood loss, severe dehydration, or injuries that cause significant fluid shifts from the intravascular space to the interstitial space (eg, burns).

 The Older Patient. *Severe dehydration is the most common cause of hypovolemic shock in older patients.*

Pathophysiology

The pathophysiology of hypovolemic shock is summarized in Figure 33-2. Acute fluid volume loss does not allow the normal compensatory mechanisms to restore an appropriate circulating volume rapidly enough, resulting in cellular hypoperfusion, anaerobic metabolism, lactic acidosis, and electrolyte and acid–base disturbances. The existing blood volume is shunted to the vital organs (ie, the heart, lungs, and brain), exacerbating the hypoperfusion of other organs (eg, the liver, stomach, and kidneys) and putting the patient at risk for organ dysfunction and failure. Complications associated with hypovolemic shock depend on the length of time and the severity of the hypotensive crisis. Complications may range from renal damage to cerebral anoxia and death.

Assessment

A thorough history may reveal underlying causes of hypovolemic shock (eg, use of nonsteroidal anti-inflammatory drugs [NSAIDs], which can cause upper gastrointestinal bleeding). Clinical findings are related to the severity and acuity of volume loss (Table 33-1).

Assessment of serum lactate, arterial pH, and base deficit helps determine the presence of acidosis due to anaerobic metabolism and facilitates

TABLE 33-1 Clinical Findings in Hypovolemic Shock

Estimated Blood Loss	Tachycardia	Hypotension	Urine Output	Pulses	Hemodynamics
500–1,000 mL	↑ HR > 20% patient's baseline	↓ SBP > 10% patient's baseline	Decreased	Weaker	Within normal limits CO, ↑ SVR
1,000–2,000 mL	↑ HR > 20%–30% patient's baseline	↓ SBP > 10%–20% patient's baseline	Decreased (< 30 mL/hr)	Poor peripheral pulses	↓ CO, ↑ SVR
2,000–3,000 mL	↑ HR > 20%–30% patient's baseline	↓ SBP > 10%–20% patient's baseline	Oliguria → anuria	Poor peripheral pulses	↓ CO, ↑ SVR

SBP, systolic blood pressure; SVR, systemic vascular resistance; CO, cardiac output; RR, respirations; HR, heart rate.

monitoring the effectiveness of fluid replacement therapy. In the presence of metabolic acidosis, lactic acid levels are increased and the base deficit becomes greater. A normalization of the base deficit is a good indicator of improvement of metabolic acidosis and tissue perfusion. Serial hemoglobin and hematocrit and coagulation panels are used to assess the need for blood product replacement. However, for several reasons (eg, delayed decrease in the hematocrit following acute blood loss, hemoconcentration caused by dehydration, or hemodilution caused by IV fluid therapy), the hemoglobin and hematocrit may not directly reflect the severity of blood loss.

Management

Management of hypovolemic shock focuses on resolving the cause of volume loss and restoring circulating volume through volume administration. Ideally, a large-bore (16-gauge or larger) IV catheter is used for the rapid infusion of fluids. Fluids are warmed during infusion to limit the negative effects of hypothermia. Isotonic crystalloid solutions (eg, lactated Ringer's solution, 0.9% normal saline) are used primarily as first-line therapy. Blood products and other colloid solutions (albumin and synthetic volume expanders) may be used to assist in the resuscitation process, especially if blood loss is the primary cause. Complications associated with fluid resuscitation are given in Table 33-2.

Cardiogenic Shock

Cardiogenic shock, which results from loss of contractility of the heart, is an extreme form of heart failure. The most common cause of cardiogenic shock is extensive left ventricular damage from myocardial infarction. Other causes of cardiogenic shock include papillary muscle rupture, ventricular septal rupture, cardiomyopathy, acute myocarditis, valvular disease, and dysrrhythmias.

RED FLAG! *Factors associated with the development of cardiogenic shock include advanced age, left ventricular ejection fraction less than 35%, large anterior wall myocardial infarction, history of diabetes mellitus, and previous myocardial infarction. Patients with all five of these risk factors have a greater than 50% chance of developing cardiogenic shock.*

Pathophysiology

The pathophysiology of cardiogenic shock is shown in Figure 33-3. Loss of ventricular contractility decreases stroke volume and cardiac output. In response to the decreased cardiac output, neuroendocrine compensatory mechanisms (see Fig. 33-1, p. 458) are activated, increasing preload through retention of sodium and water and afterload (systemic vascular resistance [SVR]) through vasoconstriction.

TABLE 33-2 Complications Associated with Volume Resuscitation

Fluid Type	Potential Complications
Crystalloid and colloid	Dilutional coagulopathy Dilutional thrombocytopenia Hypothermia Increased hemorrhage Decreased blood viscosity Pulmonary edema Intracranial hypertension (in patients with traumatic brain injury)
Packed red blood cells (PRBCs)	Acidosis (pH of banked blood is 6.9–7.1) Left shift on the oxyhemoglobin dissociation curve (banked blood is deficient in 2,3-DPG, causing an increased affinity of hemoglobin for oxygen) Hyperkalemia Immunologic and infectious complications

Acidosis	Skin	Tachypnea	Oxygen Saturation	SvO$_2$	Level of Consciousness
Mild	Cool to touch	...	...	...	...
Progressive	Cool, diaphoretic	↑ RR > 10% patient's baseline	May not be altered depending on percentage of exogenous O$_2$ patient is receiving	< 60%	Restlessness, agitation, confusion, obtunded
Severe	Cold, pallor	↑ RR > 10%–20% patient's baseline	Decreased	<55%–60%	Stuporous

These compensatory mechanisms further impair cardiac output, exacerbating the problem.

Assessment

Cardiogenic shock commonly develops within a few hours after the onset of myocardial infarction symptoms; therefore, patients admitted with a diagnosis of myocardial infarction require close monitoring. Hallmarks of cardiogenic shock are progressive hemodynamic compromise and clinical deterioration (Box 33-1).

Management

The goals of patient management for cardiogenic shock are to optimize cardiac output and decrease left ventricular workload.

Optimizing Cardiac Output

Careful monitoring and interpretation of hemodynamic parameters is necessary to achieve the goal of optimizing cardiac output. Optimal filling pressures assist in restoring cardiac output but must be attained cautiously. In general, a preload (left ventricular end-diastolic pressure [LVEDP]) of 14 to 18 mm Hg should be maintained. If the left ventricular filling pressure is too low, fluids may be used to optimize cardiac output; if it is too high, diuresis may be necessary.

Pharmacological agents (Table 33-3) can be used to augment cardiac output by increasing contractility, but they, too, must be used cautiously. Many agents can increase cardiac output but have an appreciable effect on myocardial oxygen demand.

Dysrhythmias often occur with acute myocardial infarction, ischemia, or acid–base imbalances

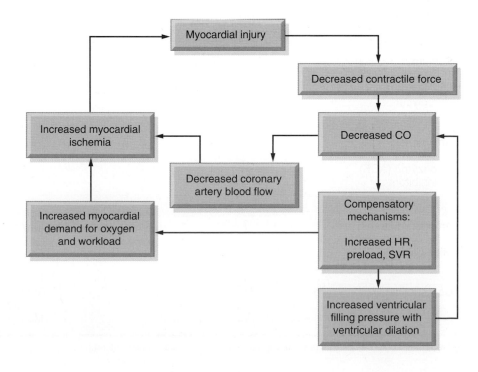

FIGURE 33-3 Pathophysiology of cardiogenic shock. CO, cardiac output; HR, heart rate; SVR, systemic vascular resistance.

BOX 33-1 Clinical Manifestations of Cardiogenic Shock

Hemodynamic Findings
- Systolic blood pressure less than 90 mm Hg
- Mean arterial pressure (MAP) less than 70 mm Hg
- Cardiac index less than 2.2 L/min/m²
- Pulmonary artery occlusion pressure (PAOP) greater than 18 mm Hg

History and Physical Examination Findings
- Thready, rapid pulse
- Narrow pulse pressure
- Distended neck veins
- Dyspnea
- Increased respiratory rate
- Inspiratory crackles, possible wheezing
- Dysrhythmias

- Chest pain
- Cool, pale, moist skin
- Oliguria
- Decreased mentation

Laboratory Findings
- Decreased arterial oxygen saturation (PaO_2)
- Respiratory alkalosis
- Elevated myocardial tissue markers, such as creatine kinase (CK-MB), cardiac troponin, and brain-type natriuretic peptide (BNP)

Radiographic Findings
- Enlarged heart
- Pulmonary congestion

TABLE 33-3 Medications Used in the Treatment of Shock[a]

Drug Category	Heart Rate	Contractility	Systemic Venous Resistance	Nursing Implications
Vasoconstrictors				
Dopamine (Intropin)	↑	↑↑	↑	Hemodynamic effects are dose dependent
Epinephrine (Adrenaline)	↑↑	↑↑	↑	May induce ventricular dysrhythmias; May increase myocardial oxygen demands; β_2 Activity may dilate peripheral beds
Norepinephrine (levarterenol [Levophed])	↑	↑	↑↑↑	Monitor peripheral circulation and urine output closely; may increase myocardial oxygen demands
Phenylephrine (Neosynephrine)			↑↑	May induce dysrhythmias
Vasopressin (Pitressin)		↑	↑↑	Monitor peripheral circulation closely; may increase myocardial oxygen demands
Vasodilators				
Sodium nitroprusside (Nipride)	↑		↓↓	Hemodynamic effects are dose dependent; adjust dosage slowly
Nitroglycerine (Tridil)	↑		↓	Hemodynamic effects are dose dependent; adjust dosage slowly; tolerance may develop
Angiotensin-converting enzyme (ACE) inhibitors	↑		↓	Initial dose may be less than goal dose to prevent hypotension
Inotropic Agents				
Amrinone (Inocor)	↑	↑	↓	May exacerbate myocardial oxygen demands
Milrinone (Primacor)	↑	↑↑	↓	May exacerbate myocardial oxygen demands; Monitor for tachyarrhythmias
Dobutamine (Dobutrex)	↑	↑↑	↓	May exacerbate myocardial oxygen demands; Monitor for tachyarrhythmias

[a]All agents should be administered through a great vein (central access) using a volumetric pump.

and can further decrease cardiac output. Correction with antidysrhythmic agents, cardioversion, or pacing can help to restore a stable heart rhythm and enhance cardiac output. Potassium, calcium, and magnesium may need to be replaced to provide optimal conditions for the damaged myocardial muscle.

Decreasing Left Ventricular Workload

Management of cardiogenic shock also focuses on conserving myocardial energy and decreasing the demands on the heart. Decreasing left ventricular workload can be accomplished in a variety of ways:

- **Pharmacotherapy.** Vasodilators may be administered to reduce SVR and LVEDP. Narcotic analgesics and sedatives may also be used to decrease myocardial oxygen demand.
- **Mechanical support devices,** such as an intra-aortic balloon pump (IABP) or left ventricular assist device, supplement the heart's ability to pump, reducing workload.
- **Mechanical ventilation** may be necessary to increase oxygen saturation, improving oxygen delivery to the tissues.
- **Scheduling physical care** to ensure periods of rest also helps to minimize myocardial energy expenditure.

Distributive Shock

The mechanism underlying all distributive shock states is vasodilation that causes decreased venous return. Distributive shock states include neurogenic shock, anaphylactic shock, and septic shock. In neurogenic shock, vasodilation results from a loss of sympathetic innervation to the blood vessels. In both anaphylactic shock and septic shock, vasodilation results from the presence of vasodilating substances in the blood.

Neurogenic Shock

Neurogenic shock results from loss or disruption of sympathetic tone, most often due to severe cervical or upper thoracic spinal cord injury. Because the sympathetic system is impaired, signs and symptoms of neurogenic shock are indicative of parasympathetic stimulation and include hypotension, severe bradycardia, and warm, dry skin. Initial management includes volume resuscitation to refill the vascular space with fluids. If the patient remains hypotensive despite the fluid resuscitation, then vasoconstrictors may be used. Typically, the bradycardia does not need to be treated. If the patient is symptomatic due to the bradycardia, external pacing may be used.

Anaphylactic Shock

Anaphylaxis is an allergic reaction to a specific allergen that evokes a life-threatening hypersensitivity response. Many different antigens (ie, substances that elicit the allergic response) are capable of evoking

anaphylaxis in humans (Box 33-2). Anaphylaxis may be either immunoglobulin E (IgE)– or non–IgE mediated:

- **IgE-mediated anaphylaxis** occurs as a result of the immune response to a specific antigen. The first time the immune system is exposed to the antigen, a very specific IgE antibody is formed and circulates in the blood. When a second exposure to this antigen occurs, the antigen binds to this circulating IgE, which then activates the immune system, triggering the release of chemical mediators that initiate anaphylaxis.
- **Non-IgE responses (anaphylactoid reactions)** occur without the presence of IgE antibodies, and can occur the first time the person is exposed to the antigen. Direct activation of mediators causes this response. Anaphylactoid reactions are commonly associated with NSAIDs, including aspirin.

The antibody–antigen reaction causes the white blood cells (WBCs) to secrete chemical mediators that cause systemic vasodilation, increased capillary permeability, bronchoconstriction, coronary vasoconstriction, and urticaria (hives). The diffuse arterial vasodilation causes maldistribution of blood volume to tissues, and venous dilation decreases preload, thus decreasing cardiac output. Increased capillary permeability leads to loss of vascular volume, further decreasing cardiac output and subsequently impairing tissue perfusion. Death due to circulatory collapse or extreme bronchoconstriction (resulting in loss of airway) may occur within minutes or hours.

 RED FLAG! Initial symptoms of anaphylaxis include generalized erythema, itching, urticaria, and difficulty breathing due to bronchoconstriction. The earlier the symptoms of anaphylaxis appear after exposure to the antigen, the more severe the response.

Assessment

A thorough history of allergies is used to avoid known allergens and is the best way to prevent anaphylactic

BOX 33-3 Clinical Manifestations of Anaphylaxis

Early Clinical Manifestations
- Generalized erythema
- Urticaria
- Pruritus
- Anxiety and restlessness
- Dyspnea
- Wheezing
- Chest tightness
- Feeling of warmth
- Nausea and vomiting
- Angioedema
- Abdominal pain

Later Clinical Manifestations
- Stridor
- Laryngeal edema
- Severe bronchoconstriction with stridor
- Hypotension leading to circulatory collapse
- Deterioration of level of consciousness to unresponsiveness

shock. Anaphylactic shock may occur without any known predisposing factors. Clinical manifestations of anaphylaxis are summarized in Box 33-3.

Management
Early recognition of anaphylaxis and prompt intervention is critical. Therapeutic goals include removal of the offending antigen, reversal of the effects of chemical mediators, and restoration of adequate tissue perfusion. Regardless of the cause of the anaphylactic reaction, treatment depends on clinical symptoms. If the symptoms are mild, immediate therapy includes oxygen; subcutaneous or IV administration of an antihistamine to block the effects of histamine; and possibly an epinephrine injection to reverse the vasodilation and broncho-constriction (Box 33-4).[1] More severe reactions may also require the administration of corticosteroids,

BOX 33-4 Epinephrine Dosage in Anaphylaxis (Adults)

If IV Access is Not Available:
- Epinephrine, 0.01 mg/kg (maximum, 0.5 mg) IM into anterolateral thigh (absorption is greatest here)
- Proceed to obtain IV access.

If IV Access is Available:
- Administer epinephrine, 1 mg in 100 mL (10 µg/mL; 1:100,000) IV by infusion pump.
- Initiate infusion at 30 to 100 mL/h (5 to 17 µg/min) and titrate to response aiming for lowest effective infusion rate.
- Stop infusion 30 minutes after signs and symptoms have resolved.

bronchodilators, or both. In some cases, intubation and mechanical ventilation are required. If the patient is experiencing circulatory collapse, vasoconstrictors and positive inotropic agents may be administered.

Other nursing priorities include monitoring the patient's response to the treatment and providing care to relieve dermatological manifestations. Once the immediate crisis is resolved, if the agent causing the anaphylaxis is unknown, the patient should be evaluated for allergies and future risk for anaphylaxis.

Septic Shock
Sepsis, SIRS, severe sepsis, septic shock, and MODS represent progressive stages of the septic process (Box 33-5). Sepsis is initiated by an infection, which may be caused by gram-negative or gram-positive bacteria, fungi, or viruses. In many patients, there are multiple causative organisms. Both host factors and treatment-related factors put patients at risk for developing sepsis and associated

BOX 33-5 Sepsis and Other Associated Clinical Conditions

Sepsis: The systemic response to known infection, manifested by two or more of the following conditions as a result of infection:
- Temperature greater than 100.4°F (38°C) or less than 96.8°F (36°C)
- Heart rate greater than 90 beats/min
- Respiratory rate greater than 20 breaths/min or arterial carbon dioxide tension $PaCO_2$ less than 32 mm Hg
- White blood cell (WBC) count greater than 12,000 cells/mm³ or less than 4000 cells/mm³ OR more than 10% immature (band) forms

Systemic inflammatory response syndrome (SIRS): The systemic inflammatory response to a severe clinical insult, manifested by the same clinical criteria as sepsis

Severe sepsis: Sepsis associated with organ dysfunction, hypoperfusion and/or hypotension; clinical manifestations of hypoperfusion may include, but are not limited to, lactic acidosis, oliguria, or an acute alteration in mental status

Septic shock: Sepsis with hypotension, despite adequate resuscitation

Multisystem organ dysfunction syndrome (MODS): Presence of altered organ function in an acutely ill patient such that homeostasis cannot be maintained without intervention

Definitions developed by the Consensus Conferences of the Society of Critical Care Medicine and the American College of Chest Physicians. Adapted from Levy MM: Definitions of sepsis revisited: Results of the SSSM/ESICM/ACCP/ATS consensus conference. In Levy MM, Vincent JL (eds): Sepsis: Pathophysiologic Insights and Current Management. Chicago, IL: Society of Critical Care Medicine, 2003, pp 39–42.

BOX 33-6 Risk Factors for Developing Sepsis and Associated Conditions

Host Factors
- Very young or very old age
- Chronic illness
- Malnutrition
- Debilitation
- Drug or alcohol abuse
- Neutropenia
- Splenectomy
- Wounds
- Multiple organ failure

Treatment-Related Factors
- Indwelling medical devices (eg, intravascular catheters, endotracheal/tracheostomy tubes, indwelling urinary catheters, surgical wound drains, intracranial monitoring devices and catheters, orthopedic hardware, nasogastric tubes, gastrointestinal tubes)
- Surgery
- Invasive diagnostic procedures
- Medications (eg, antibiotics, cytotoxic agents, steroids)

conditions (Box 33-6). Because mortality from sepsis and related conditions is so high, preventive infection control measures (eg, adherence to aseptic techniques, thorough handwashing) are imperative.

Pathophysiology

Septic shock occurs as a result of the complex interactions among invading microorganisms and the immune system, the inflammatory system, and the coagulation system.[2] In response to the presence of microorganisms, proinflammatory cytokines such as tumor necrosis factor (TNF) are released. These proinflammatory cytokines activate the immune response, complement system, and coagulation system. The activated WBCs release mediators that cause endothelial cells to lose their tight junctions, resulting in increased vascular permeability and causing protein-rich fluid to move from the vascular space into the interstitial space. To balance the proinflammatory response, anti-inflammatory cytokines (eg, interleukin-10, protein C) are released. But in some patients, these anti-inflammatory cytokines fail to shut down or control the proinflammatory cytokines, and an "out of control" inflammatory response occurs.

- **Cardiovascular alterations** in septic shock include vasodilation, maldistribution of blood flow, and myocardial depression. Proinflammatory cytokines stimulate the release of nitric oxide (a potent vasodilator) from endothelial cells, resulting in widespread vasodilation that is often resistant to vasopressor agents.[3] Other inflammatory mediators cause vasoconstriction in some vascular beds, resulting in mixed vasodilation

and vasoconstriction and producing a maldistribution of blood flow in the microcirculation. Myocardial depression is caused by myocardial depressant factors released as part of the inflammatory cascade and the release of nitric oxide. Lactic acidosis, which decreases myocardial responsiveness to catecholamines, may also be partly responsible. Myocardial depression results in a decreased ventricular ejection fraction, dilation of the ventricles, and volume overload after fluid resuscitation.[4]

- **Pulmonary alterations.** Activation of the inflammatory response and its mediators affects the lungs both directly and indirectly. Inflammatory mediators and activated neutrophils cause capillary leakage into the pulmonary interstitium, resulting in interstitial edema, areas of poor pulmonary perfusion (shunting), pulmonary hypertension, and increased respiratory work (ie, acute respiratory distress syndrome [ARDS]). As fluid collects in the interstitium, pulmonary compliance is reduced, gas exchange is impaired, and hypoxemia occurs.

- **Hematologic alterations.** The proinflammatory cytokine TNF activates the coagulation system, inducing clotting in the microcirculation (ie, disseminated intravascular coagulation [DIC]). DIC, described in more detail in Chapter 29, is a consumptive coagulopathy— the patient clots first, consumes all of his or her clotting factors, and then bleeds.

As septic shock progresses and organ hypoperfusion persists, the organs begin to fail, putting the patient at risk for developing MODS.

Assessment

Some of the earliest signs of septic shock include changes in mental status (eg, confusion, agitation), an increased respiratory rate (as compensation for the metabolic acidosis), and either hyper- or hypothermia. Early diagnosis of sepsis is typically made on the basis of sepsis/SIRS criteria (see Box 33-5). Box 33-7 summarizes laboratory and diagnostic studies that are commonly ordered in the evaluation of sepsis states.

Management

Septic shock requires prompt, aggressive, goal-directed treatment and monitoring. Initiating therapy within the first 6 hours and establishing specific hemodynamic goals for resuscitation have been shown to slow the decompensation of patients in a septic state and decrease the risk for cardiovascular collapse.[5]

Identifying and Treating Infection. Before the causal organism has been identified by the culture results, empiric broad-spectrum antibiotic therapy is initiated, usually with multiple antibiotics providing coverage against gram-negative and gram-positive bacteria and anaerobes. However, once the infectious organism has been isolated, antibiotic therapy is changed to specific antibiotics that

BOX 33-7 Laboratory and Diagnostic Studies Ordered in the Assessment of Sepsis States

- **Cultures** (blood, sputum, urine, surgical or nonsurgical wounds, sinuses, and invasive lines): Positive results are not necessary for diagnosis.
- **Complete blood count (CBC):** White blood cells (WBCs) are usually elevated and may decrease with progression of shock.
- **Sequential multiple analysis-7 (SMA-7):** Hyperglycemia may be evident, followed by hypoglycemia in later stages.
- **Arterial blood gases (ABGs):** Metabolic acidosis with possibly compensating respiratory alkalosis ($PaCO_2$ less than 35 mm Hg) is present in sepsis, with hypoxemia (PaO_2 less than 80 mm Hg).
- **Lactate level and base deficit:** Elevated levels indicate inadequate perfusion and anaerobic metabolism.
- **End-tidal carbon dioxide ($ETCO_2$) monitoring:** May detect early indications of inadequate regional and global tissue perfusion.
- **Pulmonary artery catheterization with mixed venous oxygen (SvO_2) monitoring:** Assists in the assessment of oxygen delivery and consumption.
- **Computed tomography (CT):** May identify sites of potential abscesses.
- **Chest and abdominal radiography:** May reveal infectious processes.

are effective against that organism to minimize the development of antibiotic resistance.

Providing Supportive Care. Aspects of supportive care include the following:

- **Restoring intravascular volume.** Adequate volume replacement is important for reversing hypotension, hypoperfusion, or both. Patients may require several liters or more of fluid because of mediator-induced vasodilation and capillary leak. Fluid replacement is guided by hemodynamic parameters, urine output, and indicators of metabolic acidosis ($ETCO_2$, base deficit, and lactic acid levels).[6]
- **Maintaining adequate cardiac output.** In the early phase of septic shock, cardiac output may be elevated due to decreased SVR (as a result of vasodilation). However, because of the increase in oxygen demand and the cell's inability to use the oxygen, cardiac output is not adequate to maintain tissue oxygenation and perfusion. In addition, as septic shock progresses, cardiac output may begin to decrease because of cardiac dysfunction. If adequate volume replacement does not improve tissue perfusion, vasoactive drugs are administered to support circulation.
- **Ensuring adequate ventilation and oxygenation.** Maintaining a patent airway, augmenting

EVIDENCE-BASED PRACTICE GUIDELINES
Severe Sepsis Recognition and Resuscitation

PROBLEM: Severe sepsis is associated with an extremely high mortality rate (30% to 60%) and is the leading cause of death in noncoronary critical care units. Prompt recognition and intervention can improve patient survival.

EVIDENCE-BASED PRACTICE GUIDELINES

1. Assess all patients and immediately notify the physician when a patient presents with clinical findings suggestive of sepsis.
2. Obtain serum lactate measurements. Hyperlactatemia is defined as a lactic acid level greater than 4 mmol/L. (level D)
3. Obtain blood cultures and cultures from all potential sites of infection prior to initiating broad-spectrum antibiotic therapy and within 1 hour of sepsis diagnosis. (level D)
4. Evaluate for and remove potential sources of infection (eg, obviously infected invasive devices). (level D)
5. Maintain the following therapeutic end points during resuscitation: mean arterial pressure (MAP), greater than 65 mm Hg; central venous pressure (CVP), 8 to 12 mm Hg; central venous or mixed venous oxygen saturation, greater than 70%. (level D)
   a. Administer fluids to attain a CVP of 8 to 12 mm Hg (or greater than or equal to 12 mm Hg if the patient is on a ventilator). (level D)
   b. Administer vasopressors if necessary to achieve an MAP of 65 mm Hg if fluid replacement is not successful. (level D)
   c. If venous oxygen saturation goal is not attained, consider additional fluids, blood transfusion, dobutamine administration, or all three. (level D)
6. Maintain blood glucose levels at less than 150 mg/dL. (level D)

KEY

Level A: Meta-analysis of quantitative studies or metasynthesis of qualitative studies with results that consistently support a specific action, intervention, or treatment

Level B: Well-designed, controlled studies with results that consistently support a specific action, intervention, or treatment

Level C: Qualitative studies, descriptive or correlational studies, integrative review, systematic reviews, or randomized controlled trials with inconsistent results

Level D: Peer-reviewed professional organizational standards with clinical studies to support recommendations

Level E: Multiple case reports, theory-based evidence from expert opinions, or peer-reviewed professional organizational standards without clinical studies to support recommendations

Level M: Manufacturer's recommendations only

■ Adapted from American Association of Critical-Care Nurses (AACN) Practice Alert, revised 04/2010.

ventilation, and ensuring adequate oxygenation in the patient with septic shock usually requires endotracheal intubation and mechanical ventilation.

- **Providing nutritional support.** Supplemental nutrition is required to prevent malnutrition and to optimize cellular function. Enteral nutrition is the preferred route of nutritional support because it maintains the integrity of the gastrointestinal tract, decreases infection, and decreases mortality in patients with a septic or hypotensive event.[8] If the patient cannot tolerate enteral feeding, total parenteral nutrition (TPN) may be necessary, but ideally, a small amount of enteral nutrition can still be delivered.

Multisystem Organ Dysfunction Syndrome

MODS, an end point on the continuum of shock, is the progressive physiological failure of several organ systems in an acutely ill patient, such that homeostasis cannot be maintained without intervention.[9] No organ is independent of any other; therefore, failure of one organ makes the failure of a second or third organ more likely. The more organ systems are involved, the higher the mortality rate.

Pathophysiology

Although septic shock is a common precursor to MODS, any severe illness or injury that causes a systemic inflammatory response (ie, SIRS) can lead to MODS. The pathophysiology of MODS is similar to that of sepsis and SIRS, in that underlying mechanisms include endothelial injury, inflammatory mediators, disturbed hemostasis, and microcirculatory failure.[9] Tissue hypoxia caused by microvascular thromboses probably also contributes to MODS.

Typically, the first organs to manifest signs of dysfunction are the lungs and kidneys. If the shock state persists, eventually all vital organs fail, and death occurs.

- **Pulmonary dysfunction.** The lungs are particularly vulnerable to failure because the leaky capillaries create interstitial pulmonary edema, which impairs pulmonary gas exchange and can lead to the development of ARDS.
- **Renal dysfunction** occurs secondary to prolonged ischemia of the renal tubular cells.
- **Liver dysfunction** eventually results in hepatic failure. Hepatic failure affects multiple body systems because the liver performs so many functions, including detoxification of the blood and synthesis of albumin and clotting factors.

TABLE 33-4 Sepsis-Related Organ Failure Assessment (SOFA) Scoring System

Organ System	SOFA Score 1	2	3	4
Respiration Partial pressure of oxygen/fraction of inspired oxygen (mm Hg)	Less than 400	Less than 300	Less than 200 with respiratory support	Less than 100
Coagulation Platelets ($\times 10^3$/mm^3)	Less than 150	Less than 100	Less than 50	Less than 20
Hepatic (Liver) Bilirubin (mg/dL)	1.2–1.9	2.0–5.9	6.0–11.9	Greater than 12
Cardiovascular Hypotension	MAP less than 70 mm Hg	Dopamine less than or equal to 5 µg/kg/min or dobutamine any dose	Dopamine greater than 5 µg/kg/min or epinephrine less than or equal to 0.1 µg/min or norepinephrine less than or equal to 0.1 µg/min	Dopamine greater than 15 µg/kg/min or epinephrine greater than 0.1 µg/min or norepinephrine greater than 0.1 µg/min
Central Nervous System Glasgow Coma Scale score	13–14	10–12	6–9	Less than 6
Renal Creatinine (mg/dL) or urine output	1.2–1.9	2.0–3.4	3.5–4.9 or less than 500 mL/d	Greater than 5.0 or less than 200 mL/d

The SOFA system is used to assess patients with multiple organ failure daily. Each organ system is graded from 0 (normal) to 4 (the most abnormal), resulting in a score ranging from 0 to 24. MAP, mean arterial pressure.

- **Cardiovascular dysfunction** includes abnormalities of cardiac output (dysrhythmias, myocardial depression) as well as abnormalities in the peripheral vascular system, including hypotension unresponsive to fluid administration, increased capillary permeability, edema, and maldistribution of blood flow.
- **Hematologic dysfunction.** The most common hematologic dysfunction is DIC.
- **Neurologic dysfunction** may occur secondary to poor cerebral perfusion and is manifested as altered levels of consciousness, confusion, and psychosis.

Assessment

Assessment focuses on identifying SIRS and signs and symptoms of organ failure. Multiple scoring systems exist to determine the extent of MODS, including the sepsis-related organ failure assessment (SOFA) system (Table 33-4),[10] the acute physiology and chronic health evaluation (APACHE) system,[11] and the mortality probability models (MPM) system.[12]

Management

Early recognition and management of MODS is essential. Treatment is supportive and directed at specific organ systems.

CASE STUDY

Mr. B., a 63-year-old man, is brought to the emergency department in an ambulance after being struck by a car at a local shopping center. He has suffered no loss of consciousness, and the car was reported to be traveling at a slow speed. His past medical history is significant for chronic obstructive pulmonary disease (COPD) and a cholecystectomy 5 years ago. Home medications include an albuterol/ipratropium bromide (Combivent) inhaler. He currently works as a security officer at a local high school and lives with his wife. He drinks 1 to 2 beers per week, has smoked one pack of cigarettes per day for the past 30 years, and denies illicit drug use.

On physical examination, Mr. B. is pale and diaphoretic, with diminished pulses in his feet (capillary refill of 4 seconds). His pelvis is found to be unstable on palpation, and he complains of pain in his pelvis that he rates as a 7/10. Although he is conscious, he is confused to place and time. Two 18-gauge IV lines are started in the bilateral antecubital sites. A fluid bolus of 2 L of lactated Ringer's solution is administered. Vital signs on admission are: temperature, 97.5°F (36.4°C); RR, 24 breaths/min; HR, 156 beats/min; and BP, 78/42 mm Hg. A Foley catheter is inserted, and 18 mL of concentrated urine is obtained. Laboratory values are: hemoglobin, 7.3 g/dL; hematocrit, 23.7%; white blood cell (WBC) count, 6.8 cells/mm³; glucose, 114 mg/dL; Na⁺, 148 mEq/L; K⁺, 4.1 mEq/L; BUN, 32 mg/dL; creatinine, 1.1 mg/dL; magnesium, 1.8 mg/dL; calcium, 8.7 mg/dL; and lactate, 7.7 mmol/L. Arterial blood gasses (ABGs) show metabolic acidosis. A CT scan reveals an open-book pelvic fracture. Cervical spinal damage and other traumatic injuries are ruled out with radiography and patient assessment.

Mr. B. is admitted to the critical care unit with a diagnosis of pelvic fracture with associated hemorrhage. Serial hemoglobin and hematocrit are monitored, revealing ongoing acute blood loss anemia. A double-lumen central venous catheter is inserted for fluid resuscitation and monitoring of CVP. Over the course of 16 hours, Mr. B. requires 8 U of packed red blood cells (PRBCs) to achieve a hematocrit of greater than 28%, and 4 additional liters of lactated Ringer's solution to maintain a central venous pressure (CVP) of greater than 8 mm Hg. Fluids are warmed using an in-line fluid warmer to prevent hypothermia. Mr. B. is taken to surgery the following morning for repair of vasculature and stabilization of the fracture. The estimated blood loss in surgery is 2 L. After surgery, Mr. B. is returned to the critical care unit on a mechanical ventilator.

On postoperative day 1, Mr. B. is hemodynamically stable with a hematocrit of 32%, CVP of 13 mm Hg, mean arterial pressure (MAP) of 78 mm Hg, heart rate of 86 beats/min, temperature of 98.9°F (37.2°C), and serum lactate level of 2.2 mmol/L (from his hypovolemic shock). He is recovering from his hypovolemic shock. Morphine is used for pain control, and prophylaxis against deep venous thrombosis and gastromucosal disease is initiated. IV fluids are administered at 75 mL/h. Mr. B. is placed on a ventilator-weaning protocol, but attempts to wean are unsuccessful secondary to his COPD. He remains in the critical care unit, with daily ventilator weaning trials.

On the morning of postoperative day 4, Mr. B. is successfully extubated and placed on 4 L oxygen by nasal cannula. He is tolerating a liquid diet, and plans are made for transfer to the trauma-surgical unit in the morning. Later that afternoon, his family reports that he has suddenly become irritable and is pulling at his IV lines and indwelling urinary catheter. Vital signs are temperature, 102.0°F (38.9°C); RR, 34 breaths/min; HR, 128 beats/min; and BP, 86/52 mm Hg. Blood and urine are sent for culture. Mr. B. is electively reintubated, and CVP monitoring is reinstated. The initial CVP is 4 mm Hg. Fluid resuscitation is initiated using boluses of lactated Ringer's solution. Despite an increase in CVP to 10 mm Hg, the MAP remains 59 mm Hg. A norepinephrine infusion is started at 1.0 µg/kg/min, with orders to titrate to an MAP greater than 70 mm Hg.

ABGs reveal a metabolic acidosis and a serum lactate of 5.6 mmol/L. Broad-spectrum antibiotic therapy is initiated. The WBC count increases to 12.4/mm³, and preliminary blood cultures are positive for gram-negative rods. Antibiotic therapy is adjusted appropriately.

Mr. B. remains hypotensive (MAP less than or equal to 65 mm Hg) despite doses of norepinephrine as high as 20 µg/min. A vasopressin infusion is initiated at 2 U/h. Despite titration, the MAP remains less than or equal to 65 mm Hg. A venous blood gas is obtained, revealing a venous oxygen saturation of 62%. A dobutamine infusion is started at 5 µg/kg/min. Anti-inflammatory therapy is started with low-dose corticosteroids.

Mr. B. is not responsive to pain and is unable to follow commands. His family receives regular updates concerning his condition during meetings with the interdisciplinary healthcare team. On postoperative day 6, Mr. B. continues to require high doses of vasopressor and inotropic therapy and has developed acute respiratory distress syndrome (ARDS). In collaboration with the healthcare team, the family makes the decision to initiate a do-not-resuscitate (DNR) order, and the norepinephrine, vasopressin, and dobutamine infusions are sustained at their existing rates without any further increases. Later that day, Mr. B. develops sustained ventricular tachycardia that progresses to ventricular fibrillation. Mr. B. passes away with his family at his side.

1. Analyze the sequence of events that occurred in Mr. B.'s case.

2. Describe the management goals and nursing interventions for hypovolemic and septic shock.

3. Discuss the management of Mr. B.'s septic shock. Was evidence-based care provided?

References

1. The diagnosis and management of anaphylaxis: An updated practice parameter. J Allergy Clin Immunol 115 (3 suppl):S483–S523, 2005

2. Cinel I, Dellinger R: Advances in pathogenesis and management of sepsis. Curr Opin Infect Dis 20:345, 2007.

3. Cytokine physiology of sepsis. In Vineet N, et al. (ed): Critical Care Updates (2007). Jaypee Brothers Medical Publisher, Chapter 11

4. Bridges EJ, Dukes S: Cardiovascular aspects of septic shock: Pathophysiology, monitoring, and treatment. Crit Care Nurse 25(2):14–42, 2005

5. Nguyen H, et al: Implementation of a bundle of quality indicators for the early management of severe sepsis and septic shock is associated with a decrease mortality. Crit Care Med 35(4):1105–1112, 2007

6. Dellinger RP, Carlet JM, et al.: Surviving Sepsis Campaign international guidelines for management of severe sepsis and septic shock. Crit Care Med 36:296–327, 2008

7. Marti-Carvajal A, et al: Human recombinant activated protein C for severe sepsis. Cochrane Database Sys Rev 13(4), 2011

8. Elke G, et al: Current practice in nutritional support and its association with mortality in septic patient: Results from prospective multicenter study. Crit Care Med 36:1762, 2008

9. Marsh R, Nadel E, Brown D: Multiple system organ failure. J Emerg Med 29(3):331–334, 2005

10. Vincent JL, et al.: The SOFA (Sepsis-Related Organ Failure Assessment) score to describe organ dysfunction/failure. On behalf of the Working Group on Sepsis-Related Problems of the European Society of Intensive Care Medicine. Intens Care Med 22:707–710, 1996

11. Knaus WA, et al.: APACHE II: A severity of disease classification system. Crit Care Med 13:818–828, 1985

12. Lemeshow SD, Teres D, Klar J, et al.: Mortality Probability Models (MPM II) based on an international cohort of intensive care unit patients. JAMA 270:2478–2486, 1993

Want to know more? A wide variety of resources to enhance your learning and understanding of this chapter are available on the **Point** ✳. Visit **http://thepoint.lww.com/MortonEss1e** to access chapter review questions and more!

CHAPTER
34

Trauma

OBJECTIVES

Based on the content in this chapter, the reader should be able to:

1 Compare and contrast mechanisms of trauma injury.
2 Describe phases of initial assessment and related care of the trauma patient.
3 Discuss the assessment and management of patients with thoracic, abdominal, musculoskeletal, and maxillofacial trauma.

Injury is defined by the National Committee for Injury Prevention and Control as "unintentional or intentional damage to the body resulting from acute exposure to thermal, mechanical, electrical, or chemical energy or from the absence of such essentials as heat or oxygen."[1] Mechanical injuries, such as those resulting from motor vehicle crashes (MVCs), falls, and firearms, are the focus of this chapter.

Trauma is a leading cause of critical illness and death in the United States. One third of all trauma patients seen at level I trauma centers are admitted to critical care units, where they have a mean stay of 5 days. The risk for trauma morbidity and death is increased in older patients and those with comorbidities.[2]

 The Older Patient. *Falls are the most common cause of trauma in older people.*

Mechanism of Injury

Knowledge about the mechanism of injury can help explain the type of injury, predict the eventual outcome, and identify common injury combinations. Because the patient may not show classic signs of an injury, knowledge about the mechanism of injury is also helpful for indicating the need for additional diagnostic workup and reassessment.

Injury occurs when force deforms tissues beyond their failure limits. The effects of the injury depend on the injuring agent, the amount of force (force = mass × acceleration), and the area of contact. In penetrating injury, the concentration of force is on a small area. In blunt (nonpenetrating) injury, the force is distributed over a large area. Other factors, such as the person's age and gender and the presence or absence of underlying disease processes, also influence the effects of the injury.

Blunt Injury

Blunt trauma can be caused by MVCs, falls, assaults, and contact sports. Multiple injuries are common with blunt trauma, and these injuries are often life-threatening injuries because the extent of the injury is less obvious and the diagnosis can be more difficult to make than for penetrating injuries. Blunt injury occurs when there is direct contact between the body surface and the injuring agent. Indirect forces are transmitted internally with dissipation of energy to the internal structure. Indirect forces that can result in blunt injury include the following:

• Acceleration is an increase in the velocity (speed) of a moving object.

470

- Deceleration is a decrease in the velocity of a moving object.
- Shearing occurs across a plane when structures slip relative to each other.
- Crushing occurs when continuous pressure is applied to a body part.
- Compressive resistance is the ability of an object or structure to resist squeezing forces or inward pressure.

MVCs can involve occupants of the vehicle (Fig. 34-1) or pedestrians (Fig. 34-2). Acceleration–deceleration injuries, such as those that occur in MVCs, are the most common causes of blunt injuries. Before an MVC, the occupant and the car are traveling at the same speed. During an MVC, both the occupant and the car decelerate to zero, but not at the same rate. When the vehicle comes to an abrupt stop, the occupant's body continues to move forward until it strikes a fixed object, such as the steering column, dashboard, or windshield. Although the person's body stops moving, internal structures continue to move within their enclosed spaces. For example, the brain first strikes the front of the skull and then the back. Injury occurs when soft tissue impacts rigid structures (such as bone) and from shearing forces that cause stretching and bowing of vessels, causing them to rupture. Wearing shoulder and lap restraints and deployment of air bags reduces the incidence and severity of injury by reducing the force with which the occupant of the vehicle strikes the surfaces within the vehicle and by preventing the occupant from being ejected from the vehicle.[3]

Penetrating Injury

Penetrating injuries are produced by foreign objects (eg, bullets, knife blades, debris) entering into tissue. The external appearance of the wound does not necessarily reflect the extent of internal injury.

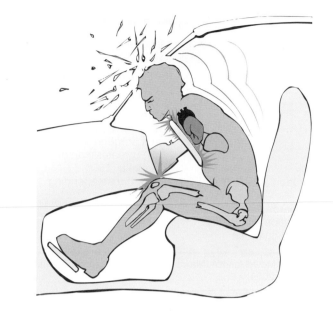

FIGURE 34-1 An unrestrained passenger in a motor vehicle crash may sustain injuries to the skull, scalp, brain, face, sternum, ribs, heart, liver, spleen, pelvis, and lower extremities.

The severity of the injury is related to the structures damaged, the amount of energy that transfers into the tissue, the amount of time it takes for the transfer to occur, and the velocity of the injuring agent. Low-velocity missiles (eg, small-caliber weapons, knife blades) cause little cavitation and blast effect, essentially only pushing the tissue aside. High-velocity missiles (eg, rifles, semiautomatic weapons) produce a greater amount of energy and cavitation.

The main injury determinants in stab wounds or impalements are the length, width, and trajectory of the penetrating object and the presence of vital organs in the area of the wound. Although the injuries tend to be localized, deep organs and multiple body cavities can be penetrated.

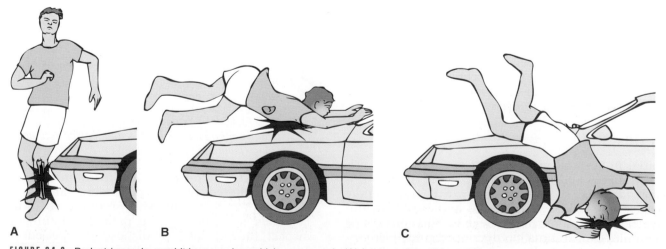

FIGURE 34-2 Pedestrians who are hit by a moving vehicle may sustain (**A**) fracture of the tibia and fibula, (**B**) fractured ribs and a ruptured spleen, or (**C**) injuries to the head and upper extremities.

TABLE 34-1 Trauma Center Designation

	Level I	Level II	Level III	Level IV
Admission requirements	1200 patients per year; 20% with an Injury Severity Score (ISS) greater than or equal to 15 or 35 patients per surgeon with an ISS greater than or equal to 15	Varies depending on geographical area, population, resources available, and system maturity	No requirement	No requirement
Surgeon availability	24-h in-house attending surgeon	Rapidly available	Promptly available	24-h emergency coverage
Research center	Required	Not required	Not required	Not required
Education, prevention, and outreach	Required	Required	Required	Required

Data from McQuillan KA, Makic MBF, Whalen E (eds): Trauma Nursing, 4th ed. Philadelphia, PA: WB Saunders, 2009.

Initial Assessment and Management

Care begins in the prehospital arena and continues in the hospital or trauma center. Trauma centers are categorized according to the resources they are able to provide and the number of annual admissions (Table 34-1).

Prehospital

Because the trauma patient has a greater chance of a positive outcome if admission to a trauma center and definitive care are initiated within 1 hour of injury, the principal factor influencing prehospital care is the transport time to the trauma center. Few interventions should be provided if transport time is short and more interventions if transport time is longer.[4]

Management during the prehospital phase focuses on maintaining the airway, ensuring adequate ventilation, controlling external bleeding and preventing shock, maintaining spine immobilization, and transporting the patient immediately to the closest appropriate facility.[4] Following assessment and management of the airway, breathing, and circulation, the patient's neurological status is assessed, including level of consciousness and pupil size and reaction. Once this primary assessment is complete, a secondary assessment is performed to determine any other injuries.

In-Hospital

Initial in-hospital management entails a rapid primary survey and resuscitation of vital functions, a more detailed secondary survey, a tertiary survey to identify specific injuries, and initiation of definitive care. The American College of Surgeons (ACS) Committee on Trauma has developed guidelines that provide an organized approach to the initial assessment of trauma patients, increasing the speed of the primary assessment and minimizing the risk that injuries will be overlooked (Table 34-2). The trauma team leader, a physician, is responsible for assessing the patient, ordering and interpreting diagnostic studies, and prioritizing the diagnostics and therapeutic concerns.

Surveys

Primary Survey
During the primary survey, life-threatening injuries are identified and managed. Each priority of care is dealt with in order (eg, a patent airway must be ensured before breathing and ventilation can be established). Other priorities during the primary survey include

- **Assessing for hypovolemia.** External or internal blood loss can lead to inadequate tissue perfusion (hemorrhagic shock). Interventions include stopping the bleeding with compression or surgery, and replacing the lost intravascular volume. Trauma patients transported to the trauma center by emergency medical services typically arrive with a large-bore IV line already in place, and IV fluid infusing rapidly.

> **RED FLAG!** Signs and symptoms of hypovolemia include pallor, poor skin turgor, diaphoresis, tachycardia, oliguria, and hypotension.

> **RED FLAG!** An extended period of hypotension and hypoperfusion increases the possibility of acute kidney failure in trauma patients.

- **Assessing for hypothermia.** Environmental factors, an altered physiological state, and interventions (such as infusing room-temperature IV fluids or removing the patient's clothing to inspect for injuries) predispose the patient to hypothermia. Hypothermia can worsen coagulopathy and increase blood loss in trauma patients.

TABLE 34-2 Initial Assessment and Management of the Patient With Trauma

Parameter	Assessment	Interventions
Airway	Air exchange Airway patency	Jaw thrust, chin lift Removal of foreign bodies Suctioning Oropharyngeal or nasopharyngeal airway Endotracheal intubation (orally or nasally) Cricothyrotomy
Breathing	Respirations (rate, depth, effort) Color Breath sounds Chest wall movement and integrity Position of trachea	Supplemental oxygen Ventilation with manual resuscitation bag (MRB) Treatment of life-threatening conditions (eg, tension pneumothorax)
Circulation	Pulse, blood pressure Capillary refill Obvious external bleeding Electrocardiogram (ECG)	Hemorrhage control: apply direct pressure, elevate extremity, pneumatic antishock garment, if indicated for tamponade effect IV therapy: crystalloids, blood transfusion Treatment of life-threatening conditions (eg, cardiac tamponade) Cardiopulmonary resuscitation (CPR)
Disability	Level of consciousness Pupils	—
Exposure	Inspection of body for injuries	—

Warm fluids and blankets are used whenever possible to increase body temperature or maintain normothermia.

The Older Patient. *Older people tend to become hypothermic more quickly than younger people.*

• **Obtaining baseline data and performing initial interventions.** The patient is placed on a monitor with pulse oximetry and end-tidal carbon dioxide ($ETCO_2$) monitoring; an electrocardiogram (ECG) is obtained; and bloodwork is sent for evaluation of electrolytes, hemoglobin and hematocrit, blood type and crossmatch, and arterial blood gases (ABGs), if the patient is believed to have a high level of injury. An indwelling urinary catheter and a nasogastric or orogastric tube are placed. Findings during the primary survey dictate which imaging studies are obtained first. Chest, abdomen, and pelvis films are generally completed at this time.

Secondary Survey
Once the primary survey is completed, a more detailed head-to-toe secondary survey is done to detect life- and limb-threatening injuries. A more detailed patient history is also obtained, including as much detail as possible about the circumstances surrounding the injury. A thorough history of the preceding events aids in assessment and treatment and can decrease morbidity and mortality. Field providers, family, and friends are valuable sources of information, especially if the patient is unable to speak or remember the event. Relevant questions include the following:

• Was the person involved in an MVC? What was the approximate speed the vehicle was traveling? Was the patient the driver or passenger? Was the

person wearing a restraining device? Was the airbag deployed? If the person was hit by a vehicle, was the person on foot or on a bike? What kind of vehicle was involved? Where was the person at the time of impact? What was the speed, point of impact, and type of impact? Was there a fatality at the scene?
• Was the person stabbed? What was the length of the knife? Was the assailant male or female?
• Was the person shot? What caliber of weapon was used? What was the distance from the assailant to the victim?
• Did the person fall? How far (approximate height)? Was the fall off a ladder, or down a flight of stairs? What part of the body impacted first?

Information obtained from the history about the mechanism of injury may raise suspicion for other injuries that require investigation. Continuous reassessment is necessary because injuries often go undetected.

Tertiary Survey
The tertiary survey is completed in the critical care unit to ensure that all of the patient's injuries have been identified, including non–life-threatening injuries. The tertiary survey entails another head-to-toe examination and assessment of the patient's response to resuscitation. Films and laboratory values are reviewed, and a preinjury medical history is completed or obtained. Although delays in injury identification are common, if the injury is found within 24 hours of admission, it is not considered a missed injury.[5]

Fluid Resuscitation
The goal of fluid resuscitation is to maintain perfusion to the vital organs without inducing complications

TABLE 34-3 Crystalloids

Type of Crystalloid	Example	Tonicity	Effect
Isotonic	0.9% normal saline	Equal to that of human body	Causes minimal shifts between intracellular and extracellular space
Hypotonic	5% dextrose in water (D_5W)	Less than that of human body	Pulls fluid into extracellular space
Hypertonic	3% saline	Greater than that of human body	Pulls fluid into intravascular space

of fluid overload (eg, generalized edema, abdominal compartment syndrome, ascites, worsening of the pulmonary status). Aggressive fluid resuscitation also puts the patient at risk for hypothermia and coagulopathy.[6]

 The Older Patient. *Older adults are more susceptible to complications of volume overload and require adequate rapid fluid replacement without excess. Consider a pulmonary artery or central venous pressure line for guidance in fluid replacement.*

The choice of fluid is based on how the volume loss occurred, the concentration of solutes, and which electrolytes need to be replaced.[7]

Crystalloids

Crystalloids may be isotonic, hypertonic, or hypotonic (Table 34-3).

- **Isotonic crystalloids** are most commonly used in trauma resuscitation. Isotonic crystalloids closely mimic the body's extracellular fluid and can be used to expand both intravascular and extravascular fluid volume.[7] Because of the equilibration of the isotonic solution outside of the vascular space, more volume is required to replace the vascular losses. A common guideline used is to administer 3 L of isotonic crystalloid for each liter of blood loss.
- **Hypertonic crystalloids** may also be used in trauma resuscitation. Hypertonic crystalloids primarily remain within the vascular space and shift water from the extravascular space into the plasma, resulting in a rapid increase in blood volume, mean arterial pressure (MAP), and cardiac output.[7] This enables a more rapid restoration of cardiac function with a smaller volume of fluid.

Colloids

Colloids (eg, albumin, dextran, hetastarch) create oncotic pressure, which encourages fluid retention and movement of fluid into the intravascular space. Colloids have a longer duration of action because they are larger molecules and stay in the intravascular compartment longer.[7] When colloids are used, less fluid volume is necessary to replace vascular losses and achieve hemodynamic stability. However, potential complications (eg, anaphylaxis, coagulopathy) and higher costs make colloids less desirable than crystalloids for use in trauma resuscitation.

Blood Products

Although there is some concern about blood-borne pathogens and transfusion reactions, blood products are an excellent resuscitation fluid.[8] Packed red blood cells (PRBCs) increase oxygen-carrying capacity and allow for volume expansion, and are the mainstay of treatment for trauma patients with hemorrhage.[8]

Blood is transfused when the patient has lost a significant amount of blood, is hemodynamically unstable, or is showing signs of tissue hypoxia despite crystalloid infusion. If the need for emergency transfusions does not allow time for type and crossmatching of the patient's blood, O-negative blood is preferred for women of childbearing age. O-positive blood may be used in men and post-menopausal women. Fresh frozen plasma (which contains coagulation factors) and platelets are transfused when the patient requires large amounts of blood.

 RED FLAG! *Massive blood transfusions increase the patient's risk for systemic inflammatory response syndrome (SIRS), acute respiratory distress syndrome (ARDS), and disseminated intravascular coagulation (DIC) due to stimulation of the inflammatory system.*

Autotransfusion is also commonly used in the hemorrhaging trauma patient. Blood is saved from a pleural chest tube via a cell saver collection bag. When ready to infuse, the cell saver is disconnected from the chest tube collection device, and the blood is transfused into the patient using a macroaggregate filter.

Damage Control

Patients who have sustained multiple traumatic injuries have a higher mortality from metabolic complications during surgery. Uncontrolled bleeding, fluid resuscitation, and surgery can result in the "lethal triad": hypothermia, acidosis, and coagulopathy. The principle of "damage control" involves performing surgery in stages to prevent metabolic complications from developing

- Stage 1: stop hemorrhage; control contamination; close wounds temporarily
- Stage 2: correct physiologic abnormalities by warming, ensuring adequate resuscitation, and

correcting coagulopathy (these interventions are continued in the critical care unit)

- Stage 3: perform definitive operative management

Definitive Care

Increasingly, stable trauma patients are managed nonoperatively. More sophisticated methods of visualizing internal structures, such as computed tomography (CT), ultrasonography, and angiography, have reduced the need for immediate surgical exploration in many cases. In addition, many of these techniques can be used for management as well as diagnosis (eg, angiographic interventions may be used to embolize a hemorrhaging internal vessel). Patients who are treated nonoperatively require close monitoring and frequent assessment in the critical care unit.

Attention is also given to managing preexisting medical conditions, identifying injuries that may have been missed earlier, providing psychosocial support for the patient and family, and monitoring for the development of complications. Situations such as prolonged extrication, prolonged hypothermia, respiratory or cardiac arrest, massive fluid resuscitation, or massive blood transfusions suggest severe injuries and a greater chance of complications (Box 34-1) and death after trauma. A Collaborative Care Guide for the patient with multisystem trauma is given in Box 34-2.

The Older Patient. *Constant monitoring is essential when caring for an older trauma patient. The threshold for invasive monitoring should be decreased with an elderly patient, secondary to predisposing conditions and past medical history.*

Assessment and Management of Specific Injuries

Although this section discusses traumatic injuries related to specific areas of the body, every trauma patient requires head-to-toe physical assessment.

Thoracic Trauma

Thoracic injuries range from simple to life-threatening (Box 34-3). In thoracic injury, the first priority is always airway management. Airway obstruction may be the primary problem or the result of another injury. Airway obstruction can be caused by the tongue, avulsed teeth, dentures, or blood, or by injuries to the trachea, thyroid cartilage, or cricoid.[9]

Tracheobronchial Trauma

Tracheobronchial injuries can be caused by blunt or penetrating trauma and frequently are accompanied by esophageal and vascular damage. Ruptured bronchi often are present in association with upper rib fractures and pneumothorax. Tracheobronchial injury is considered whenever pneumothorax persists despite management. Diagnosis usually is made with bronchoscopy or during surgery.

RED FLAG! *Signs and symptoms of tracheobronchial injuries are often subtle and may include dyspnea (occasionally the only sign), hemoptysis, cough, subcutaneous emphysema, anxiety, hoarseness, stridor, air hunger, hypoventilation, accessory muscle use, sternal and subscapular retractions, diaphragm breathing, apnea, and cyanosis.*

Small lung lacerations or pleural tears can be managed conservatively with mechanical ventilation delivered through an endotracheal tube or tracheostomy. Larger injuries may require surgical repair. Nursing responsibilities include assessing oxygenation and gas exchange and providing pulmonary care.

Bony Thorax Fractures

Rib fractures, sternal fractures, and flail chest are common in trauma patients. Rib fractures are clinically significant as markers of serious intrathoracic and abdominal injuries (Fig. 34-3, p. 478), sources of significant pain, and predictors of pulmonary deterioration. The greatest concerns for nurses caring for patients with bony thorax fractures are pain management, effective ventilation, and secretion control.

BOX 34·1 Delayed Complications of Multiple Trauma

Hematologic
- Hemorrhage, coagulopathy, disseminated intravascular coagulation (DIC)

Cardiac
- Dysrhythmia, heart failure, ventricular aneurysm

Pulmonary
- Atelectasis, pneumonia, emboli (fat or thrombotic), acute respiratory distress syndrome (ARDS)

Gastrointestinal
- Peritonitis, adynamic ileus, mechanical bowel obstruction, acalculous cholecystitis, anastomotic leak, fistula, bleeding, abdominal compartment syndrome

Hepatic
- Liver abscess, liver failure

Renal
- Hypertension, myoglobinuria, kidney failure

Orthopedic
- Compartment syndrome

Skin
- Wound infection, dehiscence, skin breakdown

Systemic
- Sepsis

BOX 34-2 COLLABORATIVE CARE GUIDE for the Patient With Multisystem Trauma

OUTCOMES	INTERVENTIONS
Oxygenation/Ventilation	
A patent airway is maintained.	• Auscultate breath sounds.
	• Perform frequent assessments.
	• Intubate if needed.
	• Provide supplemental oxygen PRN.
An arterial oxygen saturation (SaO$_2$) of 95% or more is maintained, and ABGs are within normal limits.	• Provide bronchial hygiene therapy (BHT) (chest physiotherapy and incentive spirometry).
	• Intubate.
	• Monitor ABGs.
The patient is able to take deep breaths and is free of anxiety.	• Use mechanical ventilation if necessary to support adequate ventilation.
	• Provide adequate pain medication to promote deep breathing (patient-controlled analgesia [PCA], epidural, around-the-clock medications).
	• Medicate before pain increases.
	• Use antianxiety drugs as necessary.
Circulation/Perfusion	
Adequate blood pressure, heart rate, and respiratory rate are maintained.	• Monitor respiratory rate and depth.
	• Use ECG monitor.
	• Administer IV fluids and PRBCs to ensure adequate intravascular volume and oxygen-carrying capacity.
	• Administer medications, such as vasoactive and inotropic agents, after
	• intravascular volume is restored.
	• Place pulmonary artery catheter or arterial line.
	• Assess skin color and capillary refill time.
The patient does not develop deep venous thrombosis (DVT).	• Use prophylactic anticoagulants unless contraindicated.
	• Apply antiembolic stockings.
	• Use pneumatic compression devices.
Fluids/Electrolytes	
Adequate intake and output are maintained.	• Monitor blood pressure, heart rate, central venous pressure, pulmonary artery occlusion pressure, IV fluid.
	• Use indwelling urinary catheter to monitor urine output.
	• Consider insensible fluid loss in output.
	• Monitor laboratory values.
Electrolyte balance is maintained.	• Replace electrolytes PRN.
	• Monitor ECG.
Mobility/Safety	
Range of motion is maintained.	• Consult Physical/Occupational Therapy.
	• Use splints PRN.
	• Do range-of-motion exercises q8h.
	• Out of bed as tolerated.
Skin Integrity	
The patient is without evidence of skin breakdown.	• Monitor skin q4h.
	• Turn the patient q2h and PRN.
	• Use pressure-relieving devices.
	• Remove splints to monitor skin.
	• Provide prescribed wound care.
	• Monitor wound for evidence of infection.

BOX 34-2   COLLABORATIVE CARE GUIDE (continued)

OUTCOMES	INTERVENTIONS
Nutrition Nutritional intake meets calculated metabolic need (eg, basal energy expenditure equation).	• Consult dietitian for metabolic needs assessment and recommendations. • Encourage enteral nutrition when possible. • Use TPN/lipids if enteral nutrition contraindicated. • Check prealbumin and electrolytes. • Monitor for weight loss.
Comfort/Pain Control The patient will indicate/exhibit adequate relief of discomfort/pain.	• Document pain assessment, using numerical pain rating or similar scale when possible. • Provide analgesia as appropriate, document efficacy after each dose. • Use PCA/epidural PRN. • Arrange pain consult if needed. • Use sedation as needed. • Monitor vital signs.
Psychosocial The patient will maintain as much control as possible.	• Inform the patient of procedures. • Establish a schedule with the patient if possible. • Provide an alternate means of communication if necessary, such as lip reading, writing, and a communication board.
The patient and family will cope effectively with the traumatic event.	• Provide repeated information. • Encourage use of appropriate coping. • Encourage use of support systems. • Arrange social work consult.
Teaching/Discharge Planning The patient will be involved in discharge planning.	• Discuss discharge with the patient. • Allow the patient to make decisions if possible.
The patient will understand injuries and complications of injuries.	• Provide discharge instructions accordingly with injury. • Provide the patient with list of injuries.

BOX 34-3   Life-Threatening Thoracic Injuries

Immediately life-threatening injuries (primary survey priorities)
• Airway obstruction
• Tension pneumothorax
• Cardiac tamponade
• Open pneumothorax
• Massive hemothorax
• Flail chest

Potentially life-threatening injuries (secondary survey priorities)
• Thoracic aortic disruption
• Tracheobronchial disruption
• Myocardial contusion
• Traumatic diaphragm tear
• Esophageal disruption
• Pulmonary contusion

Flail chest involves multiple adjacent rib fractures or involves sternal fracture. These fractures can be anterior, posterior, or lateral, and usually a sternal fracture is present as well. The flail segment follows pleural pressure instead of respiratory muscle activity, producing paradoxical breathing (ie, the affected portion of the chest wall moves in on inspiration and out on expiration). Ventilation is decreased, leading to hypoxia. As the patient's pulmonary status worsens, the paradoxical movement of the flail segment increases.

Initial management of flail chest and other bony thorax fractures includes airway management, pain management, and oxygen therapy to maintain adequate saturation. A patient with flail chest may be positioned with the injured side down to improve oxygenation; however, this is often difficult because of the need to maintain cervical spine immobilization. Other treatment modalities for

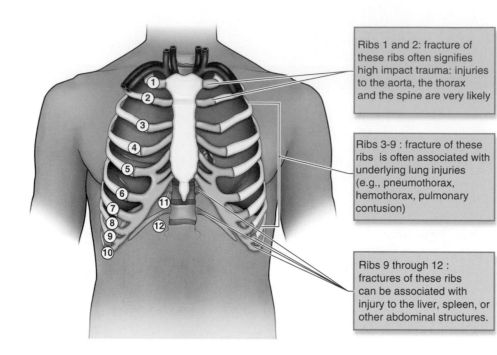

Ribs 1 and 2: fracture of these ribs often signifies high impact trauma: injuries to the aorta, the thorax and the spine are very likely

Ribs 3-9 : fracture of these ribs is often associated with underlying lung injuries (e.g., pneumothorax, hemothorax, pulmonary contusion)

Ribs 9 through 12 : fractures of these ribs can be associated with injury to the liver, spleen, or other abdominal structures.

FIGURE 34·3 Rib fractures are clinically significant as markers of serious intrathoracic and abdominal injuries.

flail chest include internal splinting (accomplished by providing positive pressure ventilation) and surgical repair.

Pleural Space Injuries

Pleural space injuries include pneumothorax (intrapleural air collection), hemothorax (intrapleural blood collection), and hemopneumothorax (interpleural air and blood collections). Normally, the pressure within the pleural space is negative, which assists with maintaining lung expansion. The introduction of air or blood into the pleural space causes the pressure in the pleural space to become positive, which causes the lung to collapse. In a patient with a pleural space injury, respiratory distress and signs of impaired gas exchange may be seen. Ongoing reassessment is necessary because even if the original pleural tear is small, it can expand, putting the patient at risk for tension pneumothorax (a life-threatening emergency).

 RED FLAG! *Signs and symptoms of impaired gas exchange include restlessness, anxiety, tachypnea, decreased oxygenation, poor color, and diaphoresis.*

Chest radiography or chest CT is usually used to diagnose pleural space injuries. Treatment entails management of the patient's airway, ventilation, and oxygenation. A large-bore chest tube is inserted to drain the air or blood from the plural space and reexpand the lung. The nurse monitors the amount of blood that drains into the chest tube drainage device. Drainage of more than 200 mL/h for 2 consecutive hours may indicate a significant injury and the need for further follow-up.

Massive Hemothorax

A massive hemothorax (1.5 to 4 L of intrathoracic blood loss) is a life-threatening injury. The source of bleeding is often a large systemic blood vessel or mediastinal structure. Left massive hemothorax is most common and is often associated with aortic rupture.

Patients with massive hemothorax may go into cardiopulmonary arrest and require immediate thoracotomy to control bleeding. Patients who are not in cardiopulmonary arrest present with signs of hypovolemic shock, dyspnea, tachypnea, and cyanosis. Initial management of these patients includes treatment of the shock state.

Tension Pneumothorax

Tension pneumothorax is caused by air continuing to enter the pleural space without being able to leave the pleural space. The resultant compression of the trachea, heart, lungs, or great vessels can result in ventilatory failure, compromised venous return, and insufficient cardiac output. Tension pneumothorax may result from primary injury to the thorax, or it may be a delayed complication related to tracheobronchial injury or mechanical ventilation.

 RED FLAG! *Signs and symptoms of tension pneumothorax include difficulty ventilating the patient despite an open airway, a decrease in oxygenation, chest asymmetry, tracheal shift, neck vein distention (unless the patient is hypovolemic), decreased breath sounds on the affected side, and evidence of decreased cardiac output (eg, decreased blood pressure and poor tissue perfusion).*

Treatment of tension pneumothorax involves the administration of supplemental oxygen and emergent decompression with chest tube placement. If a chest tube cannot be placed rapidly, the decompression can be achieved by placing a 16- or 18-gauge needle into the second intercostal space, midclavicular, to release the trapped air. After emergent decompression, the needles are changed to chest tubes to allow the lungs to expand and to prevent a reoccurrence.

Pulmonary Contusion

Pulmonary contusion (bruising of the lung parenchyma) is the most common lung injury and is potentially lethal. Rupture of the capillary cell walls causes hemorrhage and extravasation of plasma and protein into alveolar and interstitial spaces, resulting in noncardiogenic pulmonary edema that causes intrapulmonary shunting and hypoxemia. Pulmonary contusion should be anticipated in any patient who sustains significant high-energy blunt chest trauma, such as that caused by an MVC. The presence of a scapular fracture, rib fractures, or a flail chest also raises suspicion for a possible underlying pulmonary contusion. It may take 6 hours or more for a pulmonary contusion to become apparent on a chest radiograph; CT is more sensitive.

 RED FLAG! *Signs and symptoms of pulmonary contusion include dyspnea, crackles, hemoptysis, tachypnea, increasing peak airway pressures, hypoxemia, respiratory alkalosis, and poor response to high fractions of inspired oxygen (FiO$_2$).*

Treatment of pulmonary contusion is supportive. Patients with a mild contusion require close observation with frequent monitoring of ABGs and pulse oximetry. Patients with a severe contusion may require ventilatory support. Additional nursing interventions include pulmonary care, pain control, and fluid management.

The contused lung should show radiographic signs of improvement within 72 hours. The presence of persistent infiltrates may indicate complications, such as pneumonia or superimposed ARDS.

Cardiac Contusion

Cardiac contusions are usually caused by blunt chest trauma as the heart impacts the sternum during rapid deceleration or is compressed between the sternum and back. Symptoms vary in severity from none (common), to chest pain and hypotension, to heart failure and cardiogenic shock. Most patients with cardiac contusions have ECG abnormalities on admission; however, there is no correlation between the complexity of the dysrhythmia and the degree of the cardiac contusion.[10] Echocardiography may reveal myocardial depression. The patient is placed on continuous cardiac monitoring, hemodynamics are monitored, and blood is drawn for cardiac isoenzyme. Therapy is primarily aimed at supporting cardiac function and relieving symptoms.

Cardiac Tamponade

Cardiac tamponade, a life-threatening injury, can result from penetrating or blunt trauma. Cardiac tamponade is caused by blood filling the pericardial space and compressing the heart. The resultant decreased cardiac filling leads to reduced cardiac output, reduced contractility, and eventually shock. Only a small amount (50 to 100 mL) of blood in the pericardial sac can create an increase in pericardial pressure. Continued bleeding increases the pressure rapidly, leading to cardiac tamponade.

 RED FLAG! *Signs and symptoms of cardiac tamponade include Beck's triad (decreased blood pressure, muffled heart sounds, and distended neck veins) and pulsus paradoxus (an inspiratory decrease in systolic arterial pressure of 10 mm Hg or more).*

Signs and symptoms may be obscured in a hypovolemic patient. Echocardiography is most useful in making the diagnosis.[11] Definitive and life-saving treatment entails draining the blood from the pericardial sac.

Penetrating Cardiac Injury

The mortality rate associated with penetrating cardiac injury is 50% to 85%. Those who survive do so because of cardiac tamponade. Occasionally, small stab wounds to the ventricles seal themselves because of the thick ventricular musculature. For some hemodynamically stable patients, monitoring with serial CT scanning or with pericardial and pleural ultrasound is acceptable. For other patients, surgery to create a thoracoscopic pericardial window may be necessary to aid in the diagnosis of ongoing hemorrhage and to drain pericardial fluid collection. In the presence of ongoing hemorrhage and shock, the patient is immediately transported to the operating room for a median sternotomy and exploration.

After surgical repair, the nurse monitors hemodynamics, maintains blood pressure and perfusion, and corrects metabolic abnormalities. Complications include continued hemorrhage and postcardiotomy syndrome (symptoms of pericarditis, with or without fever, appearing weeks to months after cardiac surgery).

Aortic Transection

Aortic transection (tearing or rupturing of the aorta) is the leading cause of immediate death from blunt trauma; most patients die at the scene or before reaching the hospital. Aortic injury is usually associated with sudden deceleration forces, such as those sustained during an MVC or a fall. Because the thoracic aorta is very mobile, tears typically occur at points of fixation, especially at the level of the isthmus (ie, the descending portion of the arch). During a sudden deceleration, the aorta continues to travel forward but at the point of the isthmus, the ligamentum arteriosum holds the aorta back, typically causing transection of all three layers of the vessel wall. If the adventitia (outer layer) remains intact, an aneurysm or a partial circumferential hematoma (which has a tamponading effect) may form and can prolong survival, but only for a limited time. Early diagnosis and treatment are critical. Aortography is the gold standard for diagnosis.[11] A CXR identifies changes which indicate an aortic injury. These include widened mediastinum; loss aortic knob; and apical cap. Other diagnostics include CTA, MRA and echocardiogram.

 RED FLAG! *Signs and symptoms of aortic transection are related to poor perfusion beyond the aortic lesion and include pulse deficit in the lower extremities or left arm, hypotension unexplained by other injuries, upper extremity hypertension relative to lower extremities, interscapular or sternal pain, precordial or interscapular systolic murmur (caused by turbulence across the disrupted area), hoarseness (caused by hematoma pressure around the aortic arch), respiratory distress or dyspnea, and lower extremity neuromuscular or sensory deficit. However, many patients are asymptomatic.*

Surgical repair may involve placement of a synthetic graft. Cardiopulmonary bypass may be necessary for repair of the ascending aorta or the aortic arch. Nursing care focuses on hemodynamic monitoring and blood pressure management. Postoperative nursing care includes monitoring for complications of distal organ ischemia.

Abdominal Trauma

Abdominal trauma can be blunt or penetrating, and can rapidly lead to death secondary to hemorrhage, shock, and sepsis. In abdominal trauma, single-organ injuries are rare; usually, several abdominal organs are involved. Detection of injuries caused by blunt abdominal trauma can be difficult, especially if other injuries are present, and missed abdominal injuries are a frequent cause of death.[5]

 RED FLAG! *Abdominal injuries should be suspected if the patient has abdominal tenderness or guarding, hemodynamic instability, lumbar spine injury, pelvic fracture, retroperitoneal or intraperitoneal air, or unilateral loss of the psoas shadow on radiography.*

In blunt abdominal trauma, compression forces lead to fractures of solid organ capsules and parenchyma, whereas hollow organs collapse and absorb the force. Solid organs usually respond to trauma with bleeding, whereas hollow organs rupture and release their contents into the peritoneal cavity, causing inflammation and infection Penetrating trauma can result in "dirty" wounds, which are associated with high mortality rates secondary to infection caused by bacterial contamination and subsequent multisystem organ failure.

Diagnostic testing may include focused abdominal sonography for trauma (FAST), diagnostic peritoneal lavage (DPL), chest radiography (to detect organ displacement or the presence of free air), and abdominal CT. FAST is performed by passing an ultrasound probe over the abdomen to detect the presence of free fluid. DPL is the instillation of normal saline or lactated Ringer's solution into the abdominal cavity; the returned lavage fluid is then analyzed for the presence of blood RBCs and WBCs, bile, bacteria, or fecal matter, which would indicate intra-abdominal injury. If the results of FAST or DPL are positive and the patient is hemodynamically unstable, an exploratory laparotomy is performed.

Clinicians divide the abdomen into three main regions to facilitate description of the location of the injury (Fig. 34-4):

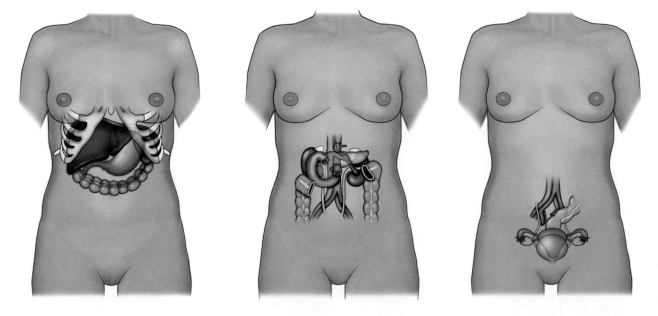

Peritoneal   Retroperitoneal   Pelvic

FIGURE 34-4 Abdominal regions.

- The peritoneal area, which includes the diaphragm, liver, spleen, stomach, transverse colon, and the portion covered by the bony thorax
- The retroperitoneal area, which includes the aorta, vena cava, pancreas, kidney, ureters, and parts of the duodenum and colon
- The pelvis, which includes the rectum, bladder, uterus, and the iliac vessels

Esophageal Trauma

Penetrating trauma is the most common cause of esophageal injury. Most often, the cervical esophagus is injured. Signs and symptoms are subtle. A hemothorax or pneumothorax without rib fractures raises suspicion for an esophageal injury. CT scan of the chest, abdomen, and pelvis with and without contrast; esophagoscopy; flexible endoscopy; and swallow studies are used in the diagnosis. Treatment is surgical repair. The patient is kept NPO with a nasogastric tube to continuously suction, and antibiotic therapy is initiated. Nursing interventions include airway, ventilation, oxygenation, and hemodynamic support.

Diaphragm Rupture

Diaphragm rupture is more common in blunt injury than in penetrating injury. A suspected diaphragm rupture raises suspicion for thoracic and abdominal injury. Movement of abdominal organs into the thorax can cause bowel strangulation. Respiratory compromise, resulting from displacement of lung tissue, may also be seen. Diagnosis is through chest radiography (often normal or nonspecific), ultrasound, CT, and exploratory laparotomy. DPL may be falsely negative. Definitive treatment is surgical repair.

 RED FLAG! *Signs and symptoms of diaphragm rupture, when herniated bowel is present, may include marked respiratory distress, dyspnea, decreased breath sounds on the affected side, positive bowel sounds in the thorax, palpation of abdominal contents when inserting a chest tube, and paradoxical movement of the abdomen when breathing.*

Stomach Trauma

Patients with blunt gastric injuries can present with blood in the nasogastric aspirate or hematemesis. Physical signs often are absent, and CT findings may be subtle and nonspecific. Close observation is required; often, the diagnosis is not made until peritonitis develops. Penetrating injuries usually cause positive results on DPL. Although a mild bowel contusion can be managed conservatively (gastric decompression and withholding oral intake), surgery usually is necessary to repair penetrating wounds. Postoperative decompression with a gastric tube is maintained until bowel function returns. In most cases, a jejunostomy tube is placed distal to the repair site, and tube feedings are initiated early in the postoperative course. Potential complications related to stomach trauma include intolerance to tube feedings, peritonitis (from irritation caused by gastric acid), and postoperative bleeding.

Pancreatic Trauma

Most injuries to the pancreas are related to penetrating trauma. Signs and symptoms of pancreatic trauma may include an acute abdomen, increased serum amylase levels, epigastric pain radiating to the back, nausea, and vomiting. Abdominal CT is most useful for diagnosis; the retroperitoneal location of the pancreas makes pancreatic injuries difficult to diagnose with DPL.

Small lacerations or contusions of the pancreas may require only the placement of drains, whereas larger wounds need surgical repair. Most pancreatic injuries require postoperative closed-suction drainage to prevent fistula formation. Postoperative nursing assessment and care involves ensuring the pancreas is rested (eg. NPO, NG tube to low wall suction). Care also involves ensuring the patency of drains and monitoring for the development of fistulas. If a cutaneous fistula does develop, skin protection is necessary because of the high enzyme content of pancreatic fluid, and ongoing assessment of fluid and electrolyte balance is required because a pancreatic fistula results in fluid, potassium, and bicarbonate loss.

Colon Trauma

Usually, injury to the colon results from penetrating trauma. Spillage of the contents of the colon predisposes the patient to intra-abdominal sepsis and abscess formation. Exploratory laparotomy is usually necessary. Whenever possible, lacerations are treated with primary repair. In some situations, an exteriorized repair or colostomy is required. The subcutaneous tissue and skin of the incision site are often left open to decrease the chance of wound infection.

Postoperative nursing care focuses on assessing for abnormal infections (eg. peritonitis). Dressing changes are necessary for open incisions, and prophylactic antibiotics may be used. The exteriorized colon must be kept moist and covered with a nonadherent dressing or bag to protect the integrity of the sutures. Because sepsis is a major complication of colon injuries, a series of radiographic and surgical procedures may be required to locate and drain abscesses.

Splenic Trauma

The spleen is the most commonly injured abdominal organ, usually as a result of blunt trauma. Because of its vascularity, the spleen has a tendency to lose blood rapidly. Injuries include hematomas and lacerations, and are graded on a scale of I to V (Box 34-4). DPL or abdominal CT is usually necessary for diagnosis.

 RED FLAG! *Signs and symptoms of splenic injury include left upper quadrant pain radiating to the left shoulder (Kehr's sign), hypovolemic shock, and increased white blood cell (WBC) count.*

Minor injuries are treated nonoperatively with observation and gastric decompression (to reduce pressure on the injured spleen). The preferred

BOX 34-4　Splenic Injury Scale

Hematomas
- **Grade I:** subcapsular, nonexpanding, involving less than 10% of surface area
- **Grade II:** subcapsular, nonexpanding, involving 10% to 50% of surface area OR intraparenchymal, less than 1 cm
- **Grade III:** subcapsular, expanding, and ruptured, with active bleeding, involving greater than 50% of surface area OR intraparenchymal, greater than or equal to 2 cm or expanding
- **Grade IV:** ruptured parenchyma with active bleeding

Lacerations
- **Grade I:** nonbleeding capsular tear less than 1 cm deep
- **Grade II:** actively bleeding capsular tear 1 to 3 cm deep without trabecular vessel involvement
- **Grade III:** greater than 3 cm deep or involving trabecular vessels
- **Grade IV:** hilar vessel involvement with greater than 25% devascularization
- **Grade V:** completely shattered spleen; hilar vascular injury with total devascularization of the spleen

BOX 34-5　Liver Injury Scale

Hematomas
- **Grade I:** subcapsular, nonexpanding, involving less than 10% of surface area OR capsular tear less than 1 cm parenchymal depth
- **Grade II:** subcapsular, nonexpanding, involving 10% to 50% of surface area OR intraparenchymal, less than 10 cm diameter
- **Grade III:** subcapsular, involving greater than 50% of surface area or expanding; ruptured subcapsular or parenchymal bleeding OR intraparenchymal, hematoma greater than or equal to 10 cm or expanding.
- **Grade IV:** ruptured parenchyma involving 25% to 75% of hepatic lobe with active bleeding

Lacerations
- **Grade I:** nonbleeding capsular tear less than 1 cm deep
- **Grade II:** actively bleeding capsular tear 1 to 3 cm deep without trabecular vessel involvement
- **Grade III:** greater than 3 cm deep
- **Grade IV:** 25% to 75% hepatic lobe parenchymal disruption
- **Grade V:** greater than 75% hepatic lobe parenchymal disruption; vascular injury includes retrohepatic vena cava and juxtahepatic venous injuries
- **Grade VI:** vascular hepatic avulsion

surgical treatment is splenorrhaphy, although in some cases splenectomy is necessary. Splenic autotransplantation (implanting splenic fragments into pockets of omentum) may be performed after splenectomy to retain normal splenic immune function.[12]

Early complications include recurrent bleeding, subphrenic abscess, and pancreatitis (from surgical trauma). Rupture of an expanding subscapular hematoma may present days or weeks later. Other late complications include thrombocytosis and overwhelming post–splenectomy sepsis (OPSS). OPSS frequently occurs with the onset of pneumococcal pneumonia, which progresses to a fulminant sepsis. Splenic autotransplantation and immunization with a polyvalent pneumococcal vaccine may decrease the patient's risk for developing OPSS.

Liver Trauma

After the spleen, the liver is the most commonly injured abdominal organ. Hepatic injury can be caused by either blunt or penetrating trauma, and may result in hematomas or lacerations (Box 34-5).

 RED FLAG! *Signs and symptoms of hepatic injury include right upper quadrant pain, rebound tenderness, hypoactive or absent bowel sounds, and signs of hypovolemic shock.*

Hepatic trauma can cause a large blood loss into the peritoneum. A hemodynamically stable patient may be managed nonoperatively with serial CT scans and hemoglobin and hematocrit levels to verify bleeding cessation. Hemodynamically unstable patients require surgery to ligate or embolize bleeding vessels, repair small lacerations, or resect and debride large areas of injured liver. When hemorrhage is uncontrollable, the liver is packed to tamponade the bleeding. After packing, the patient's abdomen may be simply covered and left open and the patient transferred to the critical care unit for management of coagulopathy. After the coagulopathy is corrected, a second surgical procedure is performed to remove the packing and repair the laceration. Patients with hepatic injuries require postoperative drainage of bile and blood with closed-suction drains.

Nursing care of patients with liver injuries includes replacing blood products and monitoring hematocrit and coagulation studies, tube drainage, and fluid balance. Potential complications include hepatic or perihepatic abscess, biliary obstruction or leak, sepsis, ARDS, and DIC.

Kidney Trauma

Trauma to the kidney may lead to a "free" hemorrhage, contained hematoma, the development of an intravascular thrombus, laceration or contusion of the renal parenchyma, or rupture of the collecting system. Signs and symptoms, when present, consist of hematuria, pain, a flank hematoma, or ecchymosis over the flank. A helical CT scan, ultrasound, or intravenous pyelography usually provides the diagnosis.

Many kidney injuries can be managed with observation and bedrest until gross hematuria resolves. However, vascular injury may necessitate surgical repair or nephrectomy. Optimal fluid balance must be maintained. Low-dose dopamine may be ordered to promote kidney perfusion. Complications may include arterial or venous thrombosis, acute kidney failure, bleeding, urinary fistula formation, and late-onset hypertension.

Bladder Trauma

The bladder can be lacerated, ruptured, or contused, most often as the consequence of blunt trauma (usually because of a full bladder at the time of injury). Bladder injuries frequently are associated with pelvic fractures. Injuries to the urethra, which may be evidenced by blood at the urethral meatus, a scrotal hematoma, or a displaced prostate gland, must be ruled out before placing a urinary catheter.[13]

A bladder injury can cause intraperitoneal or extraperitoneal urine extravasation. Extraperitoneal extravasation can often be managed with urinary catheter drainage. Intraperitoneal extravasation requires surgery and is associated with a high mortality rate because of associated injuries that occur secondary to the force involved and peritonitis. A suprapubic cystostomy tube may be placed temporarily after intraperitoneal rupture. Complications are infrequent, but infection from the urinary catheter or sepsis from extravasation of infected urine can occur. Patients may experience an inability to void or shoulder pain (caused by urine extravasation into the peritoneal space).

Musculoskeletal Injuries

Major causes of trauma-related musculoskeletal injuries include MVCs; falls; industrial, farming, and home injuries; and assaults. Musculoskeletal injuries require prompt recognition and stabilization to promote optimal recovery and function.

There are many types of musculoskeletal injuries:

- **Fractures** are classified according to type (Fig. 34-5), cause, and anatomical location. Open fractures are further classified as grade I, II, or III, depending on the tissue damage involved.
- **Dislocations** occur when the articulating surfaces of a joint are no longer in contact. Injuries to vessels, nerves, and ligaments are often associated with dislocations.
- **Amputations** are classified according to the amount of tissue, nerve, and vascular damage. A cut (guillotine) amputation has clean lines and well-defined edges, whereas a crush amputation has ill-defined edges and more soft tissue damage. An avulsion amputation occurs when part of the body is stretched and torn away.

Musculoskeletal assessment is usually part of the secondary survey. If limb swelling, ecchymosis, or deformity is noted, the nurse tests the extremities for capillary refill, pulses, crepitus, muscle spasm, movement, sensation, and pain. Physical examination for pelvic fractures includes inspection for abrasions, lacerations, contusions, and symmetry of the lower extremities, and palpation to assess for rotational and vertical instability. Rectal and vaginal examinations are performed to assess for a urethral tear in males and an open fracture in females.[13] Appropriate imaging studies (eg, radiographs, CT, magnetic resonance imaging [MRI]) are ordered according to physical examination findings.

Pelvic fractures are classified in a variety of ways (Box 34-6). Treatment goals are to control bleeding and to prevent loss of function and infection caused by open fractures. A pelvic binder or external fixator is applied for temporary stabilization and to control bleeding. Embolization of arterial bleeding in the pelvic region is indicated for hemorrhage control.[14] Permanent repair with internal fixation is usually performed within 24 to 72 hours of injury when the patient is adequately resuscitated and hemodynamically stable.

Patients with musculoskeletal trauma require continuous assessment. Infection is common in open injuries. Any musculoskeletal injury involving bone or soft tissue can cause neurological or vascular compromise because nerves and blood vessels are located in such close proximity to the bones and muscles. Serious complications of musculoskeletal injuries include compartment syndrome, fat embolus syndrome, deep venous thrombosis (DVT; see Chapter 13), and pulmonary embolus (see Chapter 16).

Compartment Syndrome

Compartment syndrome occurs when the pressure within the fascia–enclosed muscle compartment is increased, compromising blood flow to the muscles and nerves in the compartment and resulting in tissue ischemia. Prolonged elevation of compartmental pressure leads to death of the tissues involved. Patients with higher diastolic pressures are able to tolerate higher tissue pressures without ischemic damage. Hypotensive trauma patients may experience significant muscle ischemia at lower compartment pressures.

 RED FLAG! *Signs and symptoms of compartment syndrome include increased pain in the affected area that is "out of proportion" to the injury, decreased sensation and paresthesia ("pins and needles"), firmness of the affected area, and pallor and pulselessness (late signs).*

If the compartment syndrome progresses to the point that the patient is showing late signs, loss of the affected extremity is threatened. If signs or symptoms of compartment syndrome are present,

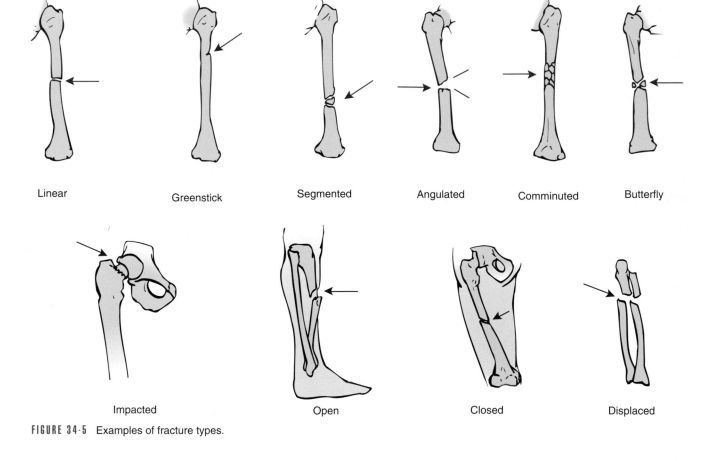

FIGURE 34-5 Examples of fracture types.

Oblique   Spiral   Transverse

Linear   Greenstick   Segmented   Angulated   Comminuted   Butterfly

Impacted   Open   Closed   Displaced

the orthopedic or general surgeon must be notified immediately. Treatment is with fasciotomy (opening of the fascia) of the involved compartment.

Fat Embolism Syndrome

Fat emboli are fat globules in the lung tissue and peripheral circulation after a long bone fracture or major trauma. Although fat emboli may not cause systemic symptoms, some patients develop fat embolism syndrome (progressive respiratory insufficiency, thrombocytopenia, and decreased mental status).

 RED FLAG! *Signs and symptoms of fat embolism syndrome usually develop within 72 hours of injury and include tachypnea, dyspnea, cyanosis, tachycardia, and fever.*

Maxillofacial Trauma

Fractures of the facial bones can be classified according to Le Fort's classification (Fig. 34-6). Maxillofacial trauma can cause airway obstruction and death if an airway and breathing are not adequately and

BOX 34-6 **Classification Schemes for Pelvic Fractures**

Tile's Classification

Type A, Stable
A1, without involvement of pelvic ring
A2, with involvement of pelvic ring

Type B, Rotationally Unstable
B1, open book
B2, ipsilateral lateral compression (LC)
B3, contralateral LC

Type C, Rotationally and Vertically Unstable
C1, rotationally and vertically unstable
C2, bilateral
C3, with associated acetabular fracture

Young and Burgess Classification

Lateral Compression (LC)
I, sacral compression on side of impact
II, iliac wing fracture on side of impact
III, LCI or LCII injury on side of impact with contralateral open-book injury

Anterior Posterior Compression (APC)
I, slight widening of pubis symphysis or anterior part of sacroiliac joint with intact anterior and posterior sacroiliac ligaments
II, widened anterior part of sacroiliac joint with disrupted anterior and intact posterior sacroiliac ligaments
III, complete disruption of the sacroiliac joint

Vertical Shear (VS)
Vertical displacement anteriorly and posteriorly

Combined Mechanism (CM)
Combination of other injury patterns

From Frakes MA, Evans T: Major pelvic fractures. Crit Care Nurse 24(2):18–32, 2004.

urgently established. When the primary survey is completed, the maxillofacial injuries are assessed. The nurse inspects the face for symmetry and then palpates systematically to observe for any movement of bony structures. Because maxillofacial injuries often coincide with head injuries, a thorough neurologic examination is necessary.

Many maxillofacial injuries require multiple surgeries before the patient is definitively treated. Because most maxillofacial injuries involve the soft tissue, measures to prevent infection and scarring are taken. The nurse continuously assesses the patient's neurological status and seeks to relieve pain and anxiety (caused by an inability to see, smell, taste, or speak secondary to the injury).

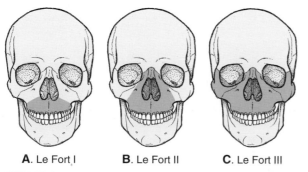

A. Le Fort I   **B.** Le Fort II   **C.** Le Fort III

FIGURE 34-6 Le Fort fractures. **A:** Le Fort I: Transverse disarticulation of the maxillary dentoalveolar process from the remaining basal bone of maxilla and midface. **B:** Le Fort II: Pyramidal fracture involving entire maxilla and nasal complex. **C:** Le Fort III: Complete craniofacial–midface disassociation. (Courtesy of Neil O. Hardy, Westpoint, Connecticut.

CASE STUDY

Mr. W., a 17-year-old man, is admitted to the trauma resuscitation unit after being involved in an motor vehicle crash (MVC). He was the driver and was wearing his seat belt. His car was broadsided. He was intubated at the scene. On arrival at the emergency department, he is unresponsive, and his vital signs are: BP, 100/70 mm Hg; HR, 110 beats/min; and RR, 12 breaths/min (on ventilator). The oxygen saturation is 100%.

After the primary and secondary survey and initial radiographs, Mr. W. is taken for a CT scan. At this time, his only apparent injury appears to be a brain injury. He is transferred to the critical care unit, where a tertiary survey is completed according to the brain injury protocol. Despite the efforts taken in the critical care unit, Mr. W.'s intracranial pressure continues to rise. He eventually goes to the operating room for a decompressive craniectomy.

After the operation, the nurse notices that Mr. W.'s ventilator requirements are increasing, his urine output is beginning to decrease, and his abdomen is firm. A bladder pressure of greater than 30 cm H_2O is obtained. Mr. W. is taken back to surgery to manage abdominal compartment syndrome by opening the abdomen (skin and fascia).

Mr. W.'s myoglobin levels continue to increase, and increased pressures in all four leg compartments are now noticeable. Four compartment fasciotomies on Mr. W.'s legs are performed. He is also placed on dialysis to prevent further renal injury from rhabdomyolysis.

1. What additional information would be helpful to gather to determine the plan of care for Mr. W.?

2. What expectations would the nurse have when caring for Mr. W. following his abdominal surgery?

3. When caring for an intubated patient with a head injury, how does the nurse handle the complication of compartment syndrome?

References

1. National Safety Council: Accident Facts. Chicago, IL: National Safety Council, 2000
2. Rushing A, Scalea T: Trauma resuscitation of the elderly patient. Clin Geriatr 34–36
3. CDC. Vital signs: nonfatal motor vehicle-occupant injuries (2009) and seat belt use (2008) among adults in United States. MMWR Morb Mortal Wkly Rep 59:1681–1686, 2011
4. Williamson K, Ramesh R, Grabinsky A: Advances in prehospital trauma care. Symposium in Trends in Trauma 1(1):44–150, 2011
5. Pfeifer R, Pape H: Missed injuries in trauma patient: A literature review. Patient Saf Surg 2:20, 2008
6. Kheinbeck T, et al.: Hypothermia in bleeding trauma patient: a friend or foe? Scand J Trauma Resusc Emerg Med 17(65), 2009
7. Ertmer C, et al.: Fluid resuscitation in multiple trauma patient. Curr Opin Anesthesiol 24(2): 202–208, 2011
8. Mitra B, et al.: Massive blood transfusion and trauma resuscitation. Injury 38(9):1023–1029, 2007
9. Salomone J: Assess and manage patient with facial trauma. J Emerg Med Serv 4, 2011
10. Karmy-Jones R, Stern E, Nathens A; Thoracic Trauma and Critical Care. New York, NY: Springer-Verlag, 2008, Chapter 6.1 Blunt Cardiac Injury
11. Holtzman S, et al.: Expert panel on vascular imaging: ACR appropriateness criteria blunt chest trauma-suspected aortic injury. Am Coll Radiol 2009
12. Doherty G (ed): Current Diagnosis and Treatment Surgery. McGraw Hill, 2009, chapter 27
13. Ingram M, et al.: Urethral injuries after pelvic trauma: evaluation with urethrography. Radiographics 28:1631–1643, 2008
14. Barentsz M, et al.: Clinical outcomes of intra-arterial embolization for treatment of patients with pelvic trauma. Radiol Res Pract 2011

Want to know more? A wide variety of resources to enhance your learning and understanding of this chapter are available on the **Point** ✳. Visit **http://thepoint.lww.com/MortonEss1e** to access chapter review questions and more!

Index

Note: Page numbers followed by b indicate boxed material; those followed by f indicate figures; those followed by t indicate tables.

Antidysrhythmics, 79–81, 80t
  adenosine, 81
  atropine, 81
  β-adrenergic blockers, 159, 160
  calcium channel blockers, 160
  class I, 79, 81
  class II, 81
  class III, 81
  class IV, 81
  digoxin, 81, 160–161
  magnesium sulfate, 81
  medications, 80t
Antiemetics, 36t
Antihyperlipidemics, 162
Anti-inflammatory agents
  corticosteroids, 225
  leukotriene receptor antagonists,
    225–226
  mast cell stabilizers, 225
Antimicrobial agents
  topical, for burns, 452, 452t
Antinuclear antibody (ANA), 406t,
  417
Antiplatelet, 188
Antithyroid drugs, 387
Anxiolytics, for pain management, 39
Aortic aneurysm, 196, 197, 197f,
  198b
  abdominal, 196, 197, 198b
  thoracic, 197, 198, 198b
Aortic dissection, 198, 198f
Aortic pulsations, abdominal,
  abnormal, 355t
Aortic regurgitation, 149t
Aortic stenosis, 149t
Aplastic anemia, 415t
Apnea test, 302b
Appropriate staffing, 3b–4b, 5
APRV. See Airway pressure release
  ventilation (APRV)
ARDS. See Acute respiratory distress
  syndrome (ARDS)
Arousal, of increased ICP and
  herniation, 306t
Arterial blood gases (ABGs), 211–
  212, 212b, 212f, 213b, 213t,
  214b, 229t, 231, 388, 446, 466b
  acid–base disorders, 213t
  interpreting, 212, 214b
  measuring oxygen in the blood
    and, 212, 212f
  measuring pH in the blood, 212,
    213b, 213t
Arterial oxygen content (CaO₂), 111t
Arterial oxygen delivery index
  (DaO₂I), 111t
Arterial pH (pHa), 111t
Arterial pressure monitoring
  complications of, 95, 97
    accidental blood loss, 95, 97
    impaired circulation, 97
    infection, 97
  of data interpretation, 95, 97f
  equipment and setup, 94, 97f
Arteriovenous malformations
  (AVMs), 332–333, 333t
  assessment, 332
  management of, 333, 333t

Artificial airways
  endotracheal tube and, 115,
    116–117, 116b, 116f, 116t, 117b
  nasopharyngeal, 114, 115, 115f
  oropharyngeal, 114, 115f
  tracheostomy, 118–119, 118b,
    118f
Ascites, 373
Aspartate aminotransferase (AST),
  356, 357t
Aspiration
  bone marrow, 404
Aspirin, 361
  for pain management, 36t
Assist-control (A/C) ventilator mode,
  123, 124t, 125f
Asthma, 232t
  acute, 250–252, 250t, 251b, 251f,
    252t, 253f
    assessment of, 251, 252t
    classification of, 250t, 252t
    management of, 252, 253f
    pathophysiology of, 251, 251f
Astrocytomas, 326t
Asynchronous pacing, 83b
Atelectasis, 232t
Atelectrauma, mechanical ventilation
  and, 122
ATN. See Acute tubular necrosis
Atrial dysrhythmias
  fibrillation, on electrocardiogram,
    73, 73f
  flutter, on electrocardiogram, 72,
    73, 73t
  paroxysmal supraventricular
    tachycardia, 72, 72t
  premature atrial contraction,
    71–72, 72f
Atrial enlargement, 66, 67, 67f
Atrial fibrillation, 73, 73f
Atrial flutter, 72, 72t, 73, 73t
Atrioventricular block (AV), 77–79,
  78b
  bundle branch block, 79, 79t
  first-degree, 77
  second-degree, 77
  third-degree, 77, 79
Atropine, 80t, 81, 139t
Auscultation, 117, 210–211, 211t
  continuous sounds, 211
  discontinuous sounds, 211
  egophony, 211
  friction rubs, 211
  in gastrointestinal assessment,
    352, 355t, 356f
  hematological and immune
    systems, 400
  whispered pectoriloquy, 211
Auscultation, in cardiovascular
  assessment, 147–150, 147f,
  148b, 149t
Authentic leadership, 4b, 5
Autolytic debridement, 439
Automated external defibrillation
  (AED), 140
Autonomic dysreflexia, with spinal
  cord injury, 344, 344b
Axial loading injuries, 341

B

Bacitracin, for burns, 452t
Band neutrophils, 403t
Barbiturate coma, for reducing
  intracranial pressure, 314
Barium enema, 358t
Barotrauma, mechanical ventilation
  and, 122
Base excess/base deficit (BE/BD),
  111t
Basophils, 403t
Beneficence, principle of, 24b
Benzodiazepines
  for pain management, 36t
BHT (bronchial hygiene therapy),
  219–221, 221f
  airway clearance adjunct therapies
    and, 220
  chest physiotherapy and, 220–221,
    221f
  coughing and deep breathing and,
    219–220
Bicarbonate replacement
  diabetic ketoacidosis, 391, 394
Bilayered dressings, 439
Bile formation and secretion, 356
Bilevel positive-pressure (BiPAP)
  ventilation mode, 124t, 127
Bilirubin, 467t
  serum, normal values for, 356t
  urine, normal values for, 356t
Biochemical markers
  brain-type natriuretic peptide, 152
  cardiac enzymes, 151, 152b
  C-reactive protein, 153
  D-dimer, 153
  myocardial proteins, 152
Bioethics. See Ethical issues
Biological valves, 201b
Biopsy, gastrointestinal, 359t
Biot's respiration, 210t
BiPAP (bilateral positive-pressure)
  ventilation mode, 124t, 127
Bipolar lead, for cardiac pacing, 83b
Birthmarks, 427
Biventricular support system, 177f
Bladder trauma, 483
Blood cholesterol, 145b
  normal values for, 356t
Blood glucose
  control of, 336
Blood loss
  anemia, 414
  arterial pressure monitoring and,
    95, 97
Blood pressure
  assessment of, 295
Blood products, 474
Blood studies, 259–260, 259t, 260b
  blood urea nitrogen, 260, 260b
  hematocrit and hemoglobin, 260
  osmolality, 260
  serum creatinine, 260
  serum electrolytes, 260
  uric acid, 260
Blood transfusion, 416
  complications of, 416b

VLDL (very-low density lipoprotein), 356t
Volume-guaranteed pressure options (VGPO) mode, 124t, 127
Volume resuscitation, 460t
Volume resuscitation, acute upper gastrointestinal bleeding, 363, 364
Volume ventilation, 121
Volutrauma, mechanical ventilation and, 122
Vomiting, in end-of-life care, 42
VTE. *See* Venous thromboembolism (VTE)

W

Warfarin, 158, 158b
WBCs. *See* White blood cells (WBCs)
Weaning
  from intra-aortic balloon pump counterpulsation, 176, 176b
  from mechanical ventilation, 130, 131–133, 132b, 133b, 133f
    for long-term ventilation, 132, 133b

methods of, 132, 133, 133f
    for short-term ventilation, 131–132, 132b
Wenckebach block, on electrocardiogram, 77
Wet-to-dry dressings, 438, 439
Wheals, 426t
Whispered pectoriloquy, 211
White blood cells (WBCs), 463
  count and differential, 401
  T-and B-lymphocyte tests, 401
  in urine, 258t
World Health Organization (WHO), 326t
Wound(s), 434–440
  arterial ulcers, 437t
  assessment of, 429, 429b, 430f
  case study of, 440
  cleansing of, 435
  closure of
    sutures, staples, and wound adhesives for, 438
    vacuum-assisted, 435, 437, 438, 438b, 438f
  cultures of, 440, 440b, 440f
  debridement of, 439–440

diabetic foot ulcers, 437t
  drainage of, 438, 439f
  dressings for, 438–439
  healing of
    methods of, 434, 435f
    phases of, 434, 435f
  high-volume draining wounds, care of, 438, 439f
  pressure ulcers. *See* Pressure ulcers
  signs and symptoms of, 440b
  skin tears, 437t
  venous stasis ulcers, 437t
Wound adhesives, 438
Wound infection, with brain tumors, 330t
Wound stressors, 437t

Y

Yeast cells, in urine, 258t

Z

Zeroing, in hemodynamic monitoring, 94, 94f